Violence in Psychiatry

Violence in Psychiatry

Edited by

Katherine D. Warburton
California Department of State Hospitals, Sacramento, and University of California, Davis, CA, USA

and

Stephen M. Stahl
University of California San Diego, CA, USA, California Department of State Hospitals, Sacramento, and University of Cambridge, UK

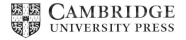

CAMBRIDGE
UNIVERSITY PRESS

University Printing House, Cambridge CB2 8BS, United Kingdom

Cambridge University Press is part of the University of Cambridge.

It furthers the University's mission by disseminating knowledge in the pursuit of education, learning and research at the highest international levels of excellence.

www.cambridge.org
Information on this title: www.cambridge.org/9781107092198

© Cambridge University Press 2016

First published 2016
Previously published in *CNS Spectrums* (Journal of the Neuroscience Education Institute, October 2014 (vol. 19, iss. 5) and June 2015, (edited by Stephen M. Stahl). ISSN: 1092–8529, www.journals.cambridge.org/cns
3rd printing 2019

Printed in the United Kingdom by TJ International Ltd. Padstow Cornwall

A catalog record for this publication is available from the British Library

Library of Congress Cataloging in Publication data
Names: Warburton, Katherine D., editor. | Stahl, Stephen M., 1951– , editor.
Title: Violence in psychiatry / edited by Katherine D. Warburton and Stephen M. Stahl.
Description: Cambridge, United Kingdom ; New York : Cambridge University Press, 2016. | Includes bibliographical references and index.
Identifiers: LCCN 2015042173 | ISBN 9781107092198 (Hardback)
Subjects: | MESH: Psychotic Disorders–drug therapy. | Violence–psychology. | Forensic Psychiatry–methods. | Neuropsychiatry–methods. | Psychotic Disorders–physiopathology.
Classification: LCC RC480.5 | NLM WM 600 | DDC 616.89/14–dc23 LC record available at http://lccn.loc.gov/2015042173

ISBN 978-1-107-09219-8 Hardback

Additional resources for this publication at www.stahlonline.org

Contents

Contributors

Mario Amore
Department of Neurosciences, Rehabilitation, Ophthalmology, Genetics and Maternal and Child Health, University of Genoa, Genoa, Italy

Allen Azizian
Coalinga State Hospital, Coalinga, and Department of Criminology, California State University, Fresno, California, USA

Shannon M. Bader
California Department of State Hospitals, and Patton State Hospital, California, USA

Michael W. Barsom
Department of State Hospitals (DSH) – Metropolitan, Norwalk, California, USA

Nicole R. Bartholomew
Psychology Services, Federal Bureau of Prisons, Big Spring, Texas, USA

Amlan Basu
Broadmoor High Secure Hospital, West London Mental Health NHS Trust, and Institute of Psychiatry, King's College, London, UK

Charles Broderick
California Department of State Hospitals, Sacramento, California, USA

Rosalie S. Brooman-White
Medical Sciences Division, John Radcliffe Hospital, University of Oxford, Oxford, UK

Darcy Brown
The School of Medicine and Dentistry, University of Aberdeen, Aberdeen, UK

Leslie Citrome
Department of Psychiatry and Behavioral Sciences, New York Medical College, Valhalla, New York, USA

Emil F. Coccaro
Clinical Neuroscience & Psychopharmacology Research Unit, Department of Psychiatry (MC#3077), Pritzker School of Medicine, University of Chicago, Chicago, Illinois, USA

Michael A. Cummings
Department of State Hospitals–Patton, Department of Psychiatry, Patton, California, USA; Department of Psychiatry and Human Behavior, University of California, Irvine, Orange, California, USA

Stephen E. Cummings
Department of Psychiatry, San Mateo Medical Center, San Mateo, California, USA

Pál Czobor
Department of Psychiatry and Psychotherapy, Semmelweis University, Budapest, Hungary

Laura J. Dardashti
California Department of State Hospitals, and Metropolitan State Hospital, California, USA

Mrigendra Das
Broadmoor Hospital, West London Mental Health Trust, Berkshire, amd School of Psychiatry, Oxford Deanery, Oxford, UK

Darci Delgado
California Department of State Hospitals, and Vacaville Psychiatric Program, California, USA

Sean E. Evans
Psychology Department, Department of State Hospitals, Patton, California, and Psychology Department, La Sierra University, Riverside, California, USA

Thomas Fahy
Department of Forensic and Neurodevelopmental Sciences, Institute of Psychiatry, Psychology and Neuroscience, King's College London, London, UK

Jennifer R. Fanning
Clinical Neuroscience & Psychopharmacology
Research Unit, Department of Psychiatry (MC#3077),
Pritzker School of Medicine, University of Chicago,
Chicago, Illinois, USA

Alan R. Felthous
Division of Forensic Psychiatry, Department of
Neurology & Psychiatry, Saint Louis University
School of Medicine, Saint Louis, Missouri, USA

E. Fuller Torrey
Department of Psychiatry, Uniformed Services
University of the Health Sciences (USUHS), Bethesda,
Maryland, USA; Stanley Medical Research Institute,
Chevy Chase, Maryland, USA

David Goldman
Laboratory of Neurogenetics, National Institute on
Alcohol Abuse and Alcoholism, National Institutes of
Health, Bethesda, Maryland, USA

Jordan H. Grafman
Rehabilitation Institute of Chicago, Chicago, Illinois, USA

Nitin Gupta
Department of Psychiatry, Government Medical
College and Hospital, Chandigarh, India

Margaret Guyer
Central Office Research Review Committee,
Massachusetts Department of Mental Health,
Massachusetts Mental Health Center Division of
Public Psychiatry, and Harvard Medical School/Beth
Israel Deaconess Medical Center, Boston,
Massachusetts, USA

Colin A. Hodgkinson
Laboratory of Neurogenetics, National Institute on
Alcohol Abuse and Alcoholism, National Institutes of
Health, Bethesda, Maryland, USA

Brian J. Holoyda
Department of Psychiatry and Behavioral Sciences,
University of California Davis School of Medicine,
Sacramento, California, USA

Matthew J. Hoptman
Schizophrenia Research Division, Nathan Kline
Institute for Psychiatric Research, Orangeburg,
Department of Psychiatry, New York, USA, and
University School of Medicine, and Department

of Psychology, City University of New York,
New York, USA

Deborah Horowitz
Office of Training and Development, Massachusetts
Department of Mental Health, Westborough,
Massachusetts, USA

James E. Hotham
Medical Sciences Division, John Radcliffe Hospital,
University of Oxford, Oxford, UK

Sharon A. Humphreys
Broadmoor High Secure Hospital, West London
Mental Health NHS Trust, London, UK

James L. Knoll IV
Division of Forensic Psychiatry, Department of
Psychiatry, SUNY Upstate Medical University,
Syracuse, New York, USA

Rebecca Kornbluh
California Department of State Hospitals,
Sacramento, California, USA

Frank Krueger
Molecular Neuroscience Department, George
Mason University, Fairfax, and Department of
Psychology, George Mason University, Fairfax,
Virginia, USA

Fintan Larkin
Broadmoor Hospital, West London Mental Health
Trust, Berkshire, UK

Royce Lee
Clinical Neuroscience & Psychopharmacology
Research Unit, Department of Psychiatry (MC#3077),
Pritzker School of Medicine, University of Chicago,
Chicago, Illinois, USA

K. Luan Phan
Department of Psychiatry, University of Illinois
College of Medicine, Mental Health Service Line, Jesse
Brown Veterans Administration Medical Center, and
Departments of Psychology, and Anatomy and Cell
Biology, University of Illinois at Chicago, Chicago,
Illinois, USA

Barbara E. McDermott
Department of Psychiatry and Behavioral Sciences,
University of California Davis School of Medicine,
Sacramento, California, USA

Jonathan M. Meyer
Department of Psychiatry, University of California–San Diego, San Diego, California Department of State Hospitals, and Patton State Hospital, California, USA

John Monahan
School of Law, University of Virginia, Charlottesville, Virginia, USA

Robert D. Morgan
Department of Psychological Sciences, Texas Tech University, Lubbock, Texas, USA

Debbi A. Morrissette
Neuroscience Education Institute, Carlsbad, California, Department of Biology, California State University, San Marcos, California, and Department of Biology, Palomar College, San Marcos, California, USA

Jennifer A. O'Day
California Department of State Hospitals, and Metropolitan State Hospital, California, USA

Mark E. Olver
Department of Psychology, University of Saskatchewan, Saskatoon, Saskatchewan, Canada

Matteo Pardini
Department of Neurosciences, Rehabilitation, Ophthalmology, Genetics and Maternal and Child Health, and Magnetic Resonance Research Centre on Nervous System Diseases, University of Genoa, Genoa, Italy

Debra A. Pinals
Law and Psychiatry Program, Department of Psychiatry, University of Massachusetts Medical School, Worcester, Massachusetts, USA

George J. Proctor
California Department of State Hospitals, and Patton State Hospital, California, USA

Cameron D. Quanbeck
Department of Psychiatry, San Mateo Health System, San Mateo, California, USA

Vanessa Raymont
Department of Medicine, Imperial College London, London, UK

Phillip J. Resnick
Division of Forensic Psychiatry, Case Western Reserve University School of Medicine, Cleveland, Ohio, USA

Jose L. Romero-Ureclay
Broadmoor Hospital, West London Mental Health Trust, Berkshire, UK

Benjamin Rose
California Department of State Hospitals, and Napa State Hospital, California, USA

Daniel R. Rosell
Department of Psychiatry, Icahn Medical School, Mount Sinai, New York, and Special Evaluation Program of Mood and Personality Disorders, Icahn Medical School, Mount Sinai, New York, USA

Callum C. Ross
Broadmoor Hospital, West London Mental Health Trust, Berkshire, UK

Kathy Sanders
Clinical and Professional Services, Massachusetts Department of Mental Health, and Harvard Medical School/Massachusetts General Hospital, Boston, Massachusetts, USA

Robert J. Schaufenbil
California Department of State Hospitals, Sacramento, California, USA

Marie Schur
California Department of State Hospitals, and Atascadero State Hospital, California, USA

Eric H. Schwartz
California Department of State Hospitals, and Vacaville Psychiatric Program, California, USA

Charles L. Scott
Division of Psychiatry and the Law, Department of Psychiatry and Behavioral Sciences, University of California–Davis School of Medicine, 5 Sacramento, California, USA

Samrat Sengupta
Broadmoor Hospital, West London Mental Health Trust, Berkshire, UK

Larry J. Siever
Department of Psychiatry, and Special Evaluation Program of Mood and Personality

Disorders, Icahn Medical School, Mount Sinai, New York, and Department of Psychiatry and the VISN3 Mental Illness Research, Education, and Clinical Center (MIRECC), James J. Peters VA Medical Center, Bronx, New York, USA

Patrick J. D. Simpson
Medical Sciences Division, John Radcliffe Hospital, University of Oxford, Oxford, UK

Jennifer L. Skeem
School of Social Welfare & Goldman School of Public Policy, University of California–Berkeley, Berkeley, California, USA

Stephen M. Stahl
California Department of State Hospitals, Sacramento, University of California San Diego, California, USA, and University of Cambridge, Cambridge, UK

Maren Strenziok
Department of Psychology, George Mason University, Fairfax, Virginia, USA

Katalin A. Szabo
Department of Psychiatry, San Mateo Health System, San Mateo, and Behavioral Health and Recovery Services, San Mateo, and Department of Psychiatry and Behavioral Sciences, Stanford University School of Medicine, Stanford, California, USA

John Tully
Department of Forensic and Neurodevelopmental Sciences, Institute of Psychiatry, Psychology and Neuroscience, King's College London, London, UK

Richard A. Van Dorn
Research Triangle Institute International, Research Triangle Park, Durham, North Carolina, USA

Susan Velasquez
California Department of State Hospitals, and Patton State Hospital, California, USA

Morris Vinestock
Broadmoor Hospital, West London Mental Health Trust, Berkshire, UK

Jan Volavka
Department of Psychiatry, New York University School of Medicine, New York, USA

Raziya S. Wang
Behavioral Health and Recovery Services, San Mateo, California, USA

Katherine D. Warburton
California Department of State Hospitals, Sacramento, and Division of Psychiatry and the Law, University of California, Davis, California, USA

Eric M. Wassermann
Behavioral Neurology Unit, National Institute of Neurological Disorders and Stroke, National Institutes of Health, Bethesda, Maryland, USA

Christopher L. White
Department of Psychiatry, San Mateo Health System, San Mateo, and Behavioral Health and Recovery Services, San Mateo, California, USA

Stephen C. P. Wong
Department of Psychology, University of Saskatchewan, Saskatoon, Saskatchewan, Canada, School of Medicine, University of Nottingham, Nottingham, UK, and Centre for Forensic Behavioural Science, Swinburne University of Technology, Melbourne, Australia

Chapter 1

Deinstitutionalization and the rise of violence

E. Fuller Torrey

Introduction

There have been occasional examples of violent behavior by individuals with serious mental illness for as long as there have been people with serious mental illness. In England in 1800, James Hadfield, responding to God's commands to bring about the Second Coming, fired a pistol but narrowly missed King George III. In the United States in 1835, Richard Lawrence, believing that he was the King of England, attempted to assassinate President Andrew Jackson but his gun misfired. In 1881, President James Garfield was shot to death by Charles Guiteau, who many claimed was insane. Throughout the nineteenth and first half of the twentieth centuries, there continued to be sporadic examples of violent behavior by individuals who today would be diagnosed with schizophrenia, bipolar disorder with psychotic features, or major depression with psychotic features.

A major reason why such episodes were relatively uncommon at this time is that most of the individuals with the most severe forms of serious mental illness were confined to psychiatric hospitals for much of their adult lives. In 1850, the number of such individuals who were hospitalized in the United States was less than 5000; by 1903 this number had increased to 150,151 and by 1955 to 558,922. It is believed by some that these sharply increased numbers reflected a real increase in the number of individuals affected by serious mental illness [1]. Whether this is true or not, the fact remains that during this period the majority of individuals with serious mental illness who had the potential to commit violent acts were confined to asylums.

The Emptying of State Mental Hospitals

The mass exodus of patients from state mental hospitals, known as deinstitutionalization, began in the 1960s. It was driven by four major factors. The first was public revelations following World War II that most state mental hospitals were grossly overcrowded and that patients were living in squalid conditions. Second was the introduction in 1954 of chlorpromazine (Thorazine), the first effective antipsychotic, which made it possible, for the first time, to control the symptoms of psychosis and thus to discharge some patients from the hospitals. A third factor was the creation in the 1960s of federal programs such as Supplemental Security Income (SSI), Social Security Disability Insurance (SSDI), Medicaid, and Medicare, which provided fiscal support with federal funds for mentally ill individuals who were living in the community. Patients in state hospitals, however, were not eligible (with a few exceptions) for Medicaid and SSI. Since state mental hospitals continued to be almost completely funded with state funds, the new federal programs created a huge incentive for states to discharge patients to the community and thus effectively shift the cost of their care from the state to the federal government. Fiscal conservatives in the state legislatures therefore strongly encouraged deinstitutionalization. The final factor was the emergence of young, civil libertarian lawyers in the 1960s who decided that mental patients needed to be "liberated." They implemented a series of successful lawsuits, forcing states to discharge mental patients and making rehospitalization exceedingly difficult.

The emptying of state mental hospitals has been dramatic. From the 558,922 patients confined in 1955, their number decreased to 193,436 by 1975 and to 69,177 by 1995. Today there are only 35,000 individuals with serious mental illness remaining in state psychiatric hospitals. Given the fact that the population in the United States almost doubled during those

Violence in Psychiatry, ed. Katherine D. Warburton and Stephen M. Stahl. Published by Cambridge University Press.

years, the effective rate of deinstitutionalization is over 96%. When the population increase is included in the calculation, there are today approximately more than 1 million mentally ill individuals living in the community who in the 1950s would have been confined in state mental hospitals.

In addition to these 1 million individuals with serious mental illness who would have been hospitalized in the past, there are additional individuals with serious mental illness who would not have been hospitalized in the past. According to estimates of the National Institute of Mental Health (NIMH), approximately 1.1% of the adult American population has schizophrenia and another 2.2% has severe bipolar disorder. Based on the current population of the United States, that means that 3.3% of adults, or 7.7 million people, are afflicted with these two disorders at any given time.

How many of them are receiving treatment for their illnesses? NIMH has estimated that 40% of adults with schizophrenia and 51% of adults with severe bipolar disorder receive no treatment in any given year [2]. This estimate is consistent with the 2010 study by Olfson *et al.* [3] that 41% of individuals with schizophrenia received no treatment in the month following their discharge from the hospital. Multiplying this percentage by the number of adults with schizophrenia and severe bipolar disorder means that at least 3.2 million Americans with severe mental illness who are living in the community are receiving no treatment for their illness at any given time. The vast majority of these individuals need antipsychotic and mood stabilizing medication to control the symptoms of their illness; without such medication they continue to experience delusional thinking, auditory hallucinations, mood swings, and other symptoms of their illness. In effect, the United States is a giant laboratory for an unplanned, naturalistic experiment on what will happen if you have 3.2 million people with untreated serious mental illness living in the community.

Initial Signs of Trouble: The 1970s

The results of this unplanned experiment are now obvious. They include hundreds of thousands of untreated mentally ill individuals who are homeless, confined to jails and prisons, being victimized and often living in conditions much worse than existed in the state mental hospitals. These aspects of the

outcome have been detailed elsewhere [4]; in this article, I will focus only on violent behavior as one aspect of the outcome.

California had been a leader among states in emptying its state psychiatric hospitals, and it was therefore not surprising that California showed the first signs of trouble. By the 1970s, episodes of violent behavior by individuals with untreated serious mental illness were being increasingly reported.

- 1970: John Frazier, responding to the voice of God, killed a prominent surgeon and his wife, two young sons, and secretary. Frazier's mother and wife had sought unsuccessfully to have him hospitalized.
- 1972: Herbert Mullin, responding to auditory hallucinations, killed 13 people over three months. He had been hospitalized three times but released without further treatment.
- 1973: Charles Soper killed his wife, three children, and himself two weeks after having been discharged from a state hospital.
- 1973: Edmund Kemper killed his mother and her friend and was charged with killing six others. Eight years earlier, he had killed his grandparents because he "tired of their company," but at age 21 had been released from the state hospital without further treatment.
- 1977: Edward Allaway, believing that people were trying to hurt him, killed seven people at Cal State Fullerton. Five years earlier, he had been hospitalized for paranoid schizophrenia but was released without further treatment.

Public concern about such episodes had become so widespread by 1973 that the California state legislature held hearings on this issue. Dr. Andrew Robertson, deputy director of the California Department of Mental Health, offered remarkable testimony. He said that the emptying of the state hospitals had indeed "exposed us as a society to some dangerous people."

> People whom we have released have gone out and killed other people, maimed other people, destroyed property; they have done many things of an evil nature without the ability to stop and many of them have immediately thereafter killed themselves. That sounds bad, but let's qualify it ... the odds are still in society's favor, even if it doesn't make the patients innocent or the guy who is hurt or killed feel any better [5].

At the same time as the violence issue was surfacing in California, it was also appearing in other states.

Between 1970 and 1975 in Albany County, New York, a study was done on all 48 homicides committed there. Eight homicides (17%) were committed by individuals with schizophrenia. Most of them were not being treated at the time of the crime, leading the authors to conclude that "closer follow-ups of psychotic patients, especially schizophrenia, could do a lot to improve the welfare of the patient and community" [6,7]. In 1979, Dr. Judith Rankin reviewed all the early studies on what was happening to the patients being discharged from the state hospitals. She concluded: "Arrest and conviction rates for the subcategory of violent crimes were found to exceed general population rates in every study in which they were measured" [8].

The Evidence Became Clearer: The 1980s

By 1980, the writing was on the wall regarding the outcome of deinstitutionalization for anyone who cared to look. The psychiatric profession, with rare exceptions, did not care to look and denied that there were problems.

Such denial became much more difficult in the 1980s. The decade opened ominously with three high-profile violent episodes within a 12-month period. Former congressman Allard Lowenstein was killed by Dennis Sweeney, John Lennon was killed by Mark David Chapman, and President Ronald Reagan was shot by John Hinckley. All three perpetrators had untreated schizophrenia. Sweeney, for example, believed that Lowenstein, his former mentor, had implanted a transmitter in his teeth through which he was sending harassing voices.

As the decade progressed, such widely publicized homicides became more common.

- 1985: Sylvia Seegrist, diagnosed with schizophrenia and with 12 past hospitalizations, killed three and wounded seven in a Pennsylvania shopping mall.
- 1985: Bryan Stanley, diagnosed with schizophrenia and with seven past hospitalizations, killed a priest and two others in a Wisconsin Catholic Church.
- 1985: Lois Lang, diagnosed with schizophrenia and discharged from a mental hospital three months earlier, killed the chairman of a foreign exchange firm and his receptionist in New York.

- 1986: Juan Gonzalez, diagnosed with schizophrenia and psychiatrically evaluated four days earlier, killed two and injured nine others with a sword on New York's Staten Island Ferry.
- 1988: Laurie Dann, who was known to both the police and FBI because of her threatening and psychotic behavior, killed a boy and injured five of his classmates in an Illinois elementary school.
- 1988: Dorothy Montalvo, diagnosed with schizophrenia, was accused of murdering at least seven elderly individuals and burying them in her backyard in California.
- 1988: Aaron Lindh, known to be mentally ill and threatening, killed the Dane County coroner in Madison, Wisconsin. This was one of six incidents in that county during 1988 "involving mentally ill individuals . . . [that] resulted in four homicides, three suicides, seven victims wounded by gunshots, and one victim mauled by a polar bear" when a mentally ill man climbed into its pen at the local zoo [9].
- 1989: Joseph Wesbecker, diagnosed with bipolar disorder, killed seven and wounded 13 at a printing plant in Kentucky.

Another indication that such episodes of violence were increasing was a study that compared admissions to a New York state psychiatric hospital in 1975 and 1982. It reported that "the percentage of patients who had committed violence toward persons while living in the community in the 1982 cohort was nearly double the percentage in the 1975 cohort" [10]. In addition, "the percentage of patients who had had encounters with the criminal justice system in the 1982 cohort was more than quadruple the percentage in the 1975 cohort" [10].

The Epidemiological Catchment Area (ECA) surveys carried out between 1980 and 1983 also contributed to the discussion about violence. Individuals with serious mental illness living in the community reported much higher rates of violent behavior than other community residents. For example, individuals with schizophrenia were 21 times more likely to have used weapons in a fight [11].

Finally, the question continued to be raised regarding what percentage of all homicides were attributable to individuals with serious mental illness. A study of 71 homicides committed between 1978 and 1980 in Contra Costa County, California, reported that seven of the 71 (10%) were carried out by individuals diagnosed with schizophrenia, all of whom had been psychiatrically evaluated prior to the crime and all of whom had refused medication [12].

The End of Professional Denial: The 1990s

By the early 1990s, the evidence linking violent behavior to untreated serious mental illness was becoming overwhelming. The effect of violent behavior on families became clear when the National Alliance for the Mentally Ill (NAMI) released the results of its 1990 survey of 1401 NAMI families. In the preceding year in 11% of the families, the seriously mentally ill family member had physically harmed another person [13]. In 1992, Link et al. [14] reported the results of their carefully controlled study of individuals with serious mental illness living in New York. Such individuals were found to be three times more likely to commit violent acts such as weapons use or "hurting someone badly." The sicker the individual, the more likely they were to have been violent [14]. Such studies were enough to convince John Monahan, who had been one of the skeptics regarding the causal relationship of mental illness and violent behavior, and in 1992, he published his *mea culpa*. In reviewing many of these studies in 1992, Prof. John Monahan concluded:

> The data that have recently become available, fairly read, suggest the one conclusion I did not want to reach: Whether the measure is the prevalence of violence among the disordered or the prevalence of disorder among the violent, whether the sample is people who are selected for treatment as inmates or patients in institutions or people randomly chosen from the open community, and no matter how many social and demographic factors are statistically taken into account, there appears to be a relationship between mental disorder and violent behavior [15].

Throughout the 1990s, the evidence linking serious mental illness to violent behavior continued to accumulate, and increasingly the studies pinpointed the importance of treatment. A study of 133 outpatients with schizophrenia reported that "13 percent of the study group were characteristically violent" and that "71 percent of the violent patients... had problems with medication compliance" [16].

Throughout the 1990s, the public was also repeatedly reminded of the link between mental illness and violence by a continuing series of high-profile homicides. The names of the perpetrators flashed across the evening news with predictable regularity, each story different and yet remarkably the same. If the individuals had been receiving treatment for their mental illness, such tragedies would probably not have occurred. As the decade progressed, the pace seemed to quicken: James Brady in Atlanta; Gary Rimert in South Carolina; John Kappler in Boston; Betty Madeira in Los Angeles; Keven McKiever in New York; Gary Rosenberg in Rochester; Jeanette Harper in West Virginia; Debra Jackson in Minnesota; Gian Ferri in San Francisco; James Swann in Washington, DC; Colin Ferguson in New York; Linda Scates in California; William Tager in New York; Michael Laudor in New York; John Salvi in Massachusetts; Wendell Williamson in North Carolina; Michael Vernon in New York; Reuben Harris in New York; Mark Bechard in Maine; John DuPont in Pennsylvania; Alfred Head in Virginia; Daniel Ellis in Iowa; Jorge Delgado in New York; Steve Abrams in California; Julie Rodriguez in Sacramento; Larry Ashbrook in Fort Worth; Russell Weston in Washington; Lisa Duy in Salt Lake City; Michael Oullette in Connecticut; Paul Harrington in Michigan; Salvatore Garrasi in New York; Andrew Goldstein in New York – the list seemed to stretch endlessly. After each headline, people inevitably asked why it happened; no answers were forthcoming, and then the story was gone. The only tragedy that generated sustained attention was the Weston case because he killed two guards as he stormed the U.S. Capitol, trying to reach a machine he believed could reverse time. Because several members of Congress were nearby when this happened, it did get the attention of Congress, at least briefly.

Since many of the homicides involved multiple victims, it was increasingly asked whether such mass killings were increasing. In 1999, Hempel et al. [17] identified 30 mass killings in which firearms were used and at least three persons were killed between 1949 and 1998. Even though the killings had occurred over a 50-year period, 21 of them, or 70%, had occurred during the final 13 years, from 1986 to 1998. And among the 30 perpetrators of the mass killings, 12 had definite psychotic symptoms at the time and another eight "exhibited behavior suggestive of psychosis" [17].

In 2000, Hempel et al.'s findings were validated by a detailed *New York Times* survey of 100 mass killings between 1949 and 1999. Only 10 of the

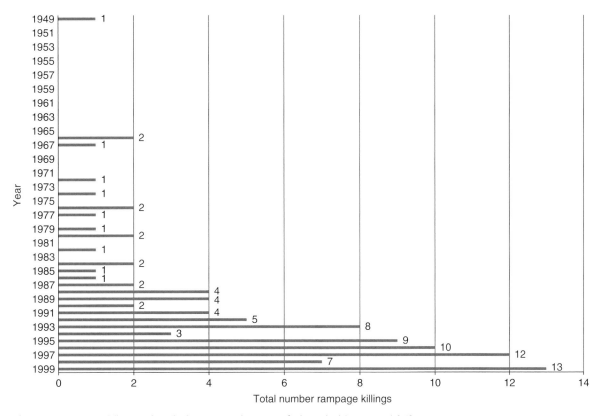

Figure 1.1 Rampage killings with multiple victims, at least one of whom died (1949–1999) [18].

mass killings occurred between 1949 and 1979, whereas 90 of them occurred between 1980 and 1999 (Figure 1.1). The survey also reported "much evidence of mental illness in its subjects. More than half had histories of serious mental health problems ... 48 killers had some kind of formal diagnosis, often schizophrenia." Among these, 24 had been prescribed psychiatric drugs but "14 had stopped taking them" [18].

Thus, by the end of the century, the violent consequences of the poorly planned deinstitutionalization of psychiatric patients were evident to everyone. Dr. John Talbott, one of the few American psychiatrists who had warned about releasing hundreds of thousands of patients without providing follow-up treatment for them, had been prophetic when he had earlier written: "With the knowledge that state hospitals required 100 years to achieve their maximum size, the precipitous attempt to move large number of their charges into settings that in fact did not exist must be seen as incompetent at best and criminal at worst" [19].

Into the Twentyfirst Century

Thus, by the beginning of the present century, the relationship between deinstitutionalization, untreated serious mental illness, and violent behavior had been clearly established. A definitive meta-analysis by Fazel *et al.* [20] identified 20 studies on violence and psychosis published between 1980 and 2009. Each of the 20 studies showed a positive association, and the authors concluded that "schizophrenia and other psychoses are associated with violence and violent offending, particularly homicide" [20]. Another seminal study by Fazel *et al.* [21] examined longitudinal data on violent crime and schizophrenia and related disorders in Sweden over 38 years, from 1972 to 2010. It reported that the rate of violent crime by individuals with these diagnoses not only increased over the 38 years but, most importantly, increased in direct proportion to the decrease of psychiatric hospitalization. Specifically, they "showed that the number of inpatient nights [in psychiatric hospitals] was negatively associated with violence ... that is, fewer annual

5

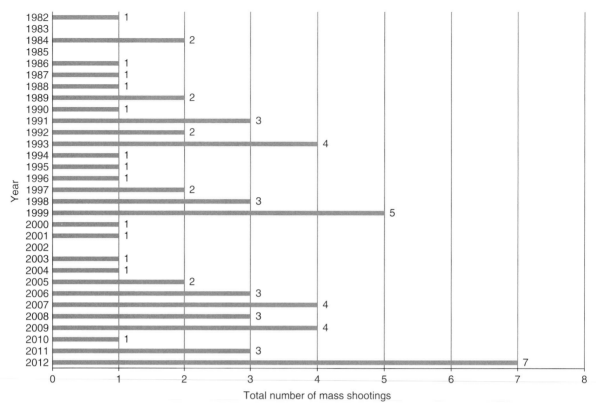

Figure 1.2 Mass shootings with >4 deaths (1982–2012), not including the person doing the shooting [26].

inpatient nights were associated with more violence ... perpetrated by those with schizophrenia and related psychoses" [21]. This strongly supported the causal relationship between deinstitutionalization and the increase in violence.

In regard to risk factors for increasing violent behavior among individuals with schizophrenia, multiple studies have shown that substance abuse is an important risk factor [20,22]. However, individuals with schizophrenia and related psychoses have been shown to have increased levels of violent behavior even when substance abuse is not involved [23]. In an Australian study, individuals with schizophrenia without substance abuse "were more than twice as likely as controls to have a violent conviction" [24].

The present century has produced additional evidence that individuals with serious mental illness are responsible for at least 10% of all homicides. A study in Indiana examined the records of 518 individuals in prison who had been convicted of homicide between 1990 and 2002. Among the 518, 53 (or 10.2%) had been diagnosed with schizophrenia (*n* = 27), bipolar

disorder (*n* = 12), or other psychotic disorders not associated with drug abuse (*n* = 14). An additional 42 individuals had been diagnosed with mania or major depressive disorder. It should be emphasized that the study included only those who had been sentenced to prison and did not include those individuals who had committed homicides and were subsequently found to be incompetent to stand trial or not guilty by reason of insanity, and therefore sent to a psychiatric facility instead of prison. Thus, the 10.2% is probably an undercount [25].

The present century has also produced additional evidence that individuals with serious mental illness are responsible for at least half of the continuing mass killings. A 2012 study suggests that such killings continue to occur regularly [26] (Figure 1.2). Virginia Tech, Tucson, Aurora, and Newtown are now synonymous with this issue. But these are merely the mass killings that receive the most public attention. In the five-year period before the Tucson tragedy, which was highly publicized because a member of Congress was involved, there had been 10 other similar tragedies, in addition to Virginia Tech, involving individuals with serious mental illness who were not being treated. Thus, Jared Loughner in Tucson became a household name after he killed six and injured 13, including Congresswoman Giffords, in Tucson. By contrast, Isaac Zamora, who killed six and injured four in Seattle in 2008, was quickly forgotten.

What is the Answer?

The answer, in a word, is treatment. The deinstitutionalization of individuals from state mental health hospitals was fundamentally a sound idea; the failure of this idea was in how it was carried out. Emptying the hospitals was thus a good idea, but failing to ensure that the individuals leaving the hospital would continue to receive the treatment necessary to keep them from again becoming psychotic has been a disaster.

Many studies have examined the relationship between medication compliance and violent behavior in mentally ill individuals. A 2002 study of 802 adults with serious mental illness reported that those who had been violent were almost twice as likely to have been noncompliant with medications [27]. A 2006 study of 1011 outpatients with serious mental illness found that "community violence was inversely related to treatment adherence" [28]. A 2007 study of 907 individuals with serious mental illness reported that those who were violent were "more likely to deny needing psychiatric treatment" [29]. A 2014 study using the Swedish national database reported that "violent crime fell by 45% in patients receiving antipsychotics" [30]. Treatment is especially important during the first episode of psychosis, at which time violent behavior is especially common [31].

There are many ways to ensure that individuals with serious mental illness receive treatment. Many patients who are aware of their own illness will accept treatment voluntarily. Others, especially those with anosognosia and are thus unaware of their own illness, will require some form of involuntary treatment. The most effective forms of outpatient involuntary treatment are assisted outpatient treatment (AOT), conditional release, and mental health courts.

Assisted outpatient treatment (AOT)

AOT is a form of outpatient commitment in which mentally ill individuals are told by court order that they can live in the community as long as they follow their treatment plan, but if they do not do so, they can be involuntarily returned to the hospital. It is available in all states except Massachusetts, Connecticut, Maryland, Tennessee, and New Mexico. The criteria for being put on AOT vary somewhat by state, but usually include having had a history of not following treatment plans and becoming dangerous to self or others when not being treated. Examples of AOT are Kendra's Law in New York and Laura's Law in California. AOT has been shown to be effective in reducing rehospitalizations, incarcerations, victimizations, episodes of violence, and homelessness [32]. A study in England claimed that the English equivalent of AOT – called community treatment disorders – was not effective in reducing psychiatric read-missions [33]. However, this study was seriously flawed in not including the patients most likely to have benefited from community treatment orders, and also insofar as it merely compared one form of mandated treatment against another form of mandated treatment (called Section 17). Thus, the fact that there was no difference in psychiatric rehospitalization was not surprising.

Conditional release

Patients who have been legally committed to a hospital can be released on the condition that they continue to be compliant with medication. Violation of the condition can result in rehospitalization. In most states the hospital director has the authority to do this without asking permission of the courts. Forty states have laws permitting conditional release. In the past, this form of assisted treatment was widely used for both civil and forensic (criminal) cases, but now it is used mostly for the latter.

Until recently, New Hampshire was the leading state using conditional release for civilly committed patients; in 1998, 27% of patients released from the New Hampshire State Hospital were put on conditional release. In a study of the effectiveness of conditional release on medication compliance, 26 severely psychiatrically ill patients were conditionally released from the New Hampshire State Hospital with assessment of various measures for the year prior to hospitalization and for the first two years on conditional release. The result was a dramatic decrease in violent behavior from 5.6 episodes in the year prior to hospitalization to 1.1 episodes in the second year on conditional release [34].

Mental Health Courts

Mental health courts are courts set up specifically to adjudicate cases in which a person with mental illness has been charged with a crime. Some mental health courts take both misdemeanors and felonies, others only the former. Mental health courts are a form of jail diversion for mentally ill individuals charged with crimes. In most cases, the judge gives the defendant the choice of going to jail or cooperation with an outpatient treatment program, including medication. If the person refuses to follow the treatment plan, he/she can be sent to jail. Mental health courts have been shown to be very effective in keeping people on medication, and in reducing rehospitalizations, incarcerations, and violent behavior. The main limitation of such courts is that a mentally ill person has to have committed a crime in order to be eligible [35,36].

Conclusion

In conclusion, the relationship between deinstitutionalization and the increasing episodes of violent behavior by individuals with serious mental illness who are not being treated has been firmly established. Until we address the treatment issue and utilize proven remedies, such as assisted outpatient treatment, conditional release, and mental health courts, we should expect these episodes of violent behavior to continue. Such violence is a major source of stigma against mentally ill individuals, thus affecting all those so affected.

Disclosures

The author has nothing to disclose.

References

1. Torrey EF, Miller J. *The Invisible Plague: The Rise of Mental Illness from 1750 to the Present*. New Brunswick, NJ: Rutgers University Press; 2002.

2. NIMH website. Prevalence of serious mental illness among U.S. adults by age, sex, and race. http://www.nimh.nih.gov/statistics/SMI_AASR.shtml.

3. Olfson M, Marcus SC, Doshi JA. Continuity of care after inpatient discharge of patients with schizophrenia in the Medicaid program: a retrospective longitudinal cohort analysis. *J. Clin. Psychiatry*. 2010; **71**(7): 831–838.

4. Torrey EF. *American Psychosis: How the Federal Government Destroyed the Mental Illness Treatment System*. New York: Oxford University Press; 2014.

5. Testimony of Dr. Andrew Robertson before the Select Committee on Proposed Phaseout of State Hospital Services, May 18–October 10, 1973, California State Archives.

6. Grunberg F, Klinger BL, Grumet B. Homicide and deinstitutionalization of the mentally ill. *Am. J. Psychiatry*. 1977; **134**(6): 685–687.

7. Grunberg F, Klinger BL, Grumet BR. Homicide and community-based psychiatry. *J. Nerv. Ment. Dis.* 1978; **166**(12): 868–874.

8. Rabkin J. Criminal behavior of discharged mental patients: a critical appraisal of the research. *Psychol. Bull.* 1979; **86**(1): 1–27.

9. Kuhlman TL. Unavoidable tragedies in Madison, WI: a third view. *Hosp. Community Psychiatry*. 1992; **43**(1): 72–73.

10. Karra A, Otis DB. A comparison of inpatients in an urban state hospital in 1975 and 1982. *Hosp. Community Psychiatry*. 1987; **38** (9): 963–967.

11. Swanson JW, Hozer CE 3rd, Ganju VK, Jono RT. Violence and psychiatric disorder in the community: evidence from the Epidemiologic Catchment Area surveys. *Hosp. Community Psychiatry*. 1990; **41**(7): 761–770.

12. Wilcox DE. The relationship of mental illness to homicide. *American Journal of Forensic Psychiatry*. 1985; **6**(1): 3–15.

13. Steinwachs DM, Kasper JD, Skinner EA. *Family Perspectives on Meeting the Needs for Care of Severely Mentally Ill Relatives: A National Survey*. Arlington, VA: National Alliance for the Mentally Ill; 1992.

14. Link BG, Andrews H, Cullen FT. The violent and illegal behavior of mental patients reconsidered. *American Sociological Review*. 1992; **57**(3): 275–292.

15. Monahan J. Mental disorder and violent behavior: perceptions and evidence. *American Psychologist*. 1992; **47**(4): 511–521.

16. Bartels J, Drake RE, Wallach MA, Freeman DH. Characteristic hostility in schizophrenic outpatients. *Schizophr. Bull.* 1991; **17**(1): 163–171.

17. Hempel AG, Meloy JR, Richards TC. Offenders and offense characteristics of a nonrandom sample of mass murders. *J. Am. Acad. Psychiatry Law*. 1999; **27**(2): 213–225.

18. Fessenden F. They threaten, seethe and unhinge, then kill in quantity. *New York Times*, April 9, 2000, pp. 1 and 20.

19. Talbott JA. Deinstitutionalization: avoiding the disasters of the past. *Hosp. Community Psychiatry*. 1979; **30**(9): 621–624.

20. Fazel S, Gulati G, Linsell L, Geddes JR, Grann M. Schizophrenia and violence: review and meta-analysis. *PLoS Med.* 2009; **6**(8): e10000120.

21. Fazel S, Wolf A, Palm C, Lichtenstein P. Violent crime, suicide, and premature mortality in patients with schizophrenia and related disorders: a 38-year total population study in Sweden. *Lancet Psychiatry.* 2014; **1**(1): 44–54.

22. Witt K, van Dorn R, Fazel S. Risk factors for violence in psychosis: systematic review and meta-regression analysis of 110 studies. *PLoS ONE.* 2013; **8**(2): e55942.

23. Van Dorn R, Volavka J, Johnson N. Mental disorder and violence: is there a relationship beyond substance abuse? *Soc. Psychiatry Psychiatr. Epidemiol.* 2012; **47**(3): 487–503.

24. Short T, Thomas S, Mullen P, Ogloff JR. Comparing violence in schizophrenia patients with and without comorbid substance-use disorders to community controls. *Acta Psychiatr. Scand.* 2013; **128**(4): 306–313.

25. Matejkowski JC, Cullen SW, Solomon PL. Characteristics of persons with severe mental illness who have been incarcerated for murder. *J. Am. Acad. Psychiatry Law.* 2008; **36**(1): 74–86.

26. Follman M, Aronsen G, Pan D. A guide to mass shootings in America. *Mother Jones,* December 15, 2012.

27. Swanson JW, Swartz MS, Essock SM, *et al.* The social–environmental context of violent behavior in persons treated for severe mental illness. *Am. J. Public Health.* 2002; **92**(9): 1523–1531.

28. Elbogen EB, van Dorn RA, Swanson JW, Swartz MS, Monahan J. Treatment engagement and violence risk in mental disorders. *Br. J. Psychiatry.* 2006; **189**(4): 354–360.

29. Elbogen EB, Mustillo S, van Dorn R, Swanson JW, Swartz MS. The impact of perceived need for treatment on risk of arrest and violence among people with severe mental illness. *Criminal Justice and Behavior.* 2007; **34**(2): 197–210.

30. Fazel S, Zetterqvist J, Larsson H, Långström N, Lichtenstein P. Antipsychotics, mood stabilisers, and risk of violent crime. *Lancet.* 2014; **384**(9949): 1167–1168.

31. Nielssen O, Large M. Rates of homicide during the first episode of psychosis and after treatment: a systematic review and meta-analysis. *Schizophr. Bull.* 2010; **36**(4): 702–712.

32. Torrey EF. *The Insanity Offense.* New York: W.W. Norton; 2008.

33. Burns T, Rugkasa J, Molodynski A, *et al.* Community treatment orders for patients with psychosis (OCTET): a randomized controlled trial. *Lancet.* 2013; **81**(9878): 1627–1633.

34. O'Keefe C, Potenza DP, Mueser KT. Treatment outcomes for severely mentally ill patients on conditional discharge to community-based treatment. *J. Nerv. Ment. Dis.* 1997; **185**(6): 409–411.

35. Lamb HR, Weinberger LE. Mental health courts as a way to provide treatment to violent persons with severe mental illness. *JAMA.* 2008; **300**(6): 722–724.

36. Steadman HJ, Redlich A, Callahan L, Robbins PC, Vesselinov R. Effect of mental health courts on arrests and jail days: a multisite study. *Arch. Gen. Psychiatry.* 2011; **68**(2): 167–172.

Chapter

2

The new mission of forensic mental health systems: managing violence as a medical syndrome in an environment that balances treatment and safety

Katherine D. Warburton

Introduction

Are psychiatric inpatient settings more violent, and if so, is it related to increasing numbers of forensic patients? The question is frequently raised in discussions regarding state hospitals, and there has been significant media attention on the issue [1–14]. Forensic psychiatric populations appear to be growing, both in terms of mentally ill inmates in correctional settings, as well as criminally committed patients in state hospital settings [15–20]. In many cases, physical aggression attributed to an underlying mental disorder is the primary reason for state hospital admission. Although anecdotal reports suggest that violence is increasing in certain inpatient psychiatric settings, varying and imprecise definitions of the term "violence," combined with limited longitudinal research, make this apparent trend of increasing violence difficult to confirm scientifically [21–25]. However, there is enough evidence to support the exploration of new conceptual models for case formulation, therapies, and therapeutic environments.

Utilization of a model where psychiatric violence is approached dimensionally, as a primary medical syndrome rather than the product of one, may allow for more effective interventions; focus on the presenting problem will allow clinicians to better understand, assess, predict, and treat physical aggression in a systematic and evidence-based manner. In this model, the collection of violent behaviors running together may stem from a variety of etiologies and diagnoses; this dimensional rather than categorical approach will provide better focus on the true presenting clinical issue, rather than the rote treatment of a categorical diagnosis.

Beyond formulations and interventions, there is a pressing need to address violent milieus. Mental health facilities have an obligation to provide appropriate physical plant security to prevent the serious injury and death of staff members and other patients, while simultaneously creating a treatment environment that maintains therapeutic value.

Is There a New Type of Patient? Mentally Ill as Well as Criminally Minded?

A society's challenge in determining which individuals will be detained in an inpatient hospital versus a correctional setting is not a new one. In 1935, Penrose [26] concluded that every society has a finite number of institutionalized persons, and that those societies with high rates of incarceration had lower rates of mental hospitalization, and vice versa. However, if the apparent trend of high (if not increasing) rates of incarcerated mental health patients, as well as increasing forensic patients, in hospitals holds correct, then Penrose's theory of a closed system is no longer viable, and the medical community has a greater task than just managing a finite and unchanging population. Furthermore, both research and clinical experience indicate that there may be a new type of patient – one who is both mentally ill and criminally minded [27,28]. This new type of patient may be due to earlier policies that resulted from noble social movements, such as deinstitutionalization of individuals with mental illness and patient-oriented outpatient commitment schemes. Additionally, the rise of

Violence in Psychiatry, ed. Katherine D. Warburton and Stephen M. Stahl. Published by Cambridge University Press.
© Cambridge University Press 2016.

methamphetamine abuse, apparent increases in incarceration of psychiatric patients, and limited access to community resources may have resulted in individuals who have bona fide psychiatric symptoms as well as criminogenic thinking [29–31]. This would further necessitate a move toward humane treatment settings that concomitantly provide adequate safety.

Historical trends demonstrating the movement of patients from hospitals to correctional facilities and back again over time indicate that society has yet to strike the correct balance between treatment and safety. Extremism in either direction has tended to cause a rapid pendulum shift toward the opposite extreme. There is some evidence that the pendulum is moving back in the direction of leveraged care over absolute patients' rights [32]. Without effective clinical intervention, the pendulum will continue to swing back in the direction of purely punitive or custodial solutions to psychiatric violence. While only a small fraction of people with mental illness are violent, our field needs to make the identification of these patients a priority and find appropriate treatment solutions. A new treatment model that balances the principles of treatment and safety may be the correct solution.

Statement of the Problem

There is a well-known association between mental illness and violence; substance abuse disorders increase violence risk the most [33,34]. Inpatient aggression can be categorized by its motivation, and further categorized by its provocation (Table 2.1) [35–37].

The three predominant motivators of inpatient violence are disordered impulse control, planned predatory behavior, and positive psychotic symptoms. Of these, psychotic violence is the least prevalent in psychiatric settings [35,36]. Individuals with high psychopathy scores perpetrate more aggression, and more severe aggression, than other groups [38]. However, research that has examined the treatability of psychopathy has led to a spectrum of conclusions, ranging from outcomes suggesting that treatment makes psychopathy worse to treatment being only mildly beneficial [39–41]. Impulsive aggression is the most prevalent type of aggression seen [35,36], but it is also the most complex and multifactorial.

There are a few possible implications from the finding that psychotic violence is the least prevalent in psychiatric inpatient settings (see Table 2.2).

- Psychiatric hospitals do their ostensible jobs very well (treating psychotic violence).
- State hospitals need to acknowledge and strategize more effectively around the issue of impulsive and predatory aggression.
- Patients are becoming more complex, and therefore violence in forensic psychiatric populations should be treated and investigated like any other type of independent medical syndrome. Targeting more categorical psychiatric syndromes has failed to remedy the problem.

This formulation of the problem leads to logical approaches to reducing the type of violence currently being seen in forensic inpatient settings.

Table 2.1 Three primary motivators of inpatient aggression

– Disordered impulse control

- Most frequent
- Most complex and multifactorial
- Requires innovative programs integrating both novel psychopharmacology and behavioral interventions

– Planned predatory behavior

- Most severe aggression
- Questionable treatability

– Positive psychotic symptoms

- Least frequent
- Most treatable

Table 2.2 Possible implications of the finding that psychotic violence is the least prevalent type in inpatient settings

1. Psychiatric hospitals do their ostensible jobs very well (treating psychotic violence).

2. State hospitals need to acknowledge and strategize more effectively around the issue of impulsive and predatory aggression.

3. Patients are becoming more complex, and therefore violence in forensic psychiatric populations should be treated and investigated like any other type of independent medical syndrome; targeting more categorical psychiatric syndromes has failed to remedy the problem.

Proposed Solutions

A dimensional conceptualization of psychiatric violence would lead to focused approach to assessment, treatment, and environment (Table 2.3).

Violence risk assessment

Training in, and implementation of, standardized violence risk assessments are the first steps in both prediction and treatment planning. More important than the selection of any particular instrument is training clinicians on the body of available tools so they know the appropriate strategy in individual situations. Mental health professionals should be familiar with the violence risk literature and trained on a variety of instruments such as the Hare Psychopathy Checklist (PCL-R); Short Term Assessment of Risk and Treatability (START); Violence Risk Screening-10 (V-RISK-10); Historical, Clinical, Risk Management-20 (HCR-20); and the Classification of Violence Risk (COVR). For patients admitted to psychiatric institutions for violent behavior, inclusion of violence risk data into the treatment planning process should be a priority [42–47].

Treatment

Psychiatry needs to prioritize the process of defining standards of care and interventions based on aggression type (e.g., dialectical behavior therapy and novel psychopharmacology for impulsive aggression; secure behavioral interventions for predatory aggression; antipsychotic medication algorithms for psychotic aggression; when and how to utilize behavioral therapies).

Addressing substance abuse

Co-occurring substance abuse diagnoses occur in the majority of the forensic patient population, and substance abuse is the diagnosis most correlated with violence [33,34]. Systems that treat violent patients should develop policies to adequately target substance abuse, diversion, and intoxication. Policy targets include random drug screening; detox/treatment protocols; and education related to/reduction of prescribed medications that are abused in this population, including not only opiates and benzodiazepines, but medications such as quetiapine and buproprion as well.

Independent forensic evaluation

There are multiple legal, ethical, clinical, and violence-related issues when treatment providers also serve as forensic evaluators [48,49]. In cases where the assessment of violence involves more than treatment planning (i.e., it impacts the evaluation of discharge readiness or placement), the evaluation should be completed by a non-treatment team member to avoid the myriad complications related to dual agency.

Data practices

The way to treat systemic aggression is to understand it. Collecting data related to all acts of physical aggression and classifying by severity and type are the best ways to understand the interventions needed and whether or not those interventions were successful.

Physical plant security

Many state hospitals were built at the turn of the twentieth century for the delivery of moral treatment. They are not appropriate treatment environments for the safe treatment of violence. Physical plant limitations include poor sight lines, large unit sizes, and aging infrastructure. Beyond just physical plant layout, a new treatment environment is required [50].

Developing a New Treatment Environment

While the above improvements will potentially bring about positive change, they alone will not solve the

Table 2.3 Dimensional approach to psychiatric violence

– *Violence risk assessment*

– *Customized treatment based on aggression type*

  Dialectical behavior therapy (DBT) and novel psychopharmacology for impulsive aggression
  Secure behavioral interventions for predatory aggression
  Antipsychotic medication algorithms for psychotic aggression
  When and how to utilize behavioral therapies

– *Addressing substance abuse*

– *Independent forensic evaluation*

– *Data collection: all acts of physical aggression, severity, and type*

  • *Outcomes of treatment intervention*

– *Physical plant security*

  • *Physical plant layout*
  • *A new treatment environment*

problem. The chasm between correctional mental health care and psychiatric hospital security is still too large. Given the increasing criminalization of the mentally ill, there may also be an increasing population of patients who are both mentally ill and dangerous, and we therefore need to develop a new treatment model that addresses both aspects, encompassing intensive treatment within a safe environment. The underlying concept of a safe treatment facility is that it will serve as a center of excellence for the assessment and treatment of violence. We need an environment that will facilitate the balance between treating patients in the least restrictive setting, and protecting our patients and staff who may be at risk of victimization. The basic need for this type facility stems from a lack of appropriate treatment environments for those patients who exhibit a high risk of severe violence who cannot be contained at traditional facilities due to physical plant limitations.

Conceptually, this type of facility will be one placement option in a stratified continuum of care – a continuum with one extreme rooted in the "moral treatment" settings of old and the other in the current correctional mental health environments. The continuum should consist of a clinical system for placement that is based on individual risk of violence to self and others in the context of treatment needs. Patients should be moved through the system based on dynamic assessment of individual risk and behavior (Table 2.4).

A new treatment model should be based heavily on the forensic literature. While academicians, politicians, and criminologists will all define aggression differently in order to understand it vis-à-vis their systemic needs, this treatment model is based on the work of Nolan and Quanbeck [35,36], who categorized violence by three broad etiologies: psychotic, impulsive, and predatory. These three broad categories serve as the foundation for the subsequent violence intervention strategies and serve as the broad basis for treatment planning for our most violent patients.

The first step in the treatment of these individuals is a violence risk assessment utilizing generally accepted methodologies. A violence risk assessment can be conceptualized as occurring in three domains: (1) history (the best predictor of future violence is past violence), (2) clinical (what is the status of the psychiatric symptoms that drive the violence?), and (3) risk management (the attempt to provide a safe environment for assessment and treatment

Table 2.4 Assessment strategies

1. Categorize violence by three broad etiologies
2. Violence risk assessment utilizing generally accepted methodologies

   a. History (the best predictor of future violence is past violence)

   b. Clinical (what is the status of the psychiatric symptoms that drive the violence?)

   c. Risk management

      i Safe environment for assessment and treatment delivery

      ii Selecting patients for enhanced treatment settings

delivery pertains to the latter domain of violence risk assessment) [42].

Once in this setting, the treatment should be highly individualized, given the complex, multifactorial nature of severe aggression. Structured clinical assessment should be utilized to delineate risk factors and gear a treatment plan accordingly. In cases of severe violence risk, careful assessment and successful treatment takes time to accomplish, and exposing other patients and staff to risk of serious injury or death is unacceptable.

Patient selection for enhanced treatment settings should be based on elevated risk, rather than diagnosis or any other singular factors. Some examples of high elevated risk in different domains illustrate the need to provide a clinical synthesis of risk rather than to rely on rigid clinical criteria. Some specific case examples follow.

- A case of psychotic aggression in a patient who had a history of strangling people to death in the night, attacks which took place in the context of specific threat/control/override delusions. In this new conceptual model, staff would have the option to contain the patient in his room during sleeping hours, until such time as he stabilized on medication. Once the specific delusions were adequately treated, his violence risk would decline precipitously and he could return to an environment with a lower safety rating. However, under current circumstances, the only option for containment of risk in the acute circumstance is seclusion or restraint, and it is questionable that he would meet the criteria. In this case, locking the door to his room is a therapeutic intervention. In this example, historical risk is high (history of murder), clinical risk is high (current symptoms match those at time of previous murder), and risk management is high (housed in a hospital with dorm-style rooms with no physical plant controls to mitigate the risk of strangling other patients). A new treatment model would provide an avenue to treat the latter domain.

- A case of predatory aggression in a patient who had previously murdered a peer. In this example, he tells staff that he did not like a peer and "you know what I do when I don't like someone." Given his history, this cold threat indicated a high risk of severe violence (murder), but current restraint and seclusion policy did not allow for containment based on a cold threat. The hospital would have no options beyond hoping that the patient did not murder someone.

- A case of a chronically assaultive patient who assaulted so frequently that he required constant restraint. He describes the assaults as impulsive, and explains that he just gets the urge to attack people and he cannot control himself. He states that he preferred the lower stimulation of a locked room when he was in prison. This treatment model could provide that; however, he would receive frequent attention and treatment interventions as his team endeavors to understand precursors and integrate him back into the milieu.

It is important to stress that each treatment plan should be individualized, staffing-enhanced, and treatment-intensive. However, the treatment model can be overly simplified for the purpose of general understanding. Patients at high risk for severe psychotic aggression require intensive psychiatric interventions with medication, low stimulation, and observation until the symptoms are stabilized. Patients at high risk of impulsive aggression require behavioral therapies, low stimulation, and physical plant controls until coping strategies to deal with the impulses are developed. Patients at high risk of predatory aggression require monitoring, physical plant barriers to potential victims, and behavioral modification therapies, including behavioral contingencies. In a sense, psychiatric systems that treat violent patients, once stratified, will provide a strong behavioral contingency intervention that will mitigate some impulsive and predatory aggressions just by virtue of existing.

Conclusion

Deinstitutionalization appears to have had two major impacts on inpatient psychiatry. First, patients who can be safely treated in the community are treated in the community; therefore, inpatient psychiatric settings treat a higher percentage of unsafe patients. Second, the criminalization of the mentally ill has contributed to the development of a new type of patient – one who is both mentally ill and dangerous. Acknowledging the issue of increasing inpatient violence is neither syntonic to the mission of psychiatry nor politically correct, but we have a duty to address the problem.

Disclosures

Katherine D. Warburton has nothing to disclose.

References

1. Finz S, King J. Napa State Hospital psychiatric worker slain. *San Francisco Chronicle*. October 25, 2010. http://www.sfgate.com/health/ article/Napa-State-Hospital-psychiatric-worker-slain-3248688.php.

2. Cohn M, Walker AK. Treatment problems, fear found in state's high-security mental hospital, workers say. *Baltimore Sun*. November 7, 2011. http://articles.baltimoresun.com/2011-11-07/health/bs-hs-perkins-fear-20111107_1_patients-maximum-security-psychiatric-hospital-susan-sachs.

3. Cohn M. Perkins patients can be the toughest to treat. *Baltimore Sun*. November 20, 2011. http://articles.baltimoresun.com/2011-11-20/health/bs-hs-perkins-treatment-20111120_1_perkins-patients-dangerous-patients-fewer-hospital-beds.

4. Violence and fear in state mental hospitals on the rise nationally. *Baltimore Sun*. November 24, 2011. http://articles.baltimoresun.com/2011-11-24/news/bs-ed-perkins-20111124_1_donna-gross-perkins-patients-mentally-ill-patients.

5. Our View: Forensic patients swamp state mental hospital. *Portland Press Herald*. August 25, 2013. http://www.pressherald.com/opinion/forensic-patients-swamp-state-mental-hospital_2013-08-25.html?pagenum = full.

6. Poindexter R. DHHS Commissioner blames growth in court ordered patients for

Riverview problems; urges passage of LePage's plan. WABI TV5. August 22, 2013. http://wabi.tv/2013/08/22/ dhhs-commissioner-blames-growth-in-court-ordered-patients-for-riverview-problems-urges-passage-of-lepages-plan/.

7. Biscobing D, LaMet M. ABC 15 investigation exposes a 'shocking' level of violence at the Arizona State Hospital. ABC15 Arizona. August 9, 2013. http://www.abc15.com/news/local-news/investigations/abc15-investigation-exposes-a-shocking-level-of-violence-at-the-arizona-state-mental-hospital.

8. Violence at Texas mental hospitals on rise. UPI. January 27, 2013. http://www.upi.com/Top_News/US/2013/01/27/Violence-at-Texas-mental-hospitals-on-rise/UPI-96021359313991/.

9. Ryan J. Violence on the rise at Western State Hospital. *Northwest Public Radio*. May 3, 2012. http://nwpr.org/post/violence-rise-western-state-hospital.

10. Ball A. Patient violence jumps at state psychiatric hospitals. Statesman.com. January 26, 2013. http://www.statesman.com/news/news/local/patient-violence-jumps-at-state-psychiatric-hospit/nT7GH/.

11. Rector K. Assaults on staff are focus of scathing report at Catonsville Psychiatric Hospital. *Baltimore Sun*. March 2, 2013. http://www.baltimoresun.com/news/maryland/baltimore-county/ catonsville/bs-md-co-spring-grove-report-20130302,0,7658971.story.

12. Hegedus N. Danger at Mid-Hudson Psych: 'I'm just waiting for a staff member to come out dead.' *Times-Herald Record*. Undated. http://www.nyscopba.org/mid-hudson-psych-center-danger.

13. Romney L. State mental hospitals remain violent, despite gains in safety. *Los Angles Times*. October

9, 2013. http://articles.latimes.com/2013/oct/09/local/la-me-mental-hospital-safety-20131010.

14. Jaffe I. Violence at Calif. mental hospitals: 'this is the norm.' NPR. July 21, 2011. http://www.npr.org/2011/07/21/137856157/ violence-at-calif-mental-hospitals-this-is-the-norm.

15. Anderson A, West SG. Violence against mental health professionals: when the treater becomes the victim. *Innov. Clin. Neurosci.* 2011; **8**(3): 34–39.

16. Lutterman T. National Association of State Mental Health Program Directors Research Institute Fiscal Year 2010 Revenues and Expenditure Study Results. 2012.

17. Lamb HR, Weinberger LE. Persons with severe mental illness in jails and prisons: a review. *Psychiatr. Serv.* 1998; **49**(4): 483–892.

18. Baillargeon J, Binswanger IA, Penn JV, Williams BA, Murray OJ. Psychiatric disorders and repeat incarcerations: the revolving prison door. *Am. J. Psychiatry.* 2009; **166** (1): 103–109.

19. Fazel S, Seewald K. Severe mental illness in 33,588 prisoners worldwide: systematic review and meta-regression analysis. *Br. J. Psychiatry.* 2012; **200**(5): 364–373.

20. Torrey EF, Kennard AD, Eslinger D, Lamb R, Pavle J. More mentally ill persons are in jails and prisons than hospitals: a survey of the states. Treatment Advocacy Center and National Sheriff's Association; 2010. http://www.treatmentadvocacycenter.org/storage/documents/final_jails_v_hospitals_study.pdf.

21. Binder RL, McNiel DE. The relationship of gender to violent behavior in acutely disturbed psychiatric patients. *J. Clin. Psychiatry.* 1990; **51**(3): 110–114.

22. Tardiff MD, Sweillam AS. Assaultive behavior among

chronic inpatients. *Am. J. Psychiatry.* 1982; **139**(2): 212–215.

23. Linhorst DM, Scott LP. Assaultive behavior in state psychiatric hospitals: differences between forensic and nonforensic patients. *J. Interpers. Violence.* 2004; **19**(8): 857–874.

24. California Department of State Hospitals Aggression Data. www.dsh.ca.gov.

25. Results from NEI Audience Survey. Neuroscience Education Institute, Audience Survey Results, Colorado Springs. 2013.

26. Penrose LS. Mental disease and crime: outline of a comparative study of European statistics. *Br. J. Med. Psychol.* 1939; **18**(1): 1–15.

27. Morgan RD, Fisher WH, Duan N, Mandracchia JT, Murray D. Prevalence of criminal thinking among state prison inmates with serious mental illness. *Law Hum. Behav.* 2010; **34**(4): 324–336.

28. Appelbaum KL, Dvoskin JA. Consultation report on the Clifton T. Perkins Hospital Center. 2012. http://www.dhmh.maryland.gov/mha/Documents/CTPHC%20Findings%20to%20Date%201-10-12.pdf.

29. Abramson MF. The criminalization of mentally disordered behavior: possible side effect of a new mental health law. *Hosp. Community Psychiatry.* 1972; **23**(4): 101–105.

30. Swank GE, Winer D. Occurrence of psychiatric disorder in a county jail population. *Am. J. Psychiatry.* 1976; **133**(11): 1331–1333.

31. Sosowsky L. Crime and violence among mental patients reconsidered in view of the new legal relationship between the state and the mentally ill. *Am. J. Psychiatry.* 1978; **135**(1): 33–42.

32. A mental health overhaul: a congressman produces a set of good ideas for a difficult problem.

Wall Street Journal. December 25, 2013. http://online.wsj.com/news/articles/SB10001424052702304367204579267030770210744.

33. Swanson JW, Holzer CE 3rd, Ganju VK, Jono RT. Violence and psychiatric disorder in the community: evidence in the Epidemiologic Catchment Area surveys. *Hosp. Community Psychiatry.* 1990; **41**(7): 761–770.

34. Steadman HJ, Mulvey EP, Monahan J, *et al.* Violence by people discharged from acute psychiatric inpatient facilities and by others in the same neighborhoods. *Arch. Gen. Psychiatry.* 1998; **55**(5): 393–401.

35. Nolan KA, Czobor P, Roy BB, *et al.* Characteristics of assaultive behavior among psychiatric inpatients. *Psychiatr. Serv.* 2003; **54**(7): 1012–1016.

36. Quanbeck CD, McDermott BE, Lam J, *et al.* Categorization of aggressive acts committed by chronically assaultive state hospital patients. *Psychiatr. Serv.* 2007; **58**(4): 521–528.

37. Maloy JR. Empirical basis and forensic application of affective and predatory violence. *Aust. N. Z. J. Psychiatry.* 2006; **40**(6–7): 539–547.

38. McDermott BE, Edens JF, Quanbeck CD, Busse D, Scott CL. Examining the role of static and dynamic risk factors in the prediction of inpatient violence: variable and person-focused analyses. *Law Hum. Behav.* 2008; **32**(4): 325–338.

39. Harris GT, Rice ME. Treatment of psychopathy: a review of empirical findings. In: Patrick CJ, ed. *Handbook of Psychopathy.* New York: The Guilford Press; 2005: 555–572.

40. Salekin RT. Psychopathy and therapeutic pessimism: clinical lore or clinical reality? *Clin. Psychol. Rev.* 2002; **22**(1): 79–112.

41. Skeem JL, Monahan J, Mulvey EP. Psychopathy, treatment involvement, and subsequent violence among civil psychiatric patients. *Law Hum. Behav.* 2002; **26**(6): 577–603.

42. Douglas KS, Hart SD, Webster CD, *et al. HCR-20V3: Assessing Risk of Violence—User Guide.* Burnaby, Canada: Mental Health, Law, and Policy Institute, Simon Fraser University; 2013.

43. Hare RD. *Manual for the Revised Psychopathy Checklist*, 2nd edn. Toronto: Multi-Health Systems; 2003.

44. Hart SD, Cox DN, Hare RD. *The Hare Psychopathy Checklist: Screening Version.* Toronto: Multi-Health Systems; 1995.

45. Monahan J, Steadman HJ, Robbins PC, *et al.* An actuarial model of violence risk assessment for persons with mental disorders. *Psychiatr. Serv.* 2005; **56**(7): 810–815.

46. Webster CD, Martin ML, Brink J, *et al. Manual for the Short-Term Assessment of Risk and Treatability (START) (Version 1.1).* Port Coquitlam, BC, Canada: Forensic Psychiatric Services Commission and St. Joseph's Healthcare; 2009.

47. Bjørkly S, Hartvig P, Heggen FA, *et al.* Development of a brief screen for violence risk (V-RISK-10) in acute and general psychiatry: an introduction with emphasis on findings from a naturalistic test of interrater reliability. *Eur. Psychiatry.* 2009; **24**(6): 388–394.

48. Strasburger LH, Gutheil TG, Brodsky A. On wearing two hats: role conflict in serving as both psychotherapist and expert witness. *Am. J. Psychiatry.* 1997; **154**(4): 448–456.

49. Greenberg SA, Shuman DA. Irreconcilable conflict between therapeutic and forensic roles. *Professional Psychology: Research and Practice.* 1997; **28**(1): 50–57.

50. Kennedy HG. Therapeutic uses of security: mapping forensic mental health services by stratifying risk. *Advances in Psychiatric Treatment.* 2002; **8**(6): 433–443.

Chapter 3

The evolution of violence risk assessment

John Monahan and Jennifer L. Skeem

Introduction

In this review, we provide a current snapshot of the field of violence risk assessment. After highlighting the contexts in which risk of violence is assessed, we describe a framework for understanding alternative approaches to risk assessment and then compare the utility of these approaches in predicting violence. Before speculating about possible future developments in the field, we draw attention to two modern debates, i.e., whether group-based instruments are useful for assessing an individual's risk, and whether the pursuits of risk assessment and risk reduction should be separated.

We wish to be clear at the outset about our terminology and scope. We endorse the general definition of risk assessment given by Kraemer *et al.* [1]: "The process of using risk factors to estimate the likelihood (i.e., probability) of an outcome occurring in a population," (p. 340). These authors define a risk factor as a correlate that precedes the outcome in time, with no implication that the risk factor and the outcome are causally related (e.g., past violence is a robust risk factor for future violence). Our outcome of focus is physical violence to others.

Legal Context

The populations in which violence risk is assessed vary across many disparate legal contexts. In the mental health system [2], civil commitment on the ground of "dangerousness," commitment as a sexually violent predator, and the tort liability of psychiatrists and psychologists for their patients' violence often turn on issues of risk assessment. In the justice system, risk assessment is increasingly being used

to inform decisions about sentencing and parole. Risk assessment for violent terrorism is also becoming increasingly common.

The law regulating the process of violence risk assessment has become much more developed in the USA in recent years. Some laws specify risk factors that may and may not be used to estimate risk (e.g., race is Constitutionally proscribed as a risk factor, whereas gender and age are generally permitted) [3]. Other laws allude to specific likelihoods of violence necessary to trigger preventive actions. For example, a Virginia statute allows for the civil commitment of a person with mental illness if "there is a substantial likelihood that, as a result of mental illness, the person will, in the near future, cause serious physical harm to himself or others." The material used to train professionals in the law elaborates on the meaning of substantial likelihood: a "'one-in-four' estimated risk of serious harm in the near future is sufficient, particularly when the harm being threatened is potentially fatal. A 'substantial risk' is not meant to mean 'more likely than not' (51%)" [4], (p. 133).

Assessment Approaches

No distinction in the history of risk assessment has been more influential than Paul Meehl's [5] cleaving the field into "clinical" and "actuarial" (or statistical) approaches. Subsequent research is fairly characterized in a comprehensive review by Ægisdóttir *et al.* [6]: "One area in which the statistical method is most clearly superior to the clinical approach is the prediction of violence." In recent years, however, a plethora of instruments has been published that are not adequately characterized by a

Violence in Psychiatry, ed. Katherine D. Warburton and Stephen M. Stahl. Published by Cambridge University Press.
© Cambridge University Press 2016.

Table 3.1 Four types of risk factors

Type of risk factor	Definition	Example
Fixed marker	Unchangeable	Male
Variable marker	Unchangeable by intervention	Young
Variable risk factor	Changeable by intervention	Unemployed
Causal risk factor	Changeable by intervention; when changed, reduces recidivism	Substance abuse

Adapted from Kraemer *et al.* [1]

simple clinical–actuarial dichotomy. Rather, the risk assessment process now exists on a continuum of rule-based structure, with completely unstructured ("clinical") assessment occupying one pole of the continuum, completely structured ("actuarial") assessment occupying the other pole, and several forms of partially structured assessment lying between the two [7].

The violence risk assessment process, in this regard, might usefully be seen as having the four components shown in Table 3.1: (1) identifying empirically valid (and legally acceptable) risk factors, (2) determining a method for measuring ("scoring") these risk factors, (3) establishing a procedure for combining scores on the risk factors, and (4) producing an estimate of violence risk. It is possible to array five current approaches to violence risk assessment according to whether the approach structures (i.e., specifies rules for generating) none, one, two, three, or all four of these components of this process. Purely "clinical" risk assessment structures none of the four components. The clinician selects, measures, and combines risk factors, and produces an estimate of violence risk, as his or her clinical experience and judgment indicate.

Performing a violence risk assessment by reference to a standard list of risk factors that have been found to be empirically valid (e.g., age, past violence, substance abuse), such as the lists provided in psychiatric texts structures one component of the process. Such lists function as an aide memoir to identify which risk factors the clinician should attend to in conducting his or her assessment, but they do not further specify a method for measuring these risk factors. As Tardiff [8] has stated, "Some factors may be more important than others for the individual patient," (p. 5).

The "structured professional judgment" approach exemplified by the HCR (Historical-Clinical-Risk Management)-20 [9] structures two components of the violence risk assessment process: the identification and measurement of risk factors, which may be scored as 0 if absent, 1 if possibly present, or 2 if definitely present. A revised version of this instrument – HCR-20 (Version 3) – has recently been released [10]. Structured professional judgment instruments do not go further and structure how the individual risk factors are to be combined in clinical practice [11]. Approaches to risk assessment that structure three components of the risk assessment process are illustrated by the Classification of Violence Risk (COVR) [12]. This instrument structures the identification, measurement, and combination of risk factors (via a classification tree design). But those who developed this instrument do not recommend that the final risk assessment reflect only the combined scores on the assessed risk factors. Given the possibility that rare factors influence the likelihood of violence in a particular case – and that, precisely because such factors rarely occur, they will never appear on an actuarial instrument – a professional review of the risk estimate is advised (while realizing that clinicians may overidentify "rare" factors). This professional review "would not revise or 'adjust' the actuarial score produced by the COVR, but would likely be of a more qualitative nature (eg, 'higher than,' or 'lower than' the COVR estimate)" [13]. A validation of the COVR in Sweden has recently been published [14].

The best known forensic instrument that structures all four of the components of the violence risk assessment process – i.e., that is completely actuarial – is the Violence Risk Appraisal Guide (VRAG). This instrument not only structures the identification, measurement, and combination of risk factors, but it also specifies that once an individual's violence risk has been actuarially characterized, the risk assessment process is complete. As Quinsey *et al.* have stated, "What we are advising is not the addition of actuarial methods to existing practice, but rather the replacement of existing practice with actuarial methods" [15], (p. 197). A revision of the VRAG has recently been published [16].

Does One Approach Predict Better than Another?

Of these five approaches, the unstructured ("clinical") one rests on the least empirical support. In one major study of this approach, Lidz *et al.* [17] concluded that

> . . . clinical judgment has been undervalued in previous research. Not only did the clinicians pick out a statistically more violent group, but the violence that the predicted group committed was more serious than the acts of the comparison group. Nonetheless, the low sensitivity and specificity of these judgments show that clinicians are relatively inaccurate predictors of violence (p.1,010).

We know of no research that systematically compares the predictive utility of strategies that structure none, one, two, three, or all four components of the process. Relevant data are available, however, on approaches that structure two or more components. Recent debates about whether it is more appropriate to structure clinical judgment (e.g., HCR-20) or replace it altogether (e.g., VRAG) have prompted a number of horse races that compare the predictive efficiency of one risk assessment instrument against another.

Taken together, these studies provide little evidence that one validated instrument predicts violence significantly better than another. In a recent meta-analysis of 28 studies that controlled well for methodological variation across studies, Yang *et al.* [18] found that the predictive efficiencies of nine risk assessment instruments (including the HCR-20 and VRAG) were essentially "interchangeable," with point estimates of accuracy falling within a narrow band (i.e., AUC = 0.65 to 0.71). This meta-analysis yields much the same message as meta-analyses of alternative psychotherapy techniques. As pronounced by the Dodo bird at the end of the race in Lewis Carroll's *Alice in Wonderland*, "Everyone has won, so all shall have prizes," (Carroll, L. *Alice's Adventures in Wonderland*. London: MacMillan; 1866, p. 34).

Why might different instruments perform equally well in predicting violence? One persuasive explanation is that they tap "common factors" or shared dimensions of risk, despite their varied items and formats. In an innovative demonstration, Kroner *et al.* [19] printed the items of several leading instruments on strips of paper, placed the strips in a coffee can, shook the can, and then randomly selected items to create four new tools. The authors found that the "coffee can instruments" predicted violent and nonviolent offenses as well as the original instruments. Factor analyses suggested that the instruments tap four overlapping dimensions: criminal history, an irresponsible lifestyle (e.g., poor engagement in school/work), psychopathy and criminal attitudes (e.g., entitlement), and substance abuse-related problems. Despite surface variation, instruments may generally tap "a longstanding pattern of dysfunctional and aggressive interpersonal interactions and antisocial and unstable lifestyle that are common to many perpetrators of violence" [18], (p. 759).

The strongest risk factors for violence seem to be shared not only among risk assessment instruments, but also across key groups. In particular, an increasing body of research suggests that only a small proportion of violence committed by people with mental illness – perhaps as little as 10% – is directly caused by symptoms [20]. Most people with mental illness share leading risk factors for violence with their relatively healthy counterparts.

Are Empirically Based Instruments Useful for Individuals?

One issue that has generated much recent controversy [21] is the argument that the margins of error surrounding individual risk assessments of violence are so wide as to make such predictions "virtually meaningless." As stated by Cooke and Michie, "On the basis of empirical findings, statistical theory, and logic, it is clear that predictions of future offending cannot be achieved, with any degree of confidence, in the individual case" [22], (p. 259).

This position has been vigorously contested, both with respect to the overall argument and application of statistics to make it. For example, Hanson and Howard [23] demonstrate that the wide margin of error for individual risk assessments is a function of having only two possible outcomes (violent or not violent), and therefore conveys nothing about the predictive utility of a risk assessment tool, which must be judged by other criteria. Because all violence risk assessment approaches, not just actuarial approaches, yield some estimate of the likelihood that a dichotomous outcome will occur, none are immune from Hart *et al.*'s [21] argument (as they recognize). Indeed, their argument "if true, . . . would be a serious challenge to the applicability of any empirically based risk procedure to any individual for anything" [23], (p. 277).

Our view is that group data theoretically can be, and in many areas empirically are, highly informative when making decisions about individual cases [24]. Consider two examples from other forms of risk assessment. In the insurance industry, "Until an individual insured is treated as a member of a group, it is impossible to know his expected loss, because for practical purposes that concept is a statistical one based on group probabilities. Without relying on such probabilities, it would be impossible to set a price for insurance coverage at all" [25], (p. 79). In weather forecasting, "Extensive statistical data are available on the average probability of the events [meteorologists] are estimating" and therefore when meteorologists "predict a 70% chance of rain, there is measurable precipitation just about 70% of the time" [26], (p. 46).

Along these lines, Faigman *et al.* [27] have recently analyzed how the law deals with what they refer to as group-to-individual (G2i) inference in scientific expert testimony, including scientific expert testimony on violence risk. They conclude as follows.

> It is customary in the ordinary practice of medicine and related fields (e.g., clinical psychology) for professionals to make individual . . . judgments derived from group-based data. Likewise, it is not customary in the ordinary practice of sociology, epidemiology, anthropology, and related fields (e.g., cognitive and social psychology) for professionals to make individual . . . judgments derived from group-based data [27].

In the view of Faigman *et al.*, evidence-based scientific expert testimony on an individual's violence risk when offered by qualified psychiatrists or clinical psychologists should have no trouble being admitted in court.

Should Risk Assessment and Reduction Be Separated?

In the USA, correctional agencies that manage a staggering number of youth and adults are increasingly endorsing structured risk assessment approaches and treatment programs that reduce reoffending by targeting risk factors such as anger, poor self-control, and antisocial attitudes. In this context, companies have begun to market complex (and poorly validated) assessment systems that explicitly include treatment-relevant variables in their risk estimates and ostensibly serve the risk reduction enterprise better than simple actuarial tools.

This has sparked debate about whether the pursuit of risk assessment and risk reduction should be separated or integrated. Baird [28] favors separation, arguing that the addition of treatment-relevant variables to otherwise parsimonious risk equations that emphasize past (mis) behavior will dilute their predictive utility. Andrews [29], on the other hand, argues that some treatment-relevant variables are risk factors and should be integrated in risk estimates. His view is that efficient prediction can be achieved by statistically selecting and combining a few highly predictive risk factors, but tools that sample risk domains more broadly and include treatment-relevant risk factors can be equally predictive.

Monahan and Skeem [30] observed that this debate has been exacerbated by confusion about what a treatment-relevant risk factor is, exactly. They differentiated among four different types of risk factors for violent re-offending or recidivism (see Table 3.2):

> A *fixed marker* is a risk factor that is unchangeable. Male gender is a fixed marker for recidivism.. . . Unlike a fixed marker, *a variable marker* or *variable risk factor* can be shown to change over time.. . . Variable markers cannot be changed through intervention, unlike variable risk factors. Young age is a variable marker for recidivism, whereas employment problems are a variable risk factor. [A] causal risk factor (a) can be changed through intervention (i.e., is a variable risk factor) and, (b) when changed through intervention, can be shown to change the risk of recidivism [30].

All four types of risk factors are relevant to risk assessment, but only causal risk factors are relevant to risk reduction. Put simply, treatment-relevant risk factors are causal risk factors. Unless a variable risk factor has been shown to be causal, there is little reason to assume that reducing the risk factor will reduce violence. This fact is rarely recognized in current discourse. Few risk factors for violence have been shown to be causal, but variable risk factors have been shown to predict proximate violence and are the best point of reference the field presently has to offer for risk reduction.

Choosing Among Valid Instruments

Given a pool of instruments that are well-validated for the groups to which an individual belongs, our view is that the choice among them should be driven by the ultimate purpose of the evaluation. If the ultimate purpose is to characterize an individual's likelihood of future violence relative to other people, then choose the most efficient instrument available. This

Table 3.2 Increasingly structured approaches to violence risk assessment

Approach/tool	Structured components of the violence risk assessment process			
	Identify risk factors	Measure risk factors	Combine risk factors	Produce final risk estimate
Clinical judgment				
Standard list of risk factors	X			
HCR-20	X	X		
COVR	X	X	X	
VRAG	X	X	X	X

Note: HCR-20 = Historical Clinical Risk-20; COVR = Classification of Violence Risk; VRAG = Violence Risk Appraisal Guide. Adapted from Skeem and Monahan [7].

is appropriate for a single event decision in which there is no real opportunity to modify the risk estimate based on future behavior [31]. If the ultimate purpose is to manage or reduce an individual's risk, then value may be added by choosing an instrument that includes treatment-relevant risk factors [32]. (Although an integrated instrument would be most parsimonious, we can easily envision a two-stage process in which a risk-assessment step was followed by an independent risk-management step.) This choice is appropriate for ongoing decisions where the risk estimate can be modified to reflect ebbs and flows in an individual's risk over time. Beyond focusing risk reduction efforts, these instruments could provide incentive for changing behavior. (A parole board cannot advise an inmate to "undo" his past commission of an assault, but can advise him to develop employment skills.)

This view comes with three important caveats. First, techniques that include treatment-relevant risk factors will add no value to simpler approaches unless the risk assessment is followed by a period of control over the individual, during which those factors are translated into an individual supervision and treatment plan (rather than simply filed away), and systematically targeted with appropriate services (rather than ignored in resource allocation). Risk reduction cannot be achieved through risk assessment alone, regardless of the approach applied. Second, treatment-relevant variables can and do appear in statistically derived risk assessment instruments [13]; an instrument's degree of structure cannot be equated with its relevance to risk reduction. Third, even well-validated instruments offer little direct validity data for the treatment-relevant

variables they include. It is not enough to demonstrate that a variable is a risk factor for violence; here, it must further be shown that the variable reduces violence risk when successfully changed by treatment (ie, is a causal risk factor) [1]. This is a crucial issue to address in future research, if tools continue to be sold on the promise of informing risk reduction [33].

Future Directions

The violence risk assessment field may be reaching a point of diminishing returns in instrument development. It has been long been argued that there may be a "sound barrier" to predictive validity in this area, such that the correlation between risk estimates and criterion measures will rarely exceed 0.40 [34]. In this regard, Paul Appelbaum [35] has stated that "predictive assessments are the most challenging evaluations performed by mental health professionals," (p. 846). He speculates on the reasons underlying this great challenge:

> The inescapable uncertainties of the course of mental disorders and their responsiveness to interventions create part of the difficulty in such assessments, but an equally important contribution is made by the unknowable contingencies of life. Will a person's spouse leave or will the person lose his job or his home? As a consequence, will the person return to drinking, stop taking medication, or reconnect with friends who have continued to engage in criminal behaviors? At best, predictive assessments can lead to general statements of probability of particular outcomes, with an acknowledgment of the uncertainties involved [35]
>
> (p. 819).

While the "sound barrier" for predictive accuracy in the case of violence may prove to be somewhat higher than it is now [36], there is no question that "the contingencies of life" will place an upper limit on what can be achieved in many risk assessment contexts. The most promising candidates for incremental advances in violence risk assessment may include violent victimization [37], implicit measures [38], patient self-perceptions [39], and the incorporation of risk factors from the neurosciences [40]. If we are approaching a "sound barrier" in the risk assessment domain, there clearly are miles to go before we can rest on the risk reduction front. We hope that in the future, psychology and psychiatry shift more of their empirical attention from predicting violence to understanding its causes and preventing its (re)occurrence.

Disclosures

John Monahan has nothing to disclose. Jennifer Skeem received research support from the National Institute of Health.

References

1. Kraemer H, Kazdin A, Offord D, *et al.* Coming to terms with the terms of risk. *Arch. Gen. Psychiatry.* 1997; **54**: 337–343.

2. Desmarais S, Van Dorn R, Johnson K, *et al.* Community violence perpetration and victimization among adults with mental illness. *Am J Public Health.* Published online ahead of print, February 13, 433 2014: e1–e8. doi:10.2105/ AJPH.2013.301680.

3. Monahan J. The inclusion of biological risk factors in violence risk assessments. In: Singh I, Sinnott-Armstrong W, Savulescu J, eds. *BioPrediction, Biomarkers, and Bad Behavior: Scientific, Legal, and Ethical Implications.* New York: Oxford University Press; 2013: 57–76, 439

4. Cohen B, Bonnie R, Monahan J. Understanding and applying Virginia's new statutory civil commitment criteria. *Developments in Mental Health Law.* 2009; **28**(1): 127–139.

5. Meehl P. *Clinical Versus Statistical Prediction: A Theoretical Analysis and a Review of the Evidence.* Minneapolis, MN: University of Minnesota; 1954.

6. Ægisdóttir S, White M, Spengler P, *et al.* The meta-analysis of clinical judgment project: fifty-six years of accumulated research on clinical versus statistical prediction. *The Counseling Psychologist.* 2006; **34** (3): 341–382.

7. Skeem J, Monahan J. Current directions in violence risk assessment. *Current Directions in Psychological Science.* 2011; **20**: 38–42.

8. Tardiff K. Clinical risk assessment of violence. In: Simon R, Tardiff K, eds. *Textbook of Violence Assessment and Management.* Washington, DC: American Psychiatric Press; 2008: 3–16.

9. Webster C, Douglas K, Eaves D, Hart S. *HCR-20: Assessing Risk for Violence (Version 2).* Vancouver: Simon Fraser University; 2007.

10. Douglas K, Hart, Webster C, Belfrage H. *HCR-20 (Version 3): Assessing Risk for Violence.* Burnaby, BC, Canada: Mental Health, Law, and Policy Institute, Simon Fraser University; 2013.

11. Douglas K, Hart S, Groscup J, Litwack T. Assessing violence risk. In: Weiner I, Otto R, eds. *The Handbook of Forensic Psychology*, 4th edn. Hoboken, NJ: John Wiley; 2014: 385–442.

12. Monahan J, Steadman H, Silver E, *et al.* Rethinking Risk Assessment: *The MacArthur Study of Mental Disorder and Violence.* New York: Oxford University Press; 2001.

13. Monahan J. The classification of violence risk. In: R. Otto R, Douglas K, eds. *Handbook of Violence Risk Assessment.* New York: Routledge; 2010: 187–198.

14. Sturup J, Kristiansson M, Monahan J. Gender and violent behavior in Swedish general psychiatric patients: a prospective clinical study. *Psychiatr. Serv.* 2013; **64**(7): 688–693.

15. Quinsey V, Harris G, Rice M, Cormier C. *Violent Offenders: Appraising and Managing Risk*, 2nd edn. Washington, DC: American Psychological Association; 2006.

16. Rice M, Harris G, Lang C. Validation of and revision to the VRAG and SORAG: the Violence Risk Appraisal Guide—Revised (VRAG-R). *Psychol. Assess.* 2013; **25**(3): 951–965.

17. Lidz C, Mulvey E, Gardner W. The accuracy of predictions of violence to others. *JAMA.* 1993; **269**(8): 1007–1011.

18. Yang M, Wong S, Coid J. The efficacy of violence prediction: a meta-analytic comparison of nine risk assessment tools. *Psychol. Bull.* 2010; **136**(5): 740–767.

19. Kroner D, Mills J, Morgan B. A coffee can, factor analysis, and prediction of antisocial behavior: the structure of criminal risk. *Int. J. Law Psychiatry.* 2005; **28**(4): 360–374.

20. Skeem J, Manchak S, Peterson J. Correctional policy for offenders with mental disorder: creating a new paradigm for recidivism reduction. *Law Hum. Behav.* 2011; **35**(2): 110–126.

21. Hart S, Michie C, Cooke D. Precision of actuarial risk assessment instruments: evaluating the 'margins of error' of group v. individual predictions

of violence. *Br. J. Psychiatry Suppl.* 2007; **49**: s60–s65.

22. Cooke D, Michie C. Limitations of diagnostic precision and predictive utility in the individual case: a challenge for forensic practice. *Law Hum. Behav.* 2010; **34**(4): 259–274.

23. Hanson R, Howard P. Individual confidence intervals do not inform decision-makers about the accuracy of risk assessment evaluations. *Law Hum. Behav.* 2010; **34**(4): 275–281.

24. Scurich N, Monahan J, John R. Innumeracy and unpacking: bridging the nomothetic/idiographic divide in violence risk assessment. *Law Hum. Behav.* 2012; **36**(6): 548–554.

25. Abraham K. *Distributing Risk: Insurance, Legal Theory, and Public Policy*. New Haven, CT: Yale University Press; 1986.

26. National Research Council. *Improving Risk Communication*. Washington, DC: National Academy Press; 1989.

27. Faigman D, Monahan J, Slobogin C. *Group to Individual (G2i) Inference in Scientific Expert Testimony*. University of Chicago Law Review. 2014; **81**(2).

28. Baird C. A question of evidence: A critique of risk assessment models used in the justice system. National Council on Crime & Delinquency website. http://www.nccdglobal.org/sites/default/files/publication_pdf/special-report-evidence.pdf. Published February 2009. Accessed November 25, 2013.

29. Andrews D. The risk-need-responsivity (RNR) model of correctional assessment and treatment. In: Dvoskin J, Skeem J, Novaco R, Douglas K, eds. *Using Social Science to Reduce Violent Offending*. New York: Oxford University Press; 2012: 127–156.

30. Monahan J, Skeem J. Risk redux: The resurgence of risk assessment in criminal sanctioning. *Federal Sentencing Reporter*. 2014; **26**(3).

31. Heilbrun K. Prediction versus management models relevant to risk assessment: the importance of legal decision-making context. *Law Hum. Behav.* 1997; **21**(4): 347–359.

32. Howard P, Dixon L. Identifying change in the likelihood of violent recidivism: causal dynamic risk factors in the OASys violence predictor. *Law Hum. Behav.* 2013; **37**(3): 163–174.

33. Kroner D, Yessine A. Changing risk factors that impact recidivism: in search of mechanisms of change. *Law Hum. Behav.* 2013; **37**(5): 321–336.

34. Menzies R, Webster C, Sepejak D. Hitting the forensic sound barrier: predictions of dangerousness in a pre-trial psychiatric clinic. In: Webster C, Ben-Aron M, Hucker S, eds. *Dangerousness: Probability and Prediction, Psychiatry and Public Policy*. New York: Cambridge University Press; 1985: 115–143.

35. Appelbaum P. Reference guide on mental health evidence. In: *Federal Judicial Center. Reference Manual on Scientific Evidence*. Washington, DC: National Academies Press; 2011: 813–896.

36. Singh J, Petrila J. Measuring and interpreting the predictive validity of violence risk assessments. *Behav. Sci. Law.* 2013; **31**(1): 1–7.

37. Sadeh N, Binder R, McNiel D. Recent victimization increases risk for violence in justice-involved persons with mental illness. *Law Hum. Behav.* Advance online publication July 15, 2013. doi:10.1037/lhb0000043.

38. Knock M, Park J, Finn C, *et al.* Measuring the suicidal mind: Implicit cognition predicts suicidal behavior. *Psychol. Sci.* 2010; **21**(4): 511–517.

39. Skeem J, Manchak S, Lidz C, Mulvey M. The utility of patients' self-perceptions of violence risk: consider asking the person who may know best. *Psychiatr. Serv.* 2013; **64**(5): 410–415.

40. Aharonia E, Vincent GM, Harenskia CL, *et al.* Neuroprediction of future rearrest. *Proc. Natl Acad. Sci. U S A.* 2013; **110**(15): 6223–6228.

Assessment of aggression in inpatient settings

Barbara E. McDermott and Brian J. Holoyda

Inpatient Violence

The threat of violence is a major concern for all individuals working or receiving treatment in an inpatient psychiatric setting [1]. For example, Silver and Yudofsky [2] recorded over 3000 episodes of aggressive behavior (both verbal and physical) in a 20-month period in just 30 psychiatric inpatients. Fellow patients are not the only victims of such assaults. According to the Bureau of Labor Statistics, in 1999, 2637 nonfatal assaults on hospital workers occurred, which translates to a rate of 8.3 assaults per 10,000 workers. This contrasts to a rate of assault of 2 per 10,000 workers in all other industries. The victims of such assaults were typically nursing staff, primarily because they spend the most time with patients. While these numbers include all healthcare employees, the Department of Justice National Crime Victimization Survey for 1993 through 1999 [3] reported that the average annual rate for nonfatal violence for mental health professionals was 68.2 per 1000 compared to a rate of 12.6 for all occupations. While the Occupational Safety and Health Administration (OSHA) provided compelling reasons for these numbers (e.g., increasing use of hospitals by police officers for the care of acutely disturbed violent individuals), the consequences are clear: many mental health professionals will at some point in their careers be the victim of an assault. The resultant loss of work and psychological trauma to both the providers and the patients is significant [4,5]. Developing methods for reducing violence on inpatient psychiatric units is of paramount importance.

The Development of Risk Assessments

One major focus in forensic psychology and psychiatry over the past several decades has been the development of risk assessments to aid in the identification of those individuals most at risk of exhibiting violent behavior. Initially, these instruments were developed primarily to make informed decisions regarding when (or if) offenders could be safely released into the community. So-called "first-generation" risk assessment consisted of unstructured, often uninformed, estimates of dangerousness, which were notoriously fallible and unreliable. This is primarily because mental health professionals placed an increased importance on idiosyncratic factors that may not bear any relationship to violence [6]. Monahan's monograph [7] documents that when using this approach, mental health professionals were inaccurate 67% of the time. "Second-generation" risk instruments were developed in the 1980s and 1990s and employed statistical analyses to assess the mathematical relationship between person variables (e.g., age, elementary school performance) and the measured outcome (violence or violent offending). Many of these instruments provided probability values that allowed mental health professionals to quantify the risk of recidivism or aggression. Aside from providing an artificial sense of accuracy (some authors suggest that these probability values, when applied to the individual, vary widely [8], although others argue that the mathematical equations to support such arguments are flawed [9]), most included primarily static or historical factors, which are not amenable to change [10,11]. One static factor that has been researched extensively is the construct of psychopathy, typically operationalized by the Hare Psychopathy Checklist–Revised (PCL-R) [12] or one of its derivatives. This construct, when included in the risk instrument, often carries the most weight. However, because many believe the primary purpose of risk

Violence in Psychiatry, ed. Katherine D. Warburton and Stephen M. Stahl. Published by Cambridge University Press.
© Cambridge University Press 2016.

assessment is risk management [13,14], static factors in theory yield little information regarding management of risk. Additionally, these second-generation risk assessments were developed to identify those individuals who are more likely to become violent in the long-term. For example, the Violence Risk Appraisal Guide (VRAG) [10,15,16] estimated the probability of violent offending at 7- and 10-year follow-up points. For inpatient psychiatry, static predictors of risk may only be useful if containment is a feasible method of risk management. The use of seclusion and restraints is often viewed as containment and nontherapeutic [17], and their use is increasingly limited in most psychiatric facilities [18]. Because psychiatric hospitals typically endeavor to focus on treatment, not containment, risk instruments with exclusively static predictors were believed to hold little utility for the management of aggressive patients. Long-term risk, which was often the focus of earlier risk instruments, is generally of importance when release is being considered. Short-term risk of aggression is much more salient to administrators of acute psychiatric units and long-term care facilities. Recent research has suggested that factors related to community violence (and therefore representative of long-term risk) may be substantially different than factors related to institutional aggression (i.e., short-term risk), although differences also may be related to the operational definition of violence [19,20].

"Third-generation" risk assessments were developed based on empirical literature describing the relationships between person variables and outcome. These tools contain both static and dynamic factors that place an individual at risk. These guided professional assessments, often termed structured professional judgment (SPJ) tools, contain items that have been empirically linked to aggression or offending (rather than statistically linked) and incorporate dynamic risk factors for two specific reasons: to provide information on how to manage risk and to provide a method for measuring change in risk as a result of treatment. As Hart [14] cogently noted, the goal of risk assessment ultimately is prevention of violence. Thus, assessment methods must include factors that are amenable to intervention [21]. Many SPJ tools include factors more traditionally associated with mental illness (e.g., diagnosis, current symptoms), which are considered more dynamic, rather than antisocial traits, which could be viewed as more historical or static. Douglas and Skeem [21] proposed

various dynamic risk factors for further investigation, including impulsivity, anger, and substance use. More recently "fourth-generation" risk tools have been proposed as superior, as these assessments contain items that are dynamic as well as potentially protective, and they place a focus on the linkage between identified risk factors and proposed interventions. However, the utility of these instruments is still unclear [22]. See Table 4.1 for a summary of the development of violence risk assessments.

The development of second- and third-generation risk instruments appears to have produced the desired results: many of these tools have been shown to provide improved accuracy over unguided clinical judgment when used in an appropriate fashion, especially as they relate to community violence. For reviews of the efficacy of risk assessment and its relationship to community violence, see for example Edens and Otto [23], Quinsey et al. [15], or Walters [24]. The strength of the relationship of these risk instruments in general, and psychopathy specifically, to community violence led investigators to extend the examination to the institutional setting. Institutional aggression is a common problem in both general and forensic psychiatric facilities, as well as in correctional facilities. While initial investigations supported a strong positive relationship between the PCL-R (a static risk factor) and institutional aggression [25,26], two meta-analyses have indicated that the PCL-R is not as robust a predictor of institutional aggression as initially believed [20,27]. In addition to concerns regarding the utility of psychopathy within institutions, concerns also have been raised regarding the predictive validity of instruments such as the VRAG and the Historical–Clinical–Risk Management (HCR-20) [28] in relation to institutional violence [19]. Compared to the community violence literature, relatively few studies have examined the efficacy of these measures in identifying violence-prone individuals in inpatient settings. McNiel et al. [29] evaluated the utility of various structured risk instruments in identifying individuals who would exhibit aggression in the short-term (mean length of stay of the sample was 9.5 days). They found that the clinical scale of the HCR-20 was most associated with inpatient violence. In a sample of 97 male offenders, Kroner and Mills [30] found that the VRAG evidenced the strongest relationship with major institutional misconduct, whereas the HCR-20 total score evidenced the lowest, although no differences were statistically significant. In contrast, Doyle et al. [31]

Table 4.1 A summary of the development of violence risk assessments

Generation	Development	Description	Example
First	Unstructured estimates of dangerousness	• Can include idiosyncratic factors • Often inaccurate	Clinical interview
Second	Actuarial developed using mathematical relationship between predictor and outcome	• Provides probability values associated with risk • Typically only includes static risk factors	VRAG, VRAG-R
Third	Structured professional judgment (SPJ) tools developed based on empirical literature	• Includes both static and dynamic risk factors • Can provide information on how to manage risk • Mechanism for measuring change in risk	HCR-20, HCR-20 Version 3 [55]
Fourth	Development based on empirical risk literature, includes protective factors as well as risk factors. Focus is on the linkage between risk and protective factors and interventions	• May be more effective at monitoring treatment • Very little research on efficacy	START

PCL-R: Hare Psychopathy Checklist–Revised; VRAG: Violence Risk Appraisal Guide; HCR-20: Historical–Clinical–Risk Management; START: Short-Term Assessment of Risk and Treatability.

found in a study of 87 mentally disordered offenders in a medium security facility that the PCL-SV was superior to the VRAG and the H scale of the HCR-20 in predicting serious aggression. In a sample of 154 forensic inpatients, McDermott *et al.* [32] found that the clinical and risk management subscales of the HCR-20, as well as hostility as measured by the Brief Psychiatric Rating Scale (BPRS), were most strongly associated with patient-directed aggression, whereas two subscales from the Novaco anger scale were most strongly associated with staff-directed aggression. Vitacco *et al.* [33] found that both static and dynamic factors predicted inpatient aggression, although none exhibited incremental validity beyond any other. In a meta-analysis of 95 studies examining the utility of the PCL in both community and institutional settings, Leistico *et al.* [34] found that the PCL exhibited greater utility in a psychiatric inpatient sample, as compared to an incarcerated correctional sample. The results of these studies suggest that there is some utility to including both static and dynamic risk factors in risk instruments as they relate to institutional aggression.

Consistent with Douglas and Skeem's suggestion [21] and McDermott *et al.*'s research [32], the extant literature offers considerable support for the contention that anger and hostility are risk factors for interpersonal aggression. For example, research has shown positive associations between anger scales and institutional misconduct among violent male offenders in prison [35,36]. In the MacArthur study of mental disorder and violence [37], anger was a potent predictor of community violence, so much so that it was incorporated into the Classification of Violence Risk (COVR) [38] as one of the 44 risk factors. More recently, Ullrich *et al.* [39] found that anger was a critical component in the pathway between delusions and violence. Impulsivity also has been associated with a greater likelihood of acting out in controlled environments [40–42]. Recently, a prospective examination of the relationship of second- and third-generation risk instruments with institutional violence [32] found that one type of patient was responsible for the majority of the aggression exhibited toward both staff and other patients in a forensic facility: patients who scored high on risk instruments (including the PCL-R, the VRAG, and the HCR-20) and who also scored high on self-report measures of anger and impulsivity. Patients who scored high only on the risk instruments but not on measures of anger and impulsivity exhibited significantly lower rates of aggression. These data provide further support that both dynamic and static risk factors are useful in identifying potentially aggressive patients.

A Typology of Aggression

In addition to categorizing aggression as staff- or patient-directed, there is also evidence that institutional aggression can be categorized according to precipitating events and that the factors associated with each type of aggression may vary. In a study conducted in a state psychiatric hospital in New York, three primary motivations for assault were described: (1) impulsive – an assault committed in response to an immediate provocation and associated with agitation and loss of emotional control; (2) planned – a controlled assault committed for a specific goal; and (3) psychotic – assaults committed as a consequence of delusions, hallucinations, and/or disordered thinking [43]. Symptoms of mental illness, especially a major mental disorder, are necessarily associated with psychotic aggression by definition; psychotic symptoms are less likely to be linked to planned/predatory aggression. Quanbeck *et al.* [44] examined almost 1000 acts of aggression exhibited by both civil and forensic patients and found that a similar trichotomy applied, which they termed impulsive, organized, and psychotic. They also were able to delineate the underlying motivation for each type of aggression. For example, an act of organized aggression may be exhibited to achieve social dominance, whereas an act of impulsive aggression may be precipitated by the patient being denied a desirable item. Using this categorization scheme, impulsive/reactive assaults comprised the largest number of observed incidents of aggression (46%) [44]. See Table 4.2 for a description of the typology of violence. Studies have been conducted to determine if traditional second- and third-generation risk instruments hold more utility in identifying individuals who are more likely to exhibit certain types of aggression. Some research suggests that planned/predatory aggression is more strongly related to psychopathic and antisocial attitudes [45,46]. In a sample of 152 male forensic patients, Vitacco *et al.* [47] found that anger and symptoms of mental illness, but not psychopathy, were associated with reactive aggression. In contrast, psychopathy, hostility, and anger were most associated with instrumental aggression. McDermott *et al.* [48] found similar results: in a sample of 238 predominantly male forensic patients, psychopathy and anger were most strongly related to predatory aggression; the clinical and risk management scales of the HCR-20 and anger were most associated with impulsive aggression. Not surprisingly, symptoms of mental illness and impulsivity were most associated with psychotically motivated aggression. Interestingly, these relationships only held true when follow-up was limited to six months; longer follow-up attenuated most of the relationships.

In psychiatric facilities, the temporal occurrence of aggression is extremely important and may, at least in part, be associated with the type of aggression exhibited. The study by McDermott *et al.* [48] demonstrated that various instruments may be differentially associated with various types of aggression at varying time points in the hospitalization. For long-term care facilities, imminent (defined as within the next 24 hours), short-term (variously defined as between one and six months), and long-term (defined in years) are all relevant in the treatment and management of psychiatric patients. For acute care inpatient psychiatric units, imminent aggression is most relevant, as most inpatient stays are extremely brief. Thus, the predictors of imminent aggression may be different from short-term aggression, which may also be quite

Table 4.2 Typology of violence

Type	Description	Risk factors
Impulsive	Assault committed in response to an immediate provocation	• Anger • Symptoms of mental illness
Planned	Controlled assault committed for specific goal	• Psychopathy • Hostility • Anger
Psychotic	Assault committed as a consequence of delusions, hallucinations, and/or disordered thinking	• Psychotic symptoms • Impulsivity

different from the predictors of longer-term recidivism and offending. As an example, Woods and Almvik [49] found that the Brøset Violence Checklist (BVC) [50], which contains six items related to patient behavior/affect, was effective in identifying individuals at higher risk of aggression in the 24-hour period following the assessment. Other authors have determined that predictors of short-term versus long-term aggression may differ widely, and are especially dependent on the type of aggression [48].

Although most standard risk instruments have been developed on forensic samples, recent research suggests that many risk instruments are applicable in both civil and forensic settings and that perhaps more important is the type of patient and the time frame under which the assessments are employed. This stands to reason, as most forensic commitments require a severe mental illness that has led to the impairment in legal reasoning. There are several validated risk assessment tools that were developed specifically to assess violence risk in the acute inpatient setting. Examples are the McNiel–Binder Violence Screening Checklist (VSC) [50], the BVC [51], and the Dynamic Appraisal of Situational Aggression (DASA) [52].

The VSC, which was developed at a university-based, locked, short-term psychiatric unit, is a screening tool that uses four variables to predict aggression and violence within 72 hours of inpatient admission. These four variables are a history of physical attacks or fear-inducing behavior within two weeks prior to admission, absence of suicidal behavior within two weeks of admission, schizophrenic or manic diagnosis, and male gender. An individual having a positive score on the VSC is 1.97 times more likely to engage in a physical attack or fear-inducing behavior. In addition, the VSC has demonstrated an ability to correctly classify 65% of patients as violent or nonviolent in a population of patients with a base rate of violent behavior of 41%.

The BVC was developed at the Norwegian maximum security unit at Brøset, which houses patients with mental disorders who were felt to be highly dangerous and difficult to manage. The checklist consists of six behaviors found to be most common during a 24-hour period prior to a violent incident, namely confusion, irritability, boisterousness, physical threats, verbal threats, and attacks on objects. The BVC has demonstrated 63% accuracy in predicting that violence will occur within the next 24 hours and 92% accuracy in predicting that violence will not

occur. A randomized, controlled trial based in a Swiss psychiatric facility utilized the BVC as part of a violence risk reduction intervention during acute admission that resulted in a 41% risk reduction in severe events of inpatient aggression and a 27% risk reduction in the need for coercive measures against patients.

The DASA is a seven-item instrument, which contains two items from the HCR-20, two from the BVC, and three based on the authors' own research. In the development study [52], the DASA evidenced an area under the curve (AUC) of 0.82 with all seven items combined. The odds ratio of a patient scoring 7 (the highest score) compared to one scoring a 0 of committing an act of aggression within 24 hours was 29 (the patient was 29 times more likely to commit an act of aggression).

Many of these instruments that are used to identify patients likely to exhibit imminent aggression rely on observation of escalating behaviors. This suggests that these tools provide the greatest utility in identifying individuals at risk of exhibiting psychotically motivated or impulsive aggression. The SPJ instruments may be of more utility in identifying those individuals who are at risk of aggression later in their course of treatment, and again, aggression that may be viewed as impulsive or psychotically motivated. Static measures of risk appear to hold the greatest utility for identifying those individuals who are most likely to exhibit predatory aggression. In a direct assessment of this, Grann et al. [53] found that static risk instruments were most efficacious in individuals with personality disorders. These same risk instruments held little utility for individuals with major mental disorders. They suggested that dynamic factors may be more useful for such individuals.

Integrating Risk, Typology, and Treatment

These data suggest that aggression exhibited in psychiatric facilities is multiply determined, and that no one intervention is likely to be effective in decreasing aggression, nor is one assessment instrument likely to be useful in delineating individuals more prone to acting aggressively. The research suggests that multiple issues are relevant with institutional aggression: the type of aggression, the time frame under which the aggression is exhibited, and patient characteristics. Consideration of all factors is necessary when developing appropriate interventions. Patients admitted with a major mental disorder and severe positive symptoms of psychosis are most appropriately evaluated with an instrument that carries utility in the short-term (within 24 hours). Interventions would necessarily be directed at reducing symptoms (e.g., medication). Individuals admitted with a psychotic disorder, but not in an active phase, may be most appropriately evaluated with a SPJ tool to inform treatment. These tools can identify dynamic factors that are associated with aggression and provide opportunities for interventions. In contrast, individuals admitted with prominent severe personality disorders may be more at risk for exhibiting predatory aggression, which often occurs later in the hospitalization. Risk instruments that contain more static factors may be most useful in identifying those individuals who might require an increase in security versus those who could be more responsive to structured behavioral approaches.

Data from Quanbeck *et al.* [44] and McDermott *et al.* [48] have consistently shown that impulsive aggression is the most common type exhibited. This type of aggression has consistently been more difficult to predict, lending support to the notion that other factors may be equally important. Johnson's [54] cogent review of the literature on inpatient aggression concluded that staff and environmental characteristics may be as important as patient characteristics. As such, a combination of behavioral and environmental interventions may be most useful in decreasing this type of aggression. Aggression driven by the symptoms of a psychotic disorder can be most effectively managed with aggressive pharmacological treatment. Predatory aggression in institutions is a serious problem, especially in long-term care facilities. This type of aggression appears to be exhibited by those patients least likely to have a major mental disorder. Data suggest that individuals with more antisocial and psychopathic tendencies are the patients responsible for the majority of predatory/instrumental aggression. Strict behavioral interventions with appropriate physical design barriers may be the most useful approach for these individuals.

Conclusion

As psychiatric institutions move toward more data-driven methods of treatment, facilities are exploring methods for identifying and treating individuals at higher risk of committing institutional infractions. Recent research has indicated that developing a typology of aggressive incidents may provide insight both into precipitants to assaults as well as appropriate interventions to reduce such aggression. Further, characteristics of patients may be as useful as categorizing types of assaults. Patients presenting with severe psychotic disorders may be most appropriately assessed for risk with an instrument that addresses the probability of aggression in the short-term. Patients presenting with severe personality disorders such as antisocial personality disorder or psychopathy may be more appropriately evaluated using instruments that capture static factors that are most associated with aggression in the long-term. The extant literature is clear: both static and dynamic risk factors are useful and may be differentially related to the type of patients exhibiting aggression as well as the type of aggression exhibited. Careful consideration of which instruments can provide the most utility for which individuals, as well as the purpose of the risk assessment, is of paramount importance.

Disclosures

Barbara McDermott and Brian Holoyda do not have anything to disclose.

References

1. Quintal SA. Violence against psychiatric nurses: an untreated epidemic? *J. Psychosoc. Nurs. Ment. Health Serv.* 2002; **40**(1): 46–53.

2. Silver JM, Yudofsky SC. Documentation of aggression in the assessment of the violent patient. *Psychiatric Annals.* 1987; **17**(6): 375–384.

3. Duhart DT. *Violence in the Workplace, 1993–99* (December 2001, NCJ 190076). Washington, DC: U.S. Department of Justice, Office of Justice Programs; 2001.

4. Hunter M, Carmel H. The cost of staff injuries from inpatient violence. *Hosp. Community Psychiatry.* 1992; **43**(6): 586–588.

5. Duxbury J, Whittington R. Causes and management of patient aggression and violence: staff and patient perspectives. *J. Adv. Nurs.* 2005; **50**(5): 469–478.

6. Skeem JL, Monahan J. Current directions in violence risk assessment. *Current Directions in Psychological Science.* 2011; **20**(1): 38–42.

7. Monahan J. *The Clinical Prediction of Violent Behavior. Crime and Delinquency Issues:*

A Monograph Series. Washington, DC: US Government Printing Office; 1981.

8. Hart SD, Michie C, Cooke DJ. Precision of actuarial risk assessment instruments: evaluating the "margins of error" of group v. individual predictions of violence. *Br. J. Psychiatry.* 2007; **190**(Suppl. 49): s60–s65.

9. Mossman D, Sellke T. Avoiding error about "margins of error." *Br. J. Psychiatry.* 2007; **191**(6): 561.

10. Harris GT, Rice ME, Quinsey VL. Violent recidivism of mentally disordered offenders: the development of a statistical prediction instrument. *Criminal Justice and Behavior.* 1993; **20**(4): 315–335.

11. Hanson RK. *The Development of a Brief Actuarial Scale for Sexual Offense Recidivism.* Ottawa, Ontario: Department of the Solicitor General; 1997.

12. Hare RD. *The Hare Psychopathy Checklist—Revised Manual,* 2nd edn. Toronto, Ontario: Multi-Health Systems; 2003.

13. Bloom H, Webster C, Hucker S, DeFreitas K. The Canadian contribution to violence risk assessment: history and implications for current psychiatric practice. *Can. J. Psychiatry.* 2005; **50**(1): 3–11.

14. Hart SD. The role of psychopathy in assessing risk for violence: conceptual and methodological issues. *Legal and Criminological Psychology.* 1998; **3**(1): 121–137.

15. Quinsey VL, Harris GT, Rice ME, Cormier CA. *Violent Offenders: Appraising and Managing Risk,* 2nd edn. Washington, DC: American Psychological Association; 2006.

16. Rice ME, Harris GT, Lang C. Validation of and revision to the VRAG and SORAG: the violence risk appraisal guide-revised (VRAG-R). *Psychol. Assess.* 2013; **25**(3): 951–965.

17. Hodgkinson P. The use of seclusion. *Med. Sci. Law.* 1985; **25**(3): 215–222.

18. Maguire T, Young R, Martin T. Seclusion reduction in a forensic mental health setting. *J. Psychiatr. Ment. Health Nurs.* 2012; **19**(2): 97–106.

19. Edens JF, Buffington-Vollum JK, Keilen A, Roskamp P, Anthony C. Predictions of future dangerousness in capital murder trials: Is it time to "disinvent the wheel?" *Law Hum. Behav.* 2005; **29**(1): 55–86.

20. Guy LS, Edens JF, Anthony C, Douglas KS. Does psychopathy predict institutional misconduct among adults? A meta-analytic investigation. *J. Consult. Clin. Psychol.* 2005; **73**(6): 1056–1064.

21. Douglas KS, Skeem JL. Violence risk assessment: getting specific about being dynamic. *Psychology, Public Policy, and Law.* 2005; **11**(3): 347–383.

22. Campbell MA, French S, Gendreau P. The prediction of violence in adult offenders: a meta-analytic comparison of instruments and methods of assessment. *Criminal Justice and Behavior.* 2009; **36**(6): 567–590.

23. Edens JF, Otto RK. Release decision making and planning. In: Ashford JB, Sales BD, Reid WH, eds. *Treating Adult and Juvenile Offenders with Special Needs.* Washington, DC: American Psychological Association; 2001: 335–371.

24. Walters GD. Risk-appraisal versus self-report in the prediction of criminal justice outcomes: a meta-analysis. *Criminal Justice and Behavior.* 2006; **33**(3): 279–304.

25. Hare RD, McPherson LM. Violent and aggressive behavior by criminal psychopaths. *Int. J. Law Psychiatry.* 1984; **7**(1): 35–50.

26. Hill CD, Rogers R, Bickford ME. Predicting aggressive and socially disruptive behavior in a maximum security forensic psychiatric hospital. *J. Forensic Sci.* 1996; **41**(1): 56–59.

27. Walters GD. Predicting institutional adjustment and recidivism with the Psychopathy Checklist factor scores: a meta-analysis. *Law Hum. Behav.* 2003; **27**(5): 541–558.

28. Webster CD, Douglas KS, Eaves D, Hart S. *HCR-20: Assessing Risk for Violence (Version 2).* Burnaby, BC, Canada: Mental Health, Law, and Policy Institute, Simon Fraser University; 1997.

29. McNiel D, Gregory A, Lam J, Binder RL, Sullivan GR. Utility of decision support tools for assessing acute risk of violence. *J. Consult. Clin. Psychol.* 2003; **71**(5): 945–953.

30. Kroner DG, Mills JF. The accuracy of five risk appraisal instruments in predicting institutional misconduct and new convictions. *Criminal Justice and Behavior.* 2001; **28**(4): 471–489.

31. Doyle M, Dolan M, McGovern J. The validity of North American risk assessment tools in predicting in-patient violent behaviour in England. *Legal and Criminological Psychology.* 2002; **7**(2): 141–154.

32. McDermott BE, Edens JF, Quanbeck CD, Busse D, Scott CL. Examining the role of static and dynamic risk factors in the prediction of inpatient violence: variable and person-focused analyses. *Law Hum. Behav.* 2008; **32**(4): 325–338.

33. Vitacco MJ, Gonsalves V, Tomony J, Smith BER, Lishner DA. Can standardized measures of risk predict inpatient violence? Combining static and dynamic variables to improve accuracy. *Criminal Justice and Behavior.* 2012; **39**(5): 589–606.

34. Leistico AMR, Salekin RT, DeCoster J, Rogers R. A large-scale meta-analysis relating the Hare measures of psychopathy to

antisocial conduct. *Law Hum. Behav.* 2008; **32**(1): 28–45.

35. Mills JF, Kroner DG. Anger as a predictor of institutional misconduct and recidivism in a sample of violent offenders. *J. Interpers. Violence.* 2003; **18**(3): 282–294.

36. Mills JF, Kroner DG, Forth A. Novaco Anger Scale: reliability and validity within an adult criminal sample. *Assessment.* 1998; **5**(3): 237–248.

37. Monahan J, Steadman H, Silver E, *et al. Rethinking Risk Assessment: The MacArthur Study of Mental Disorder and Violence.* New York: Oxford University Press; 2001.

38. Monahan J, Steadman H, Appelbaum P, *et al. Classification of Violence Risk (COVR) Professional Manual.* Lutz, FL: Psychological Assessment Resources, Inc.; 2002.

39. Ullrich S, Keers R, Coid JW. Delusions, anger, and serious violence: new findings from the MacArthur Violence Risk Assessment Study. *Schizophr. Bull.* (2013). DOI: doi: 10.1093/ schbul/ sbt126.

40. Fehon D, Grilo C, Lipschitz D. A comparison of adolescent inpatients with and without a history of violence perpetration: impulsivity, PTSD, and violence risk. *J. Nerv. Ment. Dis.* 2005; **193** (6): 405–411.

41. Wang EW, Diamond PM. Empirically identifying factors related to violence risk in corrections. *Behav. Sci. Law.* 1999; **17**(3): 377–389.

42. Barratt E. Impulsiveness and aggression. In: Monahan J, Steadman H, eds. *Violence and Mental Disorder: Developments in Risk Assessment.* Chicago: University of Chicago Press; 1994: 61–79.

43. Nolan KA, Czobor P, Roy BB, *et al.* Characteristics of assaultive behavior among psychiatric patients. *Psychiatr. Serv.* 2003; **54** (7): 1012–1016.

44. Quanbeck CD, McDermott BE, Scott CL, *et al.* Categorization of assaultive acts committed by chronically aggressive state hospital patients. *Psychiatr. Serv.* 2007; **58**(4): 521–528.

45. Cornell DG, Warren J, Hawk G, *et al.* Psychopathy in instrumental and reactive violent offenders. *J. Consult. Clin. Psychol.* 1996; **64** (4): 783–790.

46. Porter S, Woodworth M. Psychopathy and aggression. In: Patrick CJ, ed. *Handbook of Psychopathy.* New York: Guilford Press; 2006: 481–494.

47. Vitacco MJ, Van Rybroek GJ, Rogstad J, *et al.* Predicting short-term institutional aggression in forensic patients: a multi-trait method for understanding subtypes of aggression. *Law Hum. Behav.* 2009; **33**(4): 308–319.

48. McDermott BE, Quanbeck CD, Busse D, Yastro K, Scott CL. The accuracy of risk assessment instruments in the prediction of impulsive versus predatory aggression. *Behav. Sci. Law.* 2008; **26**(6): 759–777.

49. Woods P, Almvik R. The Brøset violence checklist (BVC). *Acta Psychiatr. Scand. Suppl.* 2002; **106** (412): 103–105.

50. McNiel J, Binder R. Screening for risk of inpatient violence: validation of an actuarial tool. *Law Hum. Behav.* 1994; **18**(5): 579–586.

51. Almvik R, Woods P, Rasmussen K. The Brøset Violence Checklist: sensitivity, specificity, and interrater reliability. *J. Interpers. Violence.* 2000; **15**(12): 1284–1296.

52. Ogloff JR, Daffern M. The dynamic appraisal of situational aggression: an instrument to assess risk for imminent aggression in psychiatric patients. *Behav. Sci. Law.* 2006; **24**(6): 799–813.

53. Grann M, Belfrage H, Tengstrom A. Actuarial assessment of risk for violence: predictive validity of the VRAG and the historical part of the HCR-20. *Criminal Justice and Behavior.* 2000; **27**(1): 97–114.

54. Johnson ME. Violence on inpatient psychiatric units: state of the science. *Journal of the American Psychiatric Nurses Association.* 2004; **10**(3): 113–121.

55. Douglas KS, Hart S, Webster C, Belfrage H. *HCR-20 (Version 3): Assessing Risk for Violence.* Burnaby, BC, Canada: Mental Health, Law, and Policy Institute, Simon Fraser University; 2013.

Clinical assessment of psychotic and mood disorder symptoms for risk of future violence

Charles L. Scott and Phillip J. Resnick

Introduction

Although the vast majority of individuals with mental illness are not violent [1], mental health clinicians are frequently asked to determine their patient's risk of future violence. Dangerousness assessments are required in a wide variety of situations that include involuntary commitments, emergency psychiatric evaluations, seclusion and restraint decisions, inpatient care discharges, probation/parole decisions, death penalty evaluations, domestic violence interventions, fitness for duty evaluations, and after a threat is made. The accuracy of a clinician's assessment of future violence is related to many factors, including the circumstances of the evaluation, the length of time over which violence is predicted, and the assessment of psychiatric symptoms that may increase a person's risk of dangerous behavior. Psychosis and mood symptoms are common psychiatric symptoms, and their relationship to violence risk is the focus of this article. Understanding the relationship of specific psychotic and mood symptoms to aggressive behavior can help the clinician not only provide better care but also decrease his or her own risk of malpractice when identified risk factors are more effectively targeted and treated.

Psychosis and Violence Risk

When evaluating a patient's risk of violence, the presence of psychosis is of particular concern. In their analysis of 204 studies examining the relationship between psycho-pathology and aggression, Douglas *et al.* [2] found that psychosis was the most important predictor variable of violent behavior. Witt *et al.* [3] conducted a systematic review and meta-regression analysis of 110 studies to investigate the range of risk

Table 5.1 General risk factors for violence in individuals with psychosis [3]

Poor impulse control
Hostile behavior
Lack of insight
Recent alcohol and/or drug misuse
Nonadherence with psychological therapies
Nonadherence with medication
Criminal history
History of victimization
Previous suicide attempts

factors associated with violence in 45,553 individuals with schizophrenia or other psychosis. Key findings from this study that identified risk factors specific to psychosis are summarized in Table 5.1 [3].

In addition to the dynamic and historical risk factors summarized in Table 5.1, the clinician should evaluate persecutory delusions and command auditory hallucinations when assessing a psychotic person's risk of future violence.

Evaluating persecutory delusions

Research examining the contribution of delusions to violent behavior provides mixed results. Earlier studies suggested that persecutory delusions were associated with an increased risk of aggression [4]. Delusions noted to increase the risk of violence were those characterized by threat/control-override (TCO) symptoms. TCO-type delusions are characterized by the presence of beliefs that one is being threatened (e.g., being followed or poisoned) or that one is losing control (i.e., control-override) to an external source (e.g., one's mind is dominated by forces beyond

Violence in Psychiatry, ed. Katherine D. Warburton and Stephen M. Stahl. Published by Cambridge University Press. © Cambridge University Press 2016.

the person's control) [5]. Similarly, Swanson *et al.* [6], using data from the Epidemiologic Catchment Area surveys, found that people who reported threat/control-override symptoms were about twice as likely to engage in assaultive behavior as those with other psychotic symptoms.

In contrast, results from the MacArthur Study of Mental Disorder and Violence showed that the presence of delusions did not predict higher rates of violence among recently discharged psychiatric patients [7]. In particular, a relationship between the presence of TCO delusions and violent behavior was not found. A subsequent analysis of the data indicated that men were significantly more likely than women to engage in violence during times they experience threat delusions, whereas women were significantly less likely to engage in violence due to threat delusions [8].

In a study that compared male criminal offenders with schizophrenia who had been found not guilty by reason of insanity to matched controls of non-offending schizophrenic persons, Stompe *et al.* [9] also found that TCO symptoms showed no significant association with the severity of violent behavior, nor did the prevalence of TCO symptoms differ between the two groups. However, nondelusional suspiciousness, such as misperceiving others' behavior as indicating hostile intent, has demonstrated an association with subsequent violence [7].

Nederlof *et al.* [10] conducted a cross-sectional, multi-center study to further examine whether the experience of TCO symptoms is related to aggressive behavior. The study sample included 124 psychotic patients characterized by the following diagnostic categories: 70.2% paranoid schizophrenia, 16.1% "other forms" of schizophrenia, 3.2% schizoaffective disorder, 0.8% delusional disorder, and 9.7% psychosis not otherwise specified (NOS). The authors determined that TCO symptoms were a significant correlate of aggression in their study sample. When the two domains of TCO symptoms were evaluated separately, only threat symptoms made a significant contribution to aggressive behavior. In their attempt to reconcile conflicting findings from earlier research regarding the relationship of TCO symptoms to aggressive behavior, the authors suggested that various methods of measuring TCO symptoms may underlie the seemingly contradictory findings among various studies [10].

In addition to research examining the potential relationship of particular delusional content to aggression,

Table 5.2 Specific delusions associated with serious violence when angry affect is present [15]

Being spied upon
Being followed
Being plotted against
Having thoughts inserted
Being under external control

Appelbaum *et al.* [11] utilized the MacArthur–Maudsley Delusions Assessment Schedule to examine the contribution of noncontent-related delusional material to violence. These authors found that individuals with persecutory delusions had significantly higher scores on the dimensions of "action" and "negative affect," indicating that persons with persecutory delusions may be more likely to react in response to the dysphoric aspects of their symptoms [10]. Subsequent research has demonstrated that individuals who suffer from persecutory delusions and negative affect are more likely to act on their delusions [4,12,13]. Coid *et al.* [14] found that anger due to delusions is a key factor that explains the relationship between violence and acute psychosis. Angry affect, in particular, has been shown to be an important intermediate variable in the pathway between anger delusions. When translating the various research findings into a practical examination, the psychiatrist should consider asking about five specific delusions that may increase the risk of violence, particularly when the patient presents as angry [15]. These delusions are listed in Table 5.2.

Evaluating auditory hallucinations

A careful inquiry about hallucinations is required to determine whether their presence increases the person's risk to commit a violent act. Command hallucinations are those that provide some type of directive to the patient. Command hallucinations are experienced by approximately half of hallucinating psychiatric patients [16]. The majority of command hallucinations are nonviolent in nature, and patients are more likely to obey nonviolent instructions than violent commands [17].

The research on factors that are associated with a person acting on harmful command hallucinations has been mixed. In a review of seven controlled studies examining the relationship between command hallucinations and violence, no study demonstrated a positive relationship between command hallucinations and violence, and one found an inverse relationship [18]. In contrast, McNiel *et al.* [19] reported that, in a study of 103 civil psychiatric inpatients, 33% reported having had command hallucinations to harm others during the prior year, and 22% of the patients reported that they complied with such commands. The authors concluded that patients in their study who experienced command hallucinations to harm others were more than twice as likely to be violent [19].

Much of the literature examining the relationship of a person's actions to command hallucinations has examined the person's response to all command hallucinations, without delineating factors specific to violent commands. Seven factors associated with acting due to command hallucinations include the following [16].

(1) The presence of coexisting delusions [20].
(2) Having delusions that relate to the hallucination [21].
(3) Knowing the voice's identity [21].
(4) Believing the voices to be real [22].
(5) Believing that the voices are benevolent [23].
(6) Having few coping strategies to deal with the voices [24].
(7) Not feeling in control over the voices [25].

Factors associated with acting on general command hallucinations as described above have also been found to indicate increased compliance with acting on violent command hallucinations [21,23]. Studies that have examined compliance specific to harmful command hallucinations provide additional guidance when evaluating the person's potential risk of harm. Some aspects relevant to increased compliance to violent command hallucinations include the following.

- A belief that the voice is powerful [16,24].
- A sense of personal superiority by the person evaluated [24].
- A belief that command hallucinations are of benefit to the person [16].
- Having delusions that were congruent with the action described [16].
- Experiencing hallucinations that generate negative emotions, such as anger, anxiety, and sadness [13].
- Impulsivity [25].

Schizophrenia and violence risk

Although the majority of individuals with schizophrenia do not behave violently [26], there is emerging evidence that a diagnosis of schizophrenia is associated with an increase in criminal offending. In a retrospective review of 2861 Australian patients with schizophrenia followed over a 25-year period, Wallace *et al.* [27] found that patients with schizophrenia accumulated a greater total number of criminal convictions relative to matched comparison subjects. These authors noted that the criminal behaviors committed by schizophrenic patients could not be entirely accounted for by comorbid substance use, active symptoms, or characteristics of systems of care [27]. Likewise, Short *et al.* [28] found that even schizophrenic patients without comorbid substance-use disorders were significantly more likely than controls to have been found guilty of violent offenses.

Mood Disorders and Violence Risk

Most studies examining the relationship between mood disorders and violence have not differentiated between bipolar disorder, mania, and depression [29]. To evaluate if criminal behavior and violent crimes were more common in the diagnosis of depression versus mania, Graz *et al.* [29] examined the German national crime register for 1561 patients with an affective disorder who had been released into the community. The rate of criminal behavior and violent crimes was highest in the manic disorder group (15.7%) compared to patients with major depressive disorder (1.4%). The authors concluded that different mood disorders have different risks of subsequent violence [29]. Other studies that have examined violence risk factors unique to different mood disorders are summarized below.

Depression and Violence Risk

Depression may result in violent behavior, particularly in depressed individuals who strike out against others in despair. After committing a violent act, the depressed person may attempt suicide. Depression is the most common diagnosis in murder–suicides [30]. Studies that have examined mothers who kill their children (filicide) have found that they were often suffering from severe depression. High rates of suicide following a filicide have been noted, with between 16%–29% of mothers and 40%–60% of fathers taking their life after murdering their child [30–32]. In a study of 30 family filicide–suicide files, the most common motive involved an attempt by the perpetrator to relieve real or imagined suffering of the child – a motive known as an altruistic filicide. Eighty percent of the parents in this study had evidence of a past or current psychiatric history, with nearly 60% suffering from depression, 27% with psychosis, and 20% experiencing delusional beliefs [31].

In their analysis of 386 individuals from the MacArthur Violence Risk Assessment Study with a categorical diagnosis of depression, Yang *et al.* [33] noted two important findings relevant to depression and future violence risk. First, violence that had occurred within the past 10 weeks was a strong predictor of future violence by participants with depression, but not by participants with a psychotic disorder. This finding suggests that a past history of recent violence may represent a higher risk of future violence in depressed patients than in those with psychosis. Second, this risk of future harm by depressed patients was further increased with alcohol use.

Bipolar disorder and violence risk

Patients with mania show a high percentage of assaultive or threatening behavior, but serious violence itself is rare [34]. Additionally, patients with mania show considerably less criminality of all kinds than patients with schizophrenia. Patients with mania most commonly exhibit violent behavior when they are restrained or have limits set on their behavior [35].

Active manic symptoms have been suggested as playing a substantial role in criminal behavior. In particular, Fazel *et al.* [36] compared violent crime convictions for over 3700 individuals who had been diagnosed with bipolar disorder with general population controls and unaffected full siblings. This longitudinal study had two main findings. First, although individuals with bipolar disorder exhibited an increased risk for violent crime compared to the general population, most of the excess violent crime was associated with substance abuse comorbidity. Second, unaffected siblings also had an increased risk for violent crime, which highlights the contribution of genetics or early environmental factors in families with bipolar disorder [36].

Clinical Implications and Recommendations

When conducting an assessment of current dangerousness, pay close attention to the individual's affect.

Individuals who are angry and lack empathy for others are at increased risk for violent behavior [37]. Clinicians should also assess their patients' insight into their illness and into the potential legal complications of their illness. Buckley *et al.* [38] found that violent patients with schizophrenia had more prominent lack of insight regarding their illness and legal complications of their behavior when compared with a nonviolent comparison group.

When evaluating an individual who is making a threat, the clinician should take all threats seriously and carefully elucidate the details. An important line of inquiry involves understanding the exact relationship of the person making the threat to his or her intended victim. In regard to written threats, individuals who send threats anonymously are far less likely to pursue an encounter than those who sign their names. Furthermore, the threatener who signs his true name is not trying to avoid attention; he or she is probably seeking it.

Understanding how a violent act will be carried out and the expected consequences for the patient helps the clinician in assessing the degree of danger. In addition, fully considering the consequences of an act may help the patient elect an alternative coping strategy. For example, a patient may be focused on revenge against his wife because of her infidelity. When confronted with the likelihood of spending many years in prison, he may decide to divorce his wife instead. The clinician should also assess the suicide risk in any patient making a homicidal threat. Violent suicide attempts increase the likelihood of future violence toward others [39]. One study found that 91% of psychiatric outpatients who had attempted homicide also had attempted suicide, and that 86% of patients with homicidal ideation also reported suicidal ideation [40].

Finally, the evaluator should consider asking the person to rate his or her own likelihood of future violence. Roaldset and Bjørkly [41] asked 489 patients admitted to a psychiatric hospital to rate their risk of future threatening or violent actions toward others. Moderate- or high-risk scores on self-ratings of future violence were significant predictors of violence 1 year post-discharge. However, persons who rated themselves as "no risk" or who refused to answer the question also had a considerable number of violent episodes, indicating that a self-report of low risk of violence may produce false negatives [41].

When considering strategies to decrease those risk factors that may contribute to future violence, the

Table 5.3 Example violence risk management chart

Dynamic risk factors	Recommended intervention	Status
Alcohol abuse	Refer to treatment program	Abstinent
	Obtain baseline blood labs	Complete (elevated liver enzymes)
TCO delusion	Medication adjustment and cognitive therapy as tolerated	Lessening of delusions
Suicidality	Suicide risk assessment	Completed (low risk)
	Removal of weapons	Weapons removed

clinician should distinguish static from dynamic risk factors. By definition, static factors are not subject to change by intervention. Static factors include such items as demographic information and a past history of violence. Dynamic factors are subject to change with intervention and include such factors as access to weapons, acute psychotic symptoms, active substance use, and a person's living setting. The clinician may find it helpful to organize a chart that outlines known risk factors, management and treatment strategies to address dynamic risk factors, and the current status of each risk factor. This approach will assist in the development of a violence prevention plan that addresses the specific risk factors for a particular patient. An example chart that illustrates this approach is provided in Table 5.3.

Clinical risk assessments do not typically incorporate any type of structured or standardized risk evaluation process. Unstructured clinical assessments have been criticized for having less accuracy than structured risk assessments. Structured risk assessments to assess future violence risk are based primarily on actuarial models of risks, referred to as actuarial risk assessment instruments (ARAIs). Over 120 structured instruments have been developed for the purpose of predicting violence in psychiatric or correctional populations, and many of them are relevant when evaluating individuals with psychosis or mood disorder symptoms [42]. The goals of these prediction schemes are to assist the clinician in gathering appropriate data and to anchor clinicians' assessments to established research.

Summary

A risk assessment of potential violence is important when evaluating psychiatric patients in both outpatient and inpatient settings. Identifying specific psychotic and mood disorder symptoms that increase a patient's potential for aggression provides a more structured risk assessment approach than unguided or uninformed clinical judgment. In turn, an appropriate risk assessment allows the clinician to target treatments to those identified risk factors, which is a critical component of risk management. Despite improvement in the field of risk assessment and risk management, the prediction of violence remains an inexact science. Predicting violence has been compared to forecasting the weather. Like a good weather forecaster, the clinician does not state with certainty that an event will occur. Instead, he or she estimates the likelihood that a future event will occur. Like weather forecasting, predictions of future violence will not always be correct. However, identifying those risk factors associated with psychotic and mood disorder symptoms assists the clinician in organizing the most accurate risk management approach possible.

Disclosures

Charles Scott and Phillip Resnick do not have anything to disclose.

References

1. Mulvey EP. Assessing the evidence of a link between mental illness and violence. *Hosp. Community Psychiatry*. 1994; **45**(7): 663–668.

2. Douglas KS, Guy LS, Hart SD. Psychosis as a risk factor for violence to others: a meta-analysis. *Psychol. Bull.* 2009; **135**(5): 679–706.

3. Witt K, van dorn R, Fazel S. Risk factors for violence in psychosis: systematic review and meta-regression analysis of 110 studies. *PloS One*. 2013; **8**(2): e55942.

4. Wessely S, Buchanan A, Reed A, *et al.* Acting on delusions. I: Prevalence. *Br. J. Psychiatry*. 1993; **163**(1): 69–76.

5. Link BG, Stueve A. Evidence bearing on mental illness as a possible cause of violent behavior. *Epidemiol. Rev.* 1995; **17**(1): 172–181.

6. Swanson JW, Borum R, Swartz M. Psychotic symptoms and disorders and risk of violent behavior in the community. *Crim. Behav. Ment. Health.* 1996; **6**(4): 317–338.

7. Monahan J, Steadman HJ, Silver E, *et al. Rethinking Risk Assessment: The MacArthur Study of Mental Disorder and Violence.* New York: Oxford University Press; 2001.

8. Teasdale B, Silver E, Monahan J. Gender, threat/control-override delusions and violence. *Law Hum. Behav.* 2006; **30**(6): 649–658.

9. Stompe T, Ortwein-Swoboda G, Schanda H. Schizophrenia, delusional symptoms, and violence: the threat/control override concept reexamined. *Schizophr. Bull.* 2004; **30**(1): 31–44.

10. Nederlof AF, Muris P, Hovens JE. Threat/control-override symptoms and emotional reactions to positive symptoms as correlates of aggressive behavior in psychotic patients. *J. Nerv. Ment. Dis.* 2011; **199**(5): 342–347.

11. Appelbaum PS, Robbins PC, Roth LH. Dimensional approach to delusions: comparison across types and diagnoses. *Am. J. Psychiatry.* 1999; **156**(12): 1938–1943.

12. Buchanan A, Reed A, Wessely S, *et al.* Acting on delusions. II: The phenomenological correlates of acting on delusions. *Br. J. Psychiatry.* 1993; **163**(1): 77–81.

13. Cheung P, Schweitzer I, Crowley K, Tuckwell V. Violence in schizophrenia: role of hallucinations and delusions. *Schizophr. Res.* 1997; **26**(2–3): 181–190.

14. Coid JW, Ullrich S, Kallis C, *et al.* The relationship between delusions and violence: findings from the East London first episode psychosis study. *JAMA Psychiatry.* 2013; **70**(5): 465–471.

15. Ullrich S, Robert K, Coid JW. Delusions, anger, and serious violence: new findings from the MacArthur violence risk assessment study. *Schizophr. Bull.* 2014 Sep; **40**(5): 1174–1181. Doi: 10.1093/schbul/sbt126.

16. Shawyer F, Mackinnon A, Farhall J, Trauer T, Copolov D. Command hallucinations and violence: implications for detention and treatment. *Psychiatry, Psychology and Law.* 2003; **10**(1): 97–107.

17. Chadwick P, Birchwood M. The omnipotence of voices: a cognitive approach to hallucinations. *Br. J. Psychiatry.* 1994; **164**(2): 190–201.

18. Rudnick A. Relation between command hallucinations and dangerous behavior. *J. Am. Acad. Psychiatry Law.* 1999; **27**(2): 253–257.

19. McNiel DE, Eisner JP, Binder RL. The relationship between command hallucinations and violence. *Psychiatr. Serv.* 2000; **51**(10): 1288–1292.

20. Mackinnon A, Copolov DL, Trauer T. Factors associated with compliance and resistance to command hallucinations. *J. Nerv. Ment. Dis.* 2004; **192**(5): 357–362.

21. Junginger J. Predicting compliance with command hallucinations. *Am. J. Psychiatry.* 1990; **147**(2): 245–247.

22. Erkwoh R, Willmes K, Eming-Erdmann A, Kunert HJ. Command hallucinations: who obeys and who resists them? *Psychopathology.* 2002; **35**(5): 272–279.

23. Beck-Sander A, Birchwood M, Chadwick P. Acting on command hallucinations: a cognitive approach. *Br. J. Clin. Psychol.* 1997; **36**(Pt 1): 139–148.

24. Fox JRE, Gray NS, Lewis H. Factors determining compliance with command hallucinations with violent content: the role of social rank, perceived power of the voice and voice malevolence. *The Journal of Forensic Psychiatry & Psychology.* 2004; **15**(3): 511–531.

25. Bucci S, Birchwood M, Twist L, *et al.* Predicting compliance with command hallucinations: anger, impulsivity and appraisals of voices' power and intent. *Schizophr. Res.* 2013; **147**(1): 163–168.

26. Walsh E, Buchanan A, Fahy T. Violence and schizophrenia: examining the evidence. *Br. J. Psychiatry.* 2002; **180**(6): 490–495.

27. Wallace C, Mullen PE, Burgess P. Criminal offending in schizophrenia over a 25-year period marked by deinstitutionalization and increasing prevalence of comorbid substance use disorders. *Am. J. Psychiatry.* 2004; **161**(4): 716–727.

28. Short T, Thomas S, Mullen P, Ogloff JRP. Comparing violence in schizophrenia with and without comorbid substance-use disorders to community controls. *Acta Psychiatr. Scand.* 2013; **128**(4): 306–313.

29. Graz C, Etschel E, Schoech H, Soyka M. Criminal behavior and violent crimes in former inpatients with affective disorder. *J. Affect. Disord.* 2009; **117**(1–2): 98–103.

30. Marzuk PM, Tardiff K, Hirsch CS. The epidemiology of murder-suicide. *JAMA.* 1992; **267**(23): 3179–3183.

31. Hatters Friedman S, Hrouda DR, *et al.* Filicide-suicide: common factors in parents who kill their children and themselves. *J. Am. Acad. Psychiatry Law.* 2005; **33**(4): 496–504.

32. Rodenburg M. Child murder by depressed parents. *Can. Psychiatr. Assoc. J.* 1971; **16**(1): 41–48.

33. Yang S, Mulvey EP, Loughran TA, Hanusa BH. Psychiatric symptoms and alcohol use in community violence by person with a psychotic disorder or depression. *Psychiatr. Serv.* 2012; **63**(3): 262–269.

34. Krakowski M, Volavka J, Brizer D. Psychopathology and violence: a review of literature. *Compr. Psychiatry.* 1986; **27**(2): 131–148.

35. Tardiff K, Sweillam A. Assault, suicide, and mental illness. *Arch. Gen. Psychiatry.* 1980; **37**(2): 164–169.

36. Fazel S, Lichtenstein P, Grann M, Goodwin GM, Langstrom N. Bipolar disorder in violent crime: new evidence from population-based longitudinal studies and systematic review. *Arch. Gen. Psychiatry.* 2010; **67**(9): 931–938.

37. Menzies JR, Webster CD, Sepejak DS. The dimensions of dangerousness: evaluating the accuracy of psychometric predictions of violence among forensic patients. *Law Hum. Behav.* 1985; **9**(1): 49–70.

38. Buckley PF, Hrouda DR, Friedman L, *et al.* Insight and its relationship to violent behavior in patients with schizophrenia. *Am. J. Psychiatry.* 2004; **161**(9): 1712–1714.

39. Convit A, Jaeger J, Lin SP, Meisner M, Volavka J. Predicting assaultiveness in psychiatric inpatients: a pilot study. *Hosp. Community Psychiatry.* 1988; **39**(4): 429–434.

40. Asnis GM, Kaplan ML, Hundorfean G, Saeed W. Violence and homicidal behaviors in psychiatric disorders. *Psychiatr. Clin. North Am.* 1997; **20**(2): 405–425.

41. Roaldset JO, Bjørkly S. Patients' own statements of their future risk for violent and self-harm behaviour: a prospective inpatient and post-discharge follow-up study in an acute psychiatric unit. *Psychiatry Res.* 2010; **178**(1): 153–159.

42. Singh JP, Fazel S. Forensic risk assessment: a metareview. *Criminal Justice and Behavior.* 2010; **37**(9): 965–988.

Inpatient aggression in community hospitals

Katalin A. Szabo, Christopher L. White, Stephen E. Cummings,
Raziya S. Wang, and Cameron D. Quanbeck

Introduction

A safe environment is a prerequisite for meaningful recovery for acutely hospitalized psychiatric patients, yet violence is endemic in acute psychiatric units. Threats and acts of violence jeopardize recovery and degrade the safety and effectiveness of acute psychiatric treatment programs; preventing violence is a clinical and administrative imperative.

Much of the literature has focused on development of assessment tools that accurately and reliably predict near-term violence with the hope that timely interventions may prevent violent incidents. Although most validated risk assessment instruments forecast only the long-term likelihood of future violence, structured assessments that weight current clinical factors heavily have been shown to be more successful in the prediction of violence in the short-term.

Currently the most efficacious efforts to prevent violence by psychiatric inpatients are a range of behavioral, psychopharmaceutical, and environmental interventions. Individualized, skillful behavioral management and de-escalation may serve to defuse dangerous situations, even when agitation is already overt. Judicious use of nonscheduled medications and proper psychopharmaceutical regimens often calms agitation dramatically and, thereby, forestalls violence. Further, the architectural design of a psychiatric unit can affect base rates of violence.

Methods

We conducted PubMed searches utilizing the following Medical Subject Headings (MeSH): violence, aggression, psychiatry, inpatient, hospital, community, and agitation. We identified 120 articles, and each article was reviewed to identify the most clinically relevant information. The authors utilized their discretion and best clinical judgment to determine topics in the field that are relevant to inpatient community psychiatry settings. This is not intended to be an all-inclusive review. The choice of articles and topics reflect the authors' qualitative assessment of current themes that are of the greatest clinical value to clinicians and administrators who are actively delivering care.

Discussion
Incidence of violence and aggression

Violence by patients is a common problem on acute inpatient community psychiatric units worldwide [1,2]. However, available data are unreliable as to the incidence of violence and aggression in psychiatric settings, especially in community hospitals. Systematic reviews have found that the prevalence of violence varies significantly from study to study and institution to institution [3]. This variance has been attributed to many factors, such as the great variety in incident reporting practices, a lack of clear definitions as to what constitutes violence and aggression, and lack of standard measurement instruments [4,5]. Of particular concern, evidence suggests that violent incidents are underreported [6]. Figure 6.1 lists some of the factors that may result in failure by staff to report a violent incident.

Notwithstanding these caveats, the available data demonstrate that inpatient violence is common. In a large-scale meta-analysis, Bowers et al. [5] found that the overall mean incidence of violence across seven different measurements (e.g., violent patients per month/admissions per month*100, violent patients/ total patient bed days*100, etc.) was 32.4% across

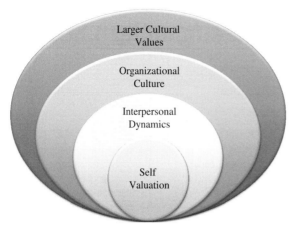

Figure 6.1 Possible spheres of influence that may contribute to an individual's decision to refrain from reporting a violent incident. Self Valuation: Individual deems his or her safety as lacking value. Interpersonal Dynamics: Individual's decision to refrain from reporting the violent act is influenced by the relationship he or she has with the assailant. Organizational Culture: An individual does not report a violent incident because of group staff pressures to normalize the incident or view it as "part of the job." Larger Cultural Values: An individual refrains from reporting violence because of religious or moral convictions from the larger culture.

different psychiatric inpatient settings in multiple countries. Forensic settings have substantially higher rates of violence (47.7%) than acute psychiatric wards (22.1%) or general psychiatric wards (26.2%). The highest rates of patient violence were found in the United States (31.92%), United Kingdom (41.73%), and Sweden (42.90%) [5]. A study of 11 psychiatric inpatient units in Australia showed that a reportable violent incident occurred in 11%–15% of all admissions in community psychiatric settings [1]. Another study conducted in the USA found similar results [7]. A minority of patients is disproportionately responsible for multiple episodes of violence: Approximately 45% of violent patients were involved in more than one incident, with each violent patient, on average, being responsible for four incidents [5].

Consequences of violence

Appreciating the impact of violence is problematic because its effects are wide ranging. Aggressive patients threaten the physical and mental well-being of other patients and of the staff. Violence has the potential to affect the therapeutic milieu in profound, negative ways, traumatizing and demoralizing all involved. A Danish study found that over 90% of staff working in psychiatric hospitals have been victims

of some form of violence by patients during their careers [8]. Psychiatric nurses are disproportionately victimized and suffer the highest incidence of violence in inpatient community psychiatric settings [9], resulting in physical, mental, and emotional distress [10].

Risk factors contributing to violence and aggression

Factors related to increased violence risk are of great interest to clinicians. An understanding of these factors informs effective risk management and enables clinical staff to select appropriate interventions. Literature focused on patient-related factors contributing to violence, such as history, symptoms, behaviors, and psychopathology, is abundant [11]. Bowers *et al.* emphasize that patient-related factors cannot be taken out of context, and interpersonal variables, such as patient–patient and patient–staff interaction, may play an even more important role [5]. Staff-related factors and environmental issues within units are also crucial [5].

Patient-related factors

A host of risk factors specific to the patient have been found to bear on the likelihood of future violence. These patient-related variables can be categorized into two major groups: (1) dynamic factors, such as acute clinical presentation, and (2) static factors, such as patient history, demographic features, and enduring character traits.

Clinical experiences inform us that acute clinical presentations are more likely to respond to clinical interventions than well-established static factors. McNiel *et al.* found that the strongest predictive relationships for aggression in the acute setting were obtained from clinical risk factors rather than historical risk factors [12,13].

Studies show that most inpatient violent outbursts do not arise abruptly, but occur after a period of escalating agitation or other change in behavior [5]. Psychomotor agitation is an established short-term risk factor for physical aggression. Acute behavioral cues often observed prior to violent incidents include boisterousness, irritability, confusion, attention-seeking behavior, and increased motor activity [5,14–16]. Threatening behaviors are often reported prior to aggressive acts; such behaviors include posturing, throwing objects, attacking or destroying property, self-harming behaviors, and direct verbal and physical threats [17], among others [18]. Some reports have identified changes in mental states including anger [19] and anxiety (75% of reported cases) [20] as antecedents to violent incidents. Triggers for violence may be highly individual, but stressors commonly associated with violence include being forced to take medications and involuntary hospitalization itself [9,21].

Static variables, including history, age, gender, and diagnosis, are well-established predictors of violence over the long term [22,23]. History of previous violence remains a vigorous static predictor of future aggression throughout most literature [24]. However, other static variables, such as sex, age, and alcohol abuse, seem to play a lesser role in acute inpatient settings, while current clinical presentation, illicit substance use, and psychopathological variables may be more significant contributors in the short-term [24]. Some studies have concluded that patients with diagnoses of schizophrenia, bipolar disorder, and mental retardation are more likely to engage in violent acts in the hospital setting than are patients with other diagnoses [3,12].

Other static factors associated with increased risk include a history of substance abuse [25–27], brain injury [28], and antisocial and other personality disorders [22,27,29]. Many of these patient-related factors are summarized in Table 6.1.

Staff-related factors

Psychiatric nurses, and staff in general, play a highly meaningful role in shaping patient experience and the social environment on the ward, interpersonally and on a group dynamic level [30,31]. Staff who are psychologically astute and who are engaged with and empathetically responsive to patients can provide a powerful stabilizing influence on patients in crisis and a milieu vulnerable to chaos. Conversely, staff who communicate negative or punitive attitudes to patients may contribute to patients' frustration or rage [32].

Bowers *et al.* found that staff–patient interactions precipitate an estimated 40% of aggressive and violent incidents [5]. Staff interventions that may lead to patient violence include limiting patients' freedom [5,33,34], administering or discussing medications [18,32,34], and placing patients in seclusion or restraints [17,18,35]. Attempts at de-escalating an already agitated patient were also found to precipitate violent outbursts [36]. Engaging in a power struggle

Table 6.1 Patient-related factors contributing to violence and aggression in inpatient settings

Dynamic factors

Mental status
- Anger
- Anxiety
- Irritability

Violent intentions
- Threatening gestures
- Verbal threats
- Self-harming

Observable behaviors
- Boisterousness
- Agitation
- Confusion
- Attention-seeking behavior
- Increased motor activity

Current involuntary admission
Current substance abuse

Static factors

Patient history
- Violence
- Multiple hospitalizations
- Substance abuse

Psychopathy
Male gender
Young
Diagnosis

has been shown to decrease therapeutic communication and trigger violence [32,33].

Of particular concern, recurrent violence on inpatient units may lead to poor job satisfaction and frank psychopathology in staff. In turn, this may result in negative staff–patient interpersonal interactions and possibly poor patient outcomes [30,31].

Patient–patient factors

Interactions with and reactions toward other patients are often found to contribute to violent incidents. Patient–patient factors include physical contact and/or intrusion into one another's "personal space" [37,38], competition [19], and retaliation [17,33].

Environmental/unit-related factors

Environmental and unit-related factors have a major role in influencing the risk of violence. Units that are overcrowded [39–41], physically restrictive [42], or inadequately staffed [43] experience higher rates of patient violence, as do those where patients experience either excessive sensory stimulation [34] or lack of stimulation and/or boredom [33,43]. A lack of psychological space, having little privacy, or not being able to spend time alone when needed may be important in triggering aggression [39].

Violence on psychiatric inpatient units appears to fluctuate throughout the day, with the highest incidence of violence occurring during staff shift changes, particularly during the swing shift (3 p.m. to 11 p.m.). Medication times and meal times were also found to be associated with higher incidence of violence [44].

Risk assessment

The ultimate goal of risk assessment is prevention of violence. The ability of clinical staff to recognize an increased likelihood of violence is crucial if interventions targeted at reducing that risk are to be deployed in time. Predictions aside, no two situations involving potential violence are ever identical; clinical skill and judgment will always inform risk assessment. Although unaided clinical judgment is notoriously inaccurate, it is more predictive than chance [45].

Formal risk assessment tools offer the hope of predicting violence more accurately and with less dependence on individual clinical acumen. Most validated instruments are actuarial in nature, and as such they reliably predict life-long risk [22,23]. Actuarial models use statistically derived static risk factors, such as age, gender, psychopathological state, diagnosis, and many other factors. However, they do not provide the near-term predictions required for treatment planning and intervention on acute units, and generally do not lend themselves readily to clinical interventions. Tools such as the Violence Risk Appraisal Guide (VRAG), Sex Offender Risk Appraisal Guide (SORAG), and Static-99 are some examples.

More recently, instruments that combine actuarial calculations of probability of violence with clinical observations and professional expertise, frequently called structured clinical instruments, have been shown to increase the accuracy and consistency of risk assessment. Instruments of this type include the Violence Prediction Scheme (VPS) and the Historical, Clinical, Risk Management-20 (HCR-20) [46,47]. A 2010 meta-review counted 126 instruments developed to assess risk in such structured forms [48].

Actuarial and structured clinical instruments are, however, time consuming, require specific training to use, and require the collection of information that may not be readily available in an acute setting [49,50]. Further, most of these instruments have been developed to assess violence risk in forensic and community settings, not for use in community inpatient psychiatric hospitals, and, moreover, have been shown to perform less well in nonforensic settings [24,51].

Few instruments are available for acute settings. In community psychiatric hospitals, risk assessments must be performed quickly, and predictions must be accurate over the short-term [23,52]. Clinicians working in acute psychiatric settings may be under time pressure to make decisions, may lack advanced training, and may not have access to predictive historical information [53]. Often, logistical constraints make it difficult to obtain much needed information, some patients may be too ill to provide accurate information, or collateral may not be available [53,54].

For these reasons, brief, simple screening tools based on immediate clinical features and readily available information prove to be more practically useful in acute hospital settings [55,56]. Examples of these types of instruments (Table 6.2) include the Brøset Violence Checklist (BVC) [14,16,55,57], the McNiel–Binder Violence Screening Checklist (VSC) [13,22], and the Dynamic Appraisal of Situation Aggression (DASA) [56]. These instruments show significantly better predictive accuracy than either structured clinical judgment or actuarial ratings in forecasting near-term violence [58].

Interventions

Behavioral, psychopharmacologic, and environmental/unit-related interventions have established roles in minimizing the incidence of patient violence on acute inpatient units. Although the available data are limited, they do support a growing consensus on best practices for preventing violence.

Behavioral management

Staff who are skilled in recognizing behavioral cues are better equipped to preempt and minimize the likelihood of a violent incident occurring. Verbal de-escalation and/or medication administration performed properly have been shown to be effective at reducing rates of containment procedures [59]. These are important findings, as these methods are

Table 6.2 Short-term risk assessment tools

	BVC	VSC	DASA
Risk assessed based on these correlates:	• Confusion • Boisterousness • Irritability • Verbal threats • Physical threats • Attacks on objects	• History of physical attacks or fear-inducing behavior within 2 weeks prior to admission • Absence of suicidal behavior within 2 weeks of admission • History of schizophrenia or mania • Male gender	• Negative attitudes • Impulsivity • Irritability • Verbal threats • Sensitive to perceived provocation • Easily angered when requests are denied • Unwillingness to follow directions
Predicts violence over the following time frame:	24 hours	72 hours	24 hours

The Brøset Violence Checklist (BVC) assesses six patient clinical correlates of imminent patient violence: confusion, boisterousness, irritability, verbal and physical threats, and attacks on objects. Sensitivity and specificity results show that the BVC accurately predicts at a rate of 85% which patients will commit violence, and which will not, over the next 24 hours. The BVC was validated in a public-sector facility, relies on observed patient behaviors, and requires documentation during each shift. The McNiel–Binder Violence Screening Checklist (VSC) is based on likely available information upon presentation, and consists of four items: (1) history of physical attacks or fear-inducing behavior within 2 weeks prior to admission, (2) absence of suicidal behavior within 2 weeks of admission, (3) history of schizophrenia or mania, and (4) male gender. Developed in a university hospital setting, these factors have been found to correlate to inpatient aggression that occurs within 72 hours of admission. The Dynamic Appraisal of Situation Aggression (DASA) assesses short-term risk of aggression by patients in psychiatric hospitals, as well as other secure settings. It consists of seven clinical items: negative attitudes, impulsivity, irritability, verbal threats, sensitive to perceived provocation, easily angered when requests are denied, and unwillingness to follow directions. DASA was shown to predict violence within 24 hours with 82% accuracy.

frequently used in response to violence and aggression. Staff therefore should receive routine, ongoing training in the use of verbal de-escalation techniques and other behavioral management approaches. The American Psychiatric Association (APA) Task Force on Psychiatric Emergency Services recommends yearly training in these methods [60].

The culture of an inpatient unit can be optimized for safety by improving the therapeutic relationship between staff and patients [43]. Patients who feel staff are accessible, listen to and advocate for them, and strive to involve them in treatment planning may be less prone to engage in violence.

Psychopharmalogical interventions

When an acutely hospitalized patient is physically agitated or threatens harm to others, clinicians often attempt to prevent a violent event by administering psychotropic medication on an as-needed basis (prn). Nonscheduled medications are also given acutely after an act of aggression has occurred to reduce time spent in seclusion and/or restraints and to prevent further violence.

Routes of administration, from most to least invasive and fastest onset of action, are intravenous (onset of action 15–30 seconds), intramuscular (20–30 minutes), and oral (60 minutes). Aside from the longer onset of action, oral administration is always preferred. However, intramuscular administration must often be resorted to when an uncooperative patient is in seclusion and/or restraints in order to assure adherence and to expedite release. Intravenous medications are typically only given in medical emergency departments.

A number of parenteral antipsychotic agents are effective in the treatment of psychotic agitation and aggression. The first-generation antipsychotic haloperidol is available in parenteral forms and has been used for decades in community hospitals. An anticholinergic agent (diphenhydramine, benztropine, or trihexyphenidyl) should always be co-administered with haloperidol in order maximize effectiveness [61], to reduce the need for additional medication intervention [62], and to prevent extrapyramidal side effects [63], primarily dystonic reactions. Of the atypical antipsychotics, only olanzapine, ziprasidone, and aripiprazole have intramuscular formulations. They are at least as effective as haloperidol alone (without an anticholinergic agent) in controlling agitation, more effective at controlling aggression [64], and carry a lower side effect burden [65]. In a study comparing the effectiveness of olanzapine and aripiprazole for the treatment of agitation in acutely ill patients with schizophrenia over a 5-day period, both were equally effective, but olanzapine was significantly more likely to increase fasting glucose and triglycerides [66].

Clinicians often use benzodiazepines alone or in combination with antipsychotics to control psychosis-induced aggression and agitation. However, a recent Cochrane Database Review found little research evidence to support this common practice [67]. Comparing benzodiazepines to placebo found little difference on most outcome measures; adding benzodiazepines to antipsychotics did not further reduce agitation and aggression 4 hours after administration, and the combination of haloperidol and midazolam actually increased aggression 12 hours after administration. In an experimental paradigm that was designed to test aggressive responding during a competitive game, male subjects given diazepam were more likely to select higher shock levels for their opponents than those given placebo [68]. Concerns have been raised regarding the safety of concurrent intramuscular administration of benzodiazepines with olanzapine due to the potential for excessive sedation, hypoxia, cardiorespiratory depression, and, in rare cases, death [69]. Benzodiazepines may be best indicated for acute nonpsychotic agitation and aggression.

In 2012, the US Food and Drug Administration (FDA) approved loxitane inhalation powder (Adusave) for the treatment of agitation in persons with schizophrenia and bipolar disorder. Inhaled loxitane results in rapid absorption through the alveoli, and maximum loxitane concentrations are reached in 2 minutes with reduced agitation seen at 10 minutes after administration [70]. Loxitane is non-invasive and simple to administer, but it requires some cooperation from the patient and is not an alternative to intramuscular injection during a psychiatric emergency [71]. Further, inhaled loxitane cannot be used in those with clinically significant pulmonary disease, and facilities administering this drug must be equipped to effectively treat broncho-spasm in the event of this potentially serious adverse effect [72].

Environmental/unit-related interventions

The architectural design of a psychiatric unit can affect base rates of violence. Environmental psychologists have identified features in the built environments of psychiatric units that are related to rates of violence. Psychiatric staff recognize that non-corridor designs, which provide good visibility, create safer environments [73]. Nursing stations that are enclosed do not protect staff from violence; no change in the prevalence of aggression is observed when enclosed nursing stations are converted into open stations [74].

Other design features that can reduce violence include single-patient rooms and personal bathrooms [75]. Private rooms give patients an opportunity to speak with caregivers without being disturbed and can be a place where they receive visits from family and friends. Psychiatric hospitals designed with sound-absorbing surfaces and that provide access to natural light and nature, such as in an outdoor garden, can help reduce the stress inherent in detention on a locked psychiatric ward [76]. From the patient perspective, an ideal psychiatric unit design would replicate a home-like environment that helps normalize their current situation, and allows the ability to move throughout a unit without excessive restriction [77].

Conclusion

An encouraging development in preventing inpatient psychiatric violence has been the validation of risk assessment tools that accurately predict violence over the short-term. For inpatient clinicians and program managers, the immediate challenge is to translate better recognition of risk into practical interventions that are focused on patients who have been identified as more likely to be violent. Violence prevention begins with a strong clinician–patient relationship to empower patients to gain recovery from mental illness. However, coupling improved risk assessment with behavioral and psychopharmacologic interventions that have established benefit offers the real hope of improved safety for patients and staff.

Inpatient violence is an extraordinarily complex problem. No risk assessment strategy is always accurate, and no clinical intervention is always effective. Although the total elimination of inpatient violence may be an unrealistic goal, addressing fundamental infrastructural weaknesses, including inadequate numbers and training of staff, and unsafe architecture, among other factors, may help to address the problem in the future.

Disclosures

Katalin Szabo, Stephen Cummings, Raziya Wang, and Cameron Quanbeck do not have anything to disclose.

Christopher White has the following disclosure: American Psychiatric Association, APA Public Psychiatry Fellow, reimbursement for accommodation and travel costs.

References

1. Carr VJ, Lewin TJ, Sly KA, *et al.* Adverse incidents in acute psychiatric inpatient units: rates, correlates and pressures. *Aust. N. Z. J. Psychiatry* 2008; **42**(4): 267–282.

2. Dack C, Ross J, Papadopoulos C, Stewart D, Bowers L. A review and meta-analysis of the patient factors associated with psychiatric inpatient aggression. *Acta Psychiatr. Scand.* 2013; **127**(4): 255–268.

3. Davis S. Violence by psychiatric inpatients: a review. *Hosp. Community Psychiatry* 1991; **42**(6): 585–590.

4. Irwin A. The nurse's role in the management of aggression. *J. Psychiatr. Ment. Health Nurs.* 2006; **13**(3): 309–318.

5. Bowers L, Stewart D, Papadopoulos C, *et al. Inpatient Violence and Aggression: A Literature Review. Report from the Conflict and Containment Reduction Research Programme.* London: Section of Mental Health Nursing, Health Service and Population Research, Institute of Psychiatry, Kings College London; 2011.

6. Khoshknab MF, Tamizi Z, Ghazanfari N, Mehrabani G. Prevalence of workplace violence in psychiatric wards, Tehran, Iran. *Pak .J. Biol. Sci.* 2012; **15**(14): 680–684.

7. Kay SR, Wolkenfeld F, Murrill LM. Profiles of aggression among psychiatric patients. I. Nature and prevalence. *J. Nerv. Ment. Dis.* 1988; **176**(9): 539–546.

8. Benjaminsen SE, Kjaerbo T. [The staff's experience of patient violence in a psychiatric department.] *Ugeskr. Laeger* 1997; **159**(12): 1768–1773.

9. Foster C, Bowers L, Nijman H. Aggressive behaviour on acute psychiatric wards: prevalence, severity and management. *J. Adv. Nurs.* 2007; **58**(2): 140–149.

10. Flannery RB Jr, Anderson E, Marks L, Uzoma LL. The Assaulted Staff Action Program (ASAP) and declines in rates of assault: mixed replicated findings. *Psychiatr. Q.* 2000; **71**(2): 165–175.

11. Johnson ME. Violence on inpatient psychiatric units: state of the science. *J. Am. Psychiatr. Nurses Assoc.* 2004; **10**(3): 113–121.

12. McNiel DE, Binder RL. The relationship between acute psychiatric symptoms, diagnosis, and short-term risk of violence. *Hosp. Community Psychiatry* 1994; **45**(2): 133–137.

13. McNiel DE, Binder RL, Greenfield TK. Predictors of violence in civilly committed acute psychiatric patients. *Am. J. Psychiatry* 1988; **145**(8): 965–970.

14. Woods P, Almvik R. The Brøset violence checklist (BVC). *Acta Psychiatr. Scand. Suppl.* 2002; **412**: 103–105.

15. Woods P, Ashley C. Violence and aggression: a literature review. *J. Psychiatr. Ment. Health Nurs.* 2007; **14**(7): 652–660.

16. Abderhalden C, Needham I, Miserez B, *et al.* Predicting inpatient violence in acute psychiatric wards using the Broset-Violence-Checklist: a multicentre prospective cohort study. *J. Psychiatr. Ment. Health Nurs.* 2004; **11**(4): 422–427.

17. Quanbeck CD, McDermott BE, Lam J, *et al.* Categorization of aggressive acts committed by chronically assaultive state hospital patients. *Psychiatr. Serv.* 2007; **58**(4): 521–528.

18. Powell G, Caan W, Crowe M. What events precede violent incidents in psychiatric hospitals? *Br. J. Psychiatry* 1994; **165**(1): 107–112.

19. Crowner ML, Peric G, Stepcic F, Lee S. Assailant and victim behaviors immediately preceding inpatient assault. *Psychiatr. Q.* 2005; **76**(3): 243–256.

20. Sheridan M, Henrion R, Robinson L, Baxter V. Precipitants of violence in a psychiatric inpatient setting. *Hosp .Community Psychiatry* 1990; **41**(7): 776–780.

21. Ketelsen R, Zechert C, Driessen M, Schulz M. Characteristics of aggression in a German psychiatric hospital and predictors of patients at risk. *J. Psychiatr. Ment. Health Nurs.* 2007; **14**(1): 92–99.

22. McNiel DE, Gregory AL, Lam JN, Binder RL, Sullivan GR. Utility of decision support tools for assessing acute risk of violence. *J. Consult. Clin. Psychol.* 2003; **71**(5): 945–953.

23. Harris GT, Rice ME. Risk appraisal and management of violent behavior. *Psychiatr. Serv.* 1997; **48**(9): 1168–1176.

24. Steinert T. Prediction of inpatient violence. *Acta Psychiatr. Scand. Suppl.* 2002; **412**: 133–141.

25. Cornaggia CM, Beghi M, Pavone F, Barale F. Aggression in psychiatry wards: a systematic review. *Psychiatry Res.* 2011; **189**(1): 10–20.

26. Serper MR, Goldberg BR, Herman KG, *et al.* Predictors of aggression on the psychiatric inpatient service. *Compr. Psychiatry* 2005; **46**(2): 121–127.

27. Fountoulakis KN, Leucht S, Kaprinis GS. Personality disorders and violence. *Curr. Opin. Psychiatry* 2008; **21**(1): 84–92.

28. McKinlay WW, Brooks DN, Bond MR, Martinage DP, Marshall MM. The short-term outcome of severe blunt head injury as reported by relatives of the injured persons. *J. Neurol. Neurosurg. Psychiatry* 1981; **44**(6): 527–533.

29. Hare RD. Psychopathy as a risk factor for violence. *Psychiatr. Q.* 1999; **70**(3): 181–197.

30. Kanerva A, Lammintakanen J, Kivinen T. Patient safety in psychiatric inpatient care: a literature review. *J. Psychiatr. Ment. Health Nurs.* 2013; **20**(6): 541–548.

31. Pulsford D, Crumpton A, Baker A, *et al.* Aggression in a high secure hospital: staff and patient attitudes. *J. Psychiatr. Ment. Health Nurs.* 2013; **20**(4): 296–304.

32. Duxbury J, Whittington R. Causes and management of patient aggression and violence: staff and patient perspectives. *J. Adv. Nurs.* 2005; **50**(5): 469–478.

33. Lavender MST. Putting aggression into context: an investigation into contextual factors influencing the rate of aggressive incidents in a psychiatric hospital. *Journal of Mental Health* 1999; **8**(2): 159–170.

34. Flannery RB Jr, Corrigan M, Hanson MA, Walker AP. Past violence, substance use, and precipitants to psychiatric patient assaults: eleven-year analysis of the Assaulted Staff Action Program (ASAP). *Int. J. Emerg. Ment. Health* 2006; **8**(3): 157–163.

35. Cooper AJ, Mendonca JD. A prospective study of patient assaults on nurses in a provincial psychiatric hospital in Canada. *Acta Psychiatr. Scand.* 1991; **84**(2): 163–166.

36. Rasmussen K, Levander S. Individual rather than situational characteristics predict violence in a maximum security hospital. *Journal of Interpersonal Violence* 1996; **11**(3): 376–390.

37. Longo DA, Bisconer SW. Treatment of aggression for an adult diagnosed with schizophrenia at a public psychiatric hospital. *Professional Psychology: Research and Practice* 2003; **34**(2): 177–179.

38. Bowers L, Allan T, Simpson A, *et al.* Identifying key factors associated with aggression on acute inpatient psychiatric wards. *Issues Ment. Health Nurs.* 2009; **30**(4): 260–271.

39. Nijman HL, Rector G. Crowding and aggression on inpatient psychiatric wards. *Psychiatr. Serv.* 1999; **50**(6): 830–831.

40. Ng B, Kumar S, Ranclaud M, Robinson E. Ward crowding and incidents of violence on an acute psychiatric inpatient unit. *Psychiatr. Serv.* 2001; **52**(4): 521–525.

41. Virtanen M, Vahtera J, Batty GD, *et al.* Overcrowding in psychiatric wards and physical assaults on staff: data-linked longitudinal study. *Br. J. Psychiatry* 2011; **198**(2): 149–155.

42. Barlow K, Grenyer B, Ilkiw-Lavalle O. Prevalence and precipitants of aggression in psychiatric inpatient units. *Aust. N. Z. J. Psychiatry* 2000; **34**(6): 967–974.

43. Hamrin V, Iennaco J, Olsen D. A review of ecological factors affecting inpatient psychiatric unit violence: implications for relational and unit cultural improvements. *Issues Ment. Health Nurs.* 2009; **30**(4): 214–226.

44. Bader S, Evans SE, Welsh E. Aggression among psychiatric inpatients: the relationship between time, place, victims, and severity ratings. *J. Am. Psychiatr. Nurses Assoc.* 2014; **20**(3): 179–186.

45. Mossman D. Assessing predictions of violence: being accurate about accuracy. *J. Consult. Clin. Psychol.* 1994; **62**(4): 783–792.

46. Douglas KS, Ogloff JR, Nicholls TL, Grant I. Assessing risk for violence among psychiatric patients: the HCR-20 violence risk assessment scheme and the Psychopathy Checklist: Screening Version. *J. Consult. Clin. Psychol.* 1999; **67**(6): 917–930.

47. Wong SCP, Gordon A. The validity and reliability of the Violence Risk Scale: a treatment-friendly violence risk assessment tool. *Psychology, Public Policy, and Law* 2006; **12**(3): 279–309.

48. Singh JP, Fazel S. Forensic risk assessment: a metareview. *Criminal Justice and Behavior* 2010; **37**(9): 965–988.

49. Steadman HJ, Silver E, Monahan J, *et al.* A classification tree approach to the development of actuarial violence risk assessment tools. *Law Hum. Behav.* 2000; **24**(1): 83–100.

50. Allen J. Assessing and managing risk of violence in the mentally disordered. *J. Psychiatr. Ment. Health Nurs.* 1997; **4**(5): 369–378.

51. Palmstierna T, Wistedt B. Risk factors for aggressive behaviour are of limited value in predicting the violent behaviour of acute involuntarily admitted patients. *Acta Psychiatr. Scand.* 1990; **81**(2): 152–155.

52. Almvik R, Woods P, Rasmussen K. The Brøset Violence Checklist: sensitivity, specificity, and interrater reliability. *Journal of Interpersonal Violence* 2000; **15**(12): 1284–1296.

53. Elbogen EB, Tomkins AJ, Pothuloori AP, Scalora MJ. Documentation of violence risk information in psychiatric hospital patient charts: an empirical examination. *J. Am. Acad. Psychiatry Law* 2003; **31**(1): 58–64.

54. Gardner W, Lidz CW, Mulvey EP, Shaw EC. Clinical versus actuarial predictions of violence of patients with mental illnesses. *J. Consult. Clin. Psychol.* 1996; **64**(3): 602–609.

55. Abderhalden C, Needham I, Dassen T, *et al.* Structured risk assessment and violence in acute psychiatric wards: randomised controlled trial. *Br. J. Psychiatry* 2008; **193**(1): 44–50.

56. Ogloff JRP, Daffern M. The dynamic appraisal of situational aggression: an instrument to assess risk for imminent aggression in psychiatric inpatients. *Behav. Sci. Law* 2006; **24**(6): 799–813.

57. Almvik R, Woods P. Predicting inpatient violence using the Brøset Violence Checklist (BVC). *Int. J. Psychiatr. Nurs. Res.* 1999; **4**(3): 498–505.

58. Chu CM, Daffern M, Ogloff JRP. Predicting aggression in acute inpatient psychiatric setting using BVC, DASA, and HCR-20 Clinical scale. *Journal of Forensic Psychiatry & Psychology* 2013; **24**(2): 269–285.

59. Beck JC, White KA, Gage B. Emergency psychiatric assessment of violence. *Am. J. Psychiatry* 1991; **148**(11): 1562–1565.

60. Allen M, Forster P, Zealberg J, *et al.* Report and recommendations regarding psychiatric emergency and crisis services: a review and model program descriptions. American Psychiatric Association Task Force. 2002. http://www .emergencypsychiatry.org/data/ tfr200201.pdf. Accessed September 1, 2014.

61. Huf G, Coutinho ESF, Adams CE. Rapid tranquillisation in psychiatric emergency settings in Brazil: pragmatic randomised controlled trial of intramuscular haloperidol versus intramuscular haloperidol plus promethazine. *BMJ* 2007; **335**: 869.

62. Raveendran NS, Thar yan P, Alexander J, Adams CE. Rapid tranquillisation in psychiatric emergency setting in India: pragmatic randomised controlled trial of intramuscular olanzapine versus intramuscular haloperidol plus promethazine. *BMJ* 2007; **335** (7625): 865–869.

63. Powney MJ, Adams CE, Jones H. Haloperidol for psychosis-induced aggression or agitation (rapid tranquillisation). *Cochrane Database Syst. Rev.* 2012; **11**: CD009377.

64. Baldaçara L, Sanches M, Cordeiro DC, Jackoswski AP. Rapid tranquilization for agitated patients in emergency psychiatric rooms: a randomized trial of olanzapine, ziprasidone, haloperidol plus promethazine, haloperidol plus midazolam and haloperidol alone. *Rev. Bras. Psiquiatr.* 2011; **33**(1): 30–39.

65. Bosanac P, Hollander Y, Castle D. The comparative efficacy of intramuscular antipsychotics for the management of acute agitation. *Australas. Psychiatry* 2013; **21**(6): 554–562.

66. Kinon BJ, Stauffer VL, Kollack-Walker S, Chen L, Sniadecki J. Olanzapine versus aripiprazole for the treatment of agitation in acutely ill patients with schizophrenia. *J. Clin. Psychopharmacol.* 2008; **28**(6): 601–607.

67. Gillies D, Sampson S, Beck A, Rathbone J. Benzodiazepines for psychosis-induced aggression or agitation. *Cochrane Database Syst. Rev.* 2013; **4**: CD003079.

68. Wallace PS, Taylor SP. Reduction of appeasement-related affect as a concomitant of diazepam-induced aggression: Evidence for a link between aggression and the expression of self-conscious emotions. *Aggress. Behav.* 2009; **35**(2): 203–212.

69. Wilson MP, MacDonald K, Vilke GM, Feifel D. Potential complications of combining intramuscular olanzapine with benzodiazepines in emergency department patients. *J. Emerg. Med.* 2012; **43**(5): 889–896.

70. Keating GM. Loxapine inhalation powder: a review of its use in the acute treatment of agitation in patients with bipolar disorder or schizophrenia. *CNS Drugs* 2013; **27**(6): 479–489.

71. Citrome L. Aerosolised antipsychotic assuages agitation: inhaled loxapine for agitation associated with schizophrenia or bipolar disorder. *Int. J. Clin. Pract.* 2011; **65**(3): 330–340.

72. Currier G, Walsh P. Safety and efficacy review of inhaled loxapine for treatment of agitation. *Clin. Schizophr. Relat .Psychoses* 2013; **7**(1): 25–32.

73. Sheehan B, Burton E, Wood S, *et al.* Evaluating the built environment in inpatient psychiatric wards. *Psychiatr. Serv.* 2013; **64**(8): 789–795.

74. Southard K, Jarrell A, Shattell MM, *et al.* Enclosed versus open nursing stations in adult acute care psychiatric settings: does the design affect the therapeutic milieu? *J. Psychosoc. Nurs. Ment. Health Serv.* 2012; **50**(5): 28–34.

75. Ulrich RS, Zimring C, Zhu X, *et al*. A review of the research literature on evidence-based healthcare design. *HERD* 2008; **1**(3): 61–125.

76. Ulrich RS, Berry LL, Quan X, Parish JT. A conceptual framework for the domain of evidence-based design. *HERD* 2011; **4**(1): 95–114.

77. Douglas CH, Douglas MR. Patient-centred improvements in healthcare built environments: perspectives and design indicators. *Health Expect*. 2005; **8**(3): 264–276.

Prevalence of physical violence in a forensic psychiatric hospital system during 2011–2013: patient assaults, staff assaults, and repeatedly violent patients

Charles Broderick, Allen Azizian, Rebecca Kornbluh, and Katherine D. Warburton

Introduction

Evidence has accumulated that shows that patients with a mental illness in a hospital setting have higher rates of violence in comparison to people with mental illness living in the community [1–3]. Investigations into patient violence in psychiatric hospitals have typically examined variables such as sex, age, ethnicity, and diagnosis. These investigations have typically found higher prevalence of violence among inpatients who are female [4–7], younger [8–10], and of ethnic minority status [11,12]. However, these findings have not been universal across all studies, as noted in the review by Bowers *et al.* [13] Their review found that of the 26 studies of psychiatric inpatients that specifically investigated the roles of age and aggression, 13 reported no significant relationship and 13 reported that aggressive patients were significantly younger.

Likewise, with regard to diagnosis, their review again found discrepancies; across 19 studies, nine reported no significant differences in diagnosis between the aggressor and non-aggressor groups, and only one study directly addressed the issue of personality disorder among aggressive and non-aggressive groups [9]. The presence and number of contradictory findings raises questions regarding methodological issues, such as the setting of the study (and subsequent generalizability to other settings), along with issues of statistical power related to the sample size of the study, which may have limited the ability of the investigators to find significance when the impact of a variable was small.

In the decade or more since many of these studies were conducted, there have been significant changes in the state psychiatric hospital system; these include a simultaneous reduction in hospital beds with an increase in the demand for beds by the criminal court system (i.e., forensic patients) [6,14]. Nationwide, as of 2012, expenditures by state psychiatric hospitals for forensic patients had grown to 36% of the total budget, with an additional 4.7% of expenditures dedicated for persons committed under sex offender commitment statutes. While several states now have a forensic population over 50% of the total inpatient population, perhaps nowhere has this impact been felt more than in the California State Hospital system, where shifts over the past decade have resulted in criminal-related, forensic inpatients comprising over 92% of the hospitalized patients.

The increasing number of forensic patients admitted to state hospitals creates a number of concerns, chief among these the concern of risk for violence. Because commitment to a state hospital in California requires an assessment of whether the patient can be safely treated in the community as an alternative to hospitalization, a patient can only be committed if the court finds that person too dangerous to treat in the community. Since the only distinguishing feature between those treated as outpatients or committed to a state hospital is that of dangerousness, in essence patients are hospitalized by courts primarily due to the issue of dangerousness and secondarily due to mental illness. Also considering the requirements of the commitment criteria in California, as the patients

Violence in Psychiatry, ed. Katherine D. Warburton and Stephen M. Stahl. Published by Cambridge University Press.

committed by the courts are presumed to be dangerous, they cannot be discharged solely by the treatment team's recommendation; the court must evaluate any treatment team discharge recommendation and can choose to follow or not follow any such recommendation based on the relevant legal issue(s) brought up at the hearing or trial. This potentially can increase the length of stay of these patients, beyond what would reasonably be expected for simple treatment of their mental illness needs. In view of previous research findings that patients who were more violent in the community are more likely to be violent while hospitalized, and those patients diagnosed with schizophrenia with recent violence or law enforcement contact have increased violence risk, there are concerns that violence by forensic patients in state hospitals may be both quantitatively and qualitatively different from violence in other psychiatric facilities that do not treat forensic patients [2,4]. Owing to these issues, and a need to develop effective methodologies to decrease violence, we decided to enumerate both the prevalence of violent assaults, as well as investigate details of the assaults that may warrant further evaluation.

Previous studies that examined prevalence of inpatient violence in psychiatric facilities typically followed one of several common methodologies. Studies conducted before 2000 routinely used questionnaire-type surveys administered to staff, asking about previous violence – a technique methodologically subject to under-reporting [15,16]. Another methodology was to conduct a one-year "look-back" at the violence committed by all patients resident in the hospital, which could systematically overlook patients resident during any part of the year but discharged prior to the study initiation [6,16]. In one such study, it is estimated that potentially up to 25% of all patients resident at any point during the year were not included [6]. More recent studies have commonly followed inpatients for a prescribed length of time and had nursing staff fill out standardized aggression surveys immediately after aggressive/violent events [7]. An issue for some of these studies is that nursing time resources are needed, if aggression ratings forms are not a routine part of nursing duties, resulting in a more limited duration for the study period.

The present study endeavored to overcome these limitations encountered by past investigations by using a computerized violent incident reporting system that is routinely used by staff to record the occurrence of every violent incident. Use of other available patient databases enabled us to cross-reference patient information with the violent incident data, and determine who was and was not violent. Additionally, the use of these databases allowed us to track and record every patient and every violent incident for three years, allowing a sufficient time period to ensure a representative portrayal of violent incidents over time. To the best of our knowledge, this is the single largest study on violent assaults in a state psychiatric hospital system.

Methods

This study was reviewed and approved by the California Health and Human Services Agency Committee for the Protection of Human Subjects (CPHS), the IRB with oversight over all research with human subjects in the California Department of State Hospitals.

Description of setting

The California Department of State Hospitals (DSH) operates five different state hospitals across the state, with current populations ranging from 600 to 1500 patients at each facility. All facilities have a mix of patients, although one hospital is the designated Sexually Violent Predator (SVP) treatment facility. Typical housing unit size at each facility ranges from 35 to 70 patients, with the majority of units being single sex, although there are several co-ed dorms exclusively for the nonforensic patients. According to California law, forensically involved patients cannot be mixed with nonforensic patients; otherwise, patients of all forensic classes (while housed on units according to legal commitment code) typically mix during daytime group and leisure activities. Treatment modalities are also similar, with a similar range of individual and group treatments available to all patients, in addition to leisure and recreational activities on evenings and weekends.

Subjects

The study subjects consisted of the entire adult (age 18 and greater) patient population in residence at, or admitted to, all five California DSH hospitals between January 1, 2011, and December 31, 2013. The total number of subjects during the entire study period was $N = 15{,}615$ and included $n = 2161$ females and $n = 13\,454$ males of various ethnicities, with a mean age of

Table 7.1 Summary of subject demographics by ethnicity

Ethnicity	Number		Age at study start		
			Mean	SD	Range
Overall study	Total	15,615	42.17	13.0	18.01–91.24
	Female	2161	41.60	12.32	18.01–85.55
	Male	13,454	42.27	13.10	18.01–91.24
African-American	Total	4525	41.81	12.61	18.01–88.76
	Female	663	41.28	12.11	18.01–85.55
	Male	3862	41.90	12.69	18.08–88.76
Asian	Total	471	42.29	12.93	19.02–87.49
	Female	71	45.04	12.39	19.03–70.42
	Male	400	41.80	12.98	19.02–87.49
Hispanic	Total	3549	38.12	12.56	18.01–90.15
	Female	423	37.63	11.59	18.04–72.28
	Male	3126	38.18	12.68	18.01–90.15
Native American	Total	117	39.75	12.12	20.38–69.91
	Female	15	36.66	8.27	24.79–56.15
	Male	102	40.20	12.55	20.38–69.91
Other/unknown	Total	244	38.64	11.92	18.32–79.86
	Female	15	42.15	15.67	20.75–79.86
	Male	229	38.41	11.64	18.32–70.07
Pacific Islander	Total	256	40.47	12.33	18.22–73.45
	Female	34	37.67	13.13	18.22–67.14
	Male	222	40.89	12.18	18.43–73.45
White	Total	6453	44.90	12.93	18.04–91.24
	Female	940	43.56	12.27	18.08–81.22
	Male	5513	45.12	13.02	18.04–91.24

42.17 years. (Table 7.1 lists the subject demographics.) At the start of the study period (January 1, 2011) there were 5499 patients in residence at the hospitals; during the study period, 2887 of these patients discharged. During the course of the study period, 10,116 patients were admitted; of these, 7220 were discharged before the study period ended, and 2896 were admitted at various points during the three-year study period and remained until the end of the study (December 31, 2013), at which point 5508 patients were residing in the hospitals.

The patients were grouped according to the overall "umbrella" legal commitment under which the exact legal code fell. (California has 39 different legal sections for holding patients in state psychiatric facilities, which can be collapsed into eight general categories.) Details and a description of the legal classes in the hospitals are shown in Box 7.1. Table 7.2 shows a summary of study subject demographics by general legal class.

Data collection

Patient demographic and legal class information were collected from system databases that are routinely used for census tracking. Data on violent incidents were collected through a computerized incident management module of the patient treatment planning database.

Study variables

Sex, ethnicity, age, and legal commitment code were collected from the patient demographic information database. Information on patient *Diagnostic and Statistical Manual of Mental Disorders*, Fourth Edition, Text Revision (DSM-IV-TR) diagnosis was collected from the patient admission diagnostic fields contained in the patient information database [17]. Since patients commonly had multiple diagnoses, only the primary diagnosis indicated on Axis I and the primary diagnosis (if any) indicated on Axis II were

Table 7.2 Summary of subject demographics by legal class

Legal class	Number		Age at study start		
			Mean	SD	Range
DJJ	Total	30	20.52	1.87	18.01–24.21
	Female	2	18.62	0.86	18.01–19.23
	Male	28	20.66	1.85	18.01–24.21
IST	Total	7587	39.62	12.95	18.08–89.12
	Female	1276	41.18	11.72	18.80–81.22
	Male	6311	39.30	13.16	18.08–89.12
LPS	Total	974	41.46	13.94	18.04–88.03
	Female	288	39.71	14.95	18.04–85.55
	Male	686	42.20	13.43	18.16–88.03
MDO	Total	2272	42.63	10.97	19.63–81.34
	Female	182	42.54	9.85	20.02–68.97
	Male	2090	42.64	11.07	19.63–81.34
MDSO	Total	32	59.25	7.69	48.68–76.52
	Female	0	N/A	N/A	N/A
	Male	32	59.25	7.69	48.68–76.52
NGI	Total	1888	46.58	12.71	18.48–91.24
	Female	275	45.97	13.07	19.80–77.40
	Male	1613	46.68	12.65	18.48–91.24
PC2684	Total	1784	41.86	11.71	19.03–83.63
	Female	137	39.64	10.92	20.97–66.28
	Male	1647	42.04	11.75	19.03–83.63
SVP	Total	1048	53.03	10.57	23.95–89.08
	Female	1	51.31	N/A	51.31
	Male	1047	53.04	10.57	23.95–89.08

See Box 7.1 for description of legal class abbreviations.

Box 7.1   Description of legal class and abbreviations

Nonforensic commitment:

LPS: short for "Lanterman-Petris-Short," i.e., nonforensically committed patients, typically patient conserved by county courts

Forensic commitments:

DJJ: Patients referred for treatment from the Division of Juvenile Justice system
IST: Patients found incompetent to stand trial
MDO: Mentally disordered offenders, i.e., parolees from the prison deemed too dangerous to allow to parole back to the community

MDSO: Mentally disordered sex offender, a since discontinued legal commitment that was a precursor to the present-day SVP commitment
NGI: Patients found not guilty by reason of insanity
PC2684: Mentally ill prisoners, i.e., prison inmates referred to DSH for treatment
SVP: Patients adjudicated under the Sexually Violent Predator law

used. Over 280 different DSM-IV-TR diagnoses were recorded for all the patients on admission; these various diagnoses were collapsed according to the DSM-IV-TR category or chapter title, with diagnoses of particular interest (such as schizophrenia, schizo-affective disorder, bipolar disorder, and psychotic disorder NOS/miscellaneous psychotic disorders) kept as separate categories.

Statistical analyses

Data preparation and analyses were performed with R version 3.1.1 [18]. Data files were provided by the centralized data management office of the California DSH for all patients who were in residence or admitted to the hospitals during the periods 2010–2014; from these were extracted the records of all patients resident or admitted to a hospital between January 1, 2011, and December 31, 2013, inclusive. Data files were also provided for all the records of physical assaults by patients during the period 2010–2014, which were again further refined to extract just the physical assaults recorded during the period between January 1, 2011, and December 31, 2013, inclusive.

The first level of data analysis consisted of a descriptive review of violence prevalence in the hospital system stratified by previously researched variables (sex, ethnicity, age, legal classification, DSM-IV-TR Axis I diagnosis and Axis II diagnosis), and calculated the prevalence of violence and approximate 95% confidence intervals (CI). Chi-squared tests were then performed to test the prevalence rates for significance. Last, a logistic regression main effects model was fitted to obtain the adjusted odds ratios (ORs) and 95% CI of violence for the different demographic and clinical diagnosis variables.

Description of aggression data

Physical violence during the study was defined as assaults directed against either another patient or a staff member, as defined in the California DSH policies (see Box 7.2). Analogous codes and definitions also existed for verbal aggression and property damage, but were not used in this study, as we examined only physical violence. There were a total of 11 302 unique recorded acts of physical violence against other patients during the study period, and a further 8482 unique recorded acts of physical violence directed against staff members. Of these total numbers, aggressors were identified in 10 958 assaults against patients, and in 8429 assaults against staff; these incidents in which aggressors were identified were used as the final count of violent assaults, as well as to determine an individual patient's aggressor and victim status.

Box 7.2 Definitions of physical violence or assault, and aggressor/victim status

Aggressive Act to Another Patient – Physical: Hitting, pushing, kicking, or similar acts directed against another individual to cause potential or actual injury

Aggressive Act to Staff – Physical: Hitting, pushing, kicking, or similar acts directed against a staff person that could cause potential or actual injury

Aggressor: One who completes acts of hostility or assault; one who starts a hostile action or exhibits hostile behavior. An aggressive act must have occurred for there to be an aggressor

Victim: Recipient of an aggressive act

Results

Overview of violent incidents and patients

The total number of subjects in the study was $N = 15$ 615. The number of unique patients having a single violent incident (whether patient assault or staff assault) was $n = 4895$, yielding an overall prevalence of violence during the study period of 31.35% (95% confidence interval (CI) 30.62%–32.08%). The number of patients having at least a single patient assault incident was $n = 4075$, yielding a violent patient assault prevalence of 26.10% (95% CI 25.54%–26.79%). The number of patients having at least a single staff assault incident was $n = 2504$, yielding a staff assault prevalence of 16.04% (95% CI 15.46%–16.62%). A simple tally showed that the top 156 aggressors (1% of the study population) were involved in 28.7% of all these violent assaults. When examining the patients still hospitalized at the conclusion of the study, those remaining ($n = 5508$) had an overall violence prevalence of 41.25% (95% CI 39.95%–42.55%), with a patient violence prevalence of 35.48% (95% CI 34.22%– 36.74%) and a staff violence prevalence of 22.97% (95% CI 21.86%–24.08%), which led us to investigate how violence impacted length of stay; these findings will be reported below.

Regarding severity of assaults, only data on patient injury severity were collected; these data showed that, for the most part, injuries suffered by patient victims were typically not severe, although one homicide did occur during the study period.

Sex differences

As shown in Table 7.3, there were no significant differences for patient assault, but there was a significant difference for staff assault [χ^2 (1, N = 15 615) = 30.51, $p < 0.001$], with assaults committed by females more prevalent (20.08%, 95% CI 18.39%–21.77%) than males (15.38%, 95% CI 14.78%–16.00%). Examining the adjusted odds ratios (ORs) in Table 7.4 shows a similar relationship, with no significant difference in the adjusted odds between females and males for patient assault, but a significant difference ($p < 0.001$) in the odds for staff assault, with females having a higher odds (OR 1.256, 95% CI 1.104–1.423).

Table 7.3 Prevalence (%) and 95% confidence interval (CI) of physical violence by demographic category

	n	Patient assaults		Staff assaults	
		n (%)	95% CI	*n* (%)	95% CI
Sex					
Females	2161	597 (27.63)	(25.74, 29.51)	434 (20.08)	(18.39, 21.77)
Males	13,454	3478 (25.85)	(25.11, 26.59)	2070 (15.38)	(14.78, 16.00)
Ethnicity					
African-American	4525	1290 (28.51)	(27.19, 29.82)	717 (15.84)	(14.78, 16.91)
Asian	471	99 (21.02)	(17.34, 24.70)	64 (13.59)	(10.49, 16.68)
Hispanic	3549	1005 (28.32)	(26.84, 29.80)	561 (15.81)	(14.61, 17.01)
Native American	117	30 (25.64)	(17.73, 33.55)	20 (17.09)	(10.27, 23.92)
Other/unknown	244	63 (25.82)	(20.33, 31.31)	36 (14.75)	(10.30, 19.20)
Pacific Islander	256	72 (28.12)	(22.62, 33.63)	42 (16.41)	(11.87, 20.94)
White	6453	1516 (23.49)	(22.46, 24.53)	1064 (16.49)	(15.58, 17.39)
Age group					
18–29	3056	986 (32.26)	(30.61, 33.92)	562 (18.39)	(17.02, 19.76)
30–39	3721	1057 (28.41)	(26.96, 29.86)	650 (17.47)	(16.25, 18.69)
40–49	3724	873 (23.44)	(22.08, 24.80)	519 (13.94)	(12.82, 15.05)
50–59	3404	784 (23.03)	(21.62, 24.45)	486 (14.28)	(13.10, 15.45)
60–69	1363	305 (22.38)	(20.16, 24.59)	232 (17.02)	(15.03, 19.02)
70 +	347	70 (20.17)	(15.95, 24.40)	55 (15.85)	(12.01, 19.69)
Legal class					
DJJ	30	15 (50.00)	(32.11, 67.89)	11 (36.67)	(19.42, 53.91)
IST	7587	1694 (22.33)	(21.39, 23.26)	949 (12.51)	(11.76, 13.25)
LPS	974	494 (50.72)	(47.58, 53.86)	422 (43.33)	(40.21, 46.44)
MDO	2272	698 (30.72)	(28.82, 32.62)	423 (18.62)	(17.02, 20.22)
MDSO	32	10 (31.25)	(15.19, 47.31)	6 (18.75)	(5.23, 32.27)
NGI	1888	559 (29.61)	(27.55, 31.67)	290 (15.36)	(13.73, 16.99)
PC2684	1784	299 (16.76)	(15.03, 18.49)	169 (9.47)	(8.11, 10.83)
SVP	1048	306 (29.20)	(26.44, 31.95)	234 (22.33)	(19.81, 24.85)

See Box 7.1 for a full description of the legal class abbreviations.

Ethnicity

There were significant differences in patient assault [χ^2 (6, N = 15 615) = 52.27, p < 0.001], but not for staff assault [χ^2 (6, N = 15 615) = 3.76, p = 0.709], among the various ethnic groups (Table 7.3). Both the prevalence of African-Americans (28.51%, 95% CI 27.19%–29.82%) and Hispanics (28.32%, 95% CI 26.84%–29.80%) for patient assault were higher than those of other ethnicities. However, there were no significant differences among the groups for staff assault. Similarly, the logistic regression model (Table 7.4) showed parallel results with the prevalence rates. Again, there were no significant differences among the various ethnicities for staff assault.

Table 7.4 Adjusted odds ratios (OR) and 95% confidence interval (CI) of physical violence by demographic variables

	Patient assault Adjusted OR (95% CI)	p-value	Staff assault Adjusted OR (95% CI)	p-value
Sex				
Females	1.037 (0.927, 1.158)	0.522	1.256 (1.104, 1.423)	<.001
Males (*reference group*)	1			
Ethnicity				
African-American	1.273 (1.161, 1.395)	<.001	0.947 (0.848, 1.057)	0.335
Asian	0.942 (0.741, 1.190)	0.625	0.914 (0.684, 1.204)	0.534
Hispanic	1.213 (1.099, 1.340)	<.001	0.939 (0.833, 1.058)	0.303
Native American	1.080 (0.690, 1.645)	0.729	1.058 (0.622, 1.714)	0.827
Other/unknown	1.148 (0.840, 1.548)	0.376	0.930 (0.630, 1.336)	0.704
Pacific Islander	1.188 (0.883, 1.578)	0.244	0.942 (0.653, 1.329)	0.741
White (*reference group*)	1		1	1
Age group				
18–29 (*reference group*)	1		1	
30–39	0.772 (0.692, 0.861)	<.001	0.881 (0.772, 1.006)	0.061
40–49	0.584 (0.520, 0.655)	<.001	0.643 (0.558, 0.739)	<.001
50–59	0.532 (0.472, 0.600)	<.001	0.612 (0.529, 0.708)	<.001
60–69	0.495 (0.421, 0.582)	<.001	0.712 (0.591, 0.857)	<.001
70 and older	0.422 (0.314, 0.561)	<.001	0.638 (0.457, 0.877)	0.007
Legal class				
DJJ	2.159 (1.031, 4.520)	0.039	3.053 (1.372, 6.484)	0.004
IST (*reference group*)	1		1	
LPS	3.562 (3.081, 4.119)	<.001	4.676 (4.011, 5.449)	<.001
MDO	1.487 (1.328, 1.664)	<.001	1.503 (1.312, 1.720)	<.001
MDSO	2.049 (0.895, 4.402)	0.074	2.106 (0.754, 5.071)	0.119
NGI	1.652 (1.465, 1.862)	<.001	1.283 (1.103, 1.490)	0.001
PC2684	0.721 (0.623, 0.833)	<.001	0.763 (0.634, 0.913)	0.003
SVP	1.650 (1.148, 2.390)	0.007	3.416 (2.158, 5.515)	<.001

See Subjects section, under Methods, for methodology of legal class assignment.

Age differences

Younger patients had a higher prevalence (Table 7.3) of violence than older patients for both patient [χ^2 (5, $N = 15\,615$) = 116.84, $p < 0.001$] and staff assault [χ^2 (5, $N = 15\,615$) = 39.25, $p < 0.001$]. The prevalence in the 18–29 age group was 32.26% (95% CI 30.61%–33.92%), and the prevalence in the 30–39 age group was 28.41% (95% CI 26.96%–29.86%), which were both higher than the prevalence rates in the older age groups. The logistic regression model showed parallel results, with younger patients having higher odds of both patient and staff assault (Table 7.4). For patient assault, with age 18–29 as the reference group, those subjects in the age 30–39 group were significantly lower (OR 0.772, 95% CI 0.692–0.861), and those in the remaining age groups lower still. For staff assault, again with age 18–29 as the reference group, the odds of staff assault for subjects in the age 30–39 group were not significantly lower ($p = 0.061$), but those in the older age groups were all significantly lower than the reference group.

Legal commitment

There were significant differences among the various groups in both patient [χ^2 (7, $N = 15\,615$) = 503.83, $p < 0.001$] and staff [χ^2 (7, $N = 15\,615$) = 728.21, $p < 0.001$] assaults (Table 7.3). Patients in the nonforensic (i.e., LPS) group had the highest prevalence of both patient assaults (50.72%, 95% CI 47.58%–53.86%) and staff assaults (43.33%, 95% CI 40.21%–46.44%), while the mentally ill prisoners (PC2684) had the lowest patient assault (16.76%, 95% CI 15.03%–18.49%) and staff assault (9.47%, 95% CI 8.11%–10.83%) prevalence. The logistic regression model (Table 7.4) showed that when taking the other variables into account, some legal commitments (both forensic and nonforensic) had a significantly higher odds of patient assault than others. Specifically regarding patient assault, those in the legal class DJJ (OR 2.159, 95% CI 1.031–4.520), LPS (OR 3.562, 95% CI 3.081–4.119), MDO (OR 1.487, 95% CI 1.328–1.664), NGI (OR 1.652, 95% CI 1.465–1.862), and SVP (OR 1.650, 95% CI 1.148–2.390) had significantly higher odds of patient assault, while one group, the mentally ill prisoners (PC2684 group), had a significantly lower odds (OR 0.721, 95% CI 0.623– 0.833). A similar pattern held for staff assault.

Axis I diagnosis

Significant differences were noted across the various diagnoses for both patient [χ^2 (15, $N = 15\,615$) = 163.61, $p < 0.001$] and staff assault [χ^2 (15, $N = 15\,615$) = 206.16, $p < 0.001$]. Focusing on the categories with the largest numbers of patients, as these results are likely the most robust (Table 7.5), those diagnosed with schizoaffective disorder (any type, $n = 3512$) had the highest prevalence of both patient assault (31.92%, 95% CI 30.37%–33.46%) and staff assault (21.38%, 95% CI 20.03%–22.74%), while those diagnosed with major depressive disorders had the lowest patient assault (16.67%, 95% CI 13.65%–19.68%) and staff assault (8.16%, 95% CI 5.95%–10.38%) prevalence. Patients diagnosed with schizophrenia, miscellaneous psychotic disorders, and bipolar disorder had prevalence rates that fell between these two groups (see Table 7.5).

Results of the logistic regression model showed that (using schizophrenia as a reference group, see Table 7.6), patients diagnosed with schizoaffective disorder had significantly higher odds of patient assault (OR 1.244, 95% CI 1.131–1.370), while those diagnosed with adjustment or miscellaneous disorders (OR 0.332, 95% CI 0.142–0.642), major depressive disorders (OR 0.629, 95% CI 0.493–0.796), miscellaneous psychotic disorders (OR 0.769, 95% CI 0.669–0.882), or a primary diagnosis of a substance use disorder (OR 0.766, 95% CI 0.604–0.965) had lower odds of patient assault. Patients diagnosed with schizoaffective disorder also had a higher odds of staff assault (OR 1.346, 95% CI 1.202–1.507), as did patients diagnosed with cognitive disorders (OR 1.606, 95% CI 1.158–2.210). Those patients diagnosed with a major depressive disorder (OR 0.459, 95% CI 0.320–0.628), miscellaneous psychotic disorders (OR 0.819, 95% CI 0.688–0.971), a primary diagnosis of a substance use disorder (OR 0.527, 95% CI 0.372–0.728), or had no diagnosis on Axis I (OR 0.385, 95% CI 0.208–0.687) all had lower odds of staff assault.

Axis II diagnosis

Significant differences in assault prevalence (Table 7.5) were noted across Axis II diagnosis for both patient [χ^2 (7, $N = 15\,615$) = 193.66, $p < 0.001$] and staff assault [χ^2 (7, $N = 15\,615$) = 197.81, $p < 0.001$)]. Most patients ($n = 9202$) did not have any diagnosis on Axis II; these

Table 7.5 Prevalence (%) and 95% confidence interval (CI) of physical violence by diagnosis

		Patient assaults		Staff assaults	
	n	*n* (%)	95% CI	*n* (%)	95% CI
Primary Axis I diagnosis					
Adjustment or misc. disorders	74	8 (10.81)	(3.74, 17.89)	7 (9.46)	(2.79, 16.13)
Anxiety/mood disorders	337	86 (25.52)	(20.86, 30.17)	50 (14.84)	(11.04, 18.63)
Bipolar disorders	1313	302 (23.00)	(20.72, 25.28)	188 (14.32)	(12.42, 16.21)
Childhood disorders	45	21 (46.67)	(32.09, 61.24)	13 (28.89)	(15.65, 42.13)
Cognitive disorders	278	74 (26.62)	(21.42, 31.82)	56 (20.14)	(15.43, 24.86)
Deferred	146	35 (23.97)	(17.05, 30.90)	25 (17.12)	(11.01, 23.23)
Major depressive disorders	588	98 (16.67)	(13.65, 19.68)	48 (8.16)	(5.95, 10.38)
Malingering	57	19 (33.33)	(21.10, 45.57)	8 (14.04)	(5.02, 23.05)
No diagnosis	223	48 (21.52)	(16.13, 26.92)	26 (11.66)	(7.45, 15.87)
Paraphilic disorders	303	104 (34.32)	(28.98, 39.67)	82 (27.06)	(22.06, 32.06)
Pedophilic disorders	518	155 (29.92)	(25.98, 33.87)	111 (21.43)	(17.90, 24.96)
Personality disorder primary	7	2 (28.57)	(4.33, 64.12)	2 (28.57)	(4.33, 64.12)
Misc. psychotic disorders	1627	338 (20.77)	(18.80, 22.74)	196 (12.05)	(10.46, 13.63)
Schizoaffective disorders	3512	1121 (31.92)	(30.37, 33.46)	751 (21.38)	(20.03, 22.74)
Schizophrenia disorders	6130	1562 (25.48)	(24.39, 26.57)	900 (14.68)	(13.80, 15.57)
Substance use disorders	457	102 (22.32)	(18.50, 26.14)	41 (8.97)	(6.35, 11.59)
Axis II or personality disorders					
Antisocial personality disorder	2404	806 (33.53)	(31.64, 35.41)	473 (19.68)	(18.09, 21.26)
Intellectual disabilities	550	193 (35.09)	(31.10, 39.08)	127 (23.09)	(19.57, 26.61)
Borderline personality disorder	290	121 (41.72)	(36.05, 47.40)	111 (38.28)	(32.68, 43.87)
All Cluster A Axis II disorders	41	11 (26.83)	(13.27, 40.39)	6 (14.63)	(3.82, 25.45)
All Cluster C Axis II disorders	347	91 (26.22)	(21.60, 30.85)	80 (23.05)	(18.62, 27.49)
Deferred Axis II diagnosis	2753	776 (28.19)	(26.51, 29.87)	435 (15.80)	(14.44, 17.16)
No Axis II diagnosis	9202	2067 (22.46)	(21.61, 23.32)	1267 (13.77)	(13.06, 14.47)
Other Cluster B disorders	28	10 (35.71)	(17.97, 53.46)	5 (17.86)	(3.67, 32.04)

See Study variables section, under Methods, for how diagnoses were grouped.

patients served as the reference group for the logistic regression model. Patients diagnosed with borderline personality disorder (*n* = 290) had the highest prevalence of both patient assault (41.72%, 95% CI 36.05%–47.40%) and staff assault (38.28%, 95% CI 32.68%–43.87%), followed by those diagnosed with intellectual disabilities (specifically, mental retardation or borderline intellectual functioning, *n* = 550; patient assault prevalence 35.09%, 95% CI 31.10%–39.08% and staff assault prevalence 23.09%, 95% CI 19.57%–26.61%), and then those diagnosed with antisocial personality disorder (n = 2404; patient assault prevalence = 33.53%, 95% CI 31.64%–35.42% and staff assault prevalence = 19.68%, 95% CI 18.09%–21.26%).

Table 7.6 Adjusted odds ratios (OR) and 95% confidence interval (CI) of physical violence by diagnosis

	Patient assault Adjusted OR (95% CI)	p-value	Staff assault Adjusted OR (95% CI)	p-value
Primary Axis I diagnosis				
Adjustment and misc. disorders	0.332 (0.142, 0.642)	0.003	0.567 (0.232, 1.179)	0.165
Anxiety/mood disorders	0.918 (0.703, 1.188)	0.523	0.830 (0.594, 1.137)	0.259
Bipolar disorders	0.900 (0.776, 1.042)	0.160	0.899 (0.750, 1.073)	0.244
Childhood disorders	1.608 (0.861, 2.980)	0.131	1.309 (0.630, 2.568)	0.449
Cognitive disorders	1.280 (0.955, 1.698)	0.092	1.606 (1.158, 2.210)	0.004
Deferred	0.957 (0.586, 1.532)	0.859	0.591 (0.320, 1.049)	0.082
Major depressive disorders	0.629 (0.493, 0.796)	<.001	0.459 (0.328, 0.628)	<.001
Malingering	1.306 (0.726, 2.271)	0.354	0.964 (0.418, 1.946)	0.924
No diagnosis	0.866 (0.547, 1.348)	0.531	0.385 (0.208, 0.687)	0.002
Paraphilic disorders	1.222 (0.797, 1.858)	0.352	0.816 (0.480, 1.359)	0.443
Pedophilic disorders	1.179 (0.808, 1.704)	0.386	0.655 (0.400, 1.046)	0.084
Personality disorder primary	1.157 (0.164, 5.458)	0.862	2.514 (0.356, 11.854)	0.275
Misc. psychotic disorders	0.769 (0.669, 0.882)	<.001	0.819 (0.688, 0.971)	0.023
Schizoaffective disorders	1.244 (1.131, 1.370)	<.001	1.346 (1.202, 1.507)	<.001
Schizophrenia disorders (reference group)	1		1	
Substance use disorders	0.766 (0.604, 0.965)	0.026	0.527 (0.372, 0.728)	<.001
Axis II or personality disorders				
Antisocial personality disorder	1.643 (1.478, 1.827)	<.001	1.526 (1.343, 1.732)	<.001
Intellectual disabilities	1.617 (1.337, 1.952)	<.001	1.698 (1.361, 2.105)	<.001
Borderline personality disorder	1.765 (1.351, 2.299)	<.001	2.402 (1.811, 3.174)	<.001
All Cluster A Axis II disorders	1.612 (0.765, 3.160)	0.183	1.498 (0.561, 3.363)	0.368
All Cluster C Axis II disorders	1.170 (0.904, 1.504)	0.225	1.771 (1.342, 2.313)	<.001
Deferred Axis II diagnosis	1.379 (1.246, 1.525)	<.001	1.237 (1.092, 1.399)	<.001
No Axis II diagnosis (reference group)	1		1	
Other Cluster B disorders	2.314 (1.013, 5.001)	0.037	1.710 (0.563, 4.274)	0.290

See Study variables section, under Methods, for how diagnoses were grouped.

The logistic regression model (Table 7.6) showed that having a personality disorder diagnosis typically meant that the patient had a significantly higher odds of both patient and staff assault when compared to the reference group (i.e., no personality or Axis II diagnosis). More specifically, regarding patient violence, having a diagnosis of antisocial personality disorder (OR 1.643, 95% CI 1.478–1.827), intellectual disabilities (OR 1.617, 95% CI 1.337–1.952), borderline personality disorder (OR 1.765, 95% CI 1.351–2.299), or a deferred diagnosis on Axis II (OR 1.379, 95% CI 1.246 to 1.525) or other Cluster B disorders (specifically, histrionic and narcissistic personality disorders, OR 2.314, 95% CI 1.013–5.001) were all associated with significantly higher odds of patient assault. Likewise, a very similar pattern for staff assault was seen as well.

Other major findings

Overall, 31.35% of patients committed at least one violent act. The top 1% of physically violent patients ($n = 156$) accounted for 28.7% of all assaults. As mentioned above, the fact that patients still hospitalized at the end of the study period ($n = 5508$) had a significantly higher prevalence of violence (41.25%, 95% CI 39.95%–42.55%) than the overall study subject violence prevalence (31.35%, 95% CI 30.62%–32.08%) led us to investigate violence and its impact on length of stay (LOS) in the hospitals. As seen in Table 7.7, when all patients in the study ($N = 15{,}615$) were categorized by number of violent incidents (grouped according to having had 0 assaults, 1 assault, 2 assaults, 3 or 4 assaults, 5–9 assaults, or 10 or more assaults), a significant difference in LOS was seen among the different groups (Kruskal–Wallis $\chi^2 = 1509.775$, df = 5, $p < 0.001$). When pairwise Mann–Whitney U-tests were carried out post-hoc with a Bonferroni correction, significant differences in LOS were found between patients with 0 violent incidents and 1 violent incident ($p < 0.001$), between 1 violent incident and 2 ($p < 0.001$), between 2 violent incidents and 3 or 4 ($p = 0.001$), between 3 or 4 violent incidents and 5–9 ($p < 0.001$), and between those with 5–9 violent incidents and the 10 or more group ($p = 0.012$).

Discussion

This study represents what we believe to be the largest single study of the prevalence of violence in a forensic psychiatric hospital setting. Given the large number of patient subjects, and also the array of diagnoses, ethnicity, and commitment types, this study allowed for a broader and more detailed analysis of the range of demographic and clinical factors related to physical violence. With these advantages, there was potential to provide further insights into physical violence in a forensic hospital setting.

Sex differences

The finding that females had a higher prevalence of violent physical assaults against staff is counter to many previous studies in the literature that focused on nonforensic settings. However, it is consistent with some previous findings that found that females engaged in proportionally more physical attacks than males [5,19]. The large sample size of this study likely afforded us more statistical power, or this may be a finding specific to forensic settings.

The finding that females had a higher rate of staff assault (but not patient assault) has interesting implications for treatment interventions. Because the female population is far less numerous in DSH hospitals, it is possible that violence reduction efforts that are effective in male patients may be less effective in female patients. DSH hospitals have already begun efforts to implement newer treatments that may have enhanced effectiveness, such as dialectical behavior therapy and trauma-informed treatments. The information here may help better target continuing risk identification and violence reduction efforts.

Age differences

These findings showed that patients in the 18–29 age group had a significantly higher prevalence and odds

Table 7.7 Length of stay (LOS), in days, by total number of violent assaults during the study period

No. incidents per patient	All incidents		LOS during study period (days)			
	n	%	Mean	Median	SD	Range
0	10,720	68.65	315.9	143	357.1	2–1097
1	1961	12.56	449.2	259	409.7	1–1097
2	930	5.96	497.3	352.5	405.7	3–1097
3–4	821	5.26	565.4	463	415.0	7–1097
5–9	677	4.34	691.3	771	397.0	12–1097
10 or more	506	3.24	754.8	880.5	361.2	24–1097

for patient violence, and that those in both the 18–29 and 30–39 age groups had a higher prevalence and odds for committing staff assault. The finding that younger patients had higher levels of violence is consistent with much of the literature on this topic [8–10]. Young age may be one of the most important risk factors to consider when determining the intensity of treatment services.

Ethnicity

Although this study showed African-American and Hispanic patients had a higher prevalence of patient assault, we suspect that, as Monahan *et al.* [20] discussed, many ethnic minority groups may have a higher risk for violence due to the fact that they have lived primarily in disadvantaged neighborhoods, where all ethnicities have a higher prevalence of violence. Our suspicion is that ethnicity is actually a proxy variable for early learning experiences associated with potentially any or all of the following: (a) early exposure to poverty, (b) low educational-attainment expectations, (c) early exposure to violence, and (d) limited social support systems. If ethnicity could instead be replaced with a variable that better captured that information, it is possible that ethnicity would then no longer be a risk factor for patient violence, just as in this study it was not a significant finding for staff assault.

These findings, in conjunction with the finding that younger males, regardless of ethnicity, have a higher prevalence of patient violence, endorse continued cultural competency efforts, and additionally suggest continued examination of issues related to male-dominance aggression – a topic usually investigated in the context of penal institutions or street gangs, but that may also apply to a forensic hospital setting.

Legal commitment

There was a wide range of prevalence associated with the eight umbrella legal classes. The finding that the nonforensic commitment (i.e., the group in California referred to as LPS) had the highest rate of violence is a consistent with previous studies from other states [6,16,21]. A peculiarity in California is that the number of hospital beds for nonforensic (LPS) patients is extremely limited, approximately 560 patients at any one time. In a state of 40 million, this likely indicates that the overwhelming majority of nonforensically involved, mentally ill patients are successfully treated in the community, and may also be an indicator that these LPS patients in this study may have been selectively placed in state hospitals due to confounding factors that could potentially include violence.

What has not been as well researched in the literature are the differing levels of violence among various forensic commitments. In this study of forensically committed patients, a wide range of violence prevalence was found (as well as differing odds of physical violence). In some cases, the prevalence or odds of physical violence almost equaled that of the nonforensic, LPS group.

We should note that the findings that the group of prison inmates committed to the forensic hospitals (the PC2684 group) had both significantly lower prevalence and significantly lower odds of patient and staff assault may be due to administrative factors, as opposed to actual prevalence. In California, mentally ill prisoners (the PC2684 group) are carefully screened by correctional staff prior to referral, with only the inmates screened as lower risk for violence sent to DSH hospitals. The remaining inmates screened as higher risk for violence are treated in special psychiatric programs on prison grounds; these inmate/patients were not included in this study.

Axis I diagnosis

The large sample size and diversity of the current population provided the opportunity to investigate prevalence among a broad range of diagnoses. Findings revealed that patients with schizoaffective disorder had higher odds of both patient and staff assault when compared to the reference group (patients diagnosed with schizophrenia), while patients diagnosed with bipolar disorder were not significantly different from those diagnosed with schizophrenia.

Another interesting area of future study concerns the finding that patients diagnosed with cognitive disorders (i.e., pathologies involving cognitive loss after age 18) had a significantly higher odds of staff assault [22]. Related disorders such as intellectual disabilities (i.e., pathologies involving intellectual deficits before age 18) were also associated with higher odds of both patient and staff assault. Given the numbers of patients with these diagnoses in the forensic setting, this indicates the need for further exploration.

Axis II or personality disorder diagnosis

Personality disorder diagnosis may be the least well-researched area of inquiry for inpatient hospital violence, although it is commonly seen as a risk factor for violence. Consistent with previous research, these results showed that having a diagnosis of a personality disorder was associated with a higher prevalence and higher odds of violence, for both patient and staff assault [9,22,23]. With patients having no diagnosis of a personality disorder as the reference group, having any personality disorder, or even being considered for a personality disorder (i.e., deferred diagnosis), was associated with higher levels of violence in the study subjects. The finding that patients with limited intellectual or cognitive functioning had higher levels of assault is of particular interest. This special population is often treated and housed with general populations. This study may add support for investigating specialized treatment programs that address violence risk in the population. Currently, DSH hospitals have in place several programs for cognitive remediation that are aimed at working with patients who have suffered cognitive losses as adults. It seems apparent, based on this current study, that these programs should be extended to patients with lifelong developmental disability diagnoses, and that specific efforts to screen for and identify these patients would be important aspects of violence reduction efforts.

The present study is not without its limitations. With the size of the staff involved, lack of inter-rater reliability training and study among the diagnosing psychiatrists is a limitation, but a reality that exists in clinical settings. The use of a locally developed special incident tracking tool limits comparability with other studies. However, the fact that the violence reporting form was integrated into regular nursing staff duties meant that the nursing staff did not view filling out this form as an extra duty, enabled the collection of data for a far longer period of time than in previous studies, and likely also reduced under-reporting. The fact that the prevalence of physical violence in this study was at levels comparable to other studies, or even higher than some other studies, provides assurance that violent incidents were routinely reported and were not systematically overlooked.

The collapsing of the patient's diagnoses into overarching DSM-IV-TR diagnostic categories undoubtedly has led to a loss of specificity. However,

given the fact that there were over 280 different primary Axis I diagnoses, few options existed to present diagnostic data in a concise, meaningful way. We plan to examine specific diagnoses in detail, as well as comorbid substance use diagnosis, as the next logical step in our programmatic study of physical violence.

This study highlights the limitations of using solely prevalence to describe violence in this population. While prevalence indicates the presence or absence of a disease in a binary "yes/no" format, when there is a subgroup of patients with an extreme amount of repeated violent acts (such as the 1% of patients who accounted for 28.7% of all assaults), a measure such as a rate measure (not employed in this study) used in conjunction with prevalence may better capture information about violence in a forensic setting than just prevalence alone.

This also brings up the issue of what can be done to address violence in this special group of repeatedly violent patients. Our review of the literature has shown that the problem of patients with repeated violent incidents during hospitalization has been an issue for decades in various settings without any apparent resolution [15,24–26]. The fact that patients with more violent incidents had a longer length of stay meant that the nonviolent patients treated alongside them had a greater exposure to victimization, a topic not addressed in this article. In the present study, patients had the greatest burden of violence, as patient assaults out-numbered staff assaults. There is a paucity of published research that directly addresses the problem of reducing incidents among repeatedly violent patients; however, a few recent studies have detailed some promising ideas, such as the use of violence risk assessment [27] or segregation in conjunction with violence risk assessment and treatment of high risk factors, to reduce physical violence in hospital settings [28].

Conclusions

This study found significant relationships between physical violence and specific demographic variables and clinical diagnoses in a forensic setting. Certain demographic and clinical variables were significantly related to higher prevalence and odds of patient assault, staff assault, or both. These findings indicate that further investigation and follow-up are warranted, especially in the areas of how specific or comorbid clinical diagnoses interact with personality disorders to impact violence. This study also pointed out the need to more closely examine the issue of patients with repeated physically violent incidents in order to identify potential treatment interventions. Further research may identify variables that could potentially provide a means of early identification of high risk factors for targeted treatment, with the ultimate goal of safety for all patients and staff.

Disclosures

None of the authors has anything to disclose.

References

1. Swanson JW. Mental disorder, substance abuse, and community violence: an epidemiological approach. In: Monahan J, Steadman HJ, eds. *Violence and Mental Disorder: Developments in Risk Assessment*. Chicago: University of Chicago Press; 1994: 101–136.

2. Swanson JW, Swartz MS, Van Dorn RA, *et al*. A national study of violent behavior in persons with schizophrenia. *Arch. Gen. Psychiatry*. 2006; **63**(5): 490–499.

3. Swanson JW, McGinty EE, Fazel S, Mays VM. Mental illness and reduction of gun violence and suicide: bringing epidemiologic research to policy. *Ann. Epidemiol*. 2015 May; **25**(5): 366–376. DOI: 10.1016/j.annepidem.2014.03.004.

4. McNiel DE, Binder RL, Greenfield TK. Predictors of violence in civilly committed acute psychiatric patients. *Am. J. Psychiatry*. 1988; **145**(8): 965–970.

5. Convit A, Isay D, Otis D, Volavka J. Characteristics of repeatedly assaultive psychiatric inpatients. *Hosp. Community Psychiatry*. 1990; **41**(10): 1112–1115.

6. Linhorst DM, Scott LP. Assaultive behavior in state psychiatric hospitals: differences between forensic and nonforensic patients. *J. Interpers. Violence*. 2004; **19**(8): 857–874.

7. Abderhalden C, Needham I, Dassen T, *et al*. Frequency and severity of aggressive incidents in acute psychiatric wards in Switzerland. *Clin. Pract. Epidemiol. Ment. Health*. 2007; **3**: 30.

8. Hoptman MJ, Yates KF, Patalinjug MB, Wack RC, Convit A. Clinical prediction of assaultive behavior among male psychiatric patients at a maximum-security forensic facility. *Psychiatr. Serv.* 1999; **50**(11): 1461–1466.

9. Soliman AE, Reza H. Risk factors and correlates of violence among acutely ill adult psychiatric inpatients. *Psychiatr. Serv.* 2001; **52**(1): 75–80.

10. Raja M, Azzoni A. Hostility and violence of acute psychiatric inpatients. *Clin. Pract. Epidemiol. Ment. Health*. 2005; **1**(1): 11.

11. Dietz PE, Rada RT. Battery incidents and batterers in a maximum security hospital. *Arch. Gen. Psychiatry*. 1982; **39**(1): 31–34.

12. Noble P, Rodger S. Violence by psychiatric in-patients. *Br. J. Psychiatry*. 1989; **155**(3): 384–390.

13. Bowers L, Stewart D, Papadopoulos C, *et al*. Inpatient violence and aggression: a literature. Report from the Conflict and Containment Reduction Research Programme. London: Kings College; 2011. http://www.kcl.ac.uk/ioppn/depts/hspr/research/ciemh/mhn/projects/litreview/LitRevAgg.pdf. Last accessed October 23, 2014.

14. Parks J, Radke AQ, Haupt MB. *The Vital Role of State Psychiatric Hospitals*. National Association of State Mental Health Program Directors (NASMHPD) Medical Directors Council: Alexandria, VA; 2014. http://www.nasmhpd.org/publications/The%20Vital%20Role%20of%20State%20Psychiatric%20Hospitals Technical%20Report_July_2014.pdf. Last accessed October 23, 2014.

15. Blow FC, Barry KL, Copeland LA, *et al*. Repeated assaults by patients in VA hospital and clinic settings. *Psychiatr. Serv.* 1999; **50**(3): 390–394.

16. Novaco R. Anger as a risk factor for violence among the mentally disordered. In: Monahan J, Steadman HJ, eds. *Violence and Mental Disorder: Developments in Risk Assessment*. Chicago, IL: University of Chicago Press; 1994: 21–60.

17. American Psychiatric Association. *Diagnostic and Statistical Manual of Mental Disorders*, 4th edn, text rev. Washington, DC: American Psychiatric Association; 2000.

18. R Core Team. R: a language and environment for statistical computing. R Foundation for Statistical Computing: Vienna, Austria. http://www.R-project.org. Last accessed October 23, 2014.

19. Binder RL, McNiel DE. The relationship of gender to violent behavior in acutely disturbed psychiatric patients. *J. Clin. Psychiatry*. 1990; **51**(3): 110–114.

20. Monahan J, Steadman HJ, Silver E, *et al. Rethinking Risk Assessment: The MacArthur Study of Mental Disorder and Violence*. New York: Oxford University Press; 2001.

21. Stokman CLJ, Heiber P. Incidents in hospitalized forensic patients. *Victimology*. 1980; **5**(2–4): 175–192.

22. Kennedy MG. Relationship between psychiatric diagnosis and patient aggression. *Issues Ment. Health Nurs*. 1993; **14**(3): 263–273.

23. Daffern M, Howells K. The prediction of imminent aggression and self-harm in personality disordered patients of a high security hospital using the HCR-20 Clinical Scale and the Dynamic Appraisal of Situational Aggression. *International Journal of Forensic Mental Health*. 2007; **6**(2): 137–143.

24. Rachlin S. On the need for a closed ward in an open hospital: the psychiatric intensive-care unit. *Hosp. Community Psychiatry*. 1973; **24**(12): 829–833.

25. Barlow K, Grenyer B, Ilkiw-Lavalle O. Prevalence and precipitants of aggression in psychiatric inpatient units. *Aust. N. Z. J. Psychiatry*. 2000; **34**(6): 967–974.

26. Lussier P, Verdun-Jones S, Deslauriers-Varin N, Nicholls T, Brink J. Chronic violent patients in an inpatient psychiatric hospital: prevalence, description, and identification. *Criminal Justice and Behavior*. 2009; **37**(1): 5–28.

27. Abderhalden C, Needham I, Dassen T, *et al*. Structured risk assessment and violence in acute psychiatric wards: randomised controlled trial. *Br. J. Psychiatry*. 2008; **193**(1): 44–50.

28. Vaaler AE, Iversen VC, Morken G, *et al*. Short-term prediction of threatening and violent behaviour in an acute psychiatric intensive care unit based on patient and environment characteristics. *BMC Psychiatry*. 2011; **11**(1): 44–50.

The psychiatrist's duty to protect

James L. Knoll IV

Introduction

Responding to the California Supreme Court's decision and its related legal obligations in *Tarasoff v. Regents of Univ. of California* over 30 years ago has become a standard part of mental health practice. This case influenced legal requirements governing therapists' duty to protect third parties in nearly every state in the country. The final ruling in Tarasoff emphasized that therapists have a *duty to protect* individuals who are being threatened with bodily harm by their patient [1]. This article provides a brief overview and update on *duty to protect* legal requirements. Clinical guidelines for addressing threats and the duty to protect will be discussed, along with risk management approaches. The article will conclude with a vignette that illustrates these principles.

Tarasoff – A Duty to Protect

Confusion may persist surrounding the meaning and proper use of the terms duty to warn vs. duty to protect, and this may in part be due to the fact that there were two Tarasoff decisions. The first Tarasoff decision in 1974 created a duty to warn in California, and was based on the special relationship between therapist and patient [2]. This first decision was not only unprecedented, but also upsetting to therapists due to its controversial expectation that therapists violate patient confidentiality. One of the most familiar quotes from "Tarasoff I" clarified that the Court was concerned with social policy: "The protective privilege ends where the public peril begins."

The California Supreme Court reheard the case, and in its 1976 ruling replaced "duty to warn" with a "duty to protect" [1]. The famous quote from "Tarasoff II," which was adapted by many states across the country, appeared to make the change clear: "When a therapist determines, or should determine, that his patient presents a serious danger of violence to another, he incurs an obligation to use reasonable care to protect the intended victim from danger." Initially, there was significant concern that this exception to confidentiality would have disastrous effects on psychiatric practice, despite the fact that most therapists had embraced such a duty before the Tarasoff ruling [3]. Over time, it became clear that the concerns about the potential loss of confidentiality did not have an adverse impact on psychiatric practice [4]. Instead, Tarasoff stimulated "greater awareness of the violent patient's potential for acting out such behavior, encouraging closer scrutiny and better documentation of the therapist's examination of this issue" [5]. More recently, after decades of misunderstanding, California passed legislation in 2013 that unambiguously established a sole duty to protect [5]. This recent California statute removed all references to duty to warn, and provides "definitive clarification" [6].

Tarasoff Expansion and Contraction

Although Tarasoff applied only in California because it was a State Supreme Court decision, the ruling "reverberated nationally" [6]. The duty to protect articulated in Tarasoff was subsequently interpreted more broadly by other courts throughout the USA. One of the broadest interpretations appears in a Nebraska federal district court's decision in the 1980 case of *Lipari v. Sears, Roebuck & Co.* [7] This case involved a VA patient who shot strangers in a crowded nightclub, without ever threatening a specific person, and one month after terminating psychiatric treatment. The court rejected the Tarasoff limitation to an

Violence in Psychiatry, ed. Katherine D. Warburton and Stephen M. Stahl. Published by Cambridge University Press. © Cambridge University Press 2016.

identified victim, imposing not only a duty on therapists to predict dangerousness, but also a duty to protect unidentified victims in the general public.

The duty was given a remarkable temporal extension in the case of the *Naidu v. Laird* [8]. This case involved a patient with schizophrenia who killed another man in a motor vehicle crash. The patient's psychiatric history included violent behavior, ramming a police car with his automobile, and driving off the road at high speed. The Supreme Court of Delaware held that 5 and 1/2 months after a hospital discharge was not too long a period to support a finding of negligence when a psychiatrist was found liable for failing to foresee a patient's potential to act violently. Despite the lengthy time since the patient's discharge, the Court stressed the "foreseeability" of harm rather than the passage of time.

The duty was extended to property in the Vermont case of *Peck v. Counseling Service of Addison County* [9]. In Peck, a counselor was told by a patient that he intended to burn down another person's barn. The court's opinion suggested that both counselors and psychiatrists had a duty to protect not only threatened victims, but their property as well. These and similar cases in the wake of Tarasoff led to significant discomfort among therapists who objected to apparent legal expectations that they foresee all dangerous situations and protect the public at large. Indeed, given psychiatry's limitations with respect to predicting violence, ethical arguments have been raised about accepting the premise of foreseeing patient violence [10].

Two decades after Tarasoff, state legislatures around the country began to reflect ambivalence about the extension of the duty to protect. As a result of therapists' success in convincing legislatures that their state courts' rulings created unreasonable expectations, state legislatures created statutes requiring that the threat be clearly foreseeable, and that the duty extended only to reasonably foreseeable victims – not to the general public. These statutes became known as "Tarasoff-limiting statutes," laying out specific criteria that typically include a credible threat made against an identifiable victim. At present, Tarasoff-limiting statutes have been passed in 39 states [11].

Some states may lack clear duty to protect statutes, leaving the psychiatrist with little guidance. In such cases, it is helpful to consult with hospital legal counsel and/or one's malpractice insurance carrier.

In those states without a clear statutory legal duty to protect, psychiatrists are often advised by legal counsel to follow the basic Tarasoff rationale and practice as though there was a legal duty. There are compelling reasons for doing so, primarily that acting in accordance with the duty to protect contributes to and improves care of one's patient.

Duty to Protect – Approach

Psychiatrists should become familiar with the specific Tarasoff duty in their locale, as well as any evolving case law that may create nuances in how the duty is properly carried out. States with duty to protect statutes contain language that can often be distilled down to two criteria: (1) an explicit, credible threat that the patient intends and is able to carry out (2) against an identifiable person [12]. If these two criteria are met, the psychiatrist then has a number of intervention options to consider, depending upon the clinical context. The options most often include those listed in Table 8.1.

Although danger to third parties can, in some cases, justify a breach of the therapist's duty to maintain confidentiality [13], breaching confidentiality should be viewed as a last option, after all other therapeutic options have been exhausted. In essence, confidentiality should be breached only if reasonable clinical efforts seem unlikely to provide adequate protection and resolution. When all reasonable options are untenable, it should be remembered that "trust," and not absolute confidentiality, is the foundation of the therapeutic alliance. Providing necessary protection "where self-control breaks down is not a breach of trust when it is not deceptive" [14]. Therefore, if circumstances permit, the psychiatrist should inform the patient about the decision to breach confidentiality.

The psychiatrist's clinical and moral duty in such situations can be viewed as transcending mere legal

Table 8.1 Duty to protect options

- Hospitalization (or escort to a hospital emergency room for evaluation)
- Warning police
- Warning the third party (intended victim)
- Asking the patient to give the warning him/herself
- Increasing the frequency of outpatient appointments

duty in that one must do what one can "to save our fellow human beings from danger" [12]. Psychiatrists should take some comfort in knowing that they have little basis "to fear being sued successfully for a bad outcome if the clinical practice has been reasonable" [11]. This is particularly the case when it is clear that the psychiatrist's actions flowed from concerns about the welfare of the patient and threatened third parties.

The psychiatrist should consider an array of options, including hospitalization, warnings, more frequent therapy sessions, starting or increasing medication, and various forms of closer monitoring. The clinical approach can be thought of as similar to the management of an acutely suicidal patient, in so far as addressing the risk of a patient acting on dangerous plans. In the performance of the clinical risk assessment, the psychiatrist should consider contacting collateral sources, such as relatives who may be able to provide important information regarding the patient's dangerousness.

Past medical records, where applicable, should be reviewed. At the very least, efforts to obtain records should be made and documented. Obtaining and reviewing medical records was at issue in the 1983 case of *Jablonski v. United States* [15]. In *Jablonski*, the duty to protect was extended to include a therapist–patient relationship limited to the emergency room setting. Mr. Jablonski was a violent man who was brought to a VA hospital by his girlfriend after he attempted to rape her mother. The psychiatrist concluded that the patient was a danger to others, but could not be committed under California's involuntary commitment statute. Jablonski's medical records revealed that he had a long history of antisocial and violent behavior; however, these records were not requested at the time of his presentation. The girlfriend was warned by emergency room psychiatrists to stay away from him if she feared him. Not long after his discharge from the ER, Jablonski killed the girlfriend. The 9th Circuit Court of Appeals concluded that the hospital had failed to obtain important prior records and to adequately warn the victim.

Finally, past therapists and referral sources should be queried where appropriate, and consultations may be sought [4]. Consultation with a psychiatric colleague, as well as hospital legal counsel, should be routine in difficult cases. If this type of careful, reasonable approach is taken (including documentation of the assessment of the pertinent issues and treatment plan), liability becomes unlikely even if harm should occur to a third party.

Evaluation of Credible Threats in Tarasoff Situations

The clinical process of violence risk assessment is beyond the scope of this article, and psychiatrists are encouraged to review the literature on this subject [16,17]. A "threat" may be defined as a declaration of intent to harm [18]. While threats are common, most are not carried out [19,20]. In contrast to a clinical risk assessment done by a treating psychiatrist, a threat assessment is ideally done by an expert with special training and experience in the field of threat assessment who has familiarity with the current literature, research, and actuarial instruments. A treating psychiatrist would not reasonably be expected to perform a formal threat assessment. When a patient makes a credible threat that he can and intends to carry out, a duty to protect his target has arisen, and the psychiatrist should undertake a thoughtful assessment to address the risk of harm.

There is only a weak association between threats and violence; nevertheless, there is an association. In a study of clinic patients who made threats to kill, assaults were made by over 20% over a 12-month assessment period [21]. Factors found to contribute to violence risk were substance abuse, prior violence, limited education, and untreated mental disorders. The combination of history of substance abuse, not receiving mental healthcare, having minimal education, and history of violent behavior predicted violence by threateners.

It is important to first address the threat toward third persons as a therapeutic issue in alliance with the patient. For example, the psychiatrist may explore with the patient what it would mean for the patient if the threat were to be acted upon. This approach will not only produce valuable risk assessment data, but will also appropriately address relevant clinical issues. The psychiatrist may find it helpful to consider the topics of questioning listed in Table 8.2, which can be recalled by the mnemonic "ACTION," or Attitudes, Capacity, Thresholds, Intent, Others' reactions, Noncompliance [22].

When evaluating whether the patient has already crossed a "threshold" in terms of threat-related behaviors, it may be helpful to ask the patient what steps he has taken so far in furtherance of his intentions. The threat assessment literature refers to such acts as "warning behaviors," which are defined as dynamic,

Table 8.2 Lines of inquiry in Tarasoff situations [22]

A—Attitudes that support or facilitate violence: What is the nature/strength of the patient's attitude toward the behavior? Rejecting or accepting? The stronger the perceived justification, the greater the likelihood of action. Assess scenarios of provocation from others. Inquire about violent fantasies and expectations of outcome.

C—Capacity or means to carry out the violence: Does the patient have the physical or intellectual capability, access to means, access to the victim, or opportunity to commit the act? How well does the patient know the victim's routines, whereabouts, etc.?

T—Thresholds crossed: Has the patient already engaged in behaviors to further the plan? Acts committed in violation of the law suggest a willingness to engage in the ultimate act.

I—Intent: Does the patient have mere ideas/fantasies or solid intention? Level of intent may be inferred from the specificity of the plans and thresholds crossed. How committed is the patient to carrying out the act? Does he believe he has "nothing to lose"?

O—Others' reactions and responses: What reactions does the patient anticipate? Does the social network reduce or enhance the risk? Do social contacts believe the patient is serious?

N—Noncompliance with risk reduction: Is the patient willing to participate in risk management interventions? What is the patient's history of compliance with previous plans? How much insight into the situation does the patient have?

acute behaviors suggestive of impending violence [23]. For example, preparatory actions, such as purchasing a gun or rehearsing plans for an attack, are highly concerning warning behaviors that push violent ideation across a threshold into physical reality.

The psychiatrist should also be aware that warnings (to police or third parties) alone may ultimately provide no protection, because they do not address the cause of the threat [6]. In fact, it is possible that a warning made in haste may actually increase the risk of violence. This phenomenon has been called "the intervention dilemma," which posits that taking certain courses of action in response to a threat may actually increase the risk of violence, and in some cases, no direct action may be preferable [24]. In some cases, certain responses may actually enflame a threatening patient by challenging or humiliating him. For this reason, there is no single best approach to risk management. Rather, risk management approaches must consider the significance of individual-specific nuances in the totality of the circumstances of each case.

If it is ultimately decided that a warning must be made to intended victims or police, it should be as discreet as possible to protect the patient's confidentiality, and remain consistent with the requirements of the law in one's state. Warnings may include statements made by the patient that are necessary to convey the serious intent of the threat to the victim [25]. Upon deciding to notify police, the psychiatrist should call the police in the precinct nearest to the patient. In addition, it is helpful to ask for and document the name and badge number of the person taking the report. It is preferable to give oral rather than written warnings due to the fact that the psychiatrist has determined the threat to be imminent, and an oral warning is likely to be received by the police and/or the intended victim sooner than a written warning.

Documentation

The standard of care does not require the psychiatrist to predict violence or prevent all tragic outcomes. Rather, the standard of care requires the psychiatrist to "exercise the skill, knowledge, and care normally possessed and exercised by other members of their profession" [26]. Documentation showing that the psychiatrist (1) performed a reasonable assessment of risk and then (2) provided a rationale for implementing a reasonable risk management plan will be very likely to provide sufficient evidence that the standard of care was met.

The importance of good clinical documentation cannot be overstated. It is the central piece of evidence in every malpractice trial, and good documentation has stopped many malpractice cases from even proceeding to trial. Documentation serves many purposes. It informs patient treatment and management, and communicates these important data to other relevant staff for future consideration when they are tasked with the patient's care. This article focuses on how documentation can reduce liability risk. In real-world clinical practice, it is simply not possible to "document everything," and there must necessarily be limits to the amount of documentation. Nevertheless, the psychiatrist should strive to document important clinical matters contemporaneously. When the psychiatrist does not document his reasoning, there will be no evidence to show that he was thoughtful, prudent, and used reasonable professional judgment.

When documenting, one should abide by the rule of austerity. Document the important facts and conclusions in an objective tone. It is important to avoid waging battles of professional disagreement in the progress notes, as this will be seized upon by plaintiff's counsel and portrayed in a manner damaging to the defendant psychiatrist's case.

When noting an action taken in furtherance of a risk management plan (e.g., committing or not committing an individual, increased frequency of appointments, etc.), it is essential to include a statement, however brief, of the *rationale* for the action. For example, the psychiatrist should document that she considered the option of civil commitment and the clinical basis for rejecting or proceeding with that option. Whenever the clinical situation requires the involvement of family members, the psychiatrist should document instructions and information given to both the patient and the family. Consider noting whether they agree with the treatment decisions, as well as noncompliance with treatment recommendations. Unrecorded instructions or conversations with family members will likely become points of contention after a suit is filed.

The issue of how much documentation is appropriate may be a source of confusion to busy psychiatrists. It has been suggested that within appropriate bounds, the more pertinent objective findings the documentation contains, the better the portrayal of competent care will be [27]. However, this raises concerns about appropriate use of the psychiatrist's time, as well as associated issues with excessive documentation. Certain elements should always be present in the documentation; however, the psychiatrist should attempt to document smarter, not longer. Documentation should be succinct and thoughtful, yet not excessive.

The psychiatrist should document as though each note will be an exhibit in court. Indeed, in the event of a lawsuit, this is precisely what will occur. In many cases, the relevant notes are enlarged and printed out on poster board for viewing by a jury. Thus, the psychiatrist should see herself as documenting a court exhibit as opposed to a note that only she will view. To the extent possible, the psychiatrist should include direct quotes from the patient. Documented quotes such as "I haven't had any thoughts of harming (the victim)" or "I no longer have any guns in my house" convey critical clinical and risk management information. In malpractice trials, patient quotes are considered powerful evidence, as the very words/thoughts of the patient appear preserved, and must be taken at face value unless proven unreliable. It is also helpful in complex cases to document evidence that the patient is reasonably competent to handle responsibilities such as considering and weighing treatment advice, seeking emergency attention, and employing coping skills in the face of stress. This information may be necessary to counteract jurors' inclination to believe that all psychiatric patients are either incompetent or otherwise completely controlled by aberrant thoughts [27].

The use of check boxes and various template forms have become more widely used, likely due to psychiatrist time constraints and increasing use of electronic health records (EHR). These types of documentation may carry unforeseen liability risks. Check box forms are necessarily limited to the predetermined items. Thus, they may encourage psychiatrists not to "think outside the box," should the form not address areas that the psychiatrist ought to consider and document. Another type of form sometimes seen is part check box and part note. However, the space left for note taking is typically scant, while the check box section overwhelms the page. A systematic violence risk assessment remains a necessity, and the process cannot be abdicated in favor of risk assessment forms [28].

Mechanical completion of forms or "checklists" may engender a false sense of security about the patient's risk of violence, as well as preclude a more thoughtful analysis of the patient's clinical risk [29]. Another problem with check box notes involves how the note will be viewed if a box is ever left unchecked. For example, if a box is left blank, this may be portrayed by plaintiff's counsel as neglected or incomplete care. Related to the liability risks of mechanical or mindless documentation is the tendency for doctors using modern EHRs to cut and paste, instead of crafting an appropriate and contemporaneous narrative. Often done for time saving reasons, this practice may cause the psychiatrist to neglect important nuances of the clinical encounter in the documentation.

In difficult cases, appropriate consultation should be sought and documented. It will be difficult for a plaintiff's attorney to prove that "no reasonably prudent psychiatrist" would have made a decision at issue, when there are two psychiatrists arriving at the same conclusion. Another key documentation principle in cases of potential third party danger is the importance of not leaving "loose ends" in the notes. Whenever issues of risk are raised in the notes, they should be addressed – preferably with a risk management plan as described in the next section. A risk management plan should be crafted immediately after the clinical risk assessment has been completed. It may be necessary to obtain collateral data from mental health records, family members, or other social contacts. Keep in mind that in the case of a psychiatric emergency (e.g., risk of violence or suicide), the need to preserve life supersedes the need to obtain consent from the patient. In most circumstances, this will mean that obtaining the patient's consent to contact family is not necessary, but this exception to consent should be documented contemporaneously.

The Risk Management Plan

From a legal standpoint, psychiatric malpractice cases involving harm to third parties often hinge on the issue of foreseeability. Further, the law considers two basic types of error when considering the issue of foreseeability and whether or not the psychiatrist exercised professional judgment: (1) errors of fact and (2) errors of judgment. An error of fact is considered to be a "mistake about a fact that is material to a transaction" [30]. For example, an error of fact occurs when the psychiatrist bases a clinical judgment on erroneous or untrue beliefs, such as might occur when the psychiatrist fails to review a patient's history or lab results prior to making a substantive clinical decision. Psychiatrists are likely to be found negligent for errors of fact.

In contrast, an error of judgment occurs when the psychiatrist makes an informed clinical decision in good faith that turns out to have been a mistake. The psychiatrist is unlikely to be held liable for mere error in professional judgment [31]. This is sometimes referred to as judgmental immunity or the "error of judgment rule," which states, "A professional is not liable to a client for advice or an opinion given in good faith and with an honest belief the advice was in the client's best interests, but that was based on a mistake either in judgment or in analyzing an unsettled area of the professional's business" [30]. Contemporaneous documentation provides the most believable evidence that the psychiatrist was diligent in gathering facts prior to exercising clinical judgment.

The psychiatrist should document that the option of involuntary hospitalization has been considered, and the clinical basis for rejecting, or proceeding with, that option. In addition, there should be documentation of actions taken (and why) and those rejected (and why). The risk assessment documentation should include some form of analysis of risk factors, and a general estimate of overall risk level (low, moderate, or high). This should be followed by a treatment plan (or risk management plan – see below) that directly addresses the relevant dynamic risk factors.

The basic principle behind the risk management plan is to identify all those risk factors that are amenable to treatment interventions (dynamic risk factors) and to target them with reasonable treatment interventions [32,33]. The following section consists of a clinical vignette and sample violence risk management plan in the case of Mr. A. Note how each dynamic risk factor is targeted with interventions that are reasonable and appropriate to the patient's clinical situation.

Clinical Vignette – The Case of Mr. A
Synopsis

Mr. A was a 40-year-old man with bipolar disorder and substance abuse who was admitted to an inpatient unit after attempting suicide by shooting himself in the head. He had been compliant with lithium, yet had also been abusing alcohol and Oxycontin. After becoming severely depressed, he developed a plan to kill himself, but also believed he should kill his 19-year-old son to spare the son the misery and fallout from his suicide.

He traveled to see his son with the intent to shoot his son and then himself. At the last minute, Mr. A decided he could not bring himself to shoot his son, and instead went to an isolated location and shot himself in the head. By chance, a passerby saw Mr. A and called 911. Miraculously, the bullet did not take a fatal course, nor did it penetrate his brain.

He initially required neurosurgical intervention, and was then transferred to the psychiatry inpatient unit.

Mr. A had no past history of violent behavior, and had never owned a firearm until he purchased one to commit suicide. Mr. A had significant stressors in his life consisting of marital problems and prescription opioid abuse, which had resulted in the loss of his last job. After a three-week inpatient stay, his psychiatric medications were augmented, and he responded very well to treatment. He reported wanting to find a new job, enter substance use treatment, and rebuild his marriage. His mood was stable, and he reported no further suicidal or homicidal ideas. His inpatient team held several meetings with his wife in attendance to discuss his future plans and to address the issue of his suicide attempt. In particular, the issue of his plan to kill his son was addressed. His inpatient team was concerned that they might have a duty to warn Mr. A's son prior to discharging him.

Mr. A was adamant that he did not want his son to be told about his former plans for committing a homicide–suicide, as he believed it would cause serious damage to their relationship. Mr. A added that he now felt embarrassed about his former plans, and that he was not thinking clearly when he made them. He emphatically stated to his team that there was a "0% chance" he would harm his son, or anyone else.

When the treatment team persisted in discussing this issue, Mr. A became moderately upset, and said he would retain an attorney should the team go forward with its plans to warn his son. His treatment team requested a consult to address, among other things, Mr. A's clinical violence risk and their duty to warn his son. The procedure of performing clinical violence risk assessment and identifying relevant risk factors is beyond the scope of this article, and readers are encouraged to consult the evidence-based literature on this subject [32,34,35].

Risk factors

Mr. A was found to have the following factors that *increased* his risk of violence:

Static

(1) Previous homicide–suicide plan (associated with severe depression, suicidal ideas, professional crisis, ego-dystonic; approached victim but ultimately aborted homicide plan)

(2) Male gender

Dynamic

(3) Bipolar disorder

(4) Substance misuse – opioids, alcohol

(5) Marital problems

(6) Uncertain employment status

Mr. A was found to have the following factors that *reduced* his risk of violence.

(1) Absence of current violent ideas or fantasies, and his own estimation of a "0%" chance he will harm someone

(2) Absence of suicidal ideas that were associated with his past homicidal ideas

(3) Current stable mood – absence of significant mood symptoms, and reported feeling hopeful about his future

(4) Future-oriented thinking with various life plans

(5) Willingness to accept and continue with treatment

Risk Management Plan

Mr. A was found to have an overall low to low-moderate risk of violence, with dynamic factors that could easily be addressed. After three weeks of treatment, the treatment team concluded that a warning was not the best clinical approach to averting the danger. Instead, since Mr. A's clinical status no longer represented a current Tarasoff duty (i.e., specific threat against an identifiable party), more treatment was the best course. The following plan was crafted by Mr. A's team. He expressed a willingness to follow the plans, and his wife expressed her willingness to assist him.

(1) Bipolar mood disorder: Mr. A's symptoms are in remission, and he no longer meets criteria for inpatient care. He should remain adherent to his psychiatric treatment and medication regimen and follow up with his psychiatrist.

(2) Statistically significant risk period (immediate post inpatient period): Mr. A was to enter a partial hospitalization program to provide continuity of care and transition to the community.

(3) Past substance misuse: Mr. A should continue to avoid misuse of substances. He agreed to enter a substance recovery program after his partial hospitalization.

(4) Access to lethal means: Mr. A and his social network were informed that he must not have access to firearms or other lethal means. Specifically, his family members confirmed to the

treatment team that they removed firearms from the home. Both the instruction to the family and their confirmation were documented.

(5) Mr. A agreed to be involved in psychotherapy designed to help him increase his awareness of mood symptoms, and how to effectively and safely cope with life stressors.

(6) Mr. A and his wife agreed to be involved in marital therapy.

(7) Mr. A agreed to work with an employment specialist to review his prospects for part-time work after discharge from partial hospitalization.

Outcome

With Mr. A's consent, the clinical risk assessment and management plans were communicated to his outpatient providers and his partial hospitalization program. Specifically, they were made aware that Mr. A, when acutely ill, had plans to kill both himself and his son. Mr. A was told by his treatment team that communication of this information to his outpatient providers was necessary to ensure a good continuum of care. Mr. A understood this rationale, and gave his consent. Mr. A was discharged to the partial hospitalization program and did well. After several months, he was discharged to outpatient care in his community. He began marital counseling with his wife. Mr. A's son was never informed by psychiatrists about Mr. A's former homicide–suicide plans.

Through an employment specialist, Mr. A was able to find a part-time job in his field. He remained adherent to treatment and required no further inpatient hospitalizations.

Conclusions

Psychiatrists' *duty to protect* in the context of a patient's realistic threats toward identifiable third parties is a well-established exception to patient confidentiality. The psychiatrist should be familiar with the duty to protect laws in his or her state. When a potential duty to protect scenario arises, it should be first addressed as a clinical issue, and an array of options should be considered prior to breaching confidentiality. Indeed, it is quite possible that clinical interventions may eliminate the need to violate confidentiality entirely.

The protection from harm for both the patient and the threatened third party should be the primary guide for interventions. Careful clinical evaluation, consultation, and implementation of a risk management plan should be documented. Even in the event of a tragic outcome and lawsuit, "Judges and juries are likely to be more impressed by psychiatrists trying to do the most protective thing for patients as opposed to merely protecting themselves" [6].

Disclosures

The author has nothing to disclose.

References

1. *Tarasoff v. Regents of Univ. of California*, 551 P.2d 334 (Cal. 1976).

2. *Tarasoff v. Regents of University of California*, 529 P.2d 553 (Cal. 1974).

3. Slovenko R. Confidentiality and testimonial privilege. In: Rosner R. ed. *Principles & Practice of Forensic Psychiatry*. New York: Oxford University Press; 2003: 145.

4. Buckner F, Firestone M. "Where the public peril begins": 25 years after Tarasoff. *J. Leg. Med.* 2000; **21**(2): 187–222.

5. Cal. Civ. Code § 43.92 (2013).

6. Weinstock R, Bonnici D, Seroussi A, Leong G. No duty to warn in California: now unambiguously solely a duty to protect. *J. Am. Acad. Psychiatry Law.* 2014; **42**(1): 101–108.

7. *Lipari v. Sears, Roebuck & Co.*, 497 F.Supp. 185 (D.Neb. 1980).

8. *Naidu v. Laird*, 539 A.2d 1064 (Del. 1988).

9. *Peck v. Counseling Service of Addison County, Inc.* 146 Vt. 61, 499 A.2d 422 (1985).

10. Mossman D. How a rabbi's sermon resolved my Tarasoff conflict. *J. Am. Acad. Psychiatry Law.* 2004; **32**(4): 359–363.

11. Soulier M, Maislen A, Beck J. Status of the psychiatric duty to protect, circa 2006. *J. Am. Acad.* *Psychiatry Law.* 2010; **38**(4): 457–473.

12. Mossman D. Critique of pure risk assessment or, Kant meets Tarasoff. *University of Cincinnati Law Review.* 2006; **75**: 523–609.

13. Appelbaum P, Gutheil T. *Clinical Handbook of Psychiatry & the Law.* Philadelphia: Lippincott Williams & Wilkins; 2007.

14. Slovenko R. Psychotherapy and confidentiality. *Cleveland State Law Review.* 1975; **24**(3): 2 http://engagedscholarship.csuohio.edu/clevstlrev/vol24/iss3/2.

15. *Jablonski by Pahls v. United States*, 712 F.2d 391 (9th Cir. 1983).

16. Buchanan A, Binder R, Norko M, Swartz M. Psychiatric violence

risk assessment. *Am. J. Psychiatry.* 2012; **169**(3): 340.

17. Monahan J, Skeem JL. The evolution of violence risk assessment. *CNS Spectr.* 2014; **19**(5): 419–424.

18. Turner J, Gelles M. *Threat Assessment: A Risk Management Approach.* Binghamton, NY: The Haworth Press; 2003.

19. Borum R, Fein R, Vossekuil B, Berglund J. Threat assessment: defining an approach for evaluating risk of targeted violence. *Behav. Sci. Law.* 1999; **17**(3): 323–337.

20. Hinman D, Cook P. A multidisciplinary team approach to threat assessment. *Journal of Threat Assessment.* 2001; **1**(1): 17–33.

21. Warren LJ, Mullen PE, Ogloff JR. A clinical study of those who utter threats to kill. *Behav. Sci. Law.* 2011; **29**(2): 141–154.

22. Borum R, Reddy M. Assessing violence risk in Tarasoff situations: a fact-based model of inquiry. *Behav. Sci. Law.* 2001; **19**(3): 375–385.

23. Meloy JR, O'Toole ME. The concept of leakage in threat assessment. *Behav. Sci .Law.* 2011; **29**(4): 513–527.

24. White S, Cawood J. Threat management of stalking cases. In: Meloy J. ed. *The Psychology of Stalking: Clinical and Forensic Perspectives.* San Diego, CA: Academic Press; 1998: 295–314.

25. *Menendez v. Superior Court* (1992) 3 Cal.4th 435, 11 Cal. Rptr.2d 92; 834 P.2d 786.

26. Dobbs D. *The Law of Torts.* St. Paul, MN: West Group; 2000.

27. Mossman D. Tips to make documentation easier, faster, more satisfying. *Current Psychiatry.* 2008; 7(2): 80–86.

28. Simon RI. Suicide risk assessment forms: form over substance? *J. Am. Acad. Psychiatry Law.* 2009; **37**(3): 290–293.

29. Simon RI. Improving suicide risk assessment: avoiding common pitfalls. *Psychiatric Times.* December 1, 2011. http://www.psychiatrictimes.com/articles/improving-suicide-risk-assessment.

30. Black H. *Black's Law Dictionary,* 8th edn. St. Paul, MN: West Publising Co.; 2004.

31. *Ballek v. Aldana-Bernier,* NY Slip Op 02823 (2d Dept. 2012).

32. Mills J, Kroner D, Morgan R. *Clinician's Guide to Violence Risk Assessment.* New York: The Guilford Press; 2011.

33. Knoll J. Violence risk assessment for mental health professionals. In: Jamieson A., Moenssens A. eds. *Wiley Encyclopedia of Forensic Science.* Chichester, UK: John Wiley & Sons, Ltd; 2009: 2597–2602.

34. Douglas K, Hart S, Webster C, Belfrage H. *HCR-20V3: Assessing Risk of Violence— User Guide.* Burnaby, Canada: Mental Health, Law, and Policy Institute, Simon Fraser University; 2013.

35. Webster C, Haque Q, Hucker S. *Violence Risk—Assessment and Management: Advances Through Structured Professional Judgment and Sequential Redirections,* 2nd edn. Chichester, UK: Wiley-Blackwell; 2013.

Deconstructing violence as a medical syndrome: mapping psychotic, impulsive, and predatory subtypes to malfunctioning brain circuits

Stephen M. Stahl

Introduction

Violence reduction is the new mission of forensic mental health systems, as it defines who enters these settings, who has the most disruptive symptoms in these settings, and whether an individual can leave these settings [1,2]. Unfortunately, almost all large, randomized, controlled trials of psychotropic agents exclude patients who are violent [3] because such trials are often impractical or even unethical in violent forensic patients. Thus, establishing the best treatment strategy for violent patients who exhibit psychotic and impulsive symptoms due to major mental illnesses is difficult, and must necessarily rely on smaller trials, open trials, expert consensus, and case-based evidence [4–35]. Discussed here are both the hypothesized dysfunctional neural circuitry underlying violence in forensic settings, as well as treatment strategies based on rational targeting of brain circuits that may mediate this violent behavior.

Deconstructing the Syndrome of Violence in Psychotic Patients

The RDoC approach to violence

Violence can be deconstructed into its component symptoms, as can any other psychiatric syndrome, and these symptoms can be theoretically mapped to hypothetically malfunctioning brain circuits. This idea models the dimensional approach taken to psychopathology by the Research Domain Criteria (RDoC) strategy, which complements the categorical diagnostic strategy of the *Diagnostic and Statistical Manual of Mental Disorders* (DSM) of the American Psychiatric Association [36]. Specifically, violence in

forensic settings can be approached as a medical syndrome [1,2], and can be deconstructed into three major symptom domains: psychotic, impulsive, and predatory (organized) [2,37–46], each with a hypothetically distinct neurobiological basis and different theoretically malfunctioning brain circuits (e.g., Stahl and Morrissette [43]). Although many if not most patients in forensic settings have a psychotic illness, this is actually the least common type of violence (Figure 9.1) [37–46]. Predatory violence may actually be more common than psychotic violence in forensic settings. Although predatory violence is not the most common form of violence in forensic settings, it is often the most severe, but perhaps the least treatable, and therefore requires therapeutic security measures. It is actually impulsive violence that is the most common in forensic settings, and thus the subtype of violence that is in most desperate need of treatment in terms of frequency of occurrence, as well as relative lack of evidence from large, multicenter, randomized trials [37–46]. Empiric findings from recent treatment guidelines [2,3] and from clinical experience, as well as the existing literature [4–35], suggest that novel and aggressive psychopharmacologic management may reduce impulsive violence in this population.

Psychotic violence

Psychotic violence is attributed to positive symptoms of psychosis, most commonly paranoid delusions of threat or persecution, command hallucinations, and grandiosity [2–35,47]. Such psychotic symptoms may lead to violent behavior due to the assailant misunderstanding or misinterpreting environmental stimuli. In line with this, a recent study determined that

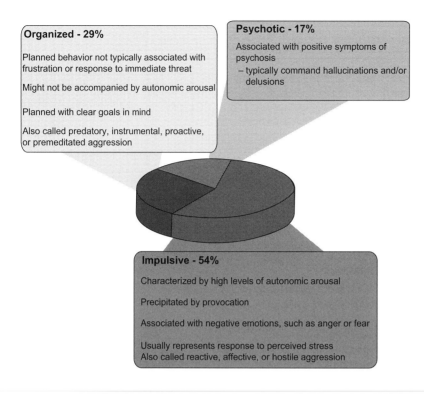

Organized - 29%

Planned behavior not typically associated with frustration or response to immediate threat

Might not be accompanied by autonomic arousal

Planned with clear goals in mind

Also called predatory, instrumental, proactive, or premeditated aggression

Psychotic - 17%

Associated with positive symptoms of psychosis
– typically command hallucinations and/or delusions

Impulsive - 54%

Characterized by high levels of autonomic arousal

Precipitated by provocation

Associated with negative emotions, such as anger or fear

Usually represents response to perceived stress
Also called reactive, affective, or hostile aggression

Figure 9.1 Heterogeneity of aggression. Identifying the type of aggression a patient is displaying may help guide the selection of appropriate treatments that target the underlying dysfunctional circuits. However, violence and aggression arise from a complex combination of neurobiological, genetic, and environmental factors, and are often presented in the context of comorbid conditions. (See plate section for color version.)

59% of individuals with schizophrenia who had committed acts of homicide were experiencing delusions, with a worsening of delusions in the months leading up to the homicidal act [19]. Psychotic violence is hypothetically linked to excessive neuronal activity in the mesolimbic dopamine pathway (Figure 9.2), where positive symptoms of psychosis are hypothetically mediated [47]. Psychotic violence linked to positive symptoms should hypothetically respond to suppression of this dopamine overactivity, and if standard doses of monotherapies or clozapine are ineffective, may be responsive to high-dosing or antipsychotic polypharmacy [2,3,37–46]. If standard doses fail to attain adequate plasma drug levels, i.e., a pharmacokinetic failure (Figure 9.3) [2,11–15,48–50], or if standard doses do attain adequate plasma drug levels but are nevertheless ineffective in reducing violence, i.e., a pharmacodynamic failure (Figure 9.3) [2,11–15,48–50], clozapine, high doses of monotherapies, or administration of two antipsychotics may be effective for positive symptoms driving psychotic violence (Figure 9.3) [2–35]. The rationale, consensus guidelines, evidence, and case-based examples are beginning to emerge from the literature for how to treat patients with psychotic violence unresponsive to standard, first-line, evidence-based treatments [2–35],

but much further research in this area remains to be done, and the positive results from the reported studies need to be replicated.

Impulsive violence

Sometimes called reactive violence, impulsive violence generally involves no planning, and is usually an immediate response to an environmental stimulus [38–43]. Impulsive violence may reflect emotional hypersensitivity and exaggerated threat perception [37–43], and may be linked with an imbalance between "top-down" cortical inhibitory controls and "bottom-up" impulsive drives (Figure 9.4) [7,43,51–58]. Both impulsive and psychotic aggression can occur in patients with schizophrenia, although impulsive violence is common in many other disorders, including mood disorders, personality disorders, substance abuse, and many more.

Both impulsive and psychotic violence have been hypothesized to involve excessive reactivity to perceived threat (bottom-up out of control) coupled with inadequate cortical regulation (top-down out of control) (Figure 9.4) [7,43,51–58]. Consistent with this, structural and functional abnormalities in frontal and temporal cortices and reduced connectivity

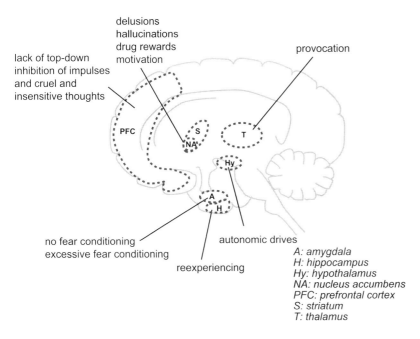

delusions
hallucinations
drug rewards
motivation

provocation

lack of top-down
inhibition of impulses
and cruel and
insensitive thoughts

PFC

S
NA

T

Hy

A
H

no fear conditioning
excessive fear conditioning

reexperiencing

autonomic drives

A: amygdala
H: hippocampus
Hy: hypothalamus
NA: nucleus accumbens
PFC: prefrontal cortex
S: striatum
T: thalamus

Figure 9.2 Brain areas related to violent and aggressive behavior. Impaired neurotransmission in various brain regions may contribute to the propensity for violent or aggressive behavior. The specific type of aggressive behavior is likely correlated with dysfunction in specific neural circuits. For example, both impulsive and psychotic aggression have been hypothesized to involve excessive reactivity to perceived threats (bottom-up out of control) and inadequate cortical regulation (top-down out of control). Although they are perhaps present in all patients with schizophrenia, structural and functional abnormalities in the frontal and temporal cortices as well as reduced connectivity between these brain areas may be more severe in aggressive patients than in those who are not aggressive. In the amygdala, fear conditioning seems to be excessive in both psychotic and impulsive aggression, whereas individuals with psychopathic aggression seem to lack fear conditioning.

between these brain areas have been reported [7,43,51–58]. Although perhaps present in all patients with schizophrenia, these findings may be more severe in aggressive patients compared with those who are nonviolent [7,43,51–58]. Impaired top-down control is most strongly associated with portions of the prefrontal cortex (PFC), including the dorsolateral PFC (DLPFC) and ventromedial PFC (VMPFC), as well as the orbitofrontal cortex (OFC) [7,43,51–58]. These regions are involved in decision making; dysfunction in these areas results in lack of recognition of consequences, inability to use previously learned information about reward and punishment, misinterpretation of emotionally neutral stimuli as being negative, and impaired recognition of social cues [7,43,51–58].

Within the temporal lobe, the amygdala is most highly implicated in violent and aggressive behaviors. The amygdala is involved in the rapid detection of threat, as well as the excitation of fight-or-flight responses. Modulation of amygdala activity comes from prefrontal brain areas; connections between these prefrontal and limbic regions may be impaired in individuals who are impulsively aggressive [7,43,51–58]. The amygdala is *hyperactive* in the case of impulsive aggression, but *hypoactive* in the case of psychopathic (predatory) aggression [43,48,51].

As in psychotic violence, impulsive violence may be responsive to antipsychotic polypharmacy or high

dosing when standard doses of monotherapies or clozapine fail to control impulsive violence [4–35]. Additional studies of impulsive violence and high-dose antipsychotics or antipsychotic polypharmacy are greatly needed.

Predatory violence

Predatory, or psychopathic, violence involves aggressive acts that are characterized by planning of assaults, predatory gain, and lack of remorse [2,37–46]. A moderate proportion of all violent acts and a high proportion of the most severe violent acts are due to psychopathy (Figure 9.4) [2,32–46]. The neurobiological basis of psychopathy is currently under intense investigation, and findings suggest that predatory/psychopathic violence may be associated with deficient fear conditioning in the amygdala [43,48,51].

Even though predatory violence in patients with psychotic illnesses may be common in forensic settings, this can occur in psychotic patients who have positive symptoms under control, and whose predatory violence will not respond to antipsychotics, including high dosing and polypharmacy. In fact, it is not clear whether predatory violence responds to any kind of treatment, least of all, psychopharmacologic interventions [2,37–46]. Psychopathic violence is not responsive to antipsychotics when comorbid psychotic symptoms are under control. Such patients

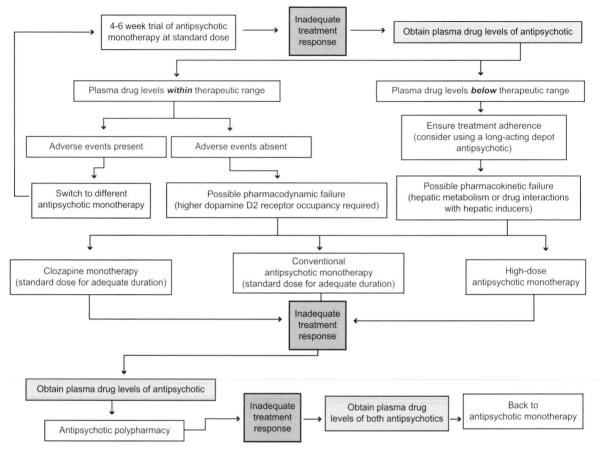

Figure 9.3 Antipsychotic treatment algorithm. Following several unsuccessful atypical antipsychotic monotherapy trials, a trial with a conventional antipsychotic or with clozapine is recommended. High-dose monotherapy may also be considered for such treatment-resistant patients. Antipsychotic polypharmacy is recommended only after antipsychotic monotherapy has failed. Note that throughout the treatment algorithm, monitoring of plasma drug levels of each antipsychotic is critical when determining the next course of action.

may require restricted housing or "therapeutic security" rather than antipsychotics [1,2].

Confounding factors

When selecting treatments for violent patients in forensic settings, it is important to consider the numerous confounding factors that may contribute to violent behavior, such as substance use disorders, personality disorders, cognitive dysfunction, mood disorders, noncompliance, etc. [2,37–46,59–61] Substance use issues are highly prevalent in patients with mental illness; approximately half of patients with schizophrenia have a comorbid substance use disorder [37–46]. Substances of abuse in particular may exacerbate symptoms of schizophrenia and lead to violence due to the effects of drugs of abuse on impulse control [16]. In fact, the risk of violent

behavior in patients with schizophrenia is four times greater if there is comorbid substance abuse [20]. Addressing substance use disorders is an integral part of the treatment plan for patients with schizophrenia, and may help prevent violence in this population [2,37–46].

Neurotransmitters and Violence

An oversimplification of the role of neurotransmitters in violence, particularly impulsive violence, involves hypothetical imbalances in the neurotransmitters dopamine (DA) and serotonin (5HT) [7,43,48]. In the prefrontal cortexes of aggressive patients, 5HT is decreased whereas DA is increased [7,43,48,62]. Dopamine is involved in the initiation and performance of aggressive behaviors, and elevated levels of striatal DA have been reported in individuals with impulsive

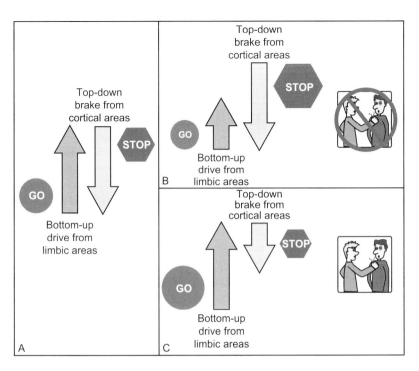

Figure 9.4 Bottom-up limbic drive and top-down cortical brake. (A) Impulsive drives in response to perceived threats stem from limbic regions, including the amygdala. Activity in limbic regions is modulated by input from cortical brain regions, including the prefrontal cortex (PFC). The balance between this limbic drive and the opposing cortical brakes determines whether one will act out an impulsive behavior such as aggression. (B) If the limbic drive is not overly strong, and/or if the cortical brake is sufficient to control impulsive drives coming from limbic areas, an individual will not act out with violent or aggressive behavior. (C) If the limbic drive is overly strong, and/or if the cortical brake system is not strong enough, an individual will be at an increased risk of violent behavior.

disorders; this hyperdopaminergia may weaken inhibitory pathways that regulate impulsivity [7,43,48,62–65]. Notably, excessive DA in mesolimbic areas of the brain is also believed to underlie psychosis; not surprisingly, antagonism of dopamine D2 receptors forms the basis of antipsychotic treatments. This may be why high degrees of blocking dopamine D2 receptors may also have therapeutic actions in impulsive violence as well.

Serotonin modulates prefrontal activity; thus the serotonergic dysfunction observed in the OFC and in the anterior cingulate of aggressive patients suggests a lack of sufficient top-down control [7,43,48,62–65]. In fact, during aggressive confrontations, 5HT levels in the PFC may decrease by as much as 80% [7]. Aggressive behavior and suicide by violent means has been correlated with low cerebrospinal fluid (CSF) levels of 5HIAA, which is a measure of 5HT concentration [51,63]. Additionally, whereas 5HT depletion increases aggressive behavior, increasing 5HT levels brings about increased activity in the PFC as well as diminished aggression [64]. This reduction in serotonergic activity observed in impulsively aggressive individuals is not found in patients with predatory aggression, which further supports the heterogeneic nature of violent behavior [23,57]. The serotonin 5HT2A receptor in particular may be implicated in aggressive behavior: a recent study showed that availability of the 5HT2A receptor is greater in aggressive patients compared to non-aggressive patients or healthy controls [64]. Contrary to the antiaggressive consequences of *antagonism* at 5HT2A receptors, *agonism* at 5HT2C receptors has also been shown to reduce impulsivity [65]. Therefore, targeting of specific serotonergic subtypes, a feature of many atypical antipsychotics, has potential for antiaggressive therapies.

Targeting Psychotic and Impulsive Violence

Once violence has been assessed in the forensic setting and a psychiatric diagnosis has been made [1–36], the next step is to deconstruct the type of violence into its psychotic, impulsive, or predatory subtypes [36]. Once the type of violence in the context of the specific DSM psychiatric diagnosis is known, the succeeding step is to find a rational treatment. The RDoC approach is to consider which brain circuits may be malfunctioning and thus hypothetically result in the unique symptom profile of an individual patient, which neurotransmitters may hypothetically regulate the efficiency of information processing in those brain circuits, and then finally, which psychopharmacologic treatments to select to rationally reduce symptoms of violence by targeting the hypothetically malfunctioning brain circuits of a given patient [36]. Interventions not only include rational psychopharmacologic measures, usually to occupy high proportions of dopamine D2 receptors, or act at serotonergic systems or ion channels, but also utilize various psychotherapies such as dialectical behavioral therapy (DBT) that can have potentially powerful therapeutic actions in selected patients [2].

In terms of empiric psychopharmacologic interventions that seem to be effective in some psychotic and impulsive patients who fail first-line, evidence-based treatments from randomized controlled trials, one current strategy is to achieve high degrees of dopamine D2 receptor occupancy by utilizing higher than normal doses of an antipsychotic, or even two concomitant antipsychotics, one often a depot formulation, while monitoring plasma drug levels [2–35].

Summary

Violence can be approached as a medical syndrome, and violence risk can be assessed as part of the psychiatric diagnostic evaluation. Specific subtypes of violence require unique treatment approaches for best outcomes. Conducting large, randomized, controlled trials is needed so that specific evidence-based treatments can be developed for subtypes of violence when first-line treatments fail. When large, randomized, controlled trials are not possible, further development of expert consensus-based and case-based treatments is needed for subtypes of violence.

References

1. Warburton K. The new mission of forensic mental health systems: managing violence as a medial syndrome in an environment that balances treatment and safety. *CNS Spectr.* 2014 Oct; **19**(5): 368–373. DOI: 10.1017/S109285291400025X.

2. Stahl SM, Morrissette DA, Cummings M, *et al.* The California Department of State Hospitals Violence Assessment and Treatment (CAL-VAT) guidelines. *CNS Spectr.* 2014; **19**(5): 357–365. DOI: 10.1017/S109285291400376.

3. Stahl SM, Morrissette DA, Citrome L, *et al.* "Metaguidelines" for the management of patients with schizophrenia. *CNS Spectr.* 2013; **18**(3): 150–162.

4. Correll CU. From receptor pharmacology to improved outcomes: individualising the selection, dosing, and switching of antipsychotics. *Eur. Psychiatry.* 2010; **25**(Suppl. 2): S12–21.

5. Davis JM, Chen N. Dose response and dose equivalence of antipsychotics. *J. Clin. Psychopharmacol.* 2004; **24**(2): 192–208.

6. Krakowski MI, Kunz M, Czobor P, Volavka J. Long-term high-dose neuroleptic treatment: who gets it and why? *Hosp. Community Psychiatry.* 1993; **44** (7): 640–644.

7. Comai S, Tau M, Gobbi G. The psychopharmacology of aggressive behavior: a translational approach: part 1:neurobiology. *J. Clin. Psychopharmacol.* 2012; **32**(1): 83–94.

8. Comai S, Tau M, Pavlovic Z, Gobbi G. The psychopharmacology of aggressive behavior: a translational approach: part 2: clinical studies using atypical antipsychotics, anticonvulsants, and lithium. *J. Clin. Psychopharmacol.* 2012; **32**(2): 237–260.

9. Citrome L, Volavka J. The psychopharmacology of violence: making sensible decisions. *CNS Spectr.* 2014 Oct; **19**(5): 411–418. DOI: 10.1017/S109285291400054.

10. Volavka J, Czobor P, Citrome L, Van Dorn RA. Effectiveness of antipsychotic drugs against hostility with schizophrenia in the Clinical Antipsychotic Trials of Intervention Effectiveness (CATIE) study. *CNS Spectr.* 2014; **0**(5): 374–381. DOI: 10.1017/S1092852913000849.

11. Meyer JM. A rational approach to employing high plasma levels of antipsychotics for violence associated with schizophrenia: case vignettes. *CNS Spectr.* 2014 Oct; **0**(5): 432–438. DOI: 10.1017/S10928514000236.

12. Morrissette DA, Stahl SM. Treating the violent patient with psychosis or impulsivity utilizing antipsychotic polypharmacy and high-dose monotherapy. *CNS Spectr.* 2014; **19**(5). DOI: 10.1017/S1092852914000388.

13. Stahl SM. Emerging guidelines for the use of antipsychotic polypharmacy. *Rev. Psiquiatr. Salud. Ment.* 2013; **6**(3): 97–100.

14. Stahl SM. Antipsychotic polypharmacy: never say never, but never say always. *Acta Psychiatr. Scand.* 2012; **125**(5): 349–351.

15. Morrissette DA, Stahl SM. Should high dose or very long-term antipsychotic monotherapy be considered before antipsychotic polypharmacy? In Ritsner MS, ed. *Polypharmacy in Psychiatric Practice, Volume 1: Multiple Medication Use Strategies.* Heidelberg: Springer; 2013: 107–125.

16. Volavka J, Citrome L. Pathways to aggression in schizophrenia affect results of treatment. *Schizophr. Bull.* 2011; **37**(5): 921–929.

17. Volavka J, Citrome L. Heterogeneity of violence in schizophrenia and implications for long-term treatment. *Int. J. Clin. Pract.* 2008; **62**(8): 1237–1245.

18. Frogley C, Taylor D, Dickens G, Picchioni M. A systematic review of the evidence of clozapine's antiaggressive effects. *Int. J. Neuropsychopharmacol.* 2012; **15**(9): 1351–1371.

19. Stilwell EN, Yates SE, Brahm NC. Violence among persons diagnosed with schizophrenia: how pharmacists can help. *Res. Social Adm. Pharm.* 2011; **7**(4): 421–429.

20. Swanson JW, Swartz MS, Van Dorn RA, *et al.* Comparison of antipsychotic medication effects on reducing violence in people with schizophrenia. *Br. J. Psychiatry.* 2008; **193**(1): 37–43.

21. Volavka J, Czobor P, Nolan K, *et al.* Overt aggression and psychotic symptoms in patients with schizophrenia treated with clozapine, olanzapine, risperidone, or haloperidol. *J. Clin. Psychopharmacol.* 2004; **24**(2): 225–228.

22. Topiwala A, Fazel S. The pharmacological management of violence in schizophrenia: a structured review. *Expert Rev. Neurother.* 2011; **11**(1): 53–63.

23. Bourget D, Labelle A. Managing pathologic aggression in people with psychotic disorders. *J. Psychiatry Neurosci.* 2012; **37**(2): E3–4.

24. Citrome L, Volavka J. Pharmacological management of acute and persistent aggression in forensic psychiatry settings. *CNS Drugs.* 2011; **25**(12): 1009–1021.

25. Roh D, Chang JG, Kim CH, *et al.* Antipsychotic polypharmacy and high-dose prescription in schizophrenia: a 5-year comparison. *Aust. N. Z. J. Psychiatry.* 2014; **48**(1): 52–60.

26. Barnes TR, Paton C. Antipsychotic polypharmacy in schizophrenia: benefits and risks. *CNS Drugs.* 2011; **25**(5): 383–399.

27. Fleischhacker WW, Uchida H. Critical review of antipsychotic polypharmacy in the treatment of schizophrenia. *Int. J. Neuropsychopharmacol.* Jul; **17**(7): 1083–1093.

28. Fujita J, Nishida A, Sakata M, Noda T, Ito H. Excessive dosing and polypharmacy of antipsychotics caused by pro re nata in agitated patients with schizophrenia. *Psychiatry Clin. Neurosci.* 2013; **67**(5): 345–351.

29. Gallego JA, Bonetti J, Zhang J, Kane JM, Correll CU. Prevalence and correlates of antipsychotic polypharmacy: a systematic review and meta-regression of global and regional trends from the 1970s to 2009. *Schizophr. Res.* 2012; **138**(1): 18–28.

30. Lochmann van Bennekom MW, Gijsman HJ, Zitman FG. Antipsychotic polypharmacy in psychotic disorders: a critical review of neurobiology, efficacy, tolerability and cost effectiveness. *J. Psychopharmacol.* 2013; **27**(4): 327–336.

31. Langle G, Steinert T, Weiser P, *et al.* Effects of polypharmacy on outcome in patients with schizophrenia in routine psychiatric treatment. *Acta Psychiatr. Scand.* 2012; **125**(5): 372–381.

32. Essock SM, Schooler NR, Stroup TS, *et al.* Effectiveness of switching from antipsychotic polypharmacy to monotherapy. *Am. J. Psychiatry.* 2011; **168**(7): 702–708.

33. Suzuki T, Uchida H, Tanaka KF, *et al.* Revising polypharmacy to a single antipsychotic regimen for patients with chronic schizophrenia. *Int. J. Neuropsychopharmacol.* 2004; **7**(2): 133–142.

34. Stahl SM, Grady MM. A critical review of atypical antipsychotic utilization: comparing monotherapy with polypharmacy and augmentation. *Curr. Med . Chem.* 2004; **11**(3): 313–327.

35. Aggarwal NK, Sernyak MJ, Rosenheck RA. Prevalence of concomitant oral antipsychotic drug use among patients treated with long-acting, intramuscular, antipsychotic medications. *J. Clin. Psychopharmacol.* 2012; **32**(3): 323–328.

36. Stahl SM. The last Diagnostic and Statistical Manual (DSM): replacing our symptom-based diagnoses with a brain circuit-based classification of mental illnesses. *CNS Spectr.* 2013; **18**(2): 65–68.

37. Singh JP, Serper M, Reinharth J, Fazel S. Structured assessment of violence risk in schizophrenia and other psychiatric disorders: a systematic review of the validity, reliability, and item content of 10 available instruments. *Schizophr. Bull.* 2011; **37**(5): 899–912.

38. Nolan KA, Czobor P, Roy BB, *et al.* Characteristics of assaultive behavior among psychiatric inpatients. *Psychiatr. Serv.* 2003; **54**(7): 1012–1016.

39. Abderhalden C, Needham I, Dassen T, *et al.* Predicting inpatient violence using an extended version of the Brøset-Violence-Checklist: instrument development and clinical application. *BMC Psychiatry.* 2006; **6**: 17.

40. Quanbeck CD, McDermott BE, Lam J, *et al.* Categorization of aggressive acts committed by chronically assaultive state hospital patients. *Psychiatr. Serv.* 2007; **58**(4): 521–528.

41. McDermott BE, Holoyda BJ. Assessment of aggression in inpatient settings. *CNS Spectr.*

2014 Oct; **0**(5): 425–431. DOI: 10.1017/S1092852914000224.

42. Monahan J, Skeem JL. The evolution of violence risk assessment. *CNS Spectr.* 2014 Oct; **0**(5): 419–424. DOI: 10.1017/ S1092852914000145.

43. Stahl SM, Morrissette DA. *Stahl's Illustrated: Violence: Neural Circuits, Genetics and Treatment.* Cambridge, UK: Cambridge University Press; 2014.

44. Wehring HJ, Carpenter WT. Violence and schizophrenia. *Schizophr. Bull.* 2011; **37**(5): 877–878.

45. Song H, Min SK. Aggressive behavior model in schizophrenic patients. *Psychiatry Res.* 2009; **167** (1–2): 58–65.

46. Serper M, Beech DR, Harvey PD, Dill C. Neuropsychological and symptom predictors of aggression on the psychiatric inpatient service. *J. Clin. Exp. Neuropsychol.* 2008; **30**(6): 700–709.

47. Stahl SM. *Stahl's Essential Psychopharmacology.* 4th edn. New York: Cambridge University Press; 2013.

48. Siever LJ. Neurobiology of aggression and violence. *Am. J. Psychiatry.* 2008; **165**(4): 429–442.

49. Nord M, Farde L. Antipsychotic occupancy of dopamine receptors in schizophrenia. *CNS Neurosci. Ther.* 2011; **17**(2): 97–103.

50. Mauri MC, Volonteri LS, Colasanti A, *et al.* Clinical pharmacokinetics of atypical antipsychotics: a critical review of the relationship between plasma concentrations and clinical response. *Clin. Pharmacokinet.* 2007; **46**(5): 359–388.

51. Coccaro EF, Sripada CS, Yanowitch RN, Phan KL. Corticolimbic function in impulsive aggressive behavior. *Biol. Psychiatry.* 2011; **69**(12): 1153–1159.

52. Coccaro EF, McCloskey MS, Fitzgerald DA, Phan KL. Amygdala and orbitofrontal reactivity to social threat in individuals with impulsive aggression. *Biol. Psychiatry.* 2007; **62**(2): 168–178.

53. Hoptman MJ, Antonius D. Neuroimaging correlates of aggression in schizophrenia: an update. *Curr. Opin. Psychiatry.* 2011; **24**(2): 100–106.

54. De Sanctis P, Foxe JJ, Czobor P, *et al.* Early sensory-perceptual processing deficits for affectively valenced inputs are more pronounced in schizophrenia patients with a history of violence than in their non-violent peers. *Soc. Cogn. Affect Neurosci.* 2013; **8** (6): 678–687.

55. Kumari V, Barkataki I, Goswami S, *et al.* Dysfunctional, but not functional, impulsivity is associated with a history of seriously violent behaviour and reduced orbitofrontal and hippocampal volumes in schizophrenia. *Psychiatry Res.* 2009; **173**(1): 39–44.

56. Coccaro EF. Intermittent explosive disorder as a disorder of impulsive aggression for DSM-5. *Am. J. Psychiatry.* 2012; **169**(6): 577–588.

57. Haller J. The neurobiology of abnormal manifestations of aggression—a review of hypothalamic mechanisms in cats, rodents, and humans. *Brain Res. Bull.* 2013; **93**: 97–109.

58. Kumari V, Aasen I, Taylor P, *et al.* Neural dysfunction and violence in schizophrenia: an fMRI investigation. *Schizophr. Res.* 2006; **84**(1): 144–164.

59. Krakowski MI, Czobor P, Nolan KA. Atypical antipsychotics, neurocognitive deficits, and aggression in schizophrenic patients. *J. Clin. Psychopharmacol.* 2008; **28**(5): 485–493.

60. Krakowski MI, Czobor P. Executive function predicts response to antiaggression treatment in schizophrenia: a randomized controlled trial. *J. Clin. Psychiatry.* 2012; **73**(1): 74–80.

61. Elie D, Poirier M, Chianetta J, *et al.* Cognitive effects of antipsychotic dosage and polypharmacy: a study with the BACS in patients with schizophrenia and schizoaffective disorder. *J. Psychopharmacol.* 2010; **24**(7): 1037–1044.

62. Singh JP, Volavka J, Czobor P, Van Dorn RA. A metaanalysis of the Val158Met COMT polymorphism and violent behavior in schizophrenia. *PLoS One.* 2012; **7**(8): e43423.

63. Pavlov KA, Chistiakov DA, Chekhonin VP. Genetic determinants of aggression and impulsivity in humans. *J. Appl. Genet.* 2012; **53**(1): 61–82.

64. Rosell DR, Thompson JL, Slifstein M, *et al.* Increased serotonin 2A receptor availability in the orbitofrontal cortex of physically aggressive personality disordered patients. *Biol. Psychiatry.* 2010; **67**(12): 1154–1162.

65. Winstanley CA, Theobald DE, Dalley JW, Glennon JC, Robbins TW. 5-HT2A and 5-HT2C receptor antagonists have opposing effects on a measure of impulsivity: interactions with global 5-HT depletion. *Psychopharmacology (Berl).* 2004; **176**(3–4): 376–385.

Chapter 10

Aggression, DRD1 polymorphism, and lesion location in penetrating traumatic brain injury

Matteo Pardini, Frank Krueger, Colin A. Hodgkinson, Vanessa Raymont, Maren Strenziok, Mario Amore, Eric M. Wassermann, David Goldman, and Jordan H. Grafman

Introduction and Aim

Pathological chronic aggressive behavior has been reported in up to 33% of patients with a traumatic brain injury (TBI) [1]. A number of different factors, including genetic predisposition, mono-aminergic system activity, and brain lesion location, are all thought to play a significant role in the development and maintenance of TBI-related aggression [2]. Regarding the symptomatic treatment options for aggression in TBI, to date most attention has been focused on the dopaminergic system [3].

Despite the widespread use of anti-dopaminergic drugs to treat aggression [4], converging evidence suggests that the relationship between dopamine and aggression is more complex than previously thought. In experimental models, for example, both D2 agonist and antagonists as well as D1 partial agonists and antagonists have been shown to reduce aggressive behaviors [5–7], while the classic pro-dopaminergic amphetamine has been shown to increase, decrease, or fail to change aggressive behavior levels depending on various factors, such as context and type of aggression [8].

Moreover, in humans, despite the consensus on the role of antipsychotics to treat aggression, pro-dopaminergic stimulants drugs have also been proposed as a possible pharmacological treatment for aggressive behaviors in specific patient groups. In attention deficit hyperactivity disorder (ADHD) patients, for example, stimulants have been shown to reduce aggressive behavior by remodulating to prefrontal cortex (PFC) dopamine levels [9], while pro-dopaminergic compounds have been proposed as a possible treatment for aggressive behavior in different dementing illnesses, such as frontotemporal dementia (FTD) [10,11].

Compared to the aforementioned clinical populations, the study of the biological basis of aggressive behavior in penetrating TBI (pTBI) presents another confounding factor, i.e., the presence of focal brain lesions, which could modulate the relationship between the dopaminergic system and aggression. Indeed, transcranial magnetic stimulation (TMS) experiments have shown that dorsolateral PFC inhibition reduces dopamine release in deep gray matter [12], while dorsolateral PFC stimulation increases striatal dopaminergic activity [13]. In animal models, medial frontal lesions have been found to increase deep gray matter dopaminergic activity [14], possibly through modulation of ventro-tegmental area activity.

In this study, we explored the relationship between lesion location, pTBI-related aggressive behaviors, and dopaminergic tone. Based on the aforementioned literature and previous studies that have shown a significant role of PFC in aggressive behaviors [2], we hypothesized that PFC lesion location significantly impacts the interaction between dopaminergic activity and aggression in pTBI. Given the key nature of PFC territories in pTBI-related aggression, we predicted a significant modulatory effect on the dopaminergic system/aggression interaction only by PFC but not non-PFC damage, and potentially a regional specificity of lesion location inside the PFC.

To test our hypotheses, we investigated, in a group of Vietnam War Veterans, the interaction between long-term pathological aggression, lesion location, and interindividual differences in endogenous dopaminergic tone due to functional single nucleotide polymorphic (SNP) differences in the main components of the dopaminergic system [15,16], i.e., the

Violence in Psychiatry, ed. Katherine D. Warburton and Stephen M. Stahl. Published by Cambridge University Press.

dopamine receptor D1 (*DRD1*), the dopamine receptor D2 (*DRD2*), and the dopamine-degrading enzyme catechol-O-methyltransferase (COMT).

We decided to focus on these components of the dopaminergic system, as *DRD1* and *DRD2* represent the prototypical members of the two groups of dopamine receptors (i.e., the *DRD1*-like and *DRD2*-like families) [15], while COMT is thought to represent the major dopamine-degrading enzyme in the synaptic cleft [16]. Evaluation of functional SNPs has been shown to be a useful tool to study the relationship between aggressive behaviors and mono-aminergic systems, both in healthy subjects and neuropsychiatric conditions [15,16], as well as a proxy-marker of baseline dopaminergic tone in pharmacological challenges studies [17].

Methods
Patient selection
Patients were drawn from Phase 3 of the Vietnam Head Injury Study (VHIS) [18], which was conducted between 2003 and 2006 (36–39 years post-injury) at the Bethesda National Naval Medical Center (Bethesda, MD, USA). Pre-injury characteristics and follow-up data of the participants (*n*=189) were available from military and Veterans Administration records. Inclusion criteria were the availability of SNP data and a negative history for treatments with drugs acting on the dopaminergic or serotoninergic system and for alcohol dependence. Eight subjects were removed due to the lack of SNP data, nine subjects due to alcohol dependence, and two subjects were excluded on the basis of previous pharmacological treatments. We thus included 141 Caucasian male veterans who suffered pTBI during their service in Vietnam and 29 healthy Caucasians male Vietnam veterans. Each subject underwent neurologic and psychiatric examinations, and pTBI subjects received a noncontrast brain CT scan.

Standard protocol approvals, registrations, and patient consents
All subjects gave informed written consent before enrollment in the study. The National Naval Medical Center and the National Institutes of Health (NIH) Institutional Review Boards approved all the study procedures.

Behavioral evaluation
Long-term aggression levels were evaluated with the agitation/aggression subscale of the Neuropsychiatric Inventory (NPI-a) [19], which was completed by the patients' caregivers. The NPI-a is based on a semi-structured interview and grades aggressive behaviors from 0 to 12, with higher values indicating more severe levels of aggression. The NPI-a has been used in clinical studies on aggression in brain injury [2] and other neurological conditions [19]. Moreover, we also used the total NPI (NPI-t) score as a global index of psychopathology. Last, we evaluated early psychological trauma by administering the Early Trauma Inventory (ETI), a validated 56-item interview that was designed for the assessment of childhood negative experiences [20].

Computed tomography (CT) scans
Axial noncontrast CT scans were acquired on a GE Medical Systems Light Speed Plus CT-scanner in helical mode as described elsewhere [18]. Briefly, images were reconstructed with an in-plane voxel size of 0.4 mm × 0.4 mm, overlapping slice thickness of 2.5 mm, and a 1-mm slice interval. Lesion location and volume were determined from CT images by manual tracing using the Analysis of Brain Lesion (ABLe) [21] software implemented in MEDx v3.44 (Medical Numerics) with enhancements to support the Automated Anatomical Labeling (AAL) atlas [22]. A trained neuropsychiatrist (V.R.) performed the tracings, which were then reviewed by an experienced observer (J.G.) who was blind to the results of the clinical evaluations. The skull and scalp were then removed from the CT images; each volume was spatially normalized to a de-skulled CT scan, which was previously spatially normalized to the T1 MNI brain (standard of the International Consortium for Brain Mapping). The ABLe software was used to exclude the manually delineated lesion from the spatial normalization process to improve registration accuracy. Spatial normalization was performed using an automated image registration algorithm using a 12-parameter affine model. The medial PFC (mPFC) region of interest was defined as those areas of the PFC medial to $x = -20$ and to $x = 20$ in the Montreal Neurological Institute (MNI) space as previously described [23]. Subjects with a PFC lesion encompassing or partially encompassing the mPFC were included in the "mPFC group," while all other subjects with PFC lesions were

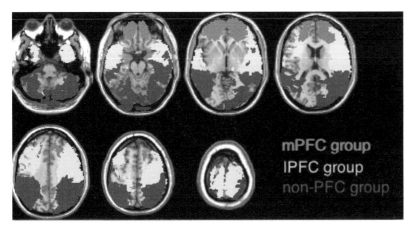

Figure 10.1 Subtraction lesions maps for the mPFC group (red), lPFC group (green), and non-PFC group (blue). For each group, the subtraction lesion map shows those brain areas that were more lesioned in 1 group compared to the other groups. Note that each subject was only included in 1 group. (See plate section for color version.)

included in the "lateral PFC (lPFC) group." Subjects with non-PFC lesions were included in the "non-PFC group."

Differences in lesion localization among the three groups are reported in Figure 10.1 using lesion subtraction maps that have been previously used in pTBI research to characterize differences in lesion localization among groups [2].

Genetic analysis

From a published SNP array [24], we selected the following functional SNPs: *DRD1* rs686 (A-to-G), *DRD2* rs4648317 (C-to-T), and COMT Val158Met rs4680 (G-to-A). Rs686 is a functional SNP located in the promoter region of the *DRD1* gene; its A allele is linked with increased transcriptional activity compared to the G allele [25]. Rs4274224 is located in the first intronic region of the *DRD2* gene; the minor allele has been linked with reduced D2 expression in healthy controls compared to the major allele [26]. Moreover, this SNP has been shown to impact behavioral inhibition [27]. COMT Val158Met rs4680 is a widely studied SNP in neuropsychiatry, and the Val allele is thought to be linked with a reduced efficiency in the degradation of dopamine [16]. Last, we decided to control for possible differences among subjects for the monoamine oxidase A (MAO-A) genotype, one of the genes more commonly linked to pathological aggression [2,28]. While the main role of the MAO-A is serotonin metabolism rather than dopamine, we decided to include it as a confounding factor since the common variable number tandem repeat (VNTR) polymorphism is known to impact aggression levels in the general population [28]. VNTR MAO-A

polymorphisms are thought to modulate MAO-A activity with the 3.5 and 4 repeats linked with MAO-A high-activity and 2, 3, and 5 repeats linked with low MAO-A activity. Genotyping for those SNPs was performed as described elsewhere [2,18,24].

Statistical analysis

Statistical threshold was set at 0.05 (2-tailed) for all first-level analyses. For each of our target SNPs (*DRD1* rs686, *DRD2* rs4648317, and COMT Val158-Met rs4680), a mixed 2×4 analysis of covariance (ANCOVA) on NPI-a (and NPI-t as a control measure) was performed with Genotype (major allele/–, minor allele/minor allele) and Group (mPFC, lPFC, non-PFC, control) as between-subjects factors and the other target genes as covariates. Based on our DRD1 results (see below), we also performed a 2×4 ANCOVA on NPI-a scores (and NPI-t scores) with *DRD1* Genotype and Group as between-subjects factors and DRD2, COMT, and MAO VNTR genotype as covariates. Follow-up independent t-tests (Bonferroni corrected for multiple comparisons) were performed for the rs686 genotypes within each lesion group.

Results
Group characteristics

All four groups did not present with significant differences in pre-injury intelligence ($F_{(3,165)}=1.2$, $p = 0.31$), early life negative experiences ($F_{(3,165)}=0.7$, $p=0.55$), education level ($F_{(3,165)}=0.8$, $p=0.50$), and age ($F_{(3,165)} = 0.4$, $p = 0.75$), and the lesion groups

Table 10.1 Demographic and clinical data for the experimental DRD1 rs686 groups

DRD1 rs686 group	NPI-a	NPI-t	Pre-injury IQ	Age	Education	% of brain volume loss	ETI
mPFC lesion group							
A/– (n = 22)	2.70 ± 0.2	5.6 ± 0.8	59.5 ± 4.6	57.5 ± 0.4	14.6 ± 0.4	3.2 ± 0.4	5.6 ± 0.4
G/G (n = 34)	0.52 ± 0.2	5.1 ± 0.7	58.0 ± 4.2	58.8 ± 0.4	14.3 ± 0.3	3.4 ± 0.4	5.9 ± 0.3
lPFC lesion group							
A/– (n = 20)	0.46 ± 0.2	5.2 ± 0.7	58.5 ± 5.6	58.8 ± 0.3	14.3 ± 0.4	4.0 ± 0.6	5.5 ± 0.5
G/G (n = 31)	2.40 ± 0.3	5.6 ± 0.9	59.6 ± 4.1	58.2 ± 0.5	15.0 ± 0.5	3.9 ± 0.7	5.8 ± 0.3
Non-PFC lesion group							
A/– (n = 14)	1.22 ± 0.3	5.6 ± 0.8	63.7 ± 5.8	58.2 ± 0.3	14.8 ± 0.4	3.0 ± 0.3	6.0 ± 0.5
G/G (n = 20)	1.44 ± 0.2	5.4 ± 0.8	62.2 ± 6.0	58.6 ± 0.5	14.9 ± 0.5	3.2 ± 0.4	5.9 ± 0.6
Control group							
A/– (n = 10)	0.93 ± 0.4	5.4 ± 0.6	60.2 ± 8.6	58.2 ± 0.6	15.4 ± 0.8	N/A	6.0 ± 0.4
G/G (n = 19)	1.12 ± 0.2	4.9 ± 0.5	61.2 ± 9.4	59.1 ± 0.3	15.5 ± 0.6	N/A	5.9 ± 0.5

Note: NPI-a: Neuropsychiatric Inventory Aggression sub-score; NPI-t: Neuropsychiatric Inventory Total score; ETI: Early Trauma Inventory Score.

were matched on percentage of brain tissue loss due to pTBI ($F_{(2,137)}$ = 0.9, p = 0.41) (Table 10.1). Lesion subtraction maps are reported in Figure 10.1. Frequency distributions for the genotyping results were as follows: DRD1: 97 A/– vs. 73 G/G subjects; DRD2: 117 C/– vs. C/– subjects vs. 53 T/T; COMT: 107 Val/– vs. 63 Met/Met subjects; MAO-A: 59 low-activity vs. 111 high-activity subjects.

DRD1

The ANCOVA on NPI-a revealed a significant interaction effect for DRD1 Genotype × Group ($F_{(3,159)}$ = 9.5, p = 0.001), but no significant main effects were found for DRD1 Genotype ($F_{(1,159)}$ = 0.4, p = 0.58) and Group ($F_{(3,159)}$ = 1.2, p = 0.35) and no covariate effect was found for COMT ($F_{(1,159)}$ = 0.45, p = 0.55), DRD2 ($F_{(1,159)}$ = 0.60, p = 0.4) or MAO-A ($F_{(1,159)}$ = 0.35, p = 0.35). Planned follow-up analyses showed that DRD1 A/– carriers had higher NPI-a scores than G/G carriers in the mPFC group (t = 2.99, p = 0.004; Cohen's d = 1.9), whereas DRD1 A/– carriers had lower NPI-a scores than G/G carriers in the lPFC group (t = 3.82, p = 0.002; Cohen's d = 1.89) (Figure 10.2). No significant differences were found between genotypes in the non-PFC (t = 0.92, p = 0.36) and control (t = 0.72, p = 0.48) groups.

The ANCOVA on NPI-t revealed no significant main effects (DRD1 Genotype: $F_{(1,159)}$ = 1.5, p = 0.25; Group: $F_{(3,159)}$ = 0.85, p = 0.38); interaction effect ($F_{(3,159)}$ = 1.1, p = 0.37); or COMT, DRD2, and MAO-A covariate effects.

DRD2

The DRD2 × Group ANCOVA performed on NPI-a scores revealed no significant main effects (DRD2 genotype: $F_{(1,159)}$=1.7, p=0.52; Group: $F_{(3,159)}$=0.5, p=0.80); interaction effect ($F_{(3,159)}$=0.15, p=0.92); or DRD1, COMT, and MAO-A covariate effects.

COMT

The COMT Genotype × Group ANCOVA performed on NPI-a scores revealed no significant main effects (COMT genotype: $F_{(1,159)}$=0.7, p=0.40; Group: $F_{(3,159)}$=0.2, p=0.89); interaction effect ($F_{(3,159)}$=0.15, p=0.92); or DRD1, DRD2, and MAO-A covariate effects.

Discussion

In this study, we studied the relationship between TBI-related aggression and the dopaminergic system and its modulation by lesion location. Our results

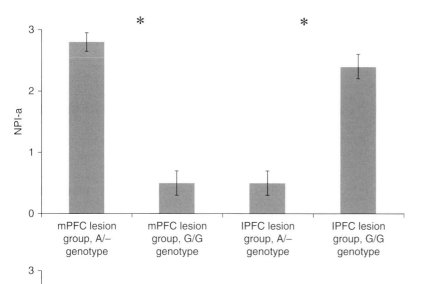

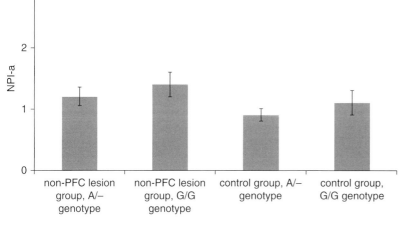

Figure 10.2 NPI-a scores (mean ± s.e.m.) for the lesion groups divided according to the functional SNP *DRD1* rs686. *Indicates a significant difference between the two genotype groups at $p < 0.05$ (Bonferroni correction).

revealed a significant interaction between aggressive behavior and the *DRD1* rs686 SNP depending upon PFC lesion location. We showed that carriers of the major and more transcriptionally active allele of *DRD1* were more aggressive compared to the minor allele homozygotes in the mPFC group, while conversely, *DRD1* major allele carriers were less aggressive than minor allele homozygotes in the lPFC group.

Moreover, we did not observe any significant interactions between lesion location and genotype for *DRD2* or COMT functional SNPs, thus suggesting a possible specificity of this effect to *DRD1* receptors. Last, no genotype effects were observed in the non-PFC and control groups or when taking into account the global index of psychopathology.

We propose that our observation of high aggression levels in two specific subsets of pTBI patients – (1) subjects with mPFC lesions and more expressed *DRD1*

receptors and (2) subjects with lPFC lesions and less expressed *DRD1* receptors – can be explained by analogy to the known relationship between impaired cognitive performance and excessively high or low levels of dopamine (i.e., the observed "U-curve" relationship between cognitive performance and dopaminergic tone) [29].

While the "U-shaped curve" relationship between function and dopamine levels was first observed at the neural level, recent years have seen its generalization to the behavioral, whole-organism setting. In rats, for example, both D1 agonists and antagonists have been shown to impair working memory performance in a dose-dependent function, leading to a U-shaped curve-like relationship (i.e., rats presented an equally pathological performance both during excessive inhibition and excessive stimulation of the D1 receptors) [30]. Moreover, in line with the proposed U-shaped curve relationship between dopamine tone and performance, a *DRD2* agonist, cabergoline, increased neural reward responses during a feedback-based reversal learning fMRI task in healthy subjects with low *DRD2* receptor density due to the A1+ Taq1A SNP, while it reduced reward responses in those subjects with higher *DRD2* receptor density due to the A– Taq1A SNP [17]. Last, a dopamine agonist, bromocriptine, has been shown to increase cognitive performance in healthy subjects with lower baseline dopamine synthesis – as quantified with fluoro-L-m-tyrosine PET scans, but showed an opposite effect (i.e., a performance reduction) in subjects with higher baseline dopaminergic tone [31].

Our findings suggest that subjects with lPFC lesions and less expressed *DRD1* represent the other extreme of the proposed "U-shaped curve" relationship between dopaminergic tone and aggression (i.e., association of high levels of aggression with reduced D1 signaling). This proposal is in line with the observed reduction of deep brain dopaminergic activity in lPFC virtual-lesion studies based on theta-burst TMS13 and an increased striatal dopaminergic tone after lPFC activation [14].

Thus, the combination of reduced dopaminergic activity with low *DRD1* expression could lead to low D1 tone in different subcortical areas linked with aggression, such as the nucleus accumbens (NA). According to pharmaco-fMRI studies, low D1 activity is linked with blunted NA responses to environmental stimuli [32]. A similar blunted NA response to environmental stimuli has been shown in subjects with ADHD, and it has been correlated with the extent of externalizing symptoms, which include aggressive conduct [33]. Interestingly, pro-dopaminergic stimulants are widely used to control externalizing aggressive behaviors in ADHD [9], as well as in some experimental models of aggression [34]. Last, a relationship between NA neuro-degeneration and disinhibited behavior has been shown in FTD in which pro-dopaminergic stimulants are used to treat aggression [35].

Our findings also indicate that subjects with mPFC lesions and more expressed *DRD1* represent the "high dopamine" end of the proposed "U-shaped curve." The mPFC territories are richly interconnected with the ventrotegmental area (the origin of the mesolimbic dopaminergic pathway to the NA), which suggests a modulatory effect of mPFC on the dopaminergic system [36], as shown in animal lesion models in which the structural lesion of medial PFC

territories was linked with an increase in NA dopaminergic activity [15]. These observations are in line with the observed activation by mPFC projections of inhibitory GABA-ergic inter-neurons in the dopaminergic mesolimbic pathway [36], as well as with the reported inverse correlation between mPFC and NA activity during immediate reward evaluation in impulsive subjects [37]. Given the relationship between D1 signaling and NA activity, the presence of mPFC lesions in subjects with highly expressed *DRD1* could lead to an excessively active NA, especially in behaviorally relevant impulsive decision-making settings, and possibly to heightened aggressive behaviors [38].

We propose that our finding of high aggression levels in pTBI subjects with mPFC lesions and more expressed *DRD1* and in subjects with lPFC lesions and less expressed *DRD1* supports a U-shaped curve modulation of the function of the mesolimbic dopaminergic system. Coincidentally, in a recent meta-analysis of striatal activation during reward anticipation tasks, a similar U-shaped curve paradigm has been proposed to link the reduced reward responsiveness of mesolimbic striatal structures observed in subjects with extremely high or extremely low impulsivity observed in ADHD and healthy control group [39]. Our findings have a potential translational application in the pharmacological treatment of behavioral disturbances in pTBI patients [40]. Lesion location could represent a low-cost, easy-to-use, para-clinical marker to help, among other factors, in the development of individualized treatment protocols.

Indeed, our findings seem to suggest that in subjects with isolated lPFC lesions D1-agonists could represent the treatment of choice for aggressive behaviors, while the compounds in this class should be avoided in subjects with isolated mPFC lesions.

Albeit indirectly, moreover, our data also advise prudence in the use of D1-active drugs in subjects with mixed mPFC/lPFC, even if our study did not directly investigate this patient group. However, while this proof-of-concept study suggests the importance of a personalized approach to aggression treatment in pTBI, future studies are needed to explore its relevance in day-to-day clinical care.

Interestingly (but unexpectedly), given the widespread use of D2-antagonists to treat behavioral disturbances in pTBI [41], we did not find any effect of the *DRD2* SNP on aggression in our target populations. We argue that this observation, while it needs to be interpreted with caution, is in line with the growing evidence of the difficulties in generalizing findings from general psychiatry to neuropsychiatry. Indeed, different studies showed that chronic reduction of D2 tone using *DRD2* inhibitors after TBIs increases the risk of stable cognitive deficits [42,43], which, given the relationship between cognitive deficits and behavioral disturbances in pTBI, could counter the potentially positive effect of D2 inhibition on aggressive behaviors in this population.

One of the key aspects of our study is the composition of our patient group. Our experimental group is highly homogeneous regarding pTBI (all subjects suffered combat-related pTBI during their service in Vietnam), their demographic characteristics (all subjects suffered pTBI during their early adulthood), and their pre-injury cognitive levels. Moreover, all subjects were matched for their early negative experience burden and their exposure to aggressive environments (i.e., all of them were exposed to infantry warfare and suffered a major injury). While this homogeneity allowed us to control for possible confounding factors (e.g., pre-injury characteristics, TBI dynamics, and exposure to significant aggressive behaviors), it also represents the main limitation of this study, which prompts the need to also evaluate our findings in non-military heterogeneous populations. Another limitation of this study is the lack of anatomical information on pTBI-related white matter damage, since retained metal fragments in the brain preclude high resolution structural MRI studies.

Moreover, in this study we focused on *DRD1* and *DRD2*, as they represent the prototypical members of the two families of dopamine receptors (i.e., the *DRD1*-like and the *DRD2*-like families) [15]. Future studies, however, are warranted to explore the role of other dopaminergic receptors in behavioral disturbances in pTBI, especially taking into account the differences in the anatomical localization of the different receptors. *DRD4*, for example, seems to be of particular interest, as it is widely expressed in the PFC [44] and been associated with interindividual differences in externalizing behaviors [45], as well as with resilience after negative life experiences [46].

The longitudinal aspect of our study allowed us to evaluate the behavioral consequences of pTBI across the patients' lifetime, which are a major determinant of quality of life levels both for our patients and their caregivers. Furthermore, the length of our follow-up suggests caution in the interpretation of our data, especially regarding their generalizability to the acute and sub-acute settings.

Conclusions

Our results suggest that pTBI modulates the relationship between pTBI-related aggression and the dopaminergic system in a lesion-location dependent way; potentially, lesion location could help in the development of individualized therapies for treatment-resistant aggression, for example, suggesting prudence in the use of D1-antagonists in subjects with lPFC lesions or of D1-agonists in subjects with mPFC damage. Pharmacological studies are warranted to explore the translational relevance of our findings.

Disclosures

Dr. Pardini received an educational grant from the nonprofit association AKWO, Lavagna (Genoa, Italy). Dr. Krueger, Dr. Hodgkinson, Dr. Raymont, Dr. Strenziok, Dr. Wassermann, and Dr. Amore report no disclosures. Dr. Goldman serves on the editorial boards of *Biological Psychiatry and Addictions Biology*. Dr. Grafman was supported by the US National Institute of Neurological Disorders and Stroke intramural research program and a project grant from the US Army Medical Research and Material Command administrated by the Henry M Jackson Foundation (Vietnam Head Injury Study Phase III: a 30-year post-injury follow-up study) and serves as co-editor of *Cortex*.

References

1. Tateno A, Jorge RE, Robinson RG. Clinical correlates of aggressive behavior after traumatic brain injury. *J. Neuropsychiatry Clin. Neurosci.* 2003; **15**(2): 155–160.

2. Pardini M, Krueger F, Hodgkinson C, *et al.* Prefrontal cortex lesions and MAO-A modulate aggression in penetrating traumatic brain injury. *Neurology.* 2011; **76**(12): 1038–1045.

3. Comai S, Tau M, Gobbi G. The psychopharmacology of aggressive behavior: a translational approach: part 1: neurobiology. *J. Clin. Psychopharmacol.* 2012; **32**(1): 83–94.

4. Goedhard LE, Stolker JJ, Heerdink ER, *et al.* Pharmacotherapy for the treatment of aggressive behavior in general adult psychiatry: a systematic review. *J. Clin. Psychiatry.* 2006; **67**(7): 1013–1024.

5. Tidey JW, Miczek KA. Effects of SKF 38393 and quinpirole on aggressive, motor and schedule-controlled behaviors in mice. *Behav. Pharmacol.* 1992; **3**(6): 553–565.

6. Rodríguez-Arias M, Miñarro J, Aguilar MA, Pinazo J, Simón VM. Effects of risperidone and SCH 23390 on isolation-induced aggression in male mice. *Eur. Neuropsychopharmacol.* 1998; **8** (2): 95–103.

7. Aguilar MA, Miñarro J, Pérez-Iranzo N, Simon VM. Behavioral profile of raclopride in agonistic encounters between male mice. *Pharmacol. Biochem. Behav.* 1994; **47**(3): 753–756.

8. Miczek KA, Tidey JW. Amphetamines: aggressive and social behavior. In: Asghar K, De Souza E, eds. *Pharmacology and Toxicology of Amphetamine and Related Designer Drugs.* Washington, DC: National Institute on Drug Abuse; 1989: 68Y100.

9. Blader JC, Pliszka SR, Jensen PS, Schooler NR, Kafantaris V. Stimulant-responsive and stimulant-refractory aggressive behavior among children with ADHD. *Pediatrics.* 2010; **126**(4): 796–806.

10. Huey ED, Putnam KT, Grafman J. A systematic review of neurotransmitter deficits and treatments in frontotemporal dementia. *Neurology.* 2006; **66**(1): 17–22.

11. Huey ED, Garcia C, Wassermann EM, Tierney MC, Grafman J. Stimulant treatment of frontotemporal dementia in 8 patients. *J. Clin. Psychiatry.* 2008; **69**(12): 1981–1982.

12. Ko JH, Monchi O, Ptito A, *et al.* Theta burst stimulation-induced inhibition of dorsolateral prefrontal cortex reveals hemispheric asymmetry in striatal dopamine release during a set-shifting task: a TMS-[(11)C]raclopride PET study. *Eur. J. Neurosci.* 2008; **28**(10): 2147–2155.

13. Strafella AP, Paus T, Barrett J, Dagher A. Repetitive transcranial magnetic stimulation of the human prefrontal cortex induces dopamine release in the caudate nucleus. *J. Neurosci.* 2001; **21**(15): RC157.

14. Jaskiw GE, Karoum FK, Weinberger DR. Persistent elevations in dopamine and its metabolites in the nucleus accumbens after mild subchronic stress in rats with ibotenic acid lesions of the medial prefrontal cortex. *Brain Res.* 1990; **534**(1–2): 321–323.

15. Seeman P, Van Tol HH. Dopamine receptor pharmacology. *Trends Pharmacol. Sci.* 1994; **15**(7): 264–270.

16. Volavka J, Bilder R, Nolan K. Catecholamines and aggression: the role of COMT and MAO polymorphisms. *Ann. N. Y. Acad. Sci.* 2004; **1036**: 393–398.

17. Cohen MX, Krohn-Grimberghe A, Elger CE, Weber B. Dopamine gene predicts the brain's response to dopaminergic drug. *Eur. J. Neurosci.* 2007; **26**(12): 3652–3660.

18. Raymont V, Greathouse A, Reding K, *et al.* Demographic, structural and genetic predictors of late cognitive decline after penetrating head injury. *Brain.* 2008; **131**(Pt 2): 543–558.

19. Cummings JL, Mega M, Gray K, *et al.* The Neuropsychiatric Inventory: comprehensive assessment of psychopathology in dementia. *Neurology.* 1994; **44** (12): 2308–2314.

20. Bremner JD, Vermetten E, Mazure CM. Development and preliminary psychometric properties of an instrument for the measurement of childhood trauma: the Early Trauma Inventory. *Depress. Anxiety.* 2000; **12**(1): 1–12.

21. Solomon J, Raymont V, Braun A, Butman JA, Grafman J. User-friendly software for the analysis of brain lesions (ABLe). *Comput. Methods Programs Biomed.* 2007; **86**(3): 245–254.

22. Tzourio-Mazoyer N, Landeau B, Papathanassiou D, *et al.* Automated anatomical labeling of activations in SPM using a macroscopic anatomical parcellation of the MNI MRI single-subject brain. *Neuroimage.* 2002; **15**(1): 273–289.

23. Koenigs M, Huey ED, Calamia M, *et al.* Distinct regions of prefrontal cortex mediate resistance and vulnerability to depression. *J. Neurosci.* 2008; **28**(47): 12,341–12,348.

24. Hodgkinson CA, Yuan Q, Xu K, *et al.* Addictions biology: haplotype-based analysis for 130 candidate genes on a single array. *Alcohol Alcohol.* 2008; **43** (5): 505–515.

25. Huang W, Ma JZ, Payne TJ, *et al.* Significant association of DRD1 with nicotine dependence. *Hum. Genet.* 2008; **123**(2): 133–140.

26. Fukui N, Suzuki Y, Sugai T, *et al.* Exploring functional polymorphisms in the dopamine receptor D2 gene using prolactin concentration in healthy subjects. *Mol. Psychiatry.* 2010; **16** (4): 356–358.

27. Hamidovic A, Dlugos A, Skol A, Palmer AA, de Wit H. Evaluation of genetic variability in the dopamine receptor D2 in relation to behavioral inhibition and impulsivity/sensation seeking: an exploratory study with d-amphetamine in healthy participants. *Exp, Clin. Psychopharmacol.* 2009; **17**(6): 374–383.

28. Shih JC, Chen K, Ridd MJ. Monoamine oxidase: from genes to behavior. *Annu. Rev. Neurosci.* 1999; **22**(1): 197–217.

29. Vijayraghavan S, Wang M, Birnbaum SG, Williams GV, Arnsten AF. Inverted-U dopamine D1 receptor actions on prefrontal neurons engaged in working memory. *Nat. Neurosci.* 2007; **10**(3): 376–384.

30. Floresco SB. Prefrontal dopamine and behavioral flexibility: shifting from an "inverted-U" toward a family of functions. *Front. Neurosci.* 2013; **7**: 62.

31. Cools R, Frank MJ, Gibbs SE, *et al.* Striatal dopamine predicts outcome-specific reversal learning and its sensitivity to dopaminergic drug administration. *J. Neurosci.* 2009; **29**(5): 1538–1543.

32. Knutson B, Gibbs SE. Linking nucleus accumbens dopamine and blood oxygenation. *Psychopharmacology (Berl.).* 2007; **191**(3): 813–822.

33. Scheres A, Milham MP, Knutson B, Castellanos FX. Ventral striatal hyporesponsiveness during reward anticipation in attention-deficit/hyperactivity disorder. *Biol .Psychiatry.* 2007; **61** (5): 720–724.

34. Couppis MH, Kennedy CH. The rewarding effect of aggression is reduced by nucleus accumbens dopamine receptor antagonism in mice. *Psychopharmacology (Berl.).* 2008; **197**(3): 449–456.

35. Zamboni G, Huey ED, Krueger F, Nichelli PF, Grafman J. Apathy and disinhibition in frontotemporal dementia: insights into their neural correlates. *Neurology.* 2008; **71**(10): 736–742.

36. Takahata R, Moghaddam B. Target-specific glutamatergic regulation of dopamine neurons in the ventral tegmental area. *J. Neurochem.* 2000; **75**(4): 1775–1778.

37. Diekhof EK, Nerenberg L, Falkai P, *et al.* Impulsive personality and the ability to resist immediate reward: an fMRI study examining interindividual differences in the neural mechanisms underlying self-control. *Hum. Brain Mapp.* 2012; **33**(12): 2768–2784.

38. Buckholtz JW, Treadway MT, Cowan RL, *et al.* Mesolimbic dopamine reward system hypersensitivity in individuals with psychopathic traits. *Nat.. Neurosci.* 2010; **13**(4): 419–421.

39. Plichta MM, Scheres A. Ventral-striatal responsiveness during reward anticipation in ADHD and its relation to trait impulsivity in the healthy population: a meta-analytic review of the fMRI literature. *Neurosci. Biobehav. Rev.* 2014; **38**: 125–134.

40. Wong TM. Brain injury and aggression: can we get some help? *Neurology.* 2011; **76**(12): 1032–1033.

41. Fowler SB, Hertzog J, Wagner BK. Pharmacological interventions for agitation in head-injured patients in the acute care setting. *J. Neurosci. Nurs.* 1995; **27**(2): 119–123.

42. Kline AE, Massucci JL, Zafonte RD, et al. Differential effects of single versus multiple administrations of haloperidol and risperidone on functional outcome after experimental brain trauma. *Crit. Care Med.* 2007; **35** (3): 919–924.

43. Hoffman AN, Cheng JP, Zafonte RD, Kline AE. Administration of haloperidol and risperidone after neurobehavioral testing hinders the recovery of traumatic brain injury-induced deficits. *Life Sci.* 2008; **83**(17–18): 602–607.

44. de Almeida J, Palacios JM, Mengod G. Distribution of 5-HT and DA receptors in primate prefrontal cortex: implications for pathophysiology and treatment. *Prog. Brain Res.* 2008; **172**: 101–115.

45. DeYoung CG, Peterson JB, Séguin JR, *et al.* The dopamine D4 receptor gene and moderation of the association between externalizing behavior and IQ. *Arch. Gen. Psychiatry.* 2006; **63** (12): 1410–1416.

46. Bakermans-Kranenburg MJ, van Ijzendoorn MH, Caspers K, Philibert R. DRD4 genotype moderates the impact of parental problems on unresolved loss or trauma. *Attach. Hum. Dev.* 2011; **13**(3): 253–269.

Is impulsive violence an addiction? The Habit Hypothesis

Stephen M. Stahl

Introduction

Violence can be deconstructed into psychotic, predatory, and impulsive subtypes [1,2], and theoretically each subtype can be mapped onto its own unique malfunctioning brain circuits [3]. In institutional settings, impulsive violence is the most frequent form of violence with the greatest unmet need for effective, evidence-based treatment [3–9]. Although not a formal diagnostic feature of any psychiatric illness, impulsive violence is nevertheless a behavioral dimension that can cut trans-diagnostically across many conditions, ranging from personality disorders (especially psychopathy and borderline personality disorder) to mood disorders and psychotic disorders [8–13]. A novel formulation of impulsive violence presented here is to conceptualize it as a behavior that lies within the impulsivity–compulsivity spectrum. Impulsive–compulsive disorders include not only drug addiction, but also behavioral addictions such as gambling, binge eating, and possibly impulsive violence [10–13]. These disorders could theoretically all share a common pathophysiology, namely an imbalance between the circuits that motivate behavior due to reward/conditioning on the one hand and circuits that control/inhibit impulsive drives on the other [8–17]. The hope is that this new formulation of impulsive violence may lead to renewed efforts to find effective treatments based on behavioral and pharmacological interventions that target the hypothetical maladaptations in these brain circuits.

Impulsive and Compulsive Behaviors Are Influenced by Multiple Areas of the Brain

Changes within four main brain circuits that control key aspects of impulsive and compulsive behavior may hypothetically underlie the pathophysiology of addiction-like behavior, from substance abuse to behavioral addictions such as gambling, binge eating, and impulsive violence [10–17]. These neuronal networks regulate the following:

- reward/saliency
- motivation/drive
- learning/conditioning
- inhibitory control/emotional regulation/executive function.

In vulnerable individuals, exposure to provocative emotional inputs (or drugs of addiction, gambling, or food) theoretically leads to a weakening of control circuits due to conditioned learning. This resets reward thresholds for reacting to the stimulus, due in part to undermining the cortical top-down networks that regulate impulses. The result is impulsivity and compulsivity [8–17]. This model has been linked extensively to the pathophysiology of drug addiction [10–17]. Applying this model to impulsive violence suggests that individuals become conditioned to having violent reactions to various provocative stimuli, so that over time, such stimuli create impulses to react violently that eventually become automatic, mindless behaviors and a compulsive habit. This hypothesis for the evolution of impulsive violence into a habit or "addiction" is analogous to how drugs of abuse theoretically lead from a rewarding "high" to the compulsive and self-destructive drug-seeking behaviors of addiction [10–17].

The Inability to Resist Urges: A Theory of Impulsive Violence

In a normal state, when a salient stimulus is presented, the reward of that stimulus is evaluated. If

Violence in Psychiatry, ed. Katherine D. Warburton and Stephen M. Stahl. Published by Cambridge University Press.
© Cambridge University Press 2016.

the stimulus is perceived to have a favorable outcome, behavior is elicited to achieve that reward. If, however, the stimulus is perceived to have an unfavorable outcome, behavior is inhibited. This type of behavior is called goal-directed behavior or action-outcome learning, such that when that same stimulus is presented again, the value of the reward will be remembered to either elicit the behavior or inhibit the behavior [14,16]. If this behavior is repeated, over time the reward of the stimulus will be devalued, such that the stimulus itself is enough to drive behavior, regardless of the outcome [14,16]. This type of behavior is called stimulus-directed behavior or stimulus-response learning (Pavlovian conditioning). It is through stimulus-response learning that habits are formed [14–16].

How does this formulation of the reward system relate to impulsive violence? Taking a rational, willful decision to commit a violent act in the absence of delusions and hallucinations is sometimes called criminogenic thinking or criminalness. More specifically, criminalness can be defined as behavior that breaks laws and social conventions and/or violates the rights and well-being of others [18]. When criminalness is impulsive, hot-blooded, characterized by high levels of autonomic arousal, precipitated by provocation, associated with negative emotions such as anger or fear, and usually representing a response to a perceived stress (reactive, affective, and hostile), it can be considered impulsive violence and can be conceptualized as an impulsive–compulsive disorder [8–13,18,19]. Analogous to other impulsive–compulsive disorders [8–13], impulsive violence can be hypothetically linked to devaluation of a salient provocative stimulus that causes an affective response, and that over time with many repetitions switches goal-directed behavior (such as removing a threat, stopping a provocation, getting one's way in a conflict situation) into stimulus-directed behavior, where a provocation immediately leads to impulsive violence without thought and as a habit. However, if criminalness is calculated, planned, premeditated, proactive, predatory, instrumental, and cold-blooded, it is psychopathic and neither impulsive nor regulated by the neural networks being discussed here [8–13,18,19]. Rather, predatory violence may preferentially involve the amygdala and its connections with prefrontal cortex [8,9]. Patients with psychopathy can have both types of criminalness [18,19].

Maladaptations in the Reward Circuitry that Could Potentially Underlie Impulsive Violence

Under normal conditions, if a salient stimulus causes a favorable outcome, this behavior will be encoded as a pleasurable reward (Figure 11.1). The reward of drug-induced euphoria is self-evident, but what is the reward of committing violence? In the context of Figure 11.1, that reward could be considered to be the removal of a threat, the termination of a provocation, or having one's demands that led to a provocative input from others nevertheless be fulfilled. Learning that the results of any given reward are pleasurable is called "liking," and is an opioid-dependent process (Figure 11.1, left) [16]. Knowledge and anticipation of these pleasurable rewards are called "wanting," and are dopamine-dependent processes (Figure 11.1, left) [16].

An increase in "wanting" is said to underlie impulsivity, such that the drive for the pleasurable reward outweighs the outcome and the behavior is repeated without forethought or weighing the favorableness of the outcome (progression of the process from Figure 11.1, left, to Figure 11.1, middle) [14–16]. In some individuals, there is a higher probability that "wanting" behavior will develop into impulsive behavior due to an underlying environmental or genetic risk.

This increased risk is deemed an "impulsivity trait," and can lead to the development of impulsive disorders such as drug addiction, binge eating, gambling, or, as hypothesized here, impulsive violence when impulsivity leads to habit, or compulsivity (progression of Figure 11.1, middle, to Figure 11.1, right) [8–17]. Repetition of the impulsive behavior, called binging, does not happen all the time; the absence of behavior, however, can lead to a stronger desire, or anticipation, for the reward. It is this cycle of binge–abstinence–anticipation that can lead to compulsivity [14–16]. When a behavior becomes compulsive, the reward no longer matters, and the behavior is strictly driven by stimulus. It is through this mechanism that habits develop, just as in the classical conditioning of Pavlovian dogs. In the case of impulsive violence, hypothetically the stimulus is an environmental provocation, and the compulsive habit is retaliatory impulsive violence.

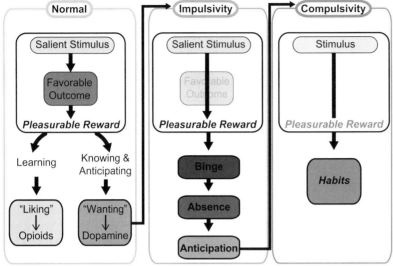

**Maladaptations of the Reward Pathway Can Shift
Behavior From Normal to Impulsive to Compulsive**

Figure 11.1 Maladaptations of the reward pathway can shift behavior from normal to impulsive to compulsive. Under normal conditions, if a salient stimulus causes a favorable outcome, this behavior will be encoded as a pleasurable reward. The learning of this pleasurable reward is called "liking," and is an opioid-dependent process. The knowledge and anticipation of this pleasurable reward is called "wanting," and is a dopamine-dependent process. An increase in "wanting" is said to underlie impulsivity, such that the drive for the pleasurable reward outweighs the outcome and the behavior is repeated without forethought. In some individuals, there is a higher probability that "wanting" behavior will develop into impulsive behavior due to an underlying environmental or genetic risk. This increased risk is deemed an "impulsivity trait" and can lead to the development of impulsive disorders such as binge eating, drug addiction, and, perhaps, impulsive violence. Repetition of the impulsive behavior, or binging, does not happen all the time; the absence of behavior, however, can lead to a stronger desire, or anticipation, for the reward. It is this cycle of binge–abstinence–anticipation that can lead to compulsivity. When a behavior becomes compulsive, the reward no longer matters and the behavior is strictly driven by stimulus. It is through this mechanism that habits develop. (See plate section for color version.)

How Do Reward Pathways Regulate the Maladaptive Shift of Normal to Impulsive to Compulsive?

In a basal, unstimulated state, in a normal individual the subcortical reward center is inhibited by inputs from the prefrontal cortex leading to an inhibition of behavior (Figure 11.2A) [14–16]. When a salient stimulus is presented, via activation of dopaminergic neurons in the midbrain, the ventral striatum becomes activated, which overrides the inhibition from the cortex and elicits goal-directed behavior (Figure 11.2B).

However, in individuals who are prone to impulsive behaviors, the subcortical reward center, in a unstimulated state, hypothetically receives less inhibitory input from the cortex, leaving these individuals more sensitive, or primed, to engage in reward-seeking behavior (Figure 11.2C) [8–16]. In response to a salient stimulus, these individuals have a greater

influx of dopamine first to the ventral striatum, which elicits a greater drive for goal-directed behavior (Figure 11.2C). If this behavior is repeated enough times, the locus of control shifts, such that dopaminergic inputs to the reward center target the area of the dorsal striatum that is important for stimulus-directed behavior (Figure 11.2D) [15]. Since the behavior is now being controlled by habit (i.e., stimulus-directed) instead of reward (i.e., goal-directed), the stimulus loses its salience and drives the behavior automatically; impulsive violence results over and again from the provocative stimulus [8–17].

Can Impulsive Violence Potentially Be Modified by Treatment?

Is there any treatment that can control impulsive violence in institutional settings across the wide range of psychiatric disorders in which it is observed? The literature suggests that treating the underlying

Normal Reward-Seeking Behavior in Response to a Salient Stimulus

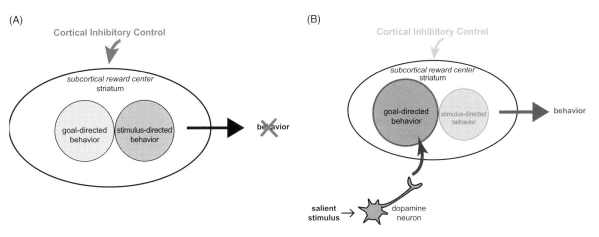

Abnormal Reward-Seeking Behavior in Response to a Salient Stimulus

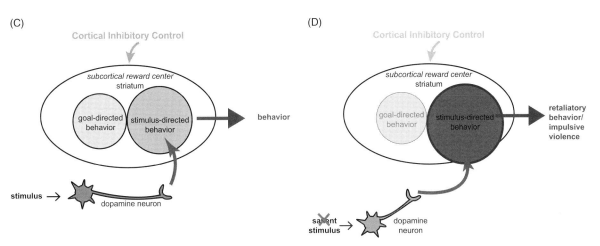

Figure 11.2 Reward-seeking behavior in response to salient stimuli. (A) In a basal, unstimulated state, the subcortical reward center is normally inhibited by inputs from the prefrontal cortex leading to an inhibition of behavior. (B) When a salient stimulus is presented, via activation of dopaminergic neurons in the midbrain, the striatum becomes activated, which overrides the inhibition from the cortex and elicits goal-directed behavior. (C) However, in individuals prone to impulsive behaviors, the subcortical reward center, in an unstimulated state, hypothetically receives less inhibitory input from the cortex, leaving these individuals more sensitive, or primed, to engage in reward-seeking behavior. In response to a salient stimulus, these individuals have a greater influx of dopamine to the striatum, which elicits a greater drive for goal-directed behavior. (D) If this goal-directed behavior is repeated enough times, the locus of control shifts, such that dopaminergic inputs to the reward center target the area of the striatum important for stimulus-directed behavior. Since the behavior is now being controlled by habit (i.e., stimulus-directed) instead of reward (i.e., goal-directed), the stimulus loses its salience and drives the behavior automatically and impulsive violence results over and again from the provocative stimulus.

psychiatric disorder is the first order of business, and in some cases, control of mood and psychosis may mitigate impulsive violence [3–9]. Psychotherapeutic interventions such as cognitive behavioral therapy (CBT) or dialectical behavioral therapy (DBT) for individuals or groups may also be effective [5]. However, in practice, such interventions have not reduced impulsive violence adequately in institutional settings.

Should control of impulsive violence be possible by "unlearning" or normalization of maladaptive behavior? Although theoretically possible with the interventions mentioned above, or empirically observed in those, for example, who are addicted to drugs following a long period of enforced abstinence, the success rate is disappointingly low and the recidivism rate disappointingly high. Perhaps it is time to direct psychotherapeutic and psychopharmacologic interventions to restoring the balance between top-down control and bottom-up drives, so that impulses that are triggered by conditioned stimuli no longer trigger habitual behavior in patients with impulsive violence. Thus, novel psychotherapeutic interventions, such as cognitive remediation, could theoretically help to restore top-down inhibitory controls [20,21]. Pro-cognitive psychopharmacologic agents may also help in this regard [22]. Aggressive antipsychotic treatment can also reduce bottom-up emotional drive [3–5], but is not commonly implemented in many institutional settings [3–5]. An optimistic note has recently been sounded by the approval of lisdexamfetamine for one of the impulsive–compulsive disorders, binge-eating disorder, in which theoretical modulation of dopaminergic neurons that feed into the reward center reset the balance of too much bottom-up drive and insufficient top-down inhibition [23]. This is consistent with shifting control away from stimulus-directed behavior, regulated by the dorsal striatum, and back toward goal-directed behavior, regulated by the ventral striatum, while also restoring adequate cortical inhibitory control. Lessons learned from emerging new targets for treatment of drug addiction may also provide leads for how to treat impulsive violence as a behavioral addiction.

References

1. Nolan KA, Czobor P, Roy BB, et al. Characteristics of assaultive behavior among psychiatric inpatients. *Psychiatr. Serv.* 2003; **54**(7): 1012–1016.

2. Quanbeck CD, McDermott BE, Lam J, et al. Categorization of aggressive acts committed by chronically assaultive state hospital patients. *Psychiatr. Serv.* 2007; **58**(4): 521–528.

3. Stahl SM. Deconstructing violence as a medical syndrome: mapping psychotic, impulsive and predatory subtypes to malfunctioning brain circuits. *CNS Spectr.* 2014; **19**(5): 357–365.

4. Stahl SM, Morrissette DA. *Stahl's Illustrated: Violence: Neural Circuits, Genetics and Treatment.* Cambridge, UK: Cambridge University Press; 2014.

5. Stahl SM, Morrissette DA, Cummings M, et al. The California Department of State Hospitals Violence Assessment and Treatment (CAL-VAT) guidelines. *CNS Spectr.* 2014; **19** (5): 449–465.

6. Dardashti L, O'Day J, Barsom M, Schwartz E, Proctor G. Illustrative cases to support Cal-VAT guidelines. *CNS Spectr.* 2015; **20**(3): 311–318. DOI: 10.1017/ S1092852915000127.

7. Morrissette DA, Stahl SM. Treating the violent patient with psychosis or impulsivity utilizing antipsychotic polypharmacy and high-dose monotherapy. *CNS Spectr.* 2014; **19**(5): 439–448.

8. Coccaro E, Fanning J, Phan KL, Lee R. Serotonin and impulsive aggression. *CNS Spectr.* 2015; **20**(3): 295–302.

9. Rosell D, Siever L. The neurobiology of violence. *CNS Spectr.* 2015; **20**(3): 1–26.

10. Grant JE, Kim SW. Brain circuitry of compulsivity and impulsivity. *CNS Spectr.* 2014; **19**(1): 21–27.

11. Fineberg NA, Chamberlain SR, Goudriaan AE, et al. New developments in human neurocognition: clinical, genetic and brain imaging correlates of impulsivity and compulsivity. *CNS Spectr.* 2014; **19**(1): 69–89.

12. Berlin GS, Hollander E. Compulsivity, impulsivity, and the DSM 5 process. *CNS Spectr.* 2014; **19**(1): 62–68.

13. Stahl SM, Grady M. *Stahl's Illustrated: Substance Use and Impulsive Disorders.* Cambridge, UK: Cambridge University Press; 2012.

14. Everitt BJ, Robbins TW. Neural systems of reinforcement for drug addiction: from actions to habits to compulsion. *Nat. Neurosci.* 2005; **8**(11): 1481–1489.

15. Everitt BJ, Robbins TW. From ventral to dorsal striatum: devolving views of their roles in drug addiction. *Neurosci. Biobehav. Rev.* 2013; 37(9 Pt A): 1946–1954.

16. Wyvell CL, Berridge KC. Intra-accumbens amphetamine increases the conditioned incentive salience of sucrose reward: enhancement of reward "wanting" without enhanced "liking" or response reinforcement. *J. Neurosci.* 2000; **20**(21): 8122–8130.

17. Volkow ND, Wang GJ, Baler RD. Reward, dopamine and the control of food intake: implications for obesity. *Trends Cogn. Sci.* 2011; **15**(1): 37–46.

18. Bartholomew N, Morgan R. Co-morbid mental illness and criminalness: implications for housing and treatment. *CNS Spectr.* 2015; **20**(3): 1–10.

19. Felthous A. The appropriateness of treating psychopathic disorders. *CNS Spectr.* 2015; **20**(3): 182–189.

20. Medalia A, Opler LA, Saperstein AM. Integrating psychopharmacology and

cognitive remediation to treat cognitive dysfunction in the psychotic disorders. *CNS Spectr.* 2014; **19**(2): 115–120.

21. Hooker CI, Bruce L, Fisher M, *et al.* Neural activity during emotion recognition after combined cognitive plus

social cognitive training in schizophrenia. *Schizophr. Res.* 2012; **139**(1–3): 53–59.

22. Stahl SM. *Stahl's Essential Psychopharmacology.* 4th edn. New York: Cambridge University Press; 2013.

23. McElroy S, Hudson JI, Mitchell JE, *et al.* Efficacy and safety of lisdexamfetamine for treatment of adults with moderate to severe binge-eating disorder: a randomized clinical trial. *JAMA Psychiatry.* 2015; **72**(3): 235–246.

Chapter 12

The neurobiology of psychopathy: recent developments and new directions in research and treatment

Michael A. Cummings

Introduction

The prevalence of significant psychopathic personality features has been estimated to be up to 1% to 2% among women and 2% to 4% among men [1]. Psychopathy is of particular clinical and forensic importance and interest, as such individuals, especially men, exhibit elevated rates of callous, remorseless, often predatory aggression [2]. To quote a particularly grandiose and narcissistic psychopathic serial killer, "I just like to kill ... You feel the last bit of breath leaving their body. You are looking into their eyes. A person in that situation is God" [3].

Recognition that the neural circuits of the frontal and temporal lobes are involved in producing personality features, including psychopathy, began with the explosive penetrating injury by a 1.1 m tamping rod of the frontal portion of Phineas Gage's brain on September 13, 1848 [4]. In the months following injury, Gage's personality changed from that of a conservative, methodical, responsible, and sober individual to a person characterized as irritable, aggressive, violent, impulsive, callous, and frequently drunken [5]. These psychopathic personality features slowly ameliorated, however, such that Gage was able to work as a coach driver in Chile before dying of status epilepticus in San Francisco in 1860 [6]. Gage's case initiated discussions in the medical community regarding the relationship between brain structure and personality, a new consideration in the nineteenth century [7]. A reconstruction of the neural circuits disrupted in Gage's brain, based on imaging studies of Gage's skull, is shown in Figure 12.1 [8].

Interest in understanding psychopathy continued from the nineteenth century into the twentieth century. Based on interviews conducted with hundreds of prisoners, Cleckley formed a narrative conceptualization and description of psychopathic personality structure and dimensions [9]. Subsequently, Hare and others organized the conceptualization of psychopathy into a 2-factor model, i.e., aggressive narcissism and deviant antisocial lifestyle [10]. This 2-factor model was later refined into 1-, 3-, and 4-factor models, with the latter composed of interpersonal deficits characterized by lack of affiliative attachment; affective deficits characterized by lack of fear and empathy; antisocial lifestyle characterized by lack of prosocial goals and behaviors; and overt antisocial acts characterized by a callous disregard for the rights and welfare of others [11].

It is worth noting that although the 4-factor model has become dominant, controversy and debate continue regarding the factor-analytic structure of psychopathy, as well as debate as to whether psychopathy should best be conceptualized in categorical versus dimensional terms. In parallel with the evolving psychological modeling of psychopathy, Raine [12] and others reported that a blunted autonomic response to frightening images during childhood was directly correlated with later criminal behavior. Conversely, increased childhood autonomic responsiveness was found to be inversely correlated with later violent and criminal behavior [12]. Taken together with prior psychological assessments indicating that diminished interpersonal affective responsiveness was a core component of psychopathy, it came to be widely hypothesized that the observed autonomic hyporeactivity was the substrate of psychopathic personality structure development [13]. This hypothesis, in turn, has driven several lines of research aimed at understanding the neurobiology of psychopathy. Such

Violence in Psychiatry, ed. Katherine D. Warburton and Stephen M. Stahl. Published by Cambridge University Press.
© Cambridge University Press 2016.

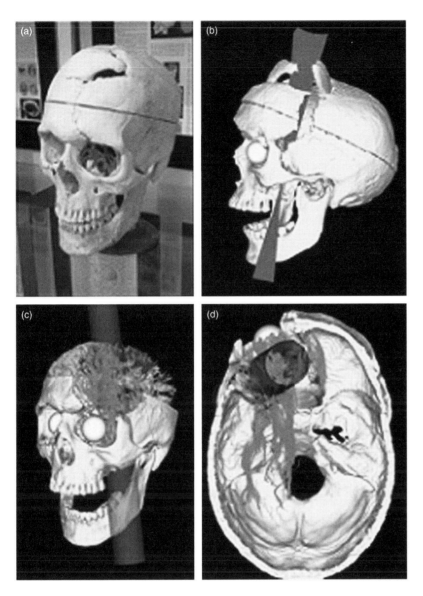

Figure 12.1 Phineas Gage – post-injury analysis of frontal connectivity. (See plate section for color version.)

understanding of the neural structures and distortions of neural circuit activity that underlie psychopathy are critical to identifying effective means of treatment to ameliorate the burden of violence and suffering imposed on others by psychopathic individuals [14].

Review of Recent Developments

Classically, it has been observed that childhood adversity or trauma can give rise to emotional and adaptive states that may go on to become persisting personality traits [15]. A recent meta-analysis of 27 peer-reviewed studies of nonclinical samples published through August 2012 found a positive correlation between childhood adversity, including trauma, and a lower transcription efficiency polymorphism of the gene for monoamine oxidase, type A (MAOA). Diminished expression of MAOA leads to diminished catabolic capacity for norepinephrine and serotonin, and was associated with the development of antisocial features (callous violence, substance abuse, and criminal behavior) in men, as well as a similar, but less robust, relationship in women [16]. Nevertheless, it is worth noting that a study of 3356 Caucasian men and 960 African-American men failed to confirm the interaction of childhood maltreatment, lesser MAOA transcriptional efficiency, and development of anti-social behavior [17]. Thus, while an interaction of childhood adversity and altered brain catechol-amine/indoleamine activity remains an attractive research area regarding the development of psycho-pathic personality characteristics, the data remain inconclusive.

Additional genes implicated, at least indirectly, in development of psychopathic personality structure include the Val-Met polymorphism of the gene coding for the amino acid sequence of brain-derived neurotrophic factor (BDNF), the oxytocin receptor gene polymorphism RS53576, and polymorphisms of the genes involved in serotonin signal transduc-tion [18–20]. More specifically, the Met-Met variant of the gene coding for BDNF made child and adoles-cent males more vulnerable to aggressive influences by peers. The RS53576 oxytocin receptor polymorph-ism was associated with diminished capacity to form affiliative attachments during periods of distress. Additionally, single nucleotide polymorphisms dimin-ishing 5HT-1B and 5HT-2A receptor serotonin signal transduction were associated with callous and unemo-tional traits in adolescent males.

Moreover, genetic studies to date underscore the importance of interactions between the inherited gen-etic polymorphisms and negative childhood and ado-lescent events and influences. These observations of the importance of genetic and environmental interactions comport with Raine's early observation that a minority of his autonomically hyporeactive children went on to develop prosocial lives and careers, e.g., police officers, bomb disposal experts, test pilots, etc., rather than becoming criminals [12]. These observations suggest that early interventions designed to limit childhood adversity and combat antisocial influences can ameli-orate the development of psychopathy. Despite this promise, it should be noted that prior attempts to extend diagnostic and intervention approaches to chil-dren and adolescents have found the developmental pathways into psychopathy and, consequently, inter-vention responses to be complex [21]. Nevertheless, it can be speculated that continued genetic research may yield future specific biological targets for the risk screening, prevention, or treatment of psychopathy.

Although not topographically precise, many electroencephalographic (EEG) studies have associ-ated forebrain circuit dysfunction and psychopathy. For example, a recent study of four men with medication-resistant medial prefrontal lobe epilepsy who exhibited antisocial behaviors found that the antisocial behaviors resolved following surgical abla-tion of the epileptiform or seizure foci [22]. Event-related investigation of psychopathic individuals has shown an inverse relationship between P3 amplitude, reflecting cortical electrical activity at c. 300 ms post event, and proneness to externalizing behaviors, sug-gesting a deficit in cortical attention in the context of introspective moral and empathetic processing [23]. Another study of psychopaths found that P3 ampli-tude was diminished in response to abrupt auditory stimuli and was directly correlated with interpersonal affective deficits [24]. These observations seem espe-cially enlightening, given recent spatiotemporal elec-troencephalographic data suggesting that in healthy controls, processing of moral decisions involves first a processing of affective interpersonal context within the temporal lobes, followed by ventromedial pre-frontal cortical processing of ethical and empathetic factors [25]. Taken together, these studies lead to the speculation that improved temporal lobe and ventro-medial prefrontal communication and cortical pro-cessing in the contexts of affiliative interpersonal affective connections and processing of moral deci-sions might ameliorate psychopathic behavior.

A variety of anatomic and functional imaging studies have implicated dysfunction of the amygdala as a core element of psychopathy [14]. In particular, although antisocial personality disorder and psycho-pathy overlap substantially, differential dysfunction in which the amygdala nuclei fail to respond to images designed to convey fear or negative emotion distin-guish psychopaths from nonpsychopathic antisocial individuals [26]. Ancillary dysfunction of the fusi-form gyrus also has been implicated in psychopaths in the context of inability to interpret negative facial expressions [27]. Finally, psychopaths exhibit a failure to activate the temporal lobe poles in response to anxiety-provoking stimuli [28]. Taken together, these studies suggest that in the psychopathic brain, the temporal lobes fail to adequately process emotional and social cues associated with negative emotions, resulting in an attenuated output signal to the ven-tromedial prefrontal cortex (VMPC). This lapse would appear to be a critical defect in initiating moral or ethical judgments [25].

As suggested, the VMPC appears to be pivotal to processing of the utilitarian or consequential aspects of moral and ethical judgments. In this context, the amygdala provides input regarding aversive affective

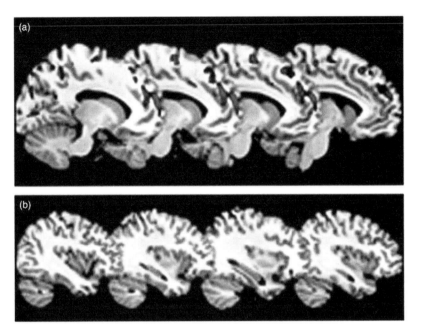

Figure 12.2 Frontal and temporal gray matter deficits in psychopathy. (See plate section for color version.)

context [29]. Recent magnetic resonance imaging (MRI) and functional magnetic resonance (fMRI) studies have affirmed prior observations of decreased amygdala and VMPC gray matter, but have gone further in identifying decreased connectivity between the amygdala nuclei, as well as other anterior temporal lobe structures and the VMPC via the uncinate fasciculus, but increased connectivity between the VMPC and the dorsolateral prefrontal cortex in psychopaths [30–32]. Moreover, it has been hypothesized that this neural circuit configuration underlies the callous, non-empathetic, unemotional, amoral, and inflexible features of psychopathic personality structure. White matter abnormalities also have been identified with respect to the genu of the corpus callosum and the fronto-occipital tract; however, the functional meaning of these observations remains to be fully investigated [33,34]. An illustration of gray matter deficits in psychopaths compared to nonpsychopathic antisocial individuals is shown in Figure 12.2 [35].

Additional forebrain and striatal structures have been found to play roles in psychopathic individuals. For example, impaired signal transduction between the VMPC and the mirror neuron network in the interhemispheric prefrontal cortex has been hypothesized to underlie the deficit observed in psychopaths to develop empathy or to appreciate the mental states of others [36]. Similarly, inadequate frontotemporal

communication with the cingulate gyrus may result in difficulty distinguishing one's egocentric desires and values from those of others, contributing to a narcissistic social perspective [37]. Also, diminished VMPC top-down suppression, coupled with hypersensitivity of the ventral tegmental area and nucleus accumbens (hypothalamus) to anticipated reward, have been hypothesized to underlie the impulsivity and increased addiction liability of psychopaths [38].

In sum, considering the 4-factor model of psychopathy derived from studies of the Psychopathy Checklist, Revised (PCLR) [39], neural structures appear to align as illustrated in Table 12.1.

To date, society has dealt with criminal psychopaths primarily via incarceration or execution; however, even in secure correctional or forensic psychiatric settings, such individuals inflict disproportionate violence on others and engage in antisocial enterprises [40–42]. In particular, it has been noted that within forensic psychiatric systems, it is likely vital to be able to match the level of security to the level of risk [43]. That is, external successful amelioration of violent and antisocial behaviors depends on being able to move the psychopathic individual into more secure settings when risks are elevated and to return the individual to lesser levels of security when levels of risk are ameliorated. As previously noted, the majority of confined psychopathic individuals return to the community.

Table 12.1 Psychopathy structural and functional associations

PCLR factor	Associated brain structures	Clinical correlates
Interpersonal deficits	VMPC	Impaired capacities to make ethical judgments about harm to others
	Mirror neuronal network	Impaired capacity to make interpersonal attachments
	Cingulate cortex	Impaired capacity to appreciate values of others
Affective deficits	Amygdala	Blunted response to fearful or negative emotional stimuli
	Temporal poles	Diminished fear response
	Uncinate fasiculus	Attenuated output of affective information to the VMPC
	Fusiform gyrus	Deficit in recognizing negative emotions in faces of others
Antisocial lifestyle	VMPC	Insensitivity to social obligations
	Cingulate gyrus	Narcissistic viewpoint
	Mirror neuronal network	Lack of empathic responses
Antisocial acts	VMPC	Impaired impulse inhibition
	Ventral striatum/nucleus accumbens	Reward hypersensitivity

PCLR = Psychopathy Checklist, Revised; VMPC = ventromedial prefrontal cortex.

Prior observations that not all persons with the biological substrate for psychopathy go on to become criminal or violent, coupled with recent observations that psychopaths can be trained to exhibit empathy, hold promise that inherent plasticity in forebrain circuits may permit development of more prosocial responses among psychopaths [12,44]. This working knowledge is the underlying basis for recent psychosocial approaches, such as risk–needs–responsivity (RNR) treatment programs [45].

Such treatment programs have shown positive preliminary treatment outcomes.

Historically, pharmacological approaches to treating violent and criminal behavior in psychopathic persons have been disappointing, as compared to pharmacological responses in other pathological personality structures [46–48]. For example, while lithium reduced impulsive violence and irritability in a group of chronically aggressive prisoners, it did not alter instrumental violence or overall criminality [49]. Similarly, a double-blind randomized trial of sertraline reduced impulsivity but increased fearlessness and dominance of others [50]. Importantly, however, preliminary data from a case series study of severely psychopathic nonpsychotic individuals treated with clozapine in a high-security forensic psychiatric hospital demonstrated impressive reductions in violence in six of seven patients at modest plasma concentrations of clozapine (mean 171 ng/ml) [51]. Recently,

there has been speculation regarding the potential benefits of electrical modulation of amygdala and nucleus accumbens activity in the context of psychiatric disorders; however, no data yet exist with respect to psychopathy or other mental disorders [52].

Conclusions

To date, no clear, reliably effective treatments for psychopathy exist; however, several lines of research hold promise. First, better understanding of relevant gene–environment interactions or epigenetic phenomena may yield more precisely targeted means to prevent psychopathy and to augment the plasticity of forebrain neural circuits during psychosocial treatments targeting psychopathy and predatory violence. That is, exploration of approaches to enhance the plasticity of circuits involving the VMPC, amygdala nuclei, and related structures may eventually be able to augment psychosocial treatments aimed at moving patients from psychopathic to prosocial. Similarly, better understanding of the electrical activity of the forebrain neural circuits of the psychopathic brain may yield treatment targets for interventions such as direct current stimulation, transcranial magnetic stimulation, or deep brain electrical stimulation. At the least, it is worth speculating that as such technologies evolve, enhanced understanding of the abnormal neural circuit activities of the psychopathic brain may yield novel treatment opportunities. Finally, while a case series can provide only limited data, the preliminary data reported for clozapine lead to a need for further research of clozapine in this context, as well as potential areas of research involving other glutamate signal transduction allosteric modulation agents, e.g., D-amino acid oxidase inhibitors, glycine reuptake transporter inhibitors, direct N-methyl D-aspartate (NMDA) allosteric modulators, etc.

In sum, the grave social and personal harm inflicted by violent criminal psychopaths warrants wide-ranging, aggressive research to refine our understanding of the neurobiology of psychopathy and to seek effective treatments. We need interventions that are more effective than confinement alone.

Disclosures

Michael A. Cummings has nothing to disclose.

References

1. Compton WM, Conway KP, Stinson FS, Colliver JD, Grant BF. Prevalence, correlates, and comorbidity of DSM-IV antisocial personality syndromes and alcohol and specific drug use disorders in the United States: results from the national epidemiologic survey on alcohol and related conditions. *J. Clin. Psychiatry.* 2005; **66**(6): 677–685.

2. Anderson NE, Kiehl KA. Psychopathy and aggression: when paralimbic dysfunction leads to violence. *Curr. Top. Behav. Neurosci.* 2014; **17**: 369–393.

3. Michaud SG, Aynesworth H. *Ted Bundy: Conversations with a Killer.* Irving, TX: Authorlink Press; 2000.

4. Macmillan MB. *An Odd Kind of Fame: Stories of Phineas Gage.* Boston, MA: The MIT Press; 2002.

5. Harlow JM. Passage of an iron rod through the head. *Boston Medical and Surgical Journal.* 1848; **39**(20): 389–393.

6. Bigelow HJ. Dr. Harlow's case of recovery from the passage of an iron bar through the head. *Am. J. Med. Sci.* 1850; **20**(39): 13–22.

7. Harlow JM. *Recovery from the Passage of an Iron Bar through the Head.* Boston: David Clapp & Son; 1869.

8. Van Horn JD, Irimia A, Torgerson CM, *et al.* Mapping connectivity damage in the case of Phineas Gage. *PLoS ONE.* 2012; **7** (5): e37454.

9. Cleckley HM. *The Mask of Sanity: An Attempt to Clarify Some Issues about the So-Called Psychopathic Personality.* 5th edn. Chicago: William A. Dolan; 1988.

10. Harpur TJ, Hare RD, Hakstain AR. Two-factor conceptualization of psychopathy: construct validity and assessment implications. *Psychol. Assess.* 1989; **11**(1): 6–17.

11. Cooke DJ, Michie C, Skeem J. Understanding the structure of the psychopathy checklist–revised: an exploration of methodological confusion. *Br. J. Psychiatry Suppl.* 2007; **49**: s39–s50.

12. Raine A. *The Psychopathology of Crime: Criminal Behavior as a Clinical Disorder.* 1st edn. San Diego, CA: Academic Press; 1997.

13. Raine A. Autonomic nervous system factors underlying disinhibited, antisocial, and violent behavior: biosocial perspectives and treatment implications. *Ann. N. Y. Acad. Sci.* 1996; **794**: 46–59.

14. Thompson DF, Ramos CL, Willett JK. Psychopathy: clinical features, developmental basis and therapeutic challenges. *J. Clin. Pharm. Ther.* 2014; **39**(5): 485–495.

15. Perry BD, Pollard R, Blakely T, Baker WL, Vigilante D. Childhood trauma, the neurobiology of adaptation and "use-dependent" development of the brain: how "states" become "traits." *Infant Mental Health Journal.* 1995; **16**(4): 271–291.

16. Byrd AL, Manuck SB. MAOA, childhood maltreatment, and antisocial behavior: meta-analysis of a gene-environment interaction. *Biol. Psychiatry.* 2014; **75**(1): 9–17.

17. Haberstick BC, Lessem JM, Hewitt JK, *et al.* MAOA genotype, childhood maltreatment, and their interaction in the etiology of adult antisocial behaviors. *Biol. Psychiatry.* 2014; **75**(1): 25–30.

18. Moul C, Dobson-Stone C, Brennan J, Hawes D, Dadds M. An exploration of the serotonin system in antisocial boys with high levels of callous-unemotional traits. *PLoS ONE.* 2013; **8**(2): e56619.

19. Kretschmer T, Vitaro F, Barker ED. The association between peer and own aggression is moderated by the BDNF Val-Met polymorphism. *J. Res. Adolesc.* 2014; **24**(1): 177–185.

20. Smearman EL, Winiarski DA, Brennan PA, Najman J, Johnson KC. Social stress and the oxytocin receptor gene interact to predict antisocial behavior in an at-risk cohort. *Dev. Psychopathol.* 2015; **27**(1): 309–318. DOI: 10.1017/ S0954579414000649.

21. Frick PJ. Extending the construct of psychopathy to youth: implications for understanding, diagnosing, and treating antisocial

children and adolescents. *Can. J. Psychiatry.* 2009; **54**(12): 803–812.

22. Trebuchon A, Bartolomei F, McGonigal A, Laguitton V, Chauvel P. Reversible antisocial behavior in ventromedial prefrontal lobe epilepsy. *Epilepsy Behav.* 2013; **29**(2): 367–373.

23. Venables NC, Patrick CJ. Reconciling discrepant findings for P3 brain response in criminal psychopathy through reference to the concept of externalizing proneness. *Psychophysiology.* 2014; **51**(5): 427–436.

24. Drislane LE, Vaidyanathan U, Patrick CJ. Reduced cortical call to arms differentiates psychopathy from antisocial personality disorder. *Psychol. Medicine.* 2013; **43**(4): 825–835.

25. Yoder KJ, Decety J. Spatiotemporal neural dynamics of moral judgment: a high-density ERP study. *Neuropsychologia.* 2014; **60**: 39–45.

26. Hyde LW, Byrd AL, Votruba-Drzal E, Hariri AR, Manuck SB. Amygdala reactivity and negative emotionality: divergent correlates of antisocial personality and psychopathy traits in a community sample. *J. Abnorm. Psychol.* 2014; **123**(1): 214–224.

27. Decety J, Skelly L, Yoder KJ, Kiehl KA. Neural processing of dynamic emotional facial expressions in psychopaths. *Soc. Neurosci.* 2014; **9**(1): 36–49.

28. Ermer E, Cope LM, Nyalakanti PK, Calhoun VD, Kiehl KA. Aberrant paralimbic gray matter in criminal psychopathy. *J. Abnorm. Psychol.* 2012; **121**(3): 649–658.

29. Shenhav A, Greene JD. Integrative moral judgment: dissociating the roles of the amygdala and ventromedial prefrontal cortex. *J. Neurosci.* 2014; **34**(13): 4741–4749.

30. Motzkin JC, Newman JP, Kiehl KA, Koenigs M. Reduced

prefrontal connectivity in psychopathy. *J. Neurosci.* 2011; **31** (48): 17,348–17,357.

31. Contreras-Rodríguez O, Pujol J, Batalla I, *et al.* Functional connectivity bias in the prefrontal cortex of psychopaths. *Biol. Psychiatry.* 2015; **78**(9): 647–655. DOI: 10.1016/j.biopsych .2014.03.007.

32. Li W, Mai X, Liu C. The default mode network and social understanding of others: what do brain connectivity studies tell us? *Front. Hum. Neurosci.* 2014; **8**: 74.

33. Raine A, Lencz T, Taylor K, *et al.* Corpus callosum abnormalities in psychopathic antisocial individuals. *Arch. Gen. Psychiatry.* 2003; **60**(11): 1134–1142.

34. Sundram F, Deeley Q, Sarkar S, *et al.* White matter microstructural abnormalities in the frontal lobe of adults with antisocial personality disorder. *Cortex.* 2012; **48**(2): 216–229.

35. Gregory S, Ffytche D, Simmons A, *et al.* The antisocial brain: psychopathy matters: a structural MRI investigation of antisocial male violent offenders. *JAMA Psychiatry.* 2012; **69**(9): 962–972.

36. Haker H, Schimansky J, Rossler W. [Sociophysiology: basic processes of empathy]. *Neuropsychiatrie.* 2010; **24**(3): 151–160.

37. Cai X, Padoa-Schioppa C. Neuronal encoding of subjective value in dorsal and ventral anterior cingulate cortex. *J. Neurosci.* 2012; **32**(11): 3791–3808.

38. Buckholtz JW, Treadway MT, Cowan RL, *et al.* Mesolimbic dopamine reward system hypersensitivity in individuals with psychopathic traits. *Nat. Neurosci.* 2010; **13**(4): 419–421.

39. Hare RD, Neumann CS. Psychopathy as a clinical and empirical construct. *Ann. Rev. Clin. Psychol.* 2008; **4**: 217–246.

40. Coid JW. Personality disorders in prisoners and their motivation for

dangerous and disruptive behaviour. *Crim. Behav. Ment. Health.* 2002; **12**(3): 209–226.

41. Sobral J, Luengo A, Gómez-Fraguela JA, Romero E, Villar P. [Personality, gender and violent criminality in prison inmates]. *Psicothema.* 2007; **19**(2): 269–275.

42. Endrass J, Urbaniok F, Gerth J, Rossegger A. [Prison violence: prevalence, manifestation and risk factors]. *Praxis (Bern 1994).* 2009; **98**(22): 1279–1283.

43. Kennedy HG. Therapeutic uses of security: mapping forensic mental health services by stratifying risk. *Advances in Psychiatric Treatment.* 2002; **8**(6): 433–443.

44. Meffert H, Gazzola V, den Boer JA, Bartels AA, Keysers C. Reduced spontaneous but relatively normal deliberate vicarious representations in psychopathy. *Brain.* 2013; **136**(8): 2550–2562.

45. Bonta J, Andrews DA. *Risk-Need-Responsivity Model for Offender Assessment and Rehabilitation 2007–06.* Ottawa: Her Majesty the Queen in Right of Canada; 2007.

46. Gitlin MJ. Pharmacotherapy of personality disorders: conceptual framework and clinical strategies. *J. Clin. Psychopharmacol.* 1993; **13** (5): 343–353.

47. Citrome L, Volavka J. Pharmacological management of acute and persistent aggression in forensic psychiatry settings. *CNS Drugs.* 2011; **25**(12): 1009–1021.

48. Ripoll LH, Triebwasser J, Siever LJ. Evidence-based pharmacotherapy for personality disorders. *Int. J. Neuropsychopharmacol.* 2011; **14**(9): 1257–1288.

49. Tupin JP, Smith DB, Clanon TL, *et al.* The long-term use of lithium in aggressive prisoners. *Compr. Psychiatry.* 1973; **14**(4): 311–317.

50. Dunlop BW, DeFife JA, Marx L, *et al.* The effects of sertraline on

psychopathic traits. *Int. Clin. Psychopharmacol.* 2011; **26**(6): 329–337.

51. Brown D, Larkin F, Sengupta S, *et al.* Clozapine: an effective treatment for seriously violent and psychopathic men with antisocial personality disorder in a UK high-security hospital. *CNS Spectr.* 2014; **19**(5): 391–402.

52. Bari A, Niu T, Langevin JP, Fried I. Limbic neuromodulation: implications for addiction, posttraumatic stress disorder, and memory. *Neurosurg. Clin. N. Am.* 2014; **25**(1): 137–145.

Chapter 13

The neurobiology of violence

Larry J. Siever and Daniel R. Rosell

Introduction

Violence and aggression are pervasive phenomena, and represent a significant public health burden [1–4]. Aggression and violence are also common symptomatic manifestations that the mental health professional is frequently called upon to identify, evaluate, and treat. While aggression and violence have multiple determinants – including social and psychological factors – characterizing neurobiological correlates of aggression may ultimately lead to the development of clinically informative biomarkers and rational treatment design.

In this review, we will discuss advances in the neurobiology of aggression and violence, addressing structural and functional neuroanatomical findings, as well as those related to neurochemistry and molecular genetics. Studies from the human literature will be our primary focus; however, preclinical or animal studies will also be discussed when there is limited human data and/or they are of a high-impact nature.

We will first examine the construct of aggression, with a specific focus on dimensional and categorical definitions, and the importance of refining the aggression phenotype under study in order to reduce neurobiological variability. The role of phenomenological heterogeneity as a potential source of inconsistencies between studies will be highlighted throughout this review. We will then review neuroanatomical findings, including volumetric, functional, and connectivity studies, with a particular emphasis on the role of the amygdala, limbic prefrontal regions, and amygdala–prefrontal circuitry. Following will be a discussion of the neurochemistry, neuropharmacology, and molecular genetics of aggression, with a primary focus on the serotonin system, as well as an examination of the less well developed literature related to dopamine, vasopressin, and the steroid hormones, cortisol and testosterone. Last, we will attempt to integrate these findings and reconcile inconsistencies in the field, and make recommendations for future studies, including potential clinical applications.

Aggression Subtypes and Dimensional Considerations
Impulsive and instrumental aggression

Aggression is a complex and heterogeneous construct, which in all likelihood serves as a significant source of variability between neurobiological studies. Therefore, it is essential to identify subtypes or classes of aggression, as well as subordinate factors and associated traits (e.g., impulsivity, callousness). A longstanding system for codifying aggression has been the impulsive/instrumental dichotomy: the former being an abrupt, "hot-headed" response to a perceived threat or provocation; and the latter being premeditated, goal-oriented, and "cold-blooded." In the clinical realm, aggression with the qualities of negative affect and impulsivity is the form that characteristically presents, whereas aggression of a more premeditated and instrumental nature is typically addressed in the forensic setting. The primary form of aggression that will be discussed in this review, and the one that has received the greatest attention in neurobiological studies, is the impulsive variant.

While highly representative manifestations of either impulsive or instrumental aggression certainly do occur, it is not uncommon that assaultive and violent acts can exhibit both impulsive and instrumental features [5]. For example, aggression can occur

Violence in Psychiatry, ed. Katherine D. Warburton and Stephen M. Stahl. Published by Cambridge University Press.
© Cambridge University Press 2016.

in a sudden and unplanned manner, in response to a perceived provocation, with a hostile or angry affect, but, nevertheless, in a highly controlled and purposeful manner, with an explicit and tangible objective, e.g., intimidation, or elevation of one's self-esteem. Thus, as we will discuss throughout this review, further refinement of the quality of aggression being studied – beyond the impulsive/instrumental distinction – we believe is critical to isolating underlying neurobiological mechanisms. Along these lines, we will next discuss the "reactive and proactive" classification of aggression.

Reactive and proactive aggression

Although similar to the impulsive/instrumental distinction, the reactive/proactive classification of aggression has been more formally operationalized and extensively validated, initially in child and adolescent populations [6–11], but more recently in adults [8,12,13]. This system does not view these two forms of aggression categorically or diametrically related, but rather, assumes that they coexist and contribute together to an individual's "total" level of aggression, and each is assessed dimensionally.

The reactive subtype best resembles what the impulsive category was originally intended to capture, i.e., aggression that (a) is invariably accompanied by anger, rage, or hostility; (b) occurs in response to frustration or perceived provocation (particularly in an interpersonal context); and (c) is motivated by the more rudimentary purpose of quelling unpleasant affect states. Proactive aggression, on the other hand, characteristically (a) does not invariably involve a negative affect state such as anger or rage; (b) is typically initiated by the offender, rather than provoked; and (c) is explicitly motivated by an expectation of obtaining something of value, e.g., an object, reward, power, status, or social dominance.

Reactive and proactive forms of aggression frequently coexist and are highly intercorrelated. Moreover, these two forms of aggression have been observed in adult populations with borderline [12] and antisocial [13] personality disorders (BPD and ASPD). Both reactive and proactive aggression subtypes have also been found to contribute to a common self-report measure of trait aggression in adults, i.e., the Buss–Perry Aggression Questionnaire (BPAQ), which is frequently used in studies of impulsive aggression [8]. Thus, both forms likely are present

to varying degrees in clinical populations as well as in research cohorts with severe/pathological aggression.

Despite the concurrence of reactive and proactive aggression, these two subtypes also exhibit important divergent properties. Reactive aggression is associated with a history of abuse [14,15], negative emotionality, and impulsivity [8,11], and it is also somewhat negatively predicted by callous-unemotional (CU) traits (a component of psychopathy) [8]. Proactive aggression, on the other hand, is associated positively with psychopathy [15], physical aggression, and violent offenses [8]. Furthermore, the tendency to over-attribute hostile intent to social cues, or hostile attribution bias, is related to reactive but not proactive aggression [16–19]. On the other hand, the belief that violence and assaultive behavior will lead to a favorable outcome, or *positive outcome expectancy*, is associated specifically with proactive aggression [20,21].

Finally, attentional interference by aggression-associated stimuli is directly and inversely correlated with reactive and proactive aggression, respectively [22]. Therefore, it is very likely that both forms are present, to varying degrees, in commonly studied, pathological manifestations of aggression, and may be a significant source of inconsistency between studies.

Aggression: Categorical Diagnoses and Intermittent Explosive Disorder

Categorical diagnoses

The role of categorical diagnoses is also a critical issue in studying the neurobiology of violence and assaultive behavior. Aggression and violence can occur as a function of a number of major psychiatric syndromal disorders, such as posttraumatic stress disorder (PTSD); attention-deficit/hyperactivity disorder (ADHD); bipolar disorder, schizophrenia (SCZ), and related psychotic illnesses; alcohol/substance abuse; and neuropsychiatric conditions (e.g., dementia, autoimmune encephalitis). Examining aggression in the context of these conditions, however, can make it difficult to differentiate the neurobiology of these disorders from that of aggression.

Intermittent explosive disorder

Clinically significant aggression also frequently manifests in a chronic and pervasive manner, independent of the above-described psychiatric syndromes, albeit, typically in the context of severe personality pathology. The syndrome of intermittent explosive disorder (IED) has been characterized in order to account for when this more chronic manifestation of aggression occurs with a frequency and intensity such that it contributes to significant subjective distress and/or functional impairment [23]. The diagnostic criteria of IED have recently undergone a number of changes that better identify a distinctly aggressive and impaired population [24,25].

Notable features of the latest iteration of IED criteria are (1) the requirement that the aggression be impulsive or reactive in nature; (2) inclusion of not only acts of severe physical aggression against other people or valuable property (including one's own property, e.g., cell phone), which typically occur at relatively low frequency, but also high-frequency occurrences of verbal assaultiveness and/ or minor physical events that do not lead to significant harm/damage (door slamming, pushing items off a table without property damage); and (3) removal of the exclusion for BPD and ASPD, as it has been demonstrated that a diagnosis of IED is associated with a distinct biological profile [26] and more severe aggression and functional impairment than these personality disorder diagnoses alone [24]. Last, there are also temporal criteria that allow for a state determination, i.e., whether IED is current or past. The development of a more valid categorical classification of chronic, clinically severe aggression has been an important advancement for neurobiological studies.

Neuroanatomy, Functional Imaging, and Neural Circuitry

As the more impulsive and reactive forms of aggression have been the focus of neurobiological studies (as opposed to purely instrumental or premeditated manifestations), not surprisingly, regions involved in affect processing, impulse control, and emotional decision making have received the greatest attention. We will primarily focus on the extensive literature regarding the amygdala, as well as limbic prefrontal regions – namely the orbitofrontal (OFC) and anterior cingulate cortex (ACC) – in aggression. We will also introduce the growing body of structural and functional findings regarding involvement of the striatum in aggression.

Amygdala: structural and functional studies

The amygdala is a medial temporal lobe structure that plays an essential role in the integration of a wide range of sensory and motivationally salient stimuli, as well as transmission of this information to various cortical and subcortical regions. These processes underlie the amygdala's essential role in emotionally valenced learning and memory, and the shaping of cognitive, affective, motor, and sympathetic representations and responses to affectively and motivationally salient stimuli [27,28].

An important consideration when examining the amygdala is its basic structure and circuitry (see Figure 13.1 for a detailed description). Briefly, the amygdala is composed of three main nuclear complexes: basolateral, central or centromedial, and superficial or cortical [29]. The circuitry and function of the basolateral and centromedial complexes have been the best characterized, whereas the superficial or cortical nuclei are less well understood. As depicted in Figure 13.1A, the basolateral complex serves as the primary locus of sensory input to the amygdala, whereas the central nucleus is considered the main output component, as it projects to numerous subcortical and brainstem structures. Intercalated cellular masses (IMs; Figure 13.1A) are clusters of inhibitory, GABAergic neurons nestled between the borders of the basolateral and centromedial complexes, which are believed to play a critical role in inhibitory control of amygdala activity [30,31]. It is worth noting that this schematic is an oversimplification, of course, and while not depicted in Figure 13.1A, sensory afferents also project directly to the central nucleus, particularly, visceral and gustatory, as opposed to visual, auditory, and polymodal information. Additionally, the basolateral complex also sends efferent projections to prefrontal and striatal regions, which will be addressed in a later section.

Owing to its relatively small size and the amorphous organization of its functional subdivisions, the amygdala has typically been assessed as a unitary structure in human imaging studies. Only until recently have the functional subdivisions of the amygdala been neuroanatomically delineated in human imaging studies (Figures 13.1B and 13.1C) [32]. As will be highlighted throughout this section, taking into account the functional subdivisions of the amygdala is critical to better resolve the relationship between amygdala structure/function and aggression.

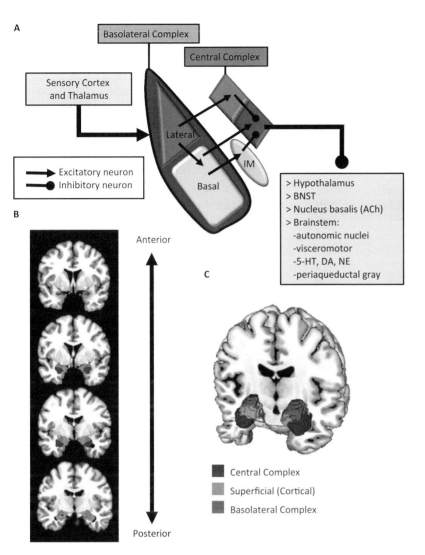

Figure 13.1 Amygdala: functional subdivisions and basic organization of flow of information. The amygdala is not a unitary structure, and consideration of its anatomical subdivisions and circuitry is essential. (A) One of the best characterized models of information flow and intra-amygdala circuitry involves the basolateral nuclear complex (which subsumes lateral and basal nuclei) and the central nuclear complex (which consists of a lateral [light red] and medial component [dark red]); these two complexes are considered the primary input and output components of this circuit, respectively. The basolateral complex receives cortical and thalamic sensory input. The lateral nucleus projects to the basal and central nuclei (lateral component); the basal nucleus projects to the central nucleus (medial component), as well as the intercalated masses (IM). The IMs are clusters of GABAergic inhibitory neurons, nestled between basolateral and central nuclei, which play a critical role in regulating central nucleus activity. The central nucleus projects to various subcortical regions, such as the hypothalamus, bed nucleus of the stria terminalis (BNST), nucleus basalis (major site of acetylcholine [ACh] ascending projection neurons), and various brainstem regions that regulate neurotransmitter systems, autonomic function, innate psychomotor and visceromotor responses, and descending pain-regulation pathways. Central nucleus efferents are believed to consist of tonically active inhibitory projection neurons that activate their downstream targets when their activity is inhibited [30,31]. (B)–(C) Studies of the amygdala in humans have typically considered it as a single functional unit, mainly due to its amorphous shape and relatively small size. Recent imaging studies have demonstrated the ability to differentiate the human amygdala in vivo into the three main nuclear complexes: basolateral, central (centromedial), and superficial (cortical) [32]. (See plate section for color version.)

A relatively consistent finding of structural imaging findings has been an association between aggression and reduced amygdala volumes. In a study of healthy, nonclinical female participants ($N = 20$) with levels of trait aggression not outside the normal range, Matthies *et al.* [33] found that both right and left whole amygdala volumes were smaller in those who scored higher than the cohort median on a commonly used measure of trait aggression (Lifetime History of Aggression; LHA) relative to those with LHA scores below the cohort median.

The volumes of both the right and left amygdala were also negatively correlated with LHA scores among all participants combined. Finally, specificity of this effect for aggression was supported by the absence of correlations between amygdala size and other clinical measures, namely general psychopathology, trait anxiety, and state depression. An important caveat of these findings, however, is their applicability to clinical populations, pathological forms of aggression, and males.

Pardini *et al.* [34] examined amygdala volumes in men (*N* = 56) who had been psychometrically assessed at three time points: (1) childhood and adolescence; (2) at the time of an MRI at 26 years of age; and (3) prospectively, approximately three years after the MRI. Notably, these participants manifested a broader range of aggression and psychopathology than in the Matthies *et al.* study, described above. Similar to what Matthies and colleagues observed, however, both the left and right whole amygdala volumes were negatively correlated with a number of measures of trait aggression performed at the time of MRI in adulthood. Remarkably, aggression that had been assessed in childhood and adolescence was also negatively related to adulthood amygdala volumes. Finally, both left and right whole amygdala volumes were found to be smaller in men who engaged in violent acts within the 3-year post-scan follow-up interval, even after adjusting for ratings of aggression prior to the post-scan assessment. Relations between amygdala volumes and psychopathy, a construct commonly associated with aggression, were somewhat mixed, however. Psychopathy assessments performed contemporaneously with the structural MRI in adulthood were not related to amygdala volumes; however, significant associations did exist between adulthood amygdala volumes and psychopathic features assessed in childhood/adolescence and at the 3-year post-scan follow-up assessment. Taking into account the different forms of aggression (namely reactive and proactive – which have different relationships with psychopathy) and characterizing amygdala subregions in future studies may allow for these complex relationships to be better resolved.

In order to enhance the specificity of the relationship between amygdala structure and aggression, studies have begun to take into account the anatomical functional subdivisions of the amygdala (described earlier, and depicted in Figures 13.1B and 13.1C). Gopal *et al.* [35] parcellated the amygdala into ventral and dorsal portions (roughly approximating the basolateral and centromedial nuclear complexes, respectively) and examined the relationship between amygdala volume and trait aggression in a mixed population of psychiatric patients with a wide range of diagnoses (*N* = 41). Unlike the two studies cited above, a relationship between *whole* amygdala volumes and trait aggression (as assessed by the LHA) was not observed. However, planned comparisons revealed that the volume of the left dorsal amygdala, specifically, was negatively correlated with the LHA. In contrast, they found that the closely related trait, (motor) impulsivity, was positively correlated with both the right and left ventral amygdalae, but not with either dorsal subdivisions. These findings highlight the importance of taking into consideration the anatomical and hemispheric specialization of the amygdala, as well as the potential confounding role of closely related traits that may in fact have contrasting neuroanatomical correlates.

Finally, Bobes *et al.* [36] reported that in a community sample of adult men (*N* = 54) whom were classified as either aggressive (*N* = 25) or non-aggressive (*N* = 29) based on a self-report measure of reactive aggression, both right and left whole amygdalae volumes were found to be smaller in the aggressive compared to the non-aggressive group. They also found that in the aggressive compared to the non-aggressive group, volumes of both the dorsal and ventral portions of the right amygdala were decreased, however, only the dorsal component of the left amygdala was reduced. Furthermore, while volumes of the left and right amygdala were negatively correlated with a general measure of trait aggression (i.e., not one specifically designed to differentiate proactive from reactive aggression), only the left amygdala correlation remained significant after correcting for multiple comparisons. Volumes of neither the left nor right amygdalae were correlated with measures of the interpersonal/affective dimensions of psychopathy. Curiously, an unexpected finding was that right amygdala volumes were found to be negatively correlated with a measure of proactive aggression.

Therefore, in a fairly wide range of populations, an inverse association between amygdala volume and trait aggression appears to be a relatively consistent finding. Further, there is growing evidence that taking the functional subdivisions of the amygdala into account is necessary in order to better resolve the amygdala–aggression relationship. Preliminarily, it appears the left, dorsal amygdala may have a distinct, albeit not exclusive, role. Preferential involvement of the dorsal amygdala points to altered amygdala output functionality; however, it will be necessary to determine the precise nature of this functional effect. Further, involvement of the left amygdala invokes a role for explicit/ conscious and effortful mechanisms of affect processing, as opposed to implicit/subconscious and automatic processes, which have been associated with the right amygdala [37].

Thus far, we have focused on the relationship between amygdala structure and trait aggression. The functional significance of these structural changes, however, remains unclear. For example, is reduced amygdala volume associated with amygdala hypoactivity or hyperactivity? Thus, we now turn to functional studies that examine the amygdala's involvement in aggression.

We recently examined patterns of regional brain metabolic activity in patients comorbid for IED and BPD ($N = 38$) in comparison to healthy control participants ($N = 36$) using [18]fluoro-deoxyglucose positron emission tomography (FDG-PET) in conjunction with a laboratory aggression task, the Point Subtraction Aggression Paradigm (PSAP) [38]. Importantly, FDG-PET was performed twice, under two different PSAP settings: a provoked condition, in which a fictitious competitor would "steal" or subtract points from the participant, and an unprovoked condition, for comparison. As expected, the BPD-IED group exhibited more aggressive behavior during the baseline (unprovoked) condition than the control group; and under the provoked condition, both groups exhibited an increased frequency of aggressive responding toward the (fictitious) competitor relative to the unprovoked state, although the level of aggressive behavior in the BPD-IED group was still greater than that of controls during provocation.

In terms of amygdala metabolic activity, we observed group differences in baseline amygdala activity, as well as in response to provocation: in the unprovoked state, amygdala metabolic activity was lower in the BPD-IED group compared to controls; and in response to provocation, amygdala activity increased in the BPD-IED group and decreased, albeit slightly, in the control group, despite the fact that both groups exhibited a similar degree of increased aggressive responding in the provoked compared to unprovoked condition [38]. Although there are important caveats to interpreting these findings, such as not accounting for amygdala functional subdivisions, they do suggest that amygdala activity is more labile, and perhaps less well modulated, in those with pathological forms of aggression.

A role for enhanced amygdala responsivity in aggression has also been demonstrated in studies employing functional magnetic resonance imaging (fMRI). For example, Coccaro et al. [39] previously described enhanced amygdala activity in response to viewing threatening facial expressions (specifically, anger and fear) in aggressive individuals relative to controls. Investigators, therefore, have taken advantage of this paradigm as a means to interrogate the neural structures and circuitry underlying aggression, without having to elicit aggressive behavior in the laboratory setting.

In addition to their analysis of amygdala volume, the study by Bobes et al. [36] discussed above, also employed fMRI to examine amygdala activation in response to fearful facial expressions. More specifically, they assessed the difference between amygdala responses to fearful and neutral faces (F/N-difference), with the neutral facing serving as a type of control stimulus. They found that in aggressive compared to non-aggressive participants, the F/N-difference was reduced, specifically, in the left dorsal amygdala. Moreover, among all participants, the amygdala F/N-difference was significantly negatively correlated with factors related to impulsive aggression, but not with the interpersonal/ affective dimensions of psychopathy.

Such a reduction in the F/N-difference potentially signifies that amygdala responses to fearful faces are reduced in aggressive individuals, which would conflict with the notion of amygdala hyperactivity in aggression. However, Bobes et al. [36] found that amygdala responses to both fearful and neutral faces were in fact increased in the aggressive group relative to the non-aggressive participants; however, the increase for neutral faces was greater than that of fearful faces. Thus, it was the increase in amygdala response to neutral faces that primarily determined the reduced F/N-difference. In other words, it is not that the aggressive group demonstrated less amygdala activity in response to fearful faces compared to the non-aggressive group, but rather, they exhibited greater amygdala activation to both fearful and neutral faces compared to the non-aggressive group. However, the neutral face-difference was even larger than that associated with fearful faces. Thus, the relatively lower F/N-difference in the aggressive group should not be equated with amygdala hypoactivity in response to socially threatening stimuli, but rather, amygdala hyperactivity in response to both fearful and neutral faces, but to a greater extent with respect to the neutral stimuli.

The last functional study we will discuss was performed Lozier *et al.* [40] in which they characterized the role of the right amygdala in proactive aggression by examining differences in the processing of fearful facial expression in adolescents with conduct problems (N = 30) compared to a healthy adolescent group (N = 16). It should be noted that this study differs from the others discussed above in that it consists of an adolescent as opposed to adult population, and is specifically focused on the right amygdala and proactive aggression.

Initially, Lozier *et al.* unexpectedly found an apparent absence of differential right amygdala activity to fearful faces in adolescents with conduct problems compared to controls; however, this was found to be due to "statistical suppressor effects" of associated pathological personality dimensions that exhibited contrasting neural correlates [40]. Specifically, they found that callous-unemotional (CU) traits (a component of psychopathy) and externalizing behaviors were negatively and positively correlated, respectively, with right amygdala responses to fearful faces. Thus, even though CU traits and externalizing behaviors commonly co-occur, they nevertheless exhibited a contradistinctive relationship with respect to right amygdala response to fearful faces. Such contrasting effects between highly covariant phenomena are a potential source of heterogeneity and inconsistency between studies.

Next, Lozier *et al.* found that, similar to CU traits, proactive aggression was also negatively correlated with amygdala response to fearful faces, while covarying for externalizing traits [40]. Further, they described that right amygdala hypoactivity to fearful faces mediated the relationship between CU traits and proactive aggression.

In other words, altered right amygdala functionality may be necessary for CU traits to manifest in terms of proactive aggression. The role of the right amygdala's differential response to fearful faces

serving as link between CU traits and proactive aggression was shown to be specific in three ways. First, right amygdala responses to angry or neutral faces did not mediate a link between CU traits and proactive aggression. Second, right amygdala responses to fearful faces did not link CU traits and reactive aggression. And last, right amygdala responses to fearful faces did not link externalizing behaviors and reactive aggression.

Prefrontal cortex and prefrontal–amygdala interactions

Studies of aggression have primarily implicated the limbic PFC, which includes portions of the orbitofrontal cortex (OFC) and the anterior cingulate cortex (ACC). Generally speaking, the OFC and ACC are both involved in the integration of affective, sensory, and cognitive processes, for the purpose of generating state representations that are coherent, nuanced, and textured, as well as behavioral, cognitive, and affective responses that are modulated, contextually appropriate, and flexible [41,42]. The OFC is considered to play more of a sensory or perceptual role, e.g., appraising the motivational value and affective valence of stimuli; the ACC, on the other hand, is more closely associated with determining "actions" or "responses."

Surprisingly, only a handful of studies have examined structural differences of the OFC and ACC in aggression. For example, smaller left OFC gray matter volume has been shown to be related to greater levels of trait aggression [43]. Similarly, greater right/left OFC volume ratios were also associated with greater trait aggression in those with a history of affective illness [44]. In child and adolescent populations, reduced right ACC volumes have been associated with increased aggression [45,46].

Early, functional studies indicated an association between aggression and reduced ventromedial PFC basal metabolic activity [47] and attenuated metabolic activation to serotonergic agents [48]. A recent study of ours, however, revealed a more complex picture. While metabolic activity of the OFC was lower under control conditions in a BPD-IED group compared to healthy controls, with provocation and increased aggressive responding, the OFC exhibited a relative increase in metabolic activity in the BPD-IED group, whereas in the healthy control group, OFC activity was reduced with provocation and increased aggressive responding [38]. The specificity of this effect for the OFC was demonstrated, as other prefrontal regions (medial, anterior, dorsolateral) did not differ between groups. Finally, we found that the correlation between medial OFC activity and aggressive responding, observed in healthy controls, was absent in the BPD-IED group. These findings suggest that the role of the OFC in the pathophysiology of aggression may not be best ascribed to a "hypoactivity" mechanism, but rather a "disconnection" one. As we will describe below, it has been useful to characterize the neural basis of aggression in terms of differential connectivity or coupling between the ventromedial PFC and the amygdala.

Coccaro *et al.* [39] described that while viewing angry faces, IED patients ($N = 10$) exhibited increased amygdala and decreased medial OFC activity compared to control participants ($N = 10$). Furthermore, it was described that among controls, amygdala activity was negatively correlated with that of the medial OFC (denoting the two regions were functionally coupled), whereas in the aggressive group, no amygdala–OFC coupling was observed [39].

We will first describe here (and in Figure 13.2) an overview of the basic neurobiology of amygdala–PFC connectivity before addressing its specific role in aggression. Work in primates has revealed a number of general principles regarding the structural basis of amygdala–PFC interconnectivity. First, the limbic portions of the PFC, namely the OFC and ACC, are the prefrontal regions that exhibit the most robust reciprocal anatomical connections with the amygdala – particularly, the posterior portion of the OFC [49,50] and the pregenual and subgenual (i.e., caudal) ACC (Figure 13.2A) [49]. Amygdala innervation is more scant and unidirectional in the more dorsal and lateral portions of the PFC [49]. Second, as illustrated in Figure 13.2A, the ACC sends more projections to the amygdala than it receives, whereas the posterior OFC receives more amygdala projections than it sends. This is consistent with the more "action"- or "response"-oriented functions of the ACC, and the "sensory" or "perceptual" role of the OFC. Finally, the termination patterns of OFC and ACC projections to the amygdala differ (see Figures 13.2C and 13.2D for details), which suggests that the former is an arbiter of central nucleus activity, whereas the latter modulates how the basal nucleus processes sensory input [51].

Human studies of amygdala–PFC connectivity, while unable to provide the same level of neuroanatomical resolution as animal studies, have been broadly consistent with the preclinical findings described above, and have offered additional functional information. As shown in Figure 13.2B, "resting state" or intrinsic functional connectivity studies have demonstrated that the basolateral nuclear complex is strongly (negatively) coupled with the ventral, pregenual PFC and (positively) coupled with the subgenual/orbital PFC. Also, there is an absence of connectivity between the basolateral complex and the dorsal and lateral portions of the PFC [52]. Notably, the negative connectivity between the ventral pregenual PFC and basolateral amygdala is consistent with a primarily "top-down," inhibitory feed-back process, whereas the positive connectivity with the subgenual/orbital PFC suggests a possible "bottom-up," feed-forward process.

We will now review specific studies in which aggression has been examined in terms of differential amygdala–PFC connectivity. As described earlier, Coccaro *et al.* [39] found that the coupling between the amygdala and medial OFC, which occurred while healthy participants viewed angry faces, was absent in patients with IED. Similarly, in a more recent study using restingstate fMRI in patients with schizophrenia ($N = 25$), Hoptman *et al.* [53] demonstrated that functional connectivity between the amygdala and ventral PFC was significantly decreased compared to healthy controls ($N = 21$), and critically, they found a significant negative correlation between trait measures of aggression and amygdalo-frontal connectivity. Similarly, studying a nonclinical male population ($N = 16$), Fulwiler *et al.* [54] observed that trait anger was inversely correlated with functional connectivity between the amygdala and contralateral medial OFC – most strongly between the right amygdala and left medial OFC. Furthermore, they found that a measure of anger control, i.e., the propensity to try to suppress one's response to angry feelings, was positively correlated with amygdala–OFC functional connectivity. An important question for future studies is to what extent altered amygdala–PFC connectivity is structural or neuromodulatory. In a recent study of a large cohort of healthy male participants ($N = 93$), Beyer *et al.* [55] did not observe a significant difference in a measure of structural connectivity between the amygdala and PFC in those with high compared to low trait-aggressiveness. It will be essential to extend such studies to clinical/pathological manifestations of aggression, however.

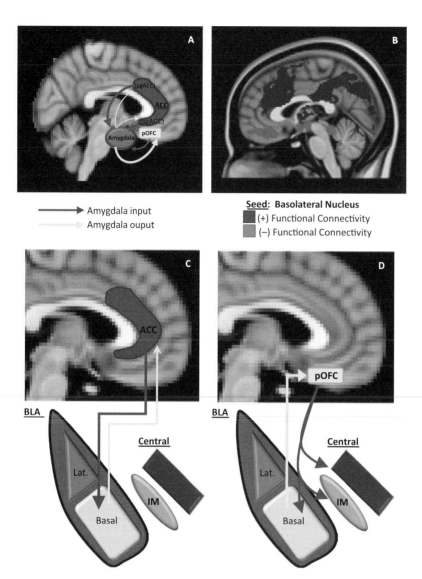

Figure 13.2 Prefrontal–amygdala circuitry. Altered prefrontal amygdala circuitry has been implicated in the neurobiology of aggression. (A) Preclinical studies in primates and rodents have demonstrated that the portions of the prefrontal cortex most robustly interconnected, anatomically, with the amygdala include two basic regions: the posterior extent of the orbitofrontal cortex (pOFC) and the caudal portions of the anterior cingulate cortex (ACC), roughly corresponding to the subgenual (sg)ACC and pregenual (pg)ACC. Anatomical connectivity between the amygdala and PFC, in general, decreases as it moves toward the dorsal and lateral aspects of the PFC (not depicted in this figure). Although there is significant bilateral anatomical connectivity between the amygdala and both the ACC and pOFC, studies in primates have also demonstrated relatively greater ACC-to-amygdala projections than amygdala-to-ACC projections; the pOFC, on the other hand, receives a greater number of projections from the amygdala compared to projections the pOFC sends to the amygdala. This has been considered to signify that the ACC is more of a sender of amygdala–PFC projections, whereas, the pOFC is more of a receiver [49,50]. (B) These structural data in primates are broadly consistent with intrinsic functional connectivity studies of the amygdala complex in humans, although the latter provides, of course, relatively less anatomical resolution. As illustrated in (B), the subgenual/orbital portion of the medial PFC exhibits positive functional connectivity (red) with the basolateral amygdala complex, which suggests a predominantly feed-forward relationship. The pregenual medial PFC, on the other hand, exhibits negative functional connectivity with the basolateral amygdala complex (blue), which indicates a feed-back role [52]. There is a general absence of functional connectivity with the more dorsal and lateral (not shown) PFC, which is similar to primate structural findings. (C)–(D) There are important anatomical differences in the termination patterns of projections from the OFC and ACC to the amygdala in the primate [51]. Projection neurons from the ACC terminate broadly throughout the basal nucleus (as well as other amygdala nuclei), whereas OFC efferents are relatively unique in that they terminate among the intercalated masses or IMs (clusters of GABAergic inhibitory neurons that regulate central nucleus activity), as well as the central nucleus itself. Therefore, the pOFC may act as a direct arbiter of central nucleus activity, and therefore, determine the extent to which a stimulus representation is infused with a visceral/autonomic or "somatic" component. The ACC, on the other hand, may influence more broadly how sensory inputs to the amygdala are processed. It remains unclear how pregenual and subgenual portions of the ACC may differ in this respect, however. (See plate section for color version.)

In terms of a neuromodulatory basis for altered amygdala–PFC connectivity, the serotonergic system is emerging as a likely candidate [56]. For example, pharmacological antagonism of 5-HT2A receptors enhances medial OFC–amygdala connectivity during the processing of fearful faces [57]. As will be discussed further below (in Receptor subtypes: 5-HT2A), this is consistent with our finding that state aggression in personality disordered patients with IED is positively correlated with 5-HT2A receptor availability in the OFC [58]. Dietary tryptophan depletion, which acutely lowers central serotonin synthesis, disrupts amygdala connectivity with the ventral ACC and ventrolateral prefrontal cortex, specifically when viewing angry faces [59]. Finally, polymorphisms of the 5-HT transporter have been associated with differential amygdala–PFC connectivity [60,61].

Therefore, it is becoming increasingly clear that while both the amygdala and ventral and medial aspects of the PFC are involved in aggression, it is essential that their concerted function be examined. Further, it is critical that the neuroanatomical specificity of amygdala–PFC interactions be taken into account, as connectivity with the amygdala differs not only between the ACC and OFC, but within functionally distinct subregions of each of these structures.

Striatum

The striatum integrates widespread, direct cortical input, and projects to pallidal structures that ultimately, via direct and indirect pathways, modulate thalamocortical activity. Through its involvement in this circuitry, the striatum plays a critical role in the appropriate selection and inhibition of various competing, motor, cognitive, and emotional response sequences [62].

The ventral and dorsomedial portions of the striatum are notable candidates for involvement in aggression, given their role in "goal-directed," "motivated," and "value-based" processes. The ventral striatum is believed to be involved in processing the anticipated value of "outcomes" or "events," whereas the dorsomedial striatum underlies the expected value of "actions."

Therefore, the ventral striatum conceivably may determine, for example, one's expectations from social interactions, and therefore contribute to phenomena, such as excessive frustration from interpersonal slights, that are common precipitants of impulsive aggression. The dorsomedial striatum, on the other hand, may be involved in determining the value of certain responses to frustration, such as assaultiveness as opposed to composed restraint.

Furthermore, striatal parameters that determine event and action values are modulated by the dopaminergic and serotonergic systems. Dopamine is believed to encode the expected value of an event or action and also the degree of increase or decrease in synaptic dopamine after an event reflects the extent to which an outcome exceeded or fell short of expectations, respectively. Through its modulation of striatal dopamine, the serotonergic system determines the temporal discount parameter, i.e., how much the delay of receiving a reward diminishes its value.

Buckholtz et al. [212] found that in a community sample of adults without a substance abuse history, the impulsive-antisocial dimension of psychopathy was positively correlated with both presynaptic dopamine release-capacity in the ventral striatum, and ventral striatal activity while waiting for a monetary reward. These findings suggest that immoderate ventral striatal function may be associated with impulsive aggression (a component of impulsive antisociality) by leaving an individual susceptible to disproportionate frustration, such as undue sensitivity to interpersonal slights and social rejection, which are common precipitants for aggression.

The dorsomedial striatum, in concert with the serotonergic system, has also been implicated in aggression. Crockett et al. [63] performed fMRI while participants engaged in a social trust paradigm in which they could accept or reject, and found that dorsomedial striatal activity was directly correlated with a participant "retaliating" by electing to reject an unfair financial offer, despite the fact that this choice was "costly" as both the participant and the offerer would not receive any money. Furthermore, they described that acute lowering of central serotonin levels with dietary tryptophan depletion led participants to reject moderately unfair offers more frequently, and take longer to accept the fairest offers. Activity of the dorsal striatum increased during rejections to a degree commensurate with the increased frequency of rejecting offers [61]. These findings of an interaction between serotonergic modulation and dorsal striatal activity in punitive, albeit costly, responses to unfair social exchanges is consistent with a finding from a recent study of ours, in which we observed that lower striatal serotonin transporter levels were related to greater state-levels of aggression in personality disordered patients [64].

Neurochemistry and Pharmacology: Serotonin

Initial studies of serotonin and aggression

One of the best studied areas of the neurobiology of aggression is the role of the serotonergic system. The first evidence for a role for serotonin (5-HT) in aggression came from animal models, in which isolation-induced aggression was shown to be reduced by numerous 5-HTergic antagonists and by pharmacological 5-HT depletion [65]. Subsequent evidence from human studies revealed a negative relationship between cerebrospinal fluid (CSF) 5-hydroxyindoleacetic acid (5-HIAA), the major metabolite of 5-HT catabolism, and aggression in patients with personality disorders [66,67]. The inverse correlation between 5-HIAA and trait aggression was interpreted as a hypo-serotonergic mechanism of impulsive aggression.

Further early findings demonstrated altered platelet 5-HT parameters, such as decreased 5-HT uptake in aggressive compared to non-aggressive participants [68] and decreased platelet imipramine binding (a measure of 5-HT transporter binding) in aggressive children with conduct disorder [69]. Attenuated hormonal responses to 5-HTergic pharmacological challenges also contributed to the initial foundation of the 5-HT hypothesis of aggression [70–72]. Finally, the selective serotonin reuptake inhibitor (SSRI) fluoxetine was shown to have an anti-aggressive therapeutic effect in personality disordered patients that was independent of antidepressant or anxiolytic effect [73,74].

Studies of 5-HT CSF metabolites, platelet measures, hormonal responses to pharmacological challenge, and the anti-aggressive effect of fluoxetine have been repeated and re-examined. There has been significant variability with respect to CSF 5-HIAA levels. While the classic finding consists of an inverse relationship [66,67,75], at least one study described a positive correlation [76], whereas another revealed no covariance, despite a reduced fenfluramine-induced prolactin response (and index of presynaptic 5-HT) in the same cohort [77]. While platelet 5-HT concentration [78] and 5-HT2A receptor levels [79] have also been shown to be related to aggression, reduced

platelet 5-HTT binding site number in aggressive patients appears to be the most consistent platelet finding [80]. It is worth noting, however, that at least two earlier studies found a positive relationship between 5-HTT platelet binding sites and aggression [81,82]; however, these studies were not done in as well-defined an aggressive population, whereas those more consistently demonstrating reductions in platelet 5-HTT have been performed in impulsive aggressive personality disordered patients either with or without a formal diagnosis of IED.

Reduced fenfluramine-induced increases in plasma prolactin also appears to be a highly reliable finding in aggression [70–72,77,83]. Change in serum prolactin after fenfluramine challenge is negatively related to trait aggression, and is lower in personality disordered patients with the more recent, integrated research criteria for IED (IED-IR); this effect is abrogated when covarying for differences in trait aggression. Moreover, prolactin level changes were not related to impulsivity; a diagnosis of BPD or ASPD; nor mood, anxiety, or alcohol/substance abuse disorders [26]. Therefore, these findings provided support for a specific involvement of 5-HT in aggression.

While these findings discussed above established the importance of the 5-HT system in aggression, further studies have been essential in more directly demonstrating the ability of the 5-HT system to modulate aggressive behavior, and address questions related to molecular genetics and pharmacology, development, and neuroanatomy. In the following sections, we will discuss the literature related to these issues.

5-HT challenges in humans: laboratory aggression, and functional neuroimaging

One of the primary methods for investigating the role of the 5-HT system in aggression is by the use of peripherally administered agents that acutely attenuate or enhance central 5-HTergic function. One of the most common and well-described interventions is dietary depletion of tryptophan, the amino acid precursor of 5-HT biosynthesis, which has been validated as a means to rapidly lower central 5-HT [84–86].

Early studies demonstrated that tryptophan depletion increased aggressive responding in nonclinical male participants in laboratory measures of aggression, which is consistent with the low-presynaptic 5-HT hypothesis [87]. However, it has become increasingly apparent that the relationship between 5-HT and aggression is complex, as a variety of factors appear to moderate how challenges to the 5-HT system affect aggressive responding.

Using a laboratory aggression paradigm, Bjork *et al.* [88] found that tryptophan depletion and tryptophan loading (which enhances central 5-HT availability) increased and decreased the frequency of aggressive responses, respectively, in those with high trait aggression. In those with low trait aggression, on the other hand, the effect was reversed, with decreases and increases in aggressive responding occurring under tryptophan-depleted and -loaded conditions, respectively [88]. Similarly, Kramer *et al.* [89] described an attenuation of aggressive responding with tryptophan depletion in a laboratory aggression paradigm, but only in those with low trait aggression, with no effect on those with high trait-aggression levels. In studies of adults and adolescents with ADHD, tryptophan depletion increased aggressive responding in a laboratory paradigm, but only in those with low trait impulsivity [90–92].

In addition to depletion/loading of dietary tryptophan, studies have also employed acute administration of SSRIs as a means to temporarily heighten synaptic 5-HT. Two studies have demonstrated that the delivery of severe, retaliatory, (laboratory-based) aggressive responses (which occurs only in those with either high levels of primary psychopathy [93] or significant histories of aggression [94], under levels of high-provocation) were reduced, acutely, after a single dose of an SSRI.

A handful of studies have begun to examine the neurobiological mechanisms involved in 5-HTergic modulation of impulse control and emotion processing relevant to aggression. Right orbitofrontal activity during inhibition of a motor response (i.e., the no-go condition of a go/no-go task) was reduced after tryptophan depletion [95]. In a laboratory aggression paradigm, tryptophan depletion was associated with reduced insula activity during selection of severity of aggressive response [89]. Acute challenges to the serotonergic system have also been shown to influence the processing of emotional faces [96] and associated neural activity. Tryptophan depletion modulated the functional connectivity that occurs between the amygdala and prefrontal regions specifically while processing angry faces, as opposed to neutral or sad faces [59].

Last, Grady *et al.* [97] compared the effects of attenuated and enhanced central 5-HT availability (with tryptophan depletion and acute citalopram administration, respectively) on the processing of neutral, angry, and fearful faces. First, they found two separate networks –one that was selective for fearful faces relative to angry and neutral expressions, and the other that distinguished between fearful and neutral faces, but with responses to angry faces that were intermediate to those of neutral and fearful ones. In both networks, tryptophan depletion specifically enhanced responses to angry faces, such that they were more like the responses to fear than neutrality. Citalopram treatment, on the other hand, led to neural network responses that were equivalent across the three emotions, yet by differing mechanisms. In the first network, increased 5-HT with citalopram decreased responses to fear equal to that of responses to neutrality. In the second network, on the other hand, citalopram increased responses to both neutral and angry faces to be similar to that of fear.

In summary, studies of acute manipulations of 5-HT availability in humans have provided strong support for a modulatory role of aggression by the 5-HTergic system. The mechanism by which 5-HT influences aggression is likely through neural networks involving the amygdala, ventro-medial prefrontal regions, and the striatum. These findings also make clear that the relationship between 5-HT and aggression is not a simple, linear function, and trait dimensions (namely aggression, impulsivity, psychopathy) and the quality of aggression (normal, pathological, reactive vs. proactive) are important moderating variables. The neural basis of the complex relationship between 5-HT and aggression likely owes to parallel neural circuits that are modulated by 5-HT, yet are differentially involved in the various facets of appraisal and response to social threat-stimuli.

Molecular biology of the 5-HT system in aggression: genetic, pharmacological, and neuroimaging studies

A wide variety of studies, methodologically speaking, have identified various molecular components of the 5-HT system involved in aggression, which can be broadly categorized as being involved in either 5-HT metabolism/turnover or 5-HT receptor signaling. Much of this work has been performed in animal genetic and pharmacological studies; however, there are also data from human genetic studies and neuro-chemical imaging.

5-HT synthesis and turnover: tryptophan hydroxylase-2

Tryptophan hydroxylase-2 (tph2) was recently found to be the brain-specific, rate-limiting enzyme mediating 5-HT synthesis [98]. The mouse tph2 single nucleotide polymorphism (SNP) C1437G has been associated with differential rates of 5-HT synthesis, and was used as a model to examine aggressive behavior, as well as depression and anxiety. Mice homozygous for the high-activity tph2 allele (1437C) were shown to exhibit greater levels of aggression compared to mice homozygous for the low-activity allele (1437G) [99]. Similarly, in a study in which highly aggressive mice were bred with a less aggressive laboratory breed, midbrain tph2 mRNA was shown to be positively correlated with the extent of severe aggression in certain resultant strains [100]. While these two former studies indicate that greater tph2 activity results in higher levels of aggression, mice with both tph2 copies deleted or "knocked out" (tph2 − / −) were found to be more aggressive than tph2(− / +) and tph2 (+ / +) mice [101]. Therefore, again, we see that the contribution of the 5-HT system to aggression is complex: "low" tph2 activity and "no" tph2 activity both affect aggression, albeit, in a contrasting manner. This is likely due to differential developmental pathways that occur in the absence of functional protein, and the development of qualitatively different forms of aggression.

To our knowledge, the human equivalent of a null tph2 mutation has not been identified. However, "risk" tph2 polymorphisms have been described in humans and nonhuman primates. Homozygosity for a functional tph2 SNP (associated with altered morning, basal cortisol levels) in rhesus monkeys was associated with attenuated aggressive behavior; however, this effect depended on a gene x environment interaction, as the anti-aggressive effect of this allele occurred only in those animals maternally reared, as opposed to being raised by peers [102]. Polymorphisms of tph2 have also been linked to anger-related personality traits [103,104]; Cluster B and C personality disorders; and the personality traits harm-avoidance [105] and reward dependence [106]. Our group recently found that a risk tph2 haplotype occurred with greater frequency in

patients with BPD compared to healthy controls, and BPD patients with the risk haplotype exhibited greater levels of aggression, as well as affective lability and suicidal/parasuicidal symptoms [107].

Polymorphisms of tph2 have also been related to structural and functional neuroanatomical differences related to aggression. Differential bilateral, dorsal amygdala reactivity to processing of angry/fearful faces (a putative biomarker of aggression) was shown to be related to tph2 polymorphism genotype [108]. In vivo 5-HT synthesis capacity, specifically, in the medial OFC – a brain region that plays a key role in aggression – has been shown to be related to tph2 polymorphisms in healthy, human control participants [109]. Moreover, carriers of a risk tph2 allele had larger medial OFC volumes [100], as well as reduced amygdala and hippocampal volumes [102].

5-HT synthesis and turnover: 5-HT transporter

The 5-HT transporter (5-HTT) is distributed along the axons and synaptic terminals of 5-HTergic neurons and plays an essential role in the clearance of extracellular 5-HT. There is a considerable mouse and human genetics literature on the role of the 5-HTT in aggression.

Attenuated aggression, as well as increased anxiety and stress-responses, were observed in mice with both 5-HTT genes knocked out (KO) [110,111]. Importantly, there appear to be interactions between genotype and the context of aggression. Homozygous 5-HTT KO mice were less aggressive than wild-type and heterozygous KO mice, specifically when in the opponent's environment as opposed to either a neutral or home setting. Heterozygous 5-HTT KO mice, on the other hand, were more aggressive than wild-type mice in their home environments, but no different than wild-type mice in a neutral setting or that of the opponent. Aggression was not affected by venue (home, neutral, or opponent's) in the wild-type. Last, no differences in aggression were found among the three genotypes in a neutral environment [110].

Mouse studies of genetically deleted 5-HTT have been complemented by those employing pharmacological antagonism of the 5-HTT (e.g., with fluoxetine treatment), which has allowed for the isolation of specific developmental periods. Interestingly, aggression in mature mice is reduced when mice are treated with fluoxetine during either an early postnatal period or a peri-adolescent one; increases in anxiety in the mature mouse, however, occur with fluoxetine treatment only during the early postnatal period, but not peri-adolescence [112]. Therefore, the developmental roles of 5-HTT in aggression and anxiety are not necessarily fully interdependent, particularly during the critical peri-adolescent period. Surprisingly, it was demonstrated that male offspring of mice treated with fluoxetine while pregnant (i.e., in utero 5-HTT inhibition) exhibited increased aggression and reduced anxiety [113], which, remarkably, is the opposite effect of postnatal fluoxetine treatment. Therefore, in addition to critical, early postnatal, and peri-adolescent developmental periods, in which 5-HTT antagonism lessens aggression in the adult, a separate, prenatal period may exist during which 5-HTT antagonism leads to increased aggression in the mature mouse.

Human genetic studies have also examined the role of the 5-HTT in aggression. The most common 5-HTT gene variant consists of the "short" and "long" forms of the 5-HTT promoter region (conventionally referred to as the 5-HTT-linked polymorphic region or 5-HTTLPR), which are associated with relatively decreased and increased expression, respectively [114]. Although at least one study, of adult males with intellectual disabilities, demonstrated an association between the long 5-HTTLPR allele and greater levels of aggression [115], the short allele has more consistently been shown to confer risk for aggression and violence in a range of populations [116–118]. Furthermore, it appears that the contribution of the short 5-HTTLPR allele to increased aggression is moderated by environmental factors, such as acute stress [119], recent, chronic stress [120], and childhood adversity [121].

In addition to the 5-HTTLPR, another risk polymorphism consists of a variable number of tandem repeats (VNTR) within intron 2 of the 5-HTT gene (STin2). The two major variants of STin2 consist of a 10- and 12-repeat, with the latter being the risk allele. Two studies have demonstrated that the contribution of risk by the 5-HTT gene for disinhibited/impulsive behavior [122] and aggression [123] was most discernible when both the 5-HTTLPR and STin2 polymorphisms were taken into account (namely, at least one short 5-HTTLPR allele and two STin2 12-repeat alleles).

In addition to assessing genotype, studies have begun to characterize the epigenetic status of the 5-HTT gene. Generally speaking, such studies have demonstrated a relationship between differential 5-HTT gene methylation and 5-HTT mRNA levels [124], vulnerability to PTSD [125], differences in depressive symptoms between monozygotic twins [126], hippocampal gray matter volume [127], and amygdala threat-related activity [128]. At least one study has demonstrated greater 5-HTT gene methylation in adults with a history of childhood aggression compared to adults without such a history; furthermore, in vivo brain 5-HT synthesis in the OFC was negatively correlated with 5-HTT gene methylation [129].

Neurochemical imaging studies, i.e., those employing PET or SPECT, have also been performed with radioligands with high affinity for 5-HTT. An early PET study of ours revealed lower 5-HTT binding in the left ACC in impulsive-aggressive personality disordered patients [130], which suggests attenuated presynaptic 5-HT in frontolimbic regions and, therefore, is consistent with the hyposerotonergic model of impulsive aggression. In a more recent study, employing a more specific radioligand and larger cohorts of personality disordered IED patients and healthy controls we did not observe the predicted inverse relationship between ACC 5-HTT availability and trait aggression until we statistically adjusted for trait callousness (a measure of the interpersonal/affective component of psychopathy), which itself was positively correlated with ACC 5-HTT availability [64].

5-HT synthesis and turnover: MAOA

Monoamine oxidase A (MAOA) is a catabolic enzyme present in the outer mitochondrial membrane of synaptic terminals of monoaminergic projection neurons; its major neurochemical substrates are 5-HT, NE, and to a lesser extent DA [131]. MAOA was one of the first genes identified as playing a role in the heritability of impulsive aggression, as a rare missense mutation was identified in a Dutch kindred with a significant history of impulsive aggression [132]. A more common human polymorphism of MAOA, consisting of a VNTR in the promoter region, has also been well characterized [133]. Carriers of the low-expressing MAOA-VNTR allele (3 repeats) exhibit greater aggression compared to those with the high-expressing allele (3.5 and 4 repeats) [134,135], and the low-expressing allele occurs more commonly in violent compared to nonviolent incarcerated males [136].

Moreover, numerous studies have demonstrated a gene x environment (GxE) effect, such that greater early-life stress increases the risk for impulsive aggression in males with the low-expressing MAOA-VNTR allele (note that this effect is most robust in men, as MAOA is an X-linked gene) [137]. This GxE effect has also been demonstrated in nonhuman primates [138,139]. Finally, using PET imaging with the MAOA radioligand [^{11}C] clorgyline, trait aggression in a healthy, nonclinical male population was negatively associated with brain MAOA availability in cortical and subcortical regions; furthermore, this effect was independent of MAOA-VNTR genotype [140].

Mouse genetic and pharmacological studies have helped to clarify the pathogenesis of MAOA-associated aggression. Increased aggression has been observed in both MAOA knockout mice [141] and mice with a naturally occurring mutation [142] that very closely mimics the rare missense mutation of the Dutch kindred (resulting, effectively, in a naturally occurring knockout). Early studies demonstrated that brain 5-HT levels, compared to NE and DA, are preferentially increased in the early postnatal phase of mice with MAOA gene deletions, thus suggesting that the increased aggression associated with loss or attenuation of MAOA activity was 5-HT-dependent [141]. However, while inhibition of 5-HT synthesis in the early postnatal period of MAOA deficient mice has been shown to abrogate certain neuroanatomical and behavioral changes [143], the development of heightened aggression, nevertheless, is unchanged [144]. Furthermore, inhibition of the dopamine transporter, but not the 5-HTT or the norepinephrine transporter, in developing mice leads to an aggressive phenotype comparable to that of MAOA deficient mice [112]. Therefore, a question for future studies will be to clarify the role of excessive 5-HT vs. DA in the pathogenesis of MAOA-dependent aggression.

Receptor subtypes: 5-HT1A

The 5-HT1A receptor plays a clear role in mood and anxiety disorders [145], and there is a growing literature examining its role in aggression, as well as the closely related construct of impulsivity. The 5-HT1A receptor is expressed on two neuronal populations: (1) as an autoreceptor, in a somato-dendritic distribution, on raphe serotonergic neurons; and (2) post-synaptically, on non-serotonergic hippocampal, septal, and cortical neurons. In both populations,

the 5-HT1A receptor promotes membrane hyperpolarization, and therefore, mediates an inhibitory action on target cells [146].

In various rodent models, pharmacological treatment with 5-HT1A agonists attenuates aggressive behaviors [147,148]; there is evidence for the importance of actions at both raphe autoreceptors and frontal postsynaptic receptors [149–152]. There is differential 5-HT1A receptor expression and 5-HT1A-dependent functional responses in rodent models of aggression [153–156]. In 5-HT1A receptor knockout mice, there is little to no evidence of altered aggression, despite a clear effect on measures related to mood and anxiety conditions. On the other hand, however, mice overexpressing the 5-HT1A receptor (specifically in raphe, 5-HTergic neurons) exhibited heightened aggression [157]. Importantly, this effect was dependent on overexpression of the 5-HT1A receptor during adulthood rather than developmentally.

In humans, agents with significant 5-HT1A receptor activity, e.g., buspirone, have not played a significant role in the pharmacotherapy of aggression and violence. Nevertheless, a consistent finding has been an inverse relationship between 5-HT1A receptor-dependent increases in serum cortisol and trait aggression in personality disordered patients [70,158,159]. In healthy participants, however, 5-HT1A receptor-dependent increases in serum cortisol were positively correlated with trait aggression, suggesting differential involvement of 5-HT1A receptor function in pathologic and "normal" forms of aggression. Polymorphisms of the 5-HT1A receptor gene have not been shown to be involved in impulsive aggression; however, they have been implicated in trait impulsivity [160] and BPD [161]. Curiously, 2 PET studies, both using the same 5-HT1A receptor radioligand ([11C]WAY100635) in healthy participants, demonstrated the opposite relation between frontal 5-HT1A receptor availability and trait aggression. One showed a positive [162] and the other an inverse correlation [163]. We speculate that the role of the 5-HT1A receptor in aggression may be due to pathophysiologic heterogeneity.

Receptor subtypes: 5-HT1B

The 5-HT1B receptor is expressed in raphe 5-HTergic neurons, as well as non-5-HTergic (namely GABAergic and glutamatergic) projection neurons originating from the striatum and hippocampus (namely, CA1 pyramidal cells). The receptors themselves are localized primarily at axonal terminals, and are believed to regulate neurotransmitter release [164]. Multiple rodent studies have demonstrated the ability of 5-HT1B agonists to mediate an anti-aggressive effect; however, which neuronal populations are responsible for this effect remains a matter of debate [150,165–172]. Mice with both copies of the 5-HT1B receptor gene knocked out have been shown to exhibit enhanced aggression [173] as well as greater impulsivity [174]. In humans, evidence for a role of the 5-HT1B receptor in aggression has been limited to genetic polymorphisms [175–178]. No PET imaging studies have been performed examining 5-HT1B receptor availability in aggression; however, such studies have been performed in externalizing or impulse control disorders, such as pathological gambling and alcohol dependence. In pathological gambling, 5-HT1B availability in the striatum and anterior cingulate was positively correlated with severity of gambling [179], and 5-HT1B availability was greater in the ventral striatum in patients with alcohol dependence compared to controls [180]. In major depression, on the other hand, 5-HT1B binding is decreased in the ventral striatum compared to controls [181]. Thus, there appear to be contrasting differences in 5-HT1B availability in impulse control disorders (increased 5-HT1B) compared to an "internalizing" condition (decreased 5-HT1B) such as major depression.

Receptor subtypes: 5-HT2A

Consistent with the important anti-aggressive and mood stabilizing effects of agents with 5-HT2A receptor antagonist activity, the 5-HT2A receptor has also been the focus of studies examining the etiology, pathogenesis, and pathophysiology of impulsive aggression. In animal pharmacological studies, the 5-HT2A receptor has been shown to promote impulsive and aggressive behavior [182–184]. A number of human genetic studies have revealed an association between 5-HT2A receptor polymorphisms and aggression [185] and impulse control disorders [186–191]. In a postmortem study of suicide victims, prefrontal 5-HT2A receptor binding was positively correlated with lifetime history of aggression [192].

A number of PET imaging studies have revealed an association between the 5-HT2A receptor and aggression and impulsivity; however, the results have been conflicting. We recently found that 5-HT2A receptor availability in the OFC was positively associated with state levels of aggression in a physically aggressive personality disordered (predominantly BPD) population meeting criteria for IED [58]. This finding was consistent with our view that OFC 5-HT2A receptor activity promotes aggression, in a dynamic, state-dependent manner, in those with IED. We suspect that increased OFC 5-HT2A receptor availability may be due to psychosocial stress [193], and that greater 5-HT2A receptor function in the OFC may promote aggression by decreasing amygdala–OFC coupling that occurs during threat processing [57]. At least two other studies found, however, that frontal 5-HT2A receptor availability was negatively correlated with trait aggression [194] in patients with BPD, and impulsivity [195] in a highly assaultive population with ASPD. Yet another study found no differences in cortical 5-HT2A receptor levels between high- and low-aggressive participants, as well as no relation to trait aggression or impulsivity [196].

These studies did not use a measure of state aggression and did not assess for whether participants met criteria for IED; therefore, it is difficult to compare these findings with our study. However, we suspect that the negative correlation between trait aggression and impulsivity and cortical 5-HT2A receptor availability may reflect a compensatory, albeit incomplete, downregulation of the 5-HT2A receptor in aggressive/impulsive individuals.

Receptor subtypes: 5-HT3

The 5-HT3 receptor is the only 5-HT receptor that functions as a ligand-gated ion channel, whereas all other known 5-HT receptors are G-protein coupled. The 5-HT3 receptor has both a pre- and postsynaptic distribution, and in the forebrain is expressed at least in part by a subpopulation of interneurons [197]. One 5-HT3-dependent mechanism of particular relevance to impulsivity and aggression is the regulation of mesolimbic dopamine release [198], which plays a key role in motivation and reward. The possibility that the 5-HT3 receptor is involved in impulsive aggression is limited to animal pharmacological studies, in which 5-HT3 receptor antagonists and agonists led to attenuated and increased aggressive behavior, respectively [199–203]. To our knowledge, no clinical studies have examined 5-HT3 receptor antagonists in aggression. In alcohol use disorders, however, 5-HT3 antagonism has been shown to lessen alcohol consumption [204], lessen subsyndromal mood symptoms [205], and attenuate alcohol cue-induced dopamine release in the ventral striatum [206]. Genetic polymorphisms of the 5-HT3 receptor have been associated with impulse control disorders, such as comorbid alcoholism and ASPD [207], and the pathological personality traits of harm avoidance and nonconformity [208]. Furthermore, 5-HT3 polymorphisms are associated with differential structure and function of limbic and prefrontal regions [209,210]. Future studies are needed to examine 5-HT3 antagonists clinically in aggressive populations, however.

Neurochemistry and Pharmacology: Dopamine

In contrast to the serotonergic system, much less has been described regarding the role of the dopaminergic (DAergic) system in aggression. Nevertheless, the DAergic system is poised to play an important role in aggression, given its involvement in decision making, reward, motivation, and higher-order cognitive processes. Additionally, the DAergic system is involved in the pathophysiology and psychopharmacology of conditions such as ADHD and schizophrenia, which commonly involve aggressive behavior.

A recent study by Schlüter et al. [211] is one of the first to use neurochemical imaging to specifically examine the role of the DAergic system in aggression in humans. Dopamine synthesis and storage capacity were assessed with PET imaging using [(18)F]DOPA in a cohort of healthy, nonclinical men who engaged in a computer-based laboratory task designed to assess aggressive reactions in response to provocation by an unseen and fictitious counterpart.

It was found that the frequency of aggressive responses by participants was inversely correlated with DA synthesis capacity, most notably in the midbrain, but also in the striatum. Additionally, DA storage capacity in the midbrain was negatively correlated with aggressive responses. These findings suggest that greater availability of dopamine may protect against non-advantageous, aggressive responses to provocation. Important questions that remain are (1) how do these findings relate to pathological forms of aggression occurring in a "real world" or non-laboratory

setting, and (2) which "down-stream," DA-modulated neuroanatomical regions are being affected and leading to differential aggressive responses?

As studies of dopaminergic neurochemistry and aggression are currently limited, comparison with findings of related constructs, such as psychopathy, may also be informative. Buckholtz et al. [212] assessed presynaptic DA release in a community sample of adults without a history of substance abuse, who were characterized with multiple self-report measures of various personality dimensions, including the Psychopathic Personality Inventory (PPI). Presynaptic DA release in the nucleus accumbens, a striatal region that plays a critical role in reward, was found to be positively correlated with the "impulsive-antisocial" component of the PPI; impulsive antisociality is related to, but is somewhat broader than, impulsive aggression. No relation between accumbal presynaptic dopamine was found with the "fearless dominance" component of the PPI, which consists of fearlessness, social influence, and stress immunity. Moreover, the relation between presynaptic DA release and impulsive antisociality remained significant even after adjusting for measures of impulsivity, extraversion, and novelty seeking.

Thus, there is an apparent conflict between the studies by Schlüter et al. [211] and Buckholtz et al. [212], with the former indicating a negative relationship between presynaptic DA and aggression and the latter suggesting the opposite. We suspect that the findings of the Schlüter et al. study may reflect the cognitive enhancing effects of adequate DAergic availability on fronto-cortical systems, which may mitigate maladaptive, aggressive responses to frustration. The increased presynaptic DA release in the ventral striatum observed in the Buckholtz et al. study, however, may reflect aberrant regulation at synaptic DA terminals in the ventral striatum, and therefore impairment of reward-related processes.

A somewhat broader literature exists regarding the molecular genetic basis of the role of the dopaminergic system in aggression. A number of studies have examined the role of catechol-O-methyltransferase (COMT), which is involved in the catabolism of DA as well as other catecholamines such as norepinephrine. The Val158Met polymorphism is a common and well-studied variant of COMT: the Met allele is the lower activity variant, resulting in higher basal levels of synaptic dopamine. Interestingly, in patients with BPD, a history of childhood sexual abuse was associated with lower levels of trait aggression, but only in those homozygous for the higher activity, Val158 COMT allele [213]. This suggests that early psychosocial adversity in those with low basal DA availability may attenuate trait aggression, at least in those predisposed to develop BPD. In patients with schizophrenia, the low activity, Met158 COMT allele has been shown to increase the risk of aggression and violence [214]. While not all studies investigating the Val158Met COMT polymorphism have demonstrated its involvement in aggression [215–217], less well-described COMT variants have been implicated in violent offenders with antisocial personality disorder [217], aggressive personality disordered patients [215], and highly aggressive children [218]. Questions for future studies are (a) to what extent is differential COMT activity involved in aggression during development as opposed to adult brain function, and (b) which catecholaminergic substrate of COMT is predominantly involved in determining aggression – DA, or others, such as norepinephrine?

At least two studies have demonstrated a role for the 48 bp repeat exon III polymorphism of the dopamine D4 receptor in aggression. The 7-repeat (7R) D4 polymorphism was found to be significantly more common in aggressive patients with schizophrenia, compared to non-aggressive schizophrenia patients and healthy controls [219]. Moreover, D4 7R allele carriers exhibited significantly greater "physical aggression against others" compared to the non-7R carriers; however, no differences in 7R allele frequency were observed with respect to other forms of aggression, namely "verbal aggression," "self-directed aggression," and "physical aggression against objects." Such a finding suggests the possibility, for example, that the D4 receptor could be related to proactive aggression, which consists of greater physical assaultiveness. In a separate study, a significant gene x environment interaction was found with the D4 receptor, such that increasing levels of prenatal stress were associated with higher levels of trait aggression manifested during young adulthood only in those with the 7R D4 allele [220]. Neither prenatal stress nor the 7R D4 allele alone was related to trait aggression during young adulthood. Moreover, this effect was specific for prenatal stress, as maternal stress up until the age of 15 of participants was not related to aggression, alone or as a function of D4 allele frequency.

These findings indicate that the DAergic system, in terms of gene x environment interactions, may be involved during development in determining an individual's propensity for aggression. Issues to be addressed in future studies include (a) whether DAergic agents, such as those targeting the D4 receptor, might have anti-aggressive therapeutic potential in the adult, and (b) whether aggression mediated by the DAergic system differs qualitatively from aggression related to 5-HTergic abnormalities.

Neurochemistry and Pharmacology: Vasopressin

While the arginine vasopressin (AVP) system has been well characterized in terms of its neuroendocrine role in the cardiovascular and renal systems, a significant number of animal studies have revealed its role as a direct neuromodulator in the CNS that regulates various social behaviors, such as aggression. Early studies in the hamster demonstrated that direct, hypothalamic administration of AVP enhanced aggressive responses [221,222], whereas AVP antagonists attenuated them [223]. More recent studies in a rat model of maternal aggression revealed that AVP release in the central nucleus of the amygdala was increased during maternal aggression, and the degree of AVP release was positively correlated with the degree of aggressive behavior. Furthermore, bilateral central amygdala administration of a vasopressin 1a receptor antagonist attenuated maternal aggression, and in a related rat strain with low levels of maternal aggression, AVP administration into the central amygdala nucleus increased aggression [224].

In mouse genetic models, knockout of the AVP 1b receptor reduced aggression [225,226], whereas deletion of the 1a receptor did not [227], despite the fact that pharmacological manipulations at the 1a receptor significantly influenced aggression and other social behaviors in animal models. A rat line with a naturally occurring deletion of the vasopressin gene also demonstrated decreased aggression and impulsivity [228].

Human studies have also lent support to the role of the AVP system in impulsive aggression. In a study of impulsive aggressive personality disordered patients, AVP obtained from the CSF was positively correlated with trait aggression, and negatively correlated with a measure of central 5-HTergic activity (i.e., fenfluramine-induced serum prolactin levels) [77].

The positive relation between CSF AVP and trait aggression persisted after covarying for fenfluramine-induced serum prolactin (an index of 5-HT activity), indicating that the relationship between AVP and aggression cannot simply be accounted for by the relationship between AVP and 5-HT. Intranasal administration of AVP has been shown to affect emotion processing in humans [229,230], and the orally available AVP V1a receptor antagonist, SRX246, was shown to block the effect of intranasal AVP on the neural responses to angry faces in the right amygdala and various other cortical regions associated with social information processing [231]. Last, a handful of human genetic studies have suggested that AVP receptor polymorphisms are associated with human aggression, particularly, the 1b receptor gene and childhood aggression [232–234].

Therefore, both genetic and pharmacological evidence in animal models and humans suggests that AVP may promote aggression in regions such as the central amygdala, and this effect may be mediated by the V1a and/or V1b receptors. Furthermore, pharmacological treatments that target the AVP system may be a novel therapeutic modality for aggressive behaviors.

Steroid Hormones: Cortisol and Testosterone

We will examine the steroid hormones cortisol and testosterone together, as there is growing evidence that these two steroid hormones may contribute to aggression and violence in an interdependent manner. Initial studies, of male adolescents with disruptive/delinquent behaviors, revealed a relationship between low baseline cortisol and heightened trait aggression [235]. Subsequently, it was found that a positive correlation between serum testosterone levels and aggression depended on the presence of low serum cortisol [236]. Thus, the effect of testosterone on aggression appeared to be moderated by serum cortisol levels.

More recent studies have revealed that the interaction between cortisol and testosterone may be more complex than a "high testosterone/low cortisol" model, and we suspect this may be related to gender and whether participants are either healthy/nonclinical, or are highly aggressive and/or exhibit psychopathic traits. For example, in nonclinical participants, trait aggression was positively associated, only in men, in those with either (a) high levels of testosterone in conjunction with high SSRI-induced cortisol, or (b) low testosterone and low SSRI-induced cortisol [237]. In a separate study, also in nonclinical participants, subclinical psychopathic traits was positively related to testosterone levels in those with high cortisol, and conversely, in those with low cortisol, subclinical psychopathy was negatively related to testosterone levels; both of these effects were only observed in the male participants [238]. In a study of a nonclinical group of women, aggressive responses after provocation in a laboratory setting were greater either in those with high testosterone/high cortisol or low testosterone/low cortisol [239]. Last, within a criminal population, morning cortisol levels were negatively correlated with psychopathy scores in psychopathic criminals, but not nonpsychopathic ones [240]. Therefore, while testosterone and cortisol appear to be inter-related with respect to aggression, the nature of this relationship likely differs as a function of variables such as gender, psychopathy, and other pathological personality dimensions.

Studies have begun to reveal potential neurobiological mechanisms that underlie the effect of cortisol and testosterone on aggression. Derntl et al. [241] demonstrated that reaction times to recognizing fearful male faces, specifically, was negatively related to morning testosterone levels in a nonclinical male population. In other words, greater testosterone levels were associated with recognizing fearful male faces more quickly. Notably, no relationship between testosterone and reaction times to recognizing other emotional facial expressions was observed [241], indicating that this effect was specific to the fear-processing circuitry associated with aggression, rather than a more global effect on facial affect processing. Amygdala responses to angry and fearful facial expressions, specifically, were directly correlated with testosterone levels [241], thus implicating the amygdala fear-processing circuitry as a potential substrate of the aggression-promoting effects of testosterone.

Hermans et al. [242] found that in a group of nonclinical, female participants, the degree of activation of the amygdala, hypothalamus, and brainstem while viewing angry faces was directly related to the baseline testosterone-to-cortisol (T/C) ratio. Interestingly, while the lateral OFC was also activated in response to angry faces in this study, its activity was not related to the T/C ratio, indicating that contribution of these steroid hormones may act on specific anger-associated brain circuits. In a nonclinical group of women, van Wingen *et al.* [243] found that intranasal testosterone administration reduced functional coupling of the left amygdala with the left OFC and with the right amygdala while performing a facial emotional processing task, indicating that testosterone may modulate amygdala–PFC circuitry involved in social threat processing. Finally, exogenous testosterone administration, after first normalizing endogenous testosterone with treatment with a gonadotropin releasing hormone antagonist in a group of nonclinical males, was associated with increased amygdala, hypothalamus, and periaqueductal gray activity, compared to placebo, while viewing angry facial expressions [244].

Collectively, these findings suggest that cortisol and testosterone influence aggression and related factors such as psychopathy in an interdependent manner; however, this relationship is complex, and likely depends on factors such as age, gender, and degree of trait aggression and psychopathy. Cortisol and testosterone likely influence aggression and psychopathy through the modulation of amygdala–PFC fear or threat circuitry. Areas of focus for future studies consist of identifying the precise loci of action of these steroid hormones, as well as the underlying cellular, molecular, and physiologic effects.

Conclusion

The studies we examined in this review have enhanced our understanding of the neurobiology of aggression and violence, but have also revealed areas of inconsistency that require clarification, as well as clues for avenues of future inquiries.

A relatively consistent and specific finding has been an association between reduced amygdala volumes and greater levels of trait aggression. Optimal resolution of this relationship appears to require analysis of a number of additional variables, such as amygdala subregion and hemisphere, aggression subtype (reactive vs. proactive), and co-variant dimensions (namely impulsivity, emotional reactivity, and psychopathy). Inconsistencies between studies – such as some demonstrating reduced whole amygdala volumes, bilaterally, and others indicating a specific involvement of the left dorsal amygdala – likely are resolvable by accounting for these anatomical and phenomenological factors. Therefore, it is likely that different processes (namely perceptual vs. motor; effortful vs.

habitual) of different aggression subtypes are a function of amygdala subregion and hemisphere.

In terms of functional abnormalities, pathological aggression is associated with a more labile range of amygdala activity, as well as differential amygdala responsivity to socially threatening stimuli. Commonly, aggression is associated with heightened amygdala reactivity to socially threatening stimuli (e.g., fearful or angry faces), and, remarkably, responses to neutral interpersonal stimuli (e.g., neutral facial expression) are also heightened. Amygdala hyporesponsiveness to threat, however, has also been observed, and this may be related to elements of aggression that are driven by the interpersonal/affective dimensions of psychopathy. Similar to the inconsistencies of amygdala volumetric changes, disentangling the role of amygdala hyper- vs. hyporesponsiveness to interpersonally salient cues will also likely require resolving the amygdala into its component functional subregions and characterizing aggression subtypes and associated dimensions. Furthermore, the 5-HTergic system also appears to be involved in determining amygdala responses to neutral and aversive interpersonal stimuli, and this effect may also be subregion- and circuit-dependent.

An important issue that remains unexamined relates to the cellular and ultrastructural basis of amygdala volumetric alterations, as well as the mechanism by which such changes yield the above-described functional differences. Animal models suggest that morphological alterations in the amygdala may reflect decreased dendritic arborization of excitatory [245–248] and local inhibitory neurons [249], which could therefore disrupt both "top-down" cortical inhibition as well as local inhibitory processes. As stress hormones or glucocorticoids are involved in dendritic remodeling in limbic regions in animal models, a potential avenue for future studies may be determining whether the cortisol abnormalities observed in aggressive individuals are related to amygdala structural changes. Such a line of inquiry would also have the potential for developing therapeutic strategies, such as those that involve pharmacological manipulation of the hypothalamic–pituitary–adrenal axis.

The OFC and ACC are limbic prefrontal regions that also play a key role in the neurobiology of aggression, particularly in terms of their interconnectivity with the amygdala. Involvement of the OFC and its coupling with the amygdala likely impairs (a) the ability to ascribe affective and motivational significance to stimuli in a manner that is integrated, moderated, and flexible; and (b) "top-down" modulation of central nucleus output, leading to an increased likelihood of a "visceral/ sympathetic" component to a stimulus representation. Altered coupling between the ACC and amygdala suggests a disruption of effortful cognitive modulation of subcortical affect processing (pregenual ACC), as well as the development of negative self-referential emotional states (subgenual ACC).

A burgeoning literature has begun to illustrate the role of the striatum in aggression. Dysfunction of the ventral striatum likely contributes to aggression, owing to disturbances in the processing of expected outcome values, and therefore, phenomena such as "frustration." Altered activity of the dorsomedial striatum may contribute to aggression by affecting the expected value or required effort associated with specific responses/actions.

Neurochemical systems are involved in aggression in at least two ways: (1) influencing central nervous system development during critical prenatal and postnatal periods, and (2) modulating developed neural system/network parameters. The relationship between 5-HT availability during development and aggression is complex. For example, the absence of 5-HT synthesis (tph2 knock-out) as well as excessive 5-HT synthesis capacity (high-activity tph2 polymorphism) can yield an aggressive phenotype in rodent genetic models. Furthermore, the prenatal and postnatal effects of 5-HTT pharmacological inhibition in animal models also appear to differ, as they lead to increased and decreased aggression, respectively. The developmental role of DA is also beginning to be elucidated, and excessive DA availability may contribute to a particularly severe form of aggression. A number of gene x environment interactions have been described, including polymorphisms of tph2, 5-HTT, MAOA, the D4 receptor and COMT, and early adversity.

Low basal levels of presynaptic 5-HT, particularly in corticolimbic regions, such as the ACC, are believed to contribute to trait levels of aggression, possibly by diminishing the efficacy of cognitive control of amygdala and striatal processes. Increased 5-HT2A receptor function in the medial OFC may influence state levels of aggression, possibly by decreasing OFC–amygdala coupling. The 5-HT1B receptor appears poised to influence aggression by its presynaptic location on 5-HTergic and GABAergic neurons projecting from the raphe and striatum, respectively, to the midbrain DAergic system. The 5-HT3 receptor also may play a role in aggression through a number of potential mechanisms, such as presynaptic modulation of DA release in the striatum. While clearly implicated in mood and anxiety disorders, the contribution of the 5-HT1A receptor in aggression is less clear; however, it may play a role in impulsivity.

Greater DAergic synthesis and storage capacity may attenuate aggression, possibly by modulating error/reward signals in striatal regions and/or by enhancing cortical cognitive processes. The neuropeptide VIP may enhance aggression through its actions in the central nucleus of the amygdala, in a manner possibly antagonistic to that of 5-HT's effect. The steroid hormones cortisol and testosterone interact to determine aggression and related constructs, such as psychopathy, possibly through their effects on amygdala–frontal connectivity. The standard view has been that low cortisol permits high testosterone to promote aggression; however, their inter-relationship appears to be more complex and dependent on a number of other variables.

There are a number of essential questions that deserve the focus of future studies. The first relates to the various forms of heterogeneity and potential confounds in the study of aggression: What are the convergent and divergent neural correlates of aggression subtypes, namely, reactive and proactive aggression? Further, how do the neural correlates of reactive and proactive aggression relate to those of their associated personality dimensions, namely negative emotionality and impulsivity, and psychopathy, respectively? How does aggression differ between nonclinical participants, and personality disordered patients with and without IED? How do the various etiopathogenetic variants of aggression differ both phenomenologically and neurobiologically? And how do different etiopathogenetic factors interact – e.g., MAOA and 5-HTT risk polymorphisms, and do these interactions possibly contribute to qualitative differences in aggression severity? In addition to these phenomenological and etiopathogenic factors, it will also be essential that neuroanatomical regions are well defined with respect to their functional subdivisions.

Future neurobiological studies will also offer the opportunity to address important clinical goals.

In this review, we described various candidate therapeutic targets that deserve further characterization, such as the 5-HT1B and 5-HT3 receptors, the D4 receptor, and the AVP V1a and V1b receptors. Therefore, PET imaging studies of these receptors may help to clarify their role in the pathophysiology of aggression, and pharmacological challenges with ligands to these targets, in combination with brain imaging and laboratory aggression paradigms, may provide initial evidence as to their anti-aggressive efficacy.

The genetic and developmental studies described here have laid the groundwork for identifying biomarkers that could be used to identify at-risk individuals and to develop potential interventions to disrupt the pathogenesis of aggression. Clarifying, for example, the differential contribution of 5-HT vs. DA in MAOA-dependent pathogenic mechanisms would allow for more rationally designed developmental interventions. Finally, as the neural circuitry of aggression is now better understood, dimensional biomarkers could be characterized that would represent sensitivity to specific treatments.

Disclosures

Daniel Rosell has the following disclosure: Dept. of Veterans Affairs, employee, salary. Larry Siever has the following disclosure: NIMH, researcher, salary/research support.

References

1. Hall JE, Simon TR, Lee RD, Mercy JA. Implications of direct protective factors for public health research and prevention strategies to reduce youth violence. *Am. J. Prev. Med.* 2012; **43**(2 Suppl 1): S76–S83.

2. Modi MN, Palmer S, Armstrong A. The role of Violence Against Women Act in addressing intimate partner violence: a public health issue. *J. Womens Health (Larchmt).* 2014; **23**(3): 253–259.

3. Ramsay SE, Bartley A, Rodger AJ. Determinants of assault-related violence in the community: potential for public health interventions in hospitals. *Emerg. Med. J.* 2014; **31**: 986–989.

4. Whitaker S. Preventing violent conflict: a revised mandate for the public health professional? *J. Public Health Policy.* 2013; **34**(1): 46–54.

5. Bushman BJ, Anderson CA. Is it time to pull the plug on the hostile versus instrumental aggression dichotomy? *Psychol. Rev.* 2001; **108**(1): 273–279.

6. Baker LA, Raine A, Liu J, Jacobson KC. Differential genetic and environmental influences on reactive and proactive aggression in children. *J. Abnorm. Child Psychol.* 2008; **36**(8): 1265–1278.

7. Bezdjian S, Tuvblad C, Raine A, Baker LA. The genetic and environmental covariation among psychopathic personality traits, and reactive and proactive aggression in childhood. *Child Dev.* 2011; **82**(4): 1267–1281.

8. Cima M, Raine A, Meesters C, Popma A. Validation of the Dutch Reactive Proactive Questionnaire (RPQ): differential correlates of reactive and proactive aggression from childhood to adulthood. *Aggress. Behav.* 2013; **39**(2): 99–113.

9. Fossati A, Raine A, Borroni S, *et al.* A cross-cultural study of the psychometric properties of the Reactive-Proactive Aggression Questionnaire among Italian nonclinical adolescents. *Psychol. Assess.* 2009; **21**(1): 131–135.

10. Fung AL, Raine A, Gao Y. Cross-cultural generalizability of the Reactive-Proactive Aggression Questionnaire (RPQ). *J. Pers. Assess.* 2009; **91**(5): 473–479.

11. Raine A, Dodge K, Loeber R, *et al.* The Reactive-Proactive Aggression Questionnaire: differential correlates of reactive and proactive aggression in adolescent boys. *Aggress .Behav.* 2006; **32**(2): 159–171.

12. Gardner KJ, Archer J, Jackson S. Does maladaptive coping mediate the relationship between borderline personality traits and reactive and proactive aggression? *Aggress. Behav.* 2012; **38**(5): 403–413.

13. Lobbestael J, Cima M, Arntz A. The relationship between adult reactive and proactive aggression, hostile interpretation bias, and antisocial personality disorder. *J. Pers. Disord.* 2013; **27**(1): 53–66.

14. Dodge KA, Lochman JE, Harnish JD, Bates JE, Pettit GS. Reactive and proactive aggression in school children and psychiatrically impaired chronically assaultive youth. *J. Abnorm. Psychol.* 1997; **106**(1): 37–51.

15. Kolla NJ, Malcolm C, Attard S, *et al.* Childhood maltreatment and aggressive behaviour in violent offenders with psychopathy. *Can. J. Psychiatry.* 2013; **58**(8): 487–494.

16. Arsenio WF, Adams E, Gold J. Social information processing, moral reasoning, and emotion attributions: relations with adolescents' reactive and proactive aggression. *Child Dev.* 2009; **80** (6): 1739–1755.

17. Crick NR, Dodge KA. Social information-processing mechanisms in reactive and proactive aggression. *Child Dev.* 1996; **67**(3): 993–1002.

18. Dodge KA, Coie JD. Social-information-processing factors in reactive and proactive aggression in children's peer groups. *J. Pers. Soc. Psychol.* 1987; **53**(6): 1146–1158.

19. Hubbard JA, Dodge KA, Cillessen AH, Coie JD, Schwartz D. The dyadic nature of social information processing in boys' reactive and proactive aggression. *J. Pers. Soc. Psychol.* 2001; **80**(2): 268–280.

20. Smithmyer CM, Hubbard JA, Simons RF. Proactive and reactive aggression in delinquent adolescents: relations to aggression outcome expectancies. *J. Clin. Child Psychol.* 2000; **29**(1): 86–93.

21. Walters GD. Measuring proactive and reactive criminal thinking with the PICTS: correlations with outcome expectancies and hostile attribution biases. *J. Interpers. Violence.* 2007; **22**(4): 371–385.

22. Brugman S, Lobbestael J, Arntz A, *et al.* Identifying cognitive predictors of reactive and proactive aggression. *Aggress. Behav.* 2014; **41**: 51–64. DOI: 10.1002/AB.21573.

23. Coccaro EF, Kavoussi RJ, Berman ME, Lish JD. Intermittent explosive disorder–revised: development, reliability, and validity of research criteria. *Compr. Psychiatry.* 1998; **39**(6): 368–376.

24. McCloskey MS, Berman ME, Noblett KL, Coccaro EF. Intermittent explosive disorder-integrated research diagnostic criteria: convergent and discriminant validity. *J. Psychiatr. Res.* 2006; **40**(3): 231–242.

25. Coccaro EF. Intermittent explosive disorder: development of integrated research criteria for Diagnostic and Statistical Manual of Mental Disorders, *Fifth Edition. Compr. Psychiatry.* 2011; **52**(2): 119–125.

26. Coccaro EF, Lee R, Kavoussi RJ. Aggression, suicidality, and intermittent explosive disorder: serotonergic correlates in personality disorder and healthy control subjects. *Neuropsychopharmacology.* 2010; **35**(2): 435–444.

27. Salzman CD, Fusi S. Emotion, cognition, and mental state representation in amygdala and prefrontal cortex. *Annu. Rev. Neurosci.* 2010; **33**: 173–202.

28. Fernando AB, Murray JE, Milton AL. The amygdala: securing pleasure and avoiding pain. *Front. Behav. Neurosci.* 2013; **7**: 190.

29. Sah P, Faber ES, Lopez De AM, Power J. The amygdaloid complex: anatomy and physiology. *Physiol. Rev.* 2003; **83**(3): 803–834.

30. John YJ, Bullock D, Zikopoulos B, Barbas H. Anatomy and computational modeling of networks underlying cognitive-emotional interaction. *Front. Hum. Neurosci.* 2013; **7**: 101.

31. Lee S, Kim SJ, Kwon OB, Lee JH, Kim JH. Inhibitory networks of the amygdala for emotional memory. *Front. Neural. Circuits.* 2013; **7**: 129.

32. Bzdok D, Laird AR, Zilles K, Fox PT, Eickhoff SB. An investigation of the structural, connectional, and functional subspecialization in the human amygdala. *Hum. Brain Mapp.* 2013; **34**(12): 3247–3266.

33. Matthies S, Rusch N, Weber M, *et al.* Small amygdala-high aggression? The role of the amygdala in modulating aggression in healthy subjects. *World J. Biol. Psychiatry.* 2012; **13**(1): 75–81.

34. Pardini DA, Raine A, Erickson K, Loeber R. Lower amygdala volume in men is associated with childhood aggression, early psychopathic traits, and future violence. *Biol. Psychiatry.* 2014; **75**(1): 73–80.

35. Gopal A, Clark E, Allgair A, *et al.* Dorsal/ventral parcellation of the amygdala: relevance to impulsivity and aggression. *Psychiatry Res.* 2013; **211**(1): 24–30.

36. Bobes MA, Ostrosky F, Diaz K, *et al.* Linkage of functional and structural anomalies in the left amygdala of reactive-aggressive men. *Soc. Cogn. Affect. Neurosci.* 2013; **8**(8): 928–936.

37. Dyck M, Loughead J, Kellermann T, *et al.* Cognitive versus automatic mechanisms of mood induction differentially activate left and right amygdala. *Neuroimage.* 2011; **54**(3): 2503–2513.

38. New AS, Hazlett EA, Newmark RE, *et al.* Laboratory induced aggression: a positron emission tomography study of aggressive individuals with borderline personality disorder. *Biol. Psychiatry.* 2009; **66**(12): 1107–1114.

39. Coccaro EF, McCloskey MS, Fitzgerald DA, Phan KL. Amygdala and orbitofrontal reactivity to social threat in individuals with impulsive aggression. *Biol. Psychiatry.* 2007; **62**(2): 168–178.

40. Lozier LM, Cardinale EM, Vanmeter JW, Marsh AA. Mediation of the relationship between callous-unemotional traits and proactive aggression by amygdala response to fear among children with conduct problems. *JAMA Psychiatry.* 2014; **71**(6): 627–636.

41. Walton ME, Croxson PL, Behrens TE, Kennerley SW, Rushworth MF. Adaptive decision making and value in the anterior cingulate cortex. *Neuroimage.* 2007; **36**(Suppl 2): T142–T154.

42. Rudebeck PH, Murray EA. The orbitofrontal oracle: cortical mechanisms for the prediction and evaluation of specific behavioral outcomes. *Neuron.* 2014; **84**(6): 1143–1156.

43. Gansler DA, McLaughlin NC, Iguchi L, et al. A multivariate approach to aggression and the orbital frontal cortex in psychiatric patients. *Psychiatry Res.* 2009; **171**(3): 145–154.

44. Antonucci AS, Gansler DA, Tan S, et al. Orbitofrontal correlates of aggression and impulsivity in psychiatric patients. *Psychiatry Res.* 2006; **147**(2–3): 213–220.

45. Boes AD, Tranel D, Anderson SW, Nopoulos P. Right anterior cingulate: a neuroanatomical correlate of aggression and defiance in boys. *Behav. Neurosci.* 2008; **122**(3): 677–684.

46. Ducharme S, Hudziak JJ, Botteron KN, et al. Right anterior cingulate cortical thickness and bilateral striatal volume correlate with child behavior checklist aggressive behavior scores in healthy children. *Biol .Psychiatry.* 2011; **70**(3): 283–290.

47. Soloff PH, Meltzer CC, Greer PJ, Constantine D, Kelly TM. A fenfluramine-activated FDG-PET study of borderline personality disorder. *Biol. Psychiatry.* 2000; **47**(6): 540–547.

48. New AS, Hazlett EA, Buchsbaum MS, et al. Blunted prefrontal cortical 18fluorodeoxyglucose positron emission tomography response to meta-chlorophenylpiperazine in impulsive aggression. *Arch. Gen. Psychiatry.* 2002; **59**(7): 621–629.

49. Ghashghaei HT, Hilgetag CC, Barbas H. Sequence of information processing for emotions based on the anatomic dialogue between prefrontal cortex and amygdala. *Neuroimage.* 2007; **34**(3): 905–923.

50. Timbie C, Barbas H. Specialized pathways from the primate amygdala to posterior orbitofrontal cortex. *J. Neurosci.* 2014; **34**(24): 8106–8118.

51. Ghashghaei HT, Barbas H. Pathways for emotion: interactions of prefrontal and anterior temporal pathways in the amygdala of the rhesus monkey. *Neuroscience.* 2002; **115**(4): 1261–1279.

52. Roy AK, Shehzad Z, Margulies DS, et al. Functional connectivity of the human amygdala using resting state fMRI. *Neuroimage.* 2009; **45**(2): 614–626.

53. Hoptman MJ, D'Angelo D, Catalano D, et al. Amygdalofrontal functional disconnectivity and aggression in schizophrenia. *Schizophr. Bull.* 2010; **36**(5): 1020–1028.

54. Fulwiler CE, King JA, Zhang N. Amygdala-orbitofrontal restingstate functional connectivity is associated with trait anger. *Neuroreport.* 2012; **23**(10): 606–610.

55. Beyer F, Munte TF, Wiechert J, Heldmann M, Kramer UM. Trait aggressiveness is not related to structural connectivity between orbitofrontal cortex and amygdala. *PLoS One.* 2014; **9**(6): e101105.

56. New AS, Hazlett EA, Buchsbaum MS, et al. Amygdala-prefrontal disconnection in borderline personality disorder. *Neuropsychopharmacology.* 2007; **32**(7): 1629–1640.

57. Hornboll B, Macoveanu J, Rowe J, et al. Acute serotonin 2A receptor blocking alters the processing of fearful faces in the orbitofrontal cortex and amygdala. *J. Psychopharmacol.* 2013; **27**(10): 903–914.

58. Rosell DR, Thompson JL, Slifstein M, et al. Increased serotonin 2A receptor availability in the orbitofrontal cortex of physically aggressive personality disordered patients. *Biol. Psychiatry.* 2010; **67**(12): 1154–1162.

59. Passamonti L, Crockett MJ, Apergis-Schoute AM, et al. Effects of acute tryptophan depletion on prefrontal-amygdala connectivity while viewing facial signals of aggression. *Biol. Psychiatry.* 2012; **71**(1): 36–43.

60. Pezawas L, Meyer-Lindenberg A, Drabant EM, et al. 5-HTTLPR polymorphism impacts human cingulate-amygdala interactions: a genetic susceptibility mechanism for depression. *Nat. Neurosci.* 2005; **8**(6): 828–834.

61. Heinz A, Braus DF, Smolka MN, et al. Amygdala-prefrontal coupling depends on a genetic variation of the serotonin transporter. *Nat. Neurosci.* 2005; **8**(1): 20–21.

62. Haber SN. The primate basal ganglia: parallel and integrative networks. *J. Chem. Neuroanat.* 2003; **26**(4): 317–330.

63. Crockett MJ, Apergis-Schoute A, Herrmann B, et al. Serotonin modulates striatal responses to fairness and retaliation in humans. *J. Neurosci.* 2013; **33**(8): 3505–3513.

64. van de Giessen E, Rosell DR, Thompson JL, et al. Serotonin transporter availability in impulsive aggressive personality disordered patients: a PET study with [(11)C]DASB. *J. Psychiatr. Res.* 2014; **58**: 147–154.

65. Malick JB, Barnett A. The role of serotonergic pathways in isolation-induced aggression in mice. *Pharmacol. Biochem. Behav.* 1976; **5**(1): 55–61.

66. Brown GL, Goodwin FK, Ballenger JC, Goyer PF, Major LF. Aggression in humans correlates with cerebrospinal fluid amine metabolites. *Psychiatry Res.* 1979; **1**(2): 131–139.

67. Brown GL, Ebert MH, Goyer PF, et al. Aggression, suicide, and serotonin: relationships to CSF amine metabolites. *Am. J. Psychiatry.* 1982; **139**(6): 741–746.

68. Brown CS, Kent TA, Bryant SG, et al. Blood platelet uptake of

serotonin in episodic aggression. *Psychiatry Res.* 1989; **27**(1): 5–12.

69. Stoff DM, Pollock L, Vitiello B, Behar D, Bridger WH. Reduction of (3H)-imipramine binding sites on platelets of conduct-disordered children. *Neuropsychopharmacology.* 1987; **1**(1): 55–62.

70. Coccaro EF, Kavoussi RJ, Hauger RL. Physiological responses to d-fenfluramine and ipsapirone challenge correlate with indices of aggression in males with personality disorder. *Int. Clin. Psychopharmacol.* 1995; **10**(3): 177–179.

71. Coccaro EF, Berman ME, Kavoussi RJ, Hauger RL. Relationship of prolactin response to d-fenfluramine to behavioral and questionnaire assessments of aggression in personality-disordered men. *Biol. Psychiatry.* 1996; **40**(3): 157–164.

72. Coccaro EF, Kavoussi RJ, Cooper TB, Hauger RL. Central serotonin activity and aggression: inverse relationship with prolactin response to d-fenfluramine, but not CSF 5-HIAA concentration, in human subjects. *Am. J. Psychiatry.* 1997; **154**(10): 1430–1435.

73. Coccaro EF, Astill JL, Herbert JL, Schut AG. Fluoxetine treatment of impulsive aggression in DSM-III-R personality disorder patients. *J. Clin. Psychopharmacol.* 1990; **10**(5): 373–375.

74. Coccaro EF, Kavoussi RJ. Fluoxetine and impulsive aggressive behavior in personality-disordered subjects. *Arch. Gen. Psychiatry.* 1997; **54**(12): 1081–1088.

75. Kruesi MJ, Rapoport JL, Hamburger S, *et al.* Cerebrospinal fluid monoamine metabolites, aggression, and impulsivity in disruptive behavior disorders of children and adolescents. *Arch. Gen. Psychiatry.* 1990; **47**(5): 419–426.

76. Coccaro EF, Lee R. Cerebrospinal fluid 5-hydroxyindolacetic acid and homovanillic acid: reciprocal relationships with impulsive aggression in human subjects. *J. Neural. Transm.* 2010; **117**(2): 241–248.

77. Coccaro EF, Kavoussi RJ, Hauger RL, Cooper TB, Ferris CF. Cerebrospinal fluid vasopressin levels: correlates with aggression and serotonin function in personality-disordered subjects. *Arch. Gen. Psychiatry.* 1998; **55**(8): 708–714.

78. Goveas JS, Csernansky JG, Coccaro EF. Platelet serotonin content correlates inversely with life history of aggression in personality-disordered subjects. *Psychiatry Res.* 2004; **126**(1): 23–32.

79. Coccaro EF, Kavoussi RJ, Sheline YI, Berman ME, Csernansky JG. Impulsive aggression in personality disorder correlates with platelet 5-HT2A receptor binding. *Neuropsychopharmacology.* 1997; **16**(3): 211–216.

80. Marseille R, Lee R, Coccaro EF. Inter-relationship between different platelet measures of 5-HT and their relationship to aggression in human subjects. *Prog. Neuropsychopharmacol. Biol. Psychiatry.* 2012; **36**(2): 277–281.

81. Modai I, Gibel A, Rauchverger B, *et al.* Paroxetine binding in aggressive schizophrenic patients. *Psychiatry Res.* 2000; **94**(1): 77–81.

82. Sarne Y, Mandel J, Goncalves MH, *et al.* Imipramine binding to blood platelets and aggressive behavior in offenders, schizophrenics and normal volunteers. *Neuropsychobiology.* 1995; **31**(3): 120–124.

83. Coccaro EF, Kavoussi RJ, Hauger RL. Serotonin function and antiaggressive response to

fluoxetine: a pilot study. *Biol. Psychiatry.* 1997; **42**(7): 546–552.

84. Carpenter LL, Anderson GM, Pelton GH, *et al.* Tryptophan depletion during continuous CSF sampling in healthy human subjects. *Neuropsychopharmacology.* 1998; **19**(1): 26–35.

85. Moreno FA, McGavin C, Malan TP, *et al.* Tryptophan depletion selectively reduces CSF 5-HT metabolites in healthy young men: results from single lumbar puncture sampling technique. *Int. J. Neuropsychopharmacol.* 2000; **3**(4): 277–283.

86. Williams WA, Shoaf SE, Hommer D, Rawlings R, Linnoila M. Effects of acute tryptophan depletion on plasma and cerebrospinal fluid tryptophan and 5-hydroxyindoleacetic acid in normal volunteers. *J. Neurochem.* 1999; **72**(4): 1641–1647.

87. Bjork JM, Dougherty DM, Moeller FG, Cherek DR, Swann AC. The effects of tryptophan depletion and loading on laboratory aggression in men: time course and a food-restricted control. *Psychopharmacology (Berl).* 1999; **142**(1): 24–30.

88. Bjork JM, Dougherty DM, Moeller FG, Swann AC. Differential behavioral effects of plasma tryptophan depletion and loading in aggressive and nonaggressive men. *Neuropsychopharmacology.* 2000; **22**(4): 357–369.

89. Kramer UM, Riba J, Richter S, Munte TF. An fMRI study on the role of serotonin in reactive aggression. *PLoS One.* 2011; **6**(11): e27668.

90. Kotting WF, Bubenzer S, Helmbold K, *et al.* Effects of tryptophan depletion on reactive aggression and aggressive decision-making in young people with ADHD. *Acta Psychiatr. Scand.* 2013; **128**(2): 114–123.

91. Stadler C, Zepf FD, Demisch L, *et al.* Influence of rapid tryptophan depletion on laboratory-provoked aggression in children with ADHD. *Neuropsychobiology.* 2007; **56** (2–3): 104–110.

92. Zimmermann M, Grabemann M, Mette C, *et al.* The effects of acute tryptophan depletion on reactive aggression in adults with attention-deficit/hyperactivity disorder (ADHD) and healthy controls. *PLoS One.* 2012; 7(3): e32023.

93. Fanning JR, Berman ME, Guillot CR, Marsic A, McCloskey MS. Serotonin (5-HT) augmentation reduces provoked aggression associated with primary psychopathy traits. *J. Pers. Disord.* 2014; **28**(3): 449–461.

94. Berman ME, McCloskey MS, Fanning JR, Schumacher JA, Coccaro EF. Serotonin augmentation reduces response to attack in aggressive individuals. *Psychol. Sci.* 2009; **20**(6): 714–720.

95. Rubia K, Lee F, Cleare AJ, *et al.* Tryptophan depletion reduces right inferior prefrontal activation during response inhibition in fast, event-related fMRI. *Psychopharmacology (Berl).* 2005; **179**(4): 791–803.

96. Lee RJ, Gill A, Chen B, McCloskey M, Coccaro EF. Modulation of central serotonin affects emotional information processing in impulsive aggressive personality disorder. *J. Clin. Psychopharmacol.* 2012; **32**(3): 329–335.

97. Grady CL, Siebner HR, Hornboll B, *et al.* Acute pharmacologically induced shifts in serotonin availability abolish emotion-selective responses to negative face emotions in distinct brain networks. *Eur. Neuropsychopharmacol.* 2013; **23**(5): 368–378.

98. Zhang X, Beaulieu JM, Sotnikova TD, Gainetdinov RR, Caron MG.

99. Osipova DV, Kulikov AV, Popova NK. C1473G polymorphism in mouse tph2 gene is linked to tryptophan hydroxylase-2 activity in the brain, intermale aggression, and depressive-like behavior in the forced swim test. *J. Neurosci. Res.* 2009; **87**(5): 1168–1174.

100. Takahashi A, Shiroishi T, Koide T. Genetic mapping of escalated aggression in wild-derived mouse strain MSM/Ms: association with serotonin-related genes. *Front. Neurosci.* 2014; **8**: 156.

101. Mosienko V, Bert B, Beis D, *et al.* Exaggerated aggression and decreased anxiety in mice deficient in brain serotonin. *Transl. Psychiatry.* 2012; **2**: e122.

102. Chen GL, Novak MA, Meyer JS, *et al.* The effect of rearing experience and TPH2 genotype on HPA axis function and aggression in rhesus monkeys: a retrospective analysis. *Horm. Behav.* 2010; **57**(2): 184–191.

103. Yang J, Lee MS, Lee SH, *et al.* Association between tryptophan hydroxylase 2 polymorphism and anger-related personality traits among young Korean women. *Neuropsychobiology.* 2010; **62**(3): 158–163.

104. Yoon HK, Lee HJ, Kim L, Lee MS, Ham BJ. Impact of tryptophan hydroxylase 2 G-703T polymorphism on anger-related personality traits and orbitofrontal cortex. *Behav. Brain Res.* 2012; **231**(1): 105–110.

105. Gutknecht L, Jacob C, Strobel A, *et al.* Tryptophan hydroxylase-2 gene variation influences personality traits and disorders related to emotional dysregulation. *Int. J. Neuropsychopharmacol.* 2007; **10**(3): 309–320.

106. Inoue H, Yamasue H, Tochigi M, *et al.* Effect of tryptophan

hydroxylase-2 gene variants on amygdalar and hippocampal volumes. *Brain Res.* 2010; **1331**: 51–57.

107. Perez-Rodriguez MM, Weinstein S, New AS, *et al.* Tryptophan-hydroxylase 2 haplotype association with borderline personality disorder and aggression in a sample of patients with personality disorders and healthy controls. *J. Psychiatr. Res.* 2010; **44**(15): 1075–1081.

108. Brown SM, Peet E, Manuck SB, *et al.* A regulatory variant of the human tryptophan hydroxylase-2 gene biases amygdala reactivity. *Mol. Psychiatry.* 2005; **10**(9): 884–888.

109. Booij L, Turecki G, Leyton M, *et al.* Tryptophan hydroxylase(2) gene polymorphisms predict brain serotonin synthesis in the orbitofrontal cortex in humans. *Mol. Psychiatry.* 2012; **17**(8): 809–817.

110. Heiming RS, Monning A, Jansen F, *et al.* To attack, or not to attack? The role of serotonin transporter genotype in the display of maternal aggression. *Behav. Brain Res.* 2013; **242**: 135–141.

111. Holmes A, Murphy DL, Crawley JN. Reduced aggression in mice lacking the serotonin transporter. *Psychopharmacology (Berl.).* 2002; **161**(2): 160–167.

112. Yu Q, Teixeira CM, Mahadevia D, *et al.* Dopamine and serotonin signaling during two sensitive developmental periods differentially impact adult aggressive and affective behaviors in mice. *Mol. Psychiatry.* 2014; **19**(6): 688–698.

113. Kiryanova V, Dyck RH. Increased aggression, improved spatial memory, and reduced anxiety-like behaviour in adult male mice exposed to fluoxetine early in life. *Dev. Neurosci.* 2014; **36**(5): 396–408.

114. Heils A, Teufel A, Petri S, *et al.* Allelic variation of human serotonin transporter gene expression. *J. Neurochem.* 1996; **66**(6): 2621–2624.

115. May ME, Lightfoot DA, Srour A, Kowalchuk RK, Kennedy CH. Association between serotonin transporter polymorphisms and problem behavior in adult males with intellectual disabilities. *Brain Res.* 2010; **1357**: 97–103.

116. Hallikainen T, Saito T, Lachman HM, *et al.* Association between low activity serotonin transporter promoter genotype and early onset alcoholism with habitual impulsive violent behavior. *Mol. Psychiatry.* 1999; **4**(4): 385–388.

117. Haberstick BC, Smolen A, Hewitt JK. Family-based association test of the 5HTTLPR and aggressive behavior in a general population sample of children. *Biol. Psychiatry.* 2006; **59**(9): 836–843.

118. Beitchman JH, Baldassarra L, Mik H, *et al.* Serotonin transporter polymorphisms and persistent, pervasive childhood aggression. *Am. J. Psychiatry.* 2006; **163**(6): 1103–1105.

119. Verona E, Joiner TE, Johnson F, Bender TW. Gender specific gene-environment interactions on laboratory-assessed aggression. *Biol. Psychol.* 2006; **71**(1): 33–41.

120. Conway CC, Keenan-Miller D, Hammen C, *et al.* Coaction of stress and serotonin transporter genotype in predicting aggression at the transition to adulthood. *J. Clin. Child Adolesc. Psychol.* 2012; **41**(1): 53–63.

121. Reif A, Rosler M, Freitag CM, *et al.* Nature and nurture predispose to violent behavior: serotonergic genes and adverse childhood environment. *Neuropsychopharmacology.* 2007; **32**(11): 2375–2383.

122. Aluja A, Garcia LF, Blanch A, De LD, Fibla J. Impulsive-disinhibited personality and serotonin transporter gene polymorphisms: association study in an inmate's sample. *J. Psychiatr. Res.* 2009; **43**(10): 906–914.

123. Payer DE, Nurmi EL, Wilson SA, McCracken JT, London ED. Effects of methamphetamine abuse and serotonin transporter gene variants on aggression and emotion-processing neurocircuitry. *Transl. Psychiatry.* 2012; **2**: e80.

124. Philibert R, Madan A, Andersen A, *et al.* Serotonin transporter mRNA levels are associated with the methylation of an upstream CpG island. *Am. J. Med. Genet. B Neuropsychiatr. Genet.* 2007; **144B**(1): 101–105.

125. Koenen KC, Uddin M, Chang SC, *et al.* SLC6A4 methylation modifies the effect of the number of traumatic events on risk for posttraumatic stress disorder. *Depress. Anxiety.* 2011; **28**(8): 639–647.

126. Zhao J, Goldberg J, Bremner JD, Vaccarino V. Association between promoter methylation of serotonin transporter gene and depressive symptoms: a monozygotic twin study. *Psychosom. Med.* 2013; **75**(6): 523–529.

127. Dannlowski U, Kugel H, Redlich R, *et al.* Serotonin transporter gene methylation is associated with hippocampal gray matter volume. *Hum. Brain Mapp.* 2014; **35**(11): 5356–5367.

128. Nikolova YS, Koenen KC, Galea S, *et al.* Beyond genotype: serotonin transporter epigenetic modification predicts human brain function. *Nat. Neurosci.* 2014; **17**(9): 1153–1155.

129. Wang D, Szyf M, Benkelfat C, *et al.* Peripheral SLC6A4 DNA methylation is associated with in vivo measures of human brain serotonin synthesis and childhood physical aggression. *PLoS One.* 2012; **7**(6): e39501.

130. Frankle WG, Lombardo I, New AS, *et al.* Brain serotonin transporter distribution in subjects with impulsive aggressivity: a positron emission study with [11C]McN 5652. *Am. J. Psychiatry.* 2005; **162**(5): 915–923.

131. Bortolato M, Chen K, Shih JC. Monoamine oxidase inactivation: from pathophysiology to therapeutics. *Adv. Drug Deliv. Rev.* 2008; **60**(13–14): 1527–1533.

132. Brunner HG, Nelen M, Breakefield XO, Ropers HH, van Oost BA. Abnormal behavior associated with a point mutation in the structural gene for monoamine oxidase A. *Science.* 1993; **262**(5133): 578–580.

133. Sabol SZ, Hu S, Hamer D. A functional polymorphism in the monoamine oxidase A gene promoter. *Hum. Genet.* 1998; **103**(3): 273–279.

134. Kuepper Y, Grant P, Wielpuetz C, Hennig J. MAOA-uVNTR genotype predicts interindividual differences in experimental aggressiveness as a function of the degree of provocation. *Behav. Brain Res.* 2013; **247**: 73–78.

135. Manuck SB, Flory JD, Ferrell RE, Mann JJ, Muldoon MF. A regulatory polymorphism of the monoamine oxidase-A gene may be associated with variability in aggression, impulsivity, and central nervous system serotonergic responsivity. *Psychiatry Res.* 2000; **95**(1): 9–23.

136. Stetler DA, Davis C, Leavitt K, *et al.* Association of low-activity MAOA allelic variants with violent crime in incarcerated offenders. *J. Psychiatr. Res.* 2014; **58**: 69–75.

137. Byrd AL, Manuck SB. MAOA, childhood maltreatment, and antisocial behavior: meta-analysis of a gene-environment interaction. *Biol. Psychiatry.* 2014; **75**(1): 9–17.

138. Karere GM, Kinnally EL, Sanchez JN, *et al.* What is an "adverse"

environment? Interactions of rearing experiences and MAOA genotype in rhesus monkeys. *Biol. Psychiatry.* 2009; **65**(9): 770–777.

139. Newman TK, Syagailo YV, Barr CS, *et al.* Monoamine oxidase A gene promoter variation and rearing experience influences aggressive behavior in rhesus monkeys. *Biol. Psychiatry.* 2005; **57**(2): 167–172.

140. Alia-Klein N, Goldstein RZ, Kriplani A, *et al.* Brain monoamine oxidase A activity predicts trait aggression. *J. Neurosci.* 2008; **28**(19): 5099–5104.

141. Cases O, Seif I, Grimsby J, *et al.* Aggressive behavior and altered amounts of brain serotonin and norepinephrine in mice lacking MAOA. *Science.* 1995; **268**(5218): 1763–1766.

142. Scott AL, Bortolato M, Chen K, Shih JC. Novel monoamine oxidase A knock out mice with human-like spontaneous mutation. *Neuroreport.* 2008; **19**(7): 739–743.

143. Cases O, Vitalis T, Seif I, *et al.* Lack of barrels in the somatosensory cortex of monoamine oxidase A-deficient mice: role of a serotonin excess during the critical period. *Neuron.* 1996; **16**(2): 297–307.

144. Bortolato M, Godar SC, Tambaro S, *et al.* Early postnatal inhibition of serotonin synthesis results in long-term reductions of perseverative behaviors, but not aggression, in MAO A-deficient mice. *Neuropharmacology.* 2013; **75**: 223–232.

145. Garcia-Garcia AL, Newman-Tancredi A, Leonardo ED. 5-HT (1A) [corrected] receptors in mood and anxiety: recent insights into autoreceptor versus heteroreceptor function. *Psychopharmacology (Berl.).* 2014; **231**(4): 623–636.

146. Polter AM, Li X. 5-HT1A receptor-regulated signal transduction pathways in brain. *Cell Signal.* 2010; **22**(10): 1406–1412.

147. Miczek KA, Hussain S, Faccidomo S. Alcohol-heightened aggression in mice: attenuation by 5-HT1A receptor agonists. *Psychopharmacology (Berl.).* 1998; **139**(1–2): 160–168.

148. Pruus K, Skrebuhhova-Malmros T, Rudissaar R, Matto V, Allikmets L. 5-HT1A receptor agonists buspirone and gepirone attenuate apomorphine-induced aggressive behaviour in adult male Wistar rats. *J. Physiol. Pharmacol.* 2000; **51**(4 Pt 2): 833–846.

149. Centenaro LA, Vieira K, Zimmermann N, *et al.* Social instigation and aggressive behavior in mice: role of 5-HT1A and 5-HT1B receptors in the prefrontal cortex. *Psychopharmacology (Berl.).* 2008; **201**(2): 237–248.

150. da Veiga CP, Miczek KA, Lucion AB, de Almeida RM. Social instigation and aggression in postpartum female rats: role of 5-Ht1A and 5-Ht1B receptors in the dorsal raphe nucleus and prefrontal cortex. *Psychopharmacology (Berl.).* 2011; **213**(2–3): 475–487.

151. de Boer SF, Lesourd M, Mocaer E, Koolhaas JM. Somatodendritic 5-HT(1A) autoreceptors mediate the anti-aggressive actions of 5-HT(1A) receptor agonists in rats: an ethopharmacological study with S-15535, alnespirone, and WAY-100635. *Neuropsychopharmacology.* 2000; **23**(1): 20–33.

152. Stein DJ, Miczek KA, Lucion AB, de Almeida RM. Aggression-reducing effects of F15599, a novel selective 5-HT1A receptor agonist, after microinjection into the ventral orbital prefrontal cortex, but not in infralimbic cortex in

male mice. *Psychopharmacology (Berl.).* 2013; **230**(3): 375–387.

153. Naumenko VS, Kozhemyakina RV, Plyusnina IF, Kulikov AV, Popova NK. Serotonin 5-HT1A receptor in infancy-onset aggression: comparison with genetically defined aggression in adult rats. *Behav. Brain Res.* 2013; **243**: 97–101.

154. Popova NK, Naumenko VS, Plyusnina IZ, Kulikov AV. Reduction in 5-HT1A receptor density, 5-HT1A mRNA expression, and functional correlates for 5-HT1A receptors in genetically defined aggressive rats. *J. Neurosci. Res.* 2005; **80**(2): 286–292.

155. Popova NK, Naumenko VS, Plyusnina IZ. Involvement of brain serotonin 5-HT1A receptors in genetic predisposition to aggressive behavior. *Neurosci. Behav. Physiol.* 2007; **37**(6): 631–635.

156. van der Vegt BJ, de Boer SF, Buwalda B, *et al.* Enhanced sensitivity of postsynaptic serotonin-1A receptors in rats and mice with high trait aggression. *Physiol. Behav.* 2001; **74**(1–2): 205–211.

157. Audero E, Mlinar B, Baccini G, *et al.* Suppression of serotonin neuron firing increases aggression in mice. *J. Neurosci.* 2013; **33**(20): 8678–8688.

158. Almeida M, Lee R, Coccaro EF. Cortisol responses to ipsapirone challenge correlate with aggression, while basal cortisol levels correlate with impulsivity, in personality disorder and healthy volunteer subjects. *J. Psychiatr. Res.* 2010; **44**(14): 874–880.

159. Coccaro EF, Gabriel S, Siever LJ. Buspirone challenge: preliminary evidence for a role for central 5-HT1a receptor function in impulsive aggressive behavior in humans.

Psychopharmacol. Bull. 1990; **26**(3): 393–405.

160. Benko A, Lazary J, Molnar E, *et al.* Significant association between the C(-1019)G functional polymorphism of the HTR1A gene and impulsivity. *Am. J. Med. Genet. B Neuropsychiatr. Genet.* 2010; **153B**(2): 592–599.

161. Joyce PR, Stephenson J, Kennedy M, Mulder RT, McHugh PC. The presence of both serotonin 1A receptor (HTR1A) and dopamine transporter (DAT1) gene variants increase the risk of borderline personality disorder. *Front. Genet.* 2014; **4**: 313.

162. Witte AV, Floel A, Stein P, *et al.* Aggression is related to frontal serotonin-1A receptor distribution as revealed by PET in healthy subjects. *Hum. Brain Mapp.* 2009; **30**(8): 2558–2570.

163. Parsey RV, Oquendo MA, Simpson NR, *et al.* Effects of sex, age, and aggressive traits in man on brain serotonin 5-HT1A receptor binding potential measured by PET using [C-11] WAY-100635. *Brain Res.* 2002; **954**(2): 173–182.

164. Sari Y. Serotonin1B receptors: from protein to physiological function and behavior. *Neurosci. Biobehav. Rev.* 2004; **28**(6): 565–582.

165. Bannai M, Fish EW, Faccidomo S, Miczek KA. Anti-aggressive effects of agonists at 5-HT1B receptors in the dorsal raphe nucleus of mice. *Psychopharmacology (Berl.).* 2007; **193**(2): 295–304.

166. de Almeida RM, Miczek KA. Aggression escalated by social instigation or by discontinuation of reinforcement ("frustration") in mice: inhibition by anpirtoline: a 5-HT1B receptor agonist. *Neuropsychopharmacology.* 2002; **27**(2): 171–181.

167. de Almeida RM, Rosa MM, Santos DM, *et al.* 5-HT(1B) receptors,

ventral orbitofrontal cortex, and aggressive behavior in mice. *Psychopharmacology (Berl.).* 2006; **185**(4): 441–450.

168. Faccidomo S, Bannai M, Miczek KA. Escalated aggression after alcohol drinking in male mice: dorsal raphe and prefrontal cortex serotonin and 5-HT(1B) receptors. *Neuropsychopharmacology.* 2008; **33**(12): 2888–2899.

169. Faccidomo S, Quadros IM, Takahashi A, Fish EW, Miczek KA. Infralimbic and dorsal raphe microinjection of the 5-HT(1B) receptor agonist CP-93,129: attenuation of aggressive behavior in CFW male mice. *Psychopharmacology (Berl.).* 2012; **222**(1): 117–128.

170. Fish EW, Faccidomo S, Miczek KA. Aggression heightened by alcohol or social instigation in mice: reduction by the 5-HT(1B) receptor agonist CP-94,253. *Psychopharmacology (Berl.).* 1999; **146**(4): 391–399.

171. Fish EW, McKenzie-Quirk SD, Bannai M, Miczek KA. 5-HT (1B) receptor inhibition of alcohol-heightened aggression in mice: comparison to drinking and running. *Psychopharmacology (Berl.).* 2008; **197**(1): 145–156.

172. Veiga CP, Miczek KA, Lucion AB, Almeida RM. Effect of 5-HT1B receptor agonists injected into the prefrontal cortex on maternal aggression in rats. *Braz. J. Med. Biol. Res.* 2007; **40**(6): 825–830.

173. Ramboz S, Saudou F, Amara DA, *et al.* 5-HT1B receptor knock out —behavioral consequences. *Behav. Brain Res.* 1996; **73**(1–2): 305–312.

174. Bouwknecht JA, Hijzen TH, van der Gugten J, *et al.* Absence of 5-HT(1B) receptors is associated with impaired impulse control in male 5-HT(1B) knockout mice. *Biol. Psychiatry.* 2001; **49**(7): 557–568.

175. Conner TS, Jensen KP, Tennen H, *et al.* Functional polymorphisms in the serotonin 1B receptor gene (HTR1B) predict self-reported anger and hostility among young men. *Am. J. Med. Genet. B Neuropsychiatr. Genet.* 2010; **153B**(1): 67–78.

176. Hakulinen C, Jokela M, Hintsanen M, *et al.* Serotonin receptor 1B genotype and hostility, anger and aggressive behavior through the lifespan: the Young Finns study. *J. Behav. Med.* 2013; **36**(6): 583–590.

177. Jensen KP, Covault J, Conner TS, *et al.* A common polymorphism in serotonin receptor 1B mRNA moderates regulation by miR-96 and associates with aggressive human behaviors. *Mol. Psychiatry.* 2009; **14**(4): 381–389.

178. Zouk H, McGirr A, Lebel V, *et al.* The effect of genetic variation of the serotonin 1B receptor gene on impulsive aggressive behavior and suicide. *Am. J. Med. Genet. B Neuropsychiatr. Genet.* 2007; **144B**(8): 996–1002.

179. Potenza MN, Walderhaug E, Henry S, *et al.* Serotonin 1B receptor imaging in pathological gambling. *World J. Biol. Psychiatry.* 2013; **14**(2): 139–145.

180. Hu J, Henry S, Gallezot JD, *et al.* Serotonin 1B receptor imaging in alcohol dependence. *Biol. Psychiatry.* 2010; **67**(9): 800–803.

181. Murrough JW, Henry S, Hu J, *et al.* Reduced ventral striatal/ventral pallidal serotonin1B receptor binding potential in major depressive disorder. *Psychopharmacology (Berl.).* 2011; **213**(2–3): 547–553.

182. Higgins GA, Enderlin M, Haman M, Fletcher PJ. The 5-HT2A receptor antagonist M100,907 attenuates motor and 'impulsive-type' behaviours produced by NMDA receptor antagonism.

Psychopharmacology (Berl.). 2003; **170**(3): 309–319.

183. Sakaue M, Ago Y, Sowa C, *et al.* Modulation by 5-hT2A receptors of aggressive behavior in isolated mice. *Jpn J. Pharmacol.* 2002; **89**(1): 89–92.

184. Winstanley CA, Theobald DE, Dalley JW, Glennon JC, Robbins TW. 5-HT2A and 5-HT2C receptor antagonists have opposing effects on a measure of impulsivity: interactions with global 5-HT depletion. *Psychopharmacology (Berl.).* 2004; **176**(3–4): 376–385.

185. Giegling I, Hartmann AM, Moller HJ, Rujescu D. Anger- and aggression-related traits are associated with polymorphisms in the 5-HT-2A gene. *J. Affect. Disord.* 2006; **96**(1–2): 75–81.

186. Bruce KR, Steiger H, Joober R, *et al.* Association of the promoter polymorphism -1438G/A of the 5-HT2A receptor gene with behavioral impulsiveness and serotonin function in women with bulimia nervosa. *Am. J. Med. Genet. B Neuropsychiatr. Genet.* 2005; **137B**(1): 40–44.

187. Jakubczyk A, Wrzosek M, Lukaszkiewicz J, *et al.* The CC genotype in HTR2A T102C polymorphism is associated with behavioral impulsivity in alcohol-dependent patients. *J. Psychiatr. Res.* 2012; **46**(1): 44–49.

188. Jakubczyk A, Klimkiewicz A, Kopera M, *et al.* The CC genotype in the T102C HTR2A polymorphism predicts relapse in individuals after alcohol treatment. *J. Psychiatr. Res.* 2013; **47**(4): 527–533.

189. Preuss UW, Koller G, Bondy B, Bahlmann M, Soyka M. Impulsive traits and 5-HT2A receptor promoter polymorphism in alcohol dependents: possible association but no influence of personality disorders.

190. Tsuang HC, Chen WJ, Lin SH, *et al.* Impaired impulse control is associated with a 5-HT2A receptor polymorphism in schizophrenia. *Psychiatry Res.* 2013; **208**(2): 105–110.

191. Bjork JM, Moeller FG, Dougherty DM, *et al.* Serotonin 2a receptor T102C polymorphism and impaired impulse control. *Am. J. Med. Genet.* 2002; **114**(3): 336–339.

192. Oquendo MA, Russo SA, Underwood MD, *et al.* Higher postmortem prefrontal 5-HT2A receptor binding correlates with lifetime aggression in suicide. *Biol. Psychiatry.* 2006; **59**(3): 235–243.

193. Dwivedi Y, Mondal AC, Payappagoudar GV, Rizavi HS. Differential regulation of serotonin (5HT)2A receptor mRNA and protein levels after single and repeated stress in rat brain: role in learned helplessness behavior. *Neuropharmacology.* 2005; **48**(2): 204–214.

194. Soloff PH, Chiappetta L, Mason NS, Becker C, Price JC. Effects of serotonin-2A receptor binding and gender on personality traits and suicidal behavior in borderline personality disorder. *Psychiatry Res.* 2014; **222**(3): 140–148.

195. Meyer JH, Wilson AA, Rusjan P, *et al.* Serotonin2A receptor binding potential in people with aggressive and violent behaviour. *J. Psychiatry Neurosci.* 2008; **33**(6): 499–508.

196. Rylands AJ, Hinz R, Jones M, *et al.* Pre- and postsynaptic serotonergic differences in males with extreme levels of impulsive aggression without callous unemotional traits: a positron emission tomography study using (11)C-DASB and (11)C-MDL100907. *Biol. Psychiatry.* 2012; **72**(12): 1004–1011.

197. Chameau P, van Hooft JA. Serotonin 5-HT(3) receptors in the central nervous system. *Cell Tissue Res.* 2006; **326**(2): 573–581.

198. De Deurwaerdère P, Moison D, Navailles S, Porras G, Spampinato U. Regionally and functionally distinct serotonin3 receptors control in vivo dopamine outflow in the rat nucleus accumbens. *J. Neurochem.* 2005; **94**(1): 140–149.

199. Cervantes MC, Delville Y. Serotonin 5-HT1A and 5-HT3 receptors in an impulsive-aggressive phenotype. *Behav. Neurosci.* 2009; **123**(3): 589–598.

200. Ricci LA, Grimes JM, Melloni RH Jr. Serotonin type 3 receptors modulate the aggression-stimulating effects of adolescent cocaine exposure in Syrian hamsters (*Mesocricetus auratus*). *Behav. Neurosci.* 2004; **118**(5): 1097–1110.

201. Ricci LA, Knyshevski I, Melloni RH Jr. Serotonin type 3 receptors stimulate offensive aggression in Syrian hamsters. *Behav. Brain Res.* 2005; **156**(1): 19–29.

202. Rudissaar R, Pruus K, Skrebuhhova T, Allikmets L, Matto V. Modulatory role of 5-HT3 receptors in mediation of apomorphine-induced aggressive behaviour in male rats. *Behav. Brain Res.* 1999; **106**(1–2): 91–96.

203. McKenzie-Quirk SD, Girasa KA, Allan AM, Miczek KA. 5-HT(3) receptors, alcohol and aggressive behavior in mice. *Behav. Pharmacol.* 2005; **16**(3): 163–169.

204. Sellers EM, Toneatto T, Romach MK, *et al.* Clinical efficacy of the 5-HT3 antagonist ondansetron in alcohol abuse and dependence. *Alcohol Clin. Exp. Res.* 1994; **18** (4): 879–885.

205. Johnson BA, Ait-Daoud N, Ma JZ, Wang Y. Ondansetron reduces mood disturbance among biologically predisposed, alcohol-dependent individuals. *Alcohol Clin. Exp. Res.* 2003; **27**(11): 1773–1779.

206. Myrick H, Anton RF, Li X, *et al.* Effect of naltrexone and ondansetron on alcohol cue-induced activation of the ventral striatum in alcohol-dependent people. *Arch. Gen. Psychiatry.* 2008; **65**(4): 466–475.

207. Ducci F, Enoch MA, Yuan Q, *et al.* HTR3B is associated with alcoholism with antisocial behavior and alpha EEG power—an intermediate phenotype for alcoholism and co-morbid behaviors. *Alcohol.* 2009; **43**(1): 73–84.

208. Melke J, Westberg L, Nilsson S, *et al.* A polymorphism in the serotonin receptor 3A (HTR3A) gene and its association with harm avoidance in women. *Arch. Gen. Psychiatry.* 2003; **60**(10): 1017–1023.

209. Gatt JM, Williams LM, Schofield PR, *et al.* Impact of the HTR3A gene with early life trauma on emotional brain networks and depressed mood. *Depress. Anxiety.* 2010; **27**(8): 752–759.

210. Iidaka T, Ozaki N, Matsumoto A, *et al.* A variant C178T in the regulatory region of the serotonin receptor gene HTR3A modulates neural activation in the human amygdala. *J. Neurosci.* 2005; **25** (27): 6460–6466.

211. Schlüter T, Winz O, Henkel K, *et al.* The impact of dopamine on aggression: an [18F]-FDOPA PET Study in healthy males. *J. Neurosci.* 2013; **33**(43): 16, 889–16, 896.

212. Buckholtz JW, Treadway MT, Cowan RL, *et al.* Mesolimbic dopamine reward system hypersensitivity in individuals with psychopathic traits. *Nat. Neurosci.* 2010; **13**(4): 419–421.

213. Wagner S, Baskaya O, Anicker NJ, *et al.* The catechol o-methyltransferase (COMT) val(158)met polymorphism modulates the association of

serious life events (SLE) and impulsive aggression in female patients with borderline personality disorder (BPD). *Acta Psychiatr. Scand.* 2010; **122**(2): 110–117.

214. Bhakta SG, Zhang JP, Malhotra AK. The COMT Met158 allele and violence in schizophrenia: a meta-analysis. *Schizophr. Res.* 2012; **140**(1–3): 192–197.

215. Flory JD, Xu K, New AS, *et al.* Irritable assault and variation in the COMT gene. *Psychiatr. Genet.* 2007; **17**(6): 344–346.

216. Soyka M, Zill P, Koller G, *et al.* Val158Met COMT polymorphism and risk of aggression in alcohol dependence. *Addict. Biol.* 2015; **20** (1): 197–204.

217. Vevera J, Stopkova R, Bes M, *et al.* COMT polymorphisms in impulsively violent offenders with antisocial personality disorder. *Neuro. Endocrinol. Lett.* 2009; **30**(6): 753–756.

218. Hirata Y, Zai CC, Nowrouzi B, Beitchman JH, Kennedy JL. Study of the catechol-o-methyltransferase (COMT) gene with high aggression in children. *Aggress. Behav.* 2013; **39**(1): 45–51.

219. Fresan A, Camarena B, Apiquian R, *et al.* Association study of MAO-A and DRD4 genes in schizophrenic patients with aggressive behavior. *Neuropsychobiology.* 2007; **55**(3–4): 171–175.

220. Buchmann AF, Zohsel K, Blomeyer D, *et al.* Interaction between prenatal stress and dopamine D4 receptor genotype in predicting aggression and cortisol levels in young adults. *Psychopharmacology (Berl.).* 2014; **231**(16): 3089–3097.

221. Delville Y, Mansour KM, Ferris CF. Serotonin blocks vasopressin-facilitated offensive aggression: interactions within the ventrolateral hypothalamus of golden hamsters. *Physiol. Behav.* 1996; **59**(4–5): 813–816.

222. Ferris CF, Melloni RH Jr, Koppel G, *et al.* Vasopressin/serotonin interactions in the anterior hypothalamus control aggressive behavior in golden hamsters. *J. Neurosci.* 1997; **17**(11): 4331–4340.

223. Ferris CF, Potegal M. Vasopressin receptor blockade in the anterior hypothalamus suppresses aggression in hamsters. *Physiol. Behav.* 1988; **44**(2): 235–239.

224. Bosch OJ, Neumann ID. Vasopressin released within the central amygdala promotes maternal aggression. *Eur. J. Neurosci.* 2010; **31**(5): 883–891.

225. Wersinger SR, Caldwell HK, Christiansen M, Young WS III. Disruption of the vasopressin 1b receptor gene impairs the attack component of aggressive behavior in mice. *Genes Brain Behav.* 2007; **6**(7): 653–660.

226. Wersinger SR, Ginns EI, O'Carroll AM, Lolait SJ, Young WS III. Vasopressin V1b receptor knockout reduces aggressive behavior in male mice. *Mol. Psychiatry.* 2002; **7**(9): 975–984.

227. Wersinger SR, Caldwell HK, Martinez L, *et al.* Vasopressin 1a receptor knockout mice have a subtle olfactory deficit but normal aggression. *Genes Brain Behav.* 2007; **6**(6): 540–551.

228. Fodor A, Barsvari B, Aliczki M, *et al.* The effects of vasopressin deficiency on aggression and impulsiveness in male and female rats. *Psychoneuroendocrinology.* 2014; **47**: 141–150.

229. Uzefovsky F, Shalev I, Israel S, Knafo A, Ebstein RP. Vasopressin selectively impairs emotion recognition in men. *Psychoneuroendocrinology.* 2012; **37**(4): 576–580.

230. Guastella AJ, Kenyon AR, Alvares GA, Carson DS, Hickie IB. Intranasal arginine vasopressin enhances the encoding of happy

and angry faces in humans. *Biol. Psychiatry.* 2010; **67**(12): 1220–1222.

231. Lee RJ, Coccaro EF, Cremers H, *et al.* A novel V1a receptor antagonist blocks vasopressin-induced changes in the CNS response to emotional stimuli: an fMRI study. *Front. Syst. Neurosci.* 2013; 7: 100.

232. Luppino D, Moul C, Hawes DJ, Brennan J, Dadds MR. Association between a polymorphism of the vasopressin 1B receptor gene and aggression in children. *Psychiatr. Genet.* 2014; **24**(5): 185–190.

233. Zai CC, Muir KE, Nowrouzi B, *et al.* Possible genetic association between vasopressin receptor 1B and child aggression. *Psychiatry Res.* 2012; **200**(2–3): 784–788.

234. Vogel F, Wagner S, Baskaya O, *et al.* Variable number of tandem repeat polymorphisms of the arginine vasopressin receptor 1A gene and impulsive aggression in patients with borderline personality disorder. *Psychiatr. Genet.* 2012; **22**(2): 105–106.

235. McBurnett K, Lahey BB, Rathouz PJ, Loeber R. Low salivary cortisol and persistent aggression in boys referred for disruptive behavior. *Arch. Gen. Psychiatry.* 2000; **57**(1): 38–43.

236. Popma A, Vermeiren R, Geluk CA, *et al.* Cortisol moderates the relationship between testosterone and aggression in delinquent male adolescents. *Biol. Psychiatry.* 2007; **61**(3): 405–411.

237. Kuepper Y, Alexander N, Osinsky R, *et al.* Aggression–interactions

of serotonin and testosterone in healthy men and women. *Behav. Brain Res.* 2010; **206**(1): 93–100.

238. Welker KM, Lozoya E, Campbell JA, Neumann CS, Carre JM. Testosterone, cortisol, and psychopathic traits in men and women. *Physiol. Behav.* 2014; **129**: 230–236.

239. Denson TF, Mehta PH, Ho TD. Endogenous testosterone and cortisol jointly influence reactive aggression in women. *Psychoneuroendocrinology.* 2013; **38**(3): 416–424.

240. Cima M, Smeets T, Jelicic M. Self-reported trauma, cortisol levels, and aggression in psychopathic and non-psychopathic prison inmates. *Biol. Psychol.* 2008; **78**(1): 75–86.

241. Derntl B, Windischberger C, Robinson S, *et al.* Amygdala activity to fear and anger in healthy young males is associated with testosterone. *Psychoneuroendocrinology.* 2009; **34**(5): 687–693.

242. Hermans EJ, Ramsey NF, van Honk J. Exogenous testosterone enhances responsiveness to social threat in the neural circuitry of social aggression in humans. *Biol. Psychiatry.* 2008; **63**(3): 263–270.

243. van Wingen G, Mattern C, Verkes RJ, Buitelaar J, Fernández G. Testosterone reduces amygdala-orbitofrontal cortex coupling. *Psychoneuroendocrinology.* 2010; **35**(1): 105–113.

244. Goetz SM, Tang L, Thomason ME, *et al.* Testosterone rapidly increases neural reactivity to

threat in healthy men: a novel two-step pharmacological challenge paradigm. *Biol. Psychiatry.* 2014; **76**(4): 324–331.

245. Grillo CA, Risher M, Macht VA, *et al.* Repeated restraint stress-induced atrophy of glutamatergic pyramidal neurons and decreases in glutamatergic efflux in the rat amygdala are prevented by the antidepressant agomelatine. *Neuroscience.* 2015; **284**: 430–443.

246. Padival MA, Blume SR, Vantrease JE, Rosenkranz JA. Qualitatively different effect of repeated stress during adolescence on principal neuron morphology across lateral and basal nuclei of the rat amygdala. *Neuroscience.* 2015; **291**: 128–145.

247. Vyas A, Mitra R, Shankaranarayana Rao BS, Chattarji S. Chronic stress induces contrasting patterns of dendritic remodeling in hippocampal and amygdaloid neurons. *J. Neurosci.* 2002; **22**(15): 6810–6818.

248. Vyas A, Bernal S, Chattarji S. Effects of chronic stress on dendritic arborization in the central and extended amygdala. *Brain Res.* 2003; **965**(1–2): 290–294.

249. Gilabert-Juan J, Castillo-Gomez E, Perez-Rando M, Molto MD, Nacher J. Chronic stress induces changes in the structure of interneurons and in the expression of molecules related to neuronal structural plasticity and inhibitory neurotransmission in the amygdala of adult mice. *Exp. Neurol.* 2011; **232**(1): 33–40.

14

Impulsivity and aggression in schizophrenia: a neural circuitry perspective with implications for treatment

Matthew J. Hoptman

Introduction

Impulsive behavior is an important feature of a number of serious mental illnesses (SMIs), including schizophrenia, bipolar disorder, substance abuse, and borderline personality disorder. In many cases, impulsive behavior can lead to other problematic behaviors, including violence or self-harm. Such violence is a highly significant public health issue because often it is a proximate cause of hospitalization and leads to increased healthcare costs [1], particularly because persistently aggressive patients can be difficult to discharge. Moreover, the media often sensationalizes violent acts associated with mental illness, which contributes to stigma [2]. It is becoming increasingly clear that increased violence risk is not fully explained by symptoms characteristic of SMI. Although aggression in SMI is heterogeneous [3], impulsivity has been posited to play an important role. This article examines the neural circuitry of impulsivity and aggression in schizophrenia, a disorder characterized by positive symptoms (e.g., hallucinations, delusions), negative symptoms (e.g., social withdrawal, blunted affect), and a wide range of cognitive deficits. Because the review focuses specifically on impulsivity and aggression, important work on psychotic and psychopathic bases of aggression is not included herein, largely due to space limitations. To set the context, I first briefly discuss the heterogeneity of violence in schizophrenia and issues related to its measurement.

Body of Review

Etiology

First and foremost, aggression in schizophrenia is multidetermined [3]. Therefore, attempts to treat aggression in schizophrenia that use a one-size-fits-all approach are doomed to fail. The literature suggests that in schizophrenia, the three primary causes of aggression are psychotic symptoms, psychopathy, and impulsivity [4]. Other factors are also important, including neurological abnormalities, substance use, and poor medication adherence [5], although these may exert their influence on aggression via the primary causes named above. Thus, in an important study, Nolan et al. [6] interviewed inpatients with schizophrenia whose violent acts were recorded on videotape. About 20% of assaults were attributed directly to positive symptoms. A factor analysis revealed two psychosis-related factors: one related to positive symptoms, and the other related to disorganization/confusion. A third factor differentiated impulsive from psychopathically based assaults. Impulsive versus psychopathically based aggression is often mapped onto a distinction between reactive and instrumental/proactive aggression [7] or impulsive versus predatory aggression [4]. An important conclusion from that study is that patients could not be characterized by the type of violence they tended to commit, and that within an incident, multiple factors are likely to play a role.

The literature consistently shows that at least a plurality of inpatient aggression has an impulsive basis [8], although it is notable that the comorbidity of psychopathy and schizophrenia is higher in violent than nonviolent patients [9]. However, the most common measures of impulsivity, such as the Barratt Impulsiveness Scale (BIS) [10], have not always shown particularly strong correlations with aggression [11]. This could be, in part, because the theory behind the BIS explicitly separates impulsivity and emotion [12].

Violence in Psychiatry, ed. Katherine D. Warburton and Stephen M. Stahl. Published by Cambridge University Press.
© Cambridge University Press 2016.

It has long been understood that impulsivity is a multifaceted construct. An important distinction in this regard is between behavioral and trait measures of impulsivity. Regarding the former, a number of studies have examined response inhibition, measured using the go/no-go and stop signal tasks, as a key aspect of impulsivity. Indeed, patients with schizophrenia show significant deficits in the ability to inhibit prepotent responses [11,13]. The circuitry for response inhibition is fairly well understood, and includes the right inferior frontal gyrus, the supplementary motor area, the globus pallidus, the striatum, the thalamus, and the subthalamic nucleus [14]. However, response inhibition is only weakly correlated with aggression [11,15], suggesting that other aspects of impulsivity may be more relevant to these behaviors in schizophrenia.

A major advance with regard to understanding trait impulsivity regarding aggression was achieved by Whiteside and Lynam [16]. They compared many different measures of impulsivity, and their factor analysis yielded five constructs: Urgency, (lack of) Premeditation, (lack of) Perseverance, and Sensation seeking (UPPS). Urgency is defined as impulsive behavior in the context of strong negative emotion. A newer subscale adds the construct of positive urgency, which is defined as impulsivity in the context of strong positive emotion, yielding the UPPS-P [17]. Urgency is elevated in a number of psychiatric populations that have affective dysregulation, including in schizophrenia [18].

The neural correlates of urgency are thought to include aberrant patterns of activity in the orbitofrontal and ventromedial prefrontal cortex, as well as in the amygdala [19]. Indeed, in a study of social drinkers, Cyders *et al.* [20] found that orbitofrontal cortex (OFC) and amygdala activation in response to negative emotional pictures correlated with negative urgency. Further, negative urgency mediated between general risk-taking and both amygdala and OFC activation to negative emotional pictures.

Behavioral and trait impulsivity measures are not strongly related in schizophrenia [21]. These measures are somewhat better correlated in healthy individuals [22]. The lack of correlation in schizophrenia may reflect other factors, including heterogeneity of symptoms or different subtypes. In healthy individuals, variable results may reflect the difference between trait and state aspects of impulsivity. More generally, trait measures (such as urgency) and the most commonly used behavioral measures (stop and go/no-go paradigms) appear to involve somewhat different neural circuitry. Relatively new behavioral tasks that include emotional conditions [23] appear to activate, among other regions, areas thought to be relevant to urgency-based circuitry. However, whether performance on these tasks correlates with trait measures of impulsivity is not yet known.

Individuals with schizophrenia appear to experience emotions at the same level as healthy individuals, albeit with reduced outward expression [24]. Patients with schizophrenia have problems in both emotional control and impulsivity – domains that are highly relevant to urgency. Moreover, urgency appears to have face validity as a correlate of aggression, and as will be discussed below, recent work suggests that it is the specific aspect of impulsivity most clearly linked to aggression in schizophrenia.

Measurement of aggression

The NIMH Research Domain Criteria (RDoC) initiative [25] points to the importance of examining different units of analysis within a domain. However, the assessment of aggression in schizophrenia so far has focused on only one or occasionally two levels of measurement. For measurement of aggressive behavior, the most relevant units would include behavior, self-reports, and paradigms. Many studies of violence in schizophrenia use direct observation of behavior [26]. Self-report measures also have been used extensively [27]. Paradigms such as the Taylor Aggression Paradigm (TAP) [28] and the Point Subtraction Aggression Paradigm (PSAP) [29] allow for fine-grained analyses of aggressive phenomena, but these have not been widely applied in schizophrenia. It is thus promising that the PSAP has been included in the RDoC matrix (http://www.nimh.nih.gov/research-priorities/rdoc/nimh-research-domain-criteria-rdoc.shtml), which may lead to a broader adoption of this online measure of aggression (classified under Frustrative Nonreward construct within the Negative Valence Systems domain).

Neural correlates of aggression in schizophrenia

Magnetic resonance imaging (MRI) studies of aggression specifically in schizophrenia have been relatively limited [30–32]. Most studies of the neurobiology of aggression have been based on findings from studies examining mixed diagnostic populations, as well as animal studies that concluded that aggression is associated with dysfunctions in ventral prefrontal and temporolimbic regions, as well as the interaction of these regions [33].

Structural MRI

Structural MRI studies have primarily focused on cortical volumetrics. Some of these studies have found that larger caudate [34], left orbitofrontal volume, and right orbitofrontal white matter volume [35] correlated with aggression in treatment-resistant patients with schizophrenia. These findings may reflect enlargement in cortical volumes due to the iatrogenic effects of long-term treatment with first-generation neuroleptics, given that these agents can increase basal ganglia volumes [36]. Similar findings with regard to orbitofrontal white matter volume were found in patients with schizophrenia who had prior suicide attempts [37]. Narayan et al. [38] found reduced cortical thickness in the ventromedial PFC (vmPFC) and lateral sensorimotor areas in violent compared to nonviolent patients. Of the violent patients, only those with antisocial personality disorder (and not schizophrenia) showed a reduction in thickness of the vmPFC. In a diffusion tensor imaging study, Hoptman et al. [39] found that increased diffusivity, which may be reflective of atrophy, was correlated with higher levels of aggressive attitudes in men with persistent, long-term forms of schizophrenia. These studies are broadly consistent with the idea that structural abnormalities in ventral prefrontal and some subcortical regions are associated with aggression in schizophrenia.

Functional studies

There are quite a few functional studies of violence in patients with SMI, although these studies have not necessarily been limited to patients with schizophrenia, and most of them have used radiological methods. For instance, Raine et al. [40] conducted an important series of studies using positron emission tomography to examine murderers judged not guilty by reason of insanity who were performing a continuous performance task. These studies found reduced glucose metabolism in prefrontal brain regions. Similarly, Volkow et al. [41] found reduced resting regional cerebral metabolism in prefrontal and medial temporal regions in a small sample of psychiatric

patients with repetitive violence. Other radiological studies have found generally similar results [42].

Task-based functional MRI (fMRI) studies of violence in schizophrenia are relatively uncommon and point to the importance of comorbid diagnoses. Joyal et al. [43] examined blood oxygen level-dependent (BOLD) responses during a go/no-go task. Patients with comorbid antisocial personality and substance use showed increased activation in motor, premotor, and anterior cingulate cortex, as well as reduced ventral prefrontal activation compared to controls and to violent patients with schizophrenia. Kumari et al. [44] used an anticipatory fear task, and found that individuals with schizophrenia and violent history showed hyperactivity in thalamostriatal regions, whereas antisocial patients showed hypoactivity in the same regions. Finally, in a small study of men with schizophrenia, Dolan and Fullam [45] found that patients with schizophrenia and high psychopathy had reduced amygdala activation to fearful faces compared to individuals with schizophrenia with low comorbid psychopathy.

A promising area of study is resting state fMRI. A major advantage of this method is that it avoids performance confounds and can thus be used in most study populations. A key measure using this approach is functional connectivity, which describes the temporal correlation of activation in different brain regions. In an initial study, Hoptman et al. [46] examined functional connectivity of the amygdala in patients with persistent forms of schizophrenia. Compared to healthy controls, individuals with schizophrenia showed reduced functional connectivity between the amygdala and ventral prefrontal regions. This reduction correlated with higher levels of aggression in the patients as measured using arrest histories and self-report measures.

In a more recent study, Hoptman et al. [18] examined impulsivity and aggression in patients with schizophrenia compared to healthy controls using the UPPS-P, as well as several aggression questionnaires. They found that on the UPPS-P, patients had a selective increase in urgency, and that this increase explained significant variance in the also-observed increase in aggressive attitudes. Moreover, the investigators found that impulsive, but not premeditated, aggression was elevated in patients. Higher levels of urgency predicted reduced cortical thickness in ventral prefrontal regions, as well as reduced functional connectivity between ventral prefrontal and both

Table 14.1 Potential neuroanatomical substrates and causes of aggression in schizophrenia

Neuroanatomical substrate	Finding(s)
Caudate and orbitofrontal cortex	Increased volume associated with higher aggression in treatment-resistant SZ [33,34]
Orbitofrontal white matter	Increased volume in patients with prior suicide attempts [36]
Ventral prefrontal cortex and lateral sensorimotor areas	Reduced cortical thickness in violent vs. nonviolent patients with SZ [37] Reduced cortical thickness and functional connectivity of ventral prefrontal cortex associated with urgency in SZ [18] Reduced activation in SZ + APD + SUD during a go/no-go task compared to SZ only [42]
Motor, premotor, anterior cingulate cortex	Increased activation in SZ + APD + SUD during a go/no-go task compared to SZ only [42]
Ventral prefrontal white matter	Greater diffusivity associated with more aggression [38]
Thalamus and striatum	Hyperactivity during an anticipatory fear task in patients with SZ and violent history [43]
Amygdala	Reduced activation to fear faces in SZ with high psychopathy [44], reduced resting state functional connectivity to frontal regions associated with aggression in SZ [45]

Note. SZ = schizophrenia, APD = antisocial personality disorder, SUD = substance use disorder.

limbic (e.g., rostral anterior cingulate) and executive brain regions. It is clear that a number of frontolimbic and subcortical regions are involved in impulsivity and aggression in schizophrenia. These are shown in Table 14.1.

Implications

These findings may have important implications for the theoretical and clinical understanding of aggression in schizophrenia [18,47]. From a theoretical perspective, the findings refine our understanding of the role of impulsivity in aggression. Thus, not all impulsivity is the same, and many aspects of impulsivity are not elevated in chronic schizophrenia. On the basis of self-report measures, only the emotional components (i.e., urgency) of the construct were elevated. Moreover, the neural circuitry related to urgency involves the structural integrity of ventral prefrontal regions and their functional connections to limbic and executive regions. Dysfunction of these circuits, which are implicated in emotional regulation, may predispose an individual toward aggression [48]. The extant literature suggests the importance of emotional dysregulation deficits in schizophrenia [49].

From a clinical perspective, the results suggest implications for treatment. Targets may include cognitive interventions to enhance regulation of impulsivity

and aggression. These could include techniques such as reappraisal of negative emotional experiences, or suppression of negative affect [50]. It is not yet known if these interventions can be used to effectively reduce aggression in patients with schizophrenia. However, their use, including techniques related to acceptance of emotional experiences [51], might lessen the impact of distress associated with strong emotional states, and thereby prevent urgency-related aggression.

The literature also points to neural targets. Some antipsychotic medications appear to have specific antiaggressive effects, particularly clozapine [52,53]. Although second-generation antipsychotic agents have mixed effects on neurotransmitters, they do affect serotonin systems. Abnormalities in these systems have been associated with violent behavior in a number of populations. Of relevance to aggressive behavior, serotonin transporter sites are selectively reduced in ventral prefrontal regions in suicide victims compared to those with depression only [54]. It would be important to examine serotonin transporter distribution patterns in violent patients with schizophrenia. Moreover, it would be interesting to examine the effects of clozapine on urgency in patients with schizophrenia. In the study by Hoptman *et al.* [18], patients taking clozapine had lower urgency ratings on the UPPS-P than patients taking other medications. Clearly, a better definition of the multidimensional construct of aggression may lead to better treatment decisions and outcomes [55].

Other treatment approaches also may be useful to reduce impulsivity-based aggression. Transcranial magnetic stimulation (TMS) has traditionally been unable to reach cortical depths of greater than 2 cm, thereby rendering it unable to stimulate ventral prefrontal regions. However, we can apply our knowledge from big data approaches such as the Functional Connectomes Project [56] to identify circuits that are functionally connected to ventral prefrontal regions. Thus, it may be efficacious to stimulate regions such as the dorsolateral prefrontal cortex or precuneus in order to modulate activation in ventral prefrontal regions. Alternatively, deep TMS has the potential to reach depths of up to 6 cm from the cortical surface. This technique has shown treatment utility in a number of disorders involving emotional dysregulation, including major depression, hallucinations and delusions in schizophrenia, bipolar depression, and Asperger's syndrome [57]. Neither of these TMS approaches has been specifically applied to impulsive aggression in schizophrenia, but such methods may prove useful from both mechanistic and treatment perspectives.

Another potentially interesting approach is the use of real-time fMRI neurofeedback [58] to modulate the neural circuitry related to impulsivity and aggression. Real-time fMRI has been applied to the "default mode network" (DMN [59]) – a set of brain regions, including medial prefrontal cortex, posterior cingulate, and lateral parietal regions, that typically shows increased activity during rest, compared to task, conditions. Studies on DMN suggest its involvement in self-directed cognition [60]. Real-time fMRI has had limited application in schizophrenia so far [61]. In principle, one could identify critical circuitry for urgency and train patients to modulate their own circuitry. Recent studies show that orbitofrontal circuitry can be manipulated in this manner in healthy subjects with contamination anxiety [62], and that anterior insula circuitry can be modulated in criminal psychopaths [63], which suggests that this approach might be applicable in other populations with abnormalities in such circuitry.

As has been stressed in this article, aggression has multiple causes, and a complete understanding of aggression in schizophrenia will extend the knowledge of impulsive, psychotic, and psychopathically based aggression, as well as interactions among these three types of aggression. For example, an important literature is emerging on the role of persecutory

delusions in aggression in schizophrenia [64]. Significantly, it appears that delusions that engender anger are those that are most likely to lead to aggression [65], suggesting a mechanism whereby urgency could interact with psychotic symptoms to yield violent behavior. Finally, the circuitry underlying psychotic, impulsive, and predatory violence likely differs, and an understanding of these distinct circuits and their interactions will inform our ability to understand the genesis of aggression in schizophrenia [4].

It should be noted that I am not arguing that all aspects of aggression in schizophrenia are determined by urgency. However, given the role that urgency may well play in aggression in schizophrenia, as well as the fact that at least a plurality of inpatient aggression is impulsive in nature, it may be that an assessment of urgency would be useful prior to intervention. Moreover, as noted above, it could be that other causal factors might interact with urgency so that changes in urgency might have as-yet-unknown effects on those factors. It would thus be important to know to what extent treatments typically used to address impulsively based aggression work through the construct of urgency and/or via related circuitry.

More generally, the literature on impulsivity and violence in schizophrenia points to the need for a better understanding of the regulation of emotionally based impulsivity and aggression in this disorder, as well as the need to better understand the regulation of other problematic behaviors associated with emotionally based impulsivity. This conceptualization places the problem in the context of a phenomenon that we know to be an issue transdiagnostically [66], in keeping with the NIMH's RDoC mission. It will be important to use information on regulation of impulsivity and aggression more broadly to help understand how it plays out in schizophrenia and other disorders.

Challenges

There are several important challenges in this line of work. First, there is no known paradigm that ideally probes urgency, which makes it difficult to objectively evaluate this construct in imaging studies. It may be that urgency has such strong trait properties that it cannot be easily modified. Alternatively, behavioral tasks that are typically used to measure impulsivity may have to be adapted to include a strong emotional component in order to better investigate this construct. Even if urgency cannot be easily manipulated, initial approaches might include (a) finding tasks that are closely related to urgency that can be modulated and/or (b) modulating urgency-related circuitry with the goal of examining its downstream effects on impulsively based aggression,

Paradigms such as the TAP or PSAP might be promising. Although the PSAP is part of the RDoC-matrix, the task requires substantial motor activity and thus might be difficult to implement in fMRI studies. The TAP has been used in some fMRI studies. In particular, Dambacher *et al.* [67] used the go/no-go task to measure response inhibition and the TAP to measure reactive aggression in healthy men. They found that both failed response inhibition (compared to go trials) and reactive aggression were associated with activation of the anterior insula, suggesting a role for that region in self-control. This same group showed that theta burst TMS in the right anterior insula and superior frontal cortex leads to impairments in both action restraint (go/no-go task) and action cancellation (stop task) in the former, and in action restraint in the latter compared to sham stimulation [68]. By identifying regions indirectly stimulated by TMS in these studies, a better understanding of the circuitry associated with reactive aggression, action restraint, and action cancellation could be derived.

Conclusion

This article focuses on impulsive aggression. In general, imaging studies point to the role of abnormalities in circuitry involving ventral prefrontal, medial temporal, and subcortical regions as playing a key role in these behaviors. The recent finding that urgency plays a special role in aggression in schizophrenia suggests several novel approaches to better understand and treat these dysfunctional behaviors, and these approaches may have utility for other problematic behaviors associated with urgency, as well. Nonetheless, aggression in schizophrenia is not homogeneous across individuals, and a complete understanding of these behaviors will consider this heterogeneity. Newer assessments and guidelines for inpatient aggression are explicitly doing just that [69,70]. By improving this understanding, we will be better equipped to manage aggressive behavior in schizophrenia, leading to reductions in harm, trauma, healthcare costs, and stigma.

Disclosures

Matthew Hoptman has the following disclosures: NIMH, researcher, research support (grants); Kessler Foundation, consultant, consulting fees.

References

1. McEvoy JP. The costs of schizophrenia. *J. Clin. Psychiatry.* 2007; **68**(Suppl 14): 4–7.

2. Torrey EF. Stigma and violence: isn't it time to connect the dots? *Schizophr. Bull.* 2011; **37**(5): 892–896.

3. Volavka J, Citrome L. Heterogeneity of violence in schizophrenia and implications for long-term treatment. *Int. J. Clin. Pract.* 2008; **62**(8): 1237–1245.

4. Stahl SM. Deconstructing violence as a medical syndrome: mapping psychotic, impulsive, and predatory subtypes to malfunctioning brain circuits. *CNS Spectr.* 2014; **19**(5): 357–365.

5. Witt K, van Dorn R, Fazel S. Risk factors for violence in psychosis: systematic review and meta-regression analysis of 110 studies. *PLoS One.* 2013; **8**(2): e55942.

6. Nolan KA, Czobor P, Roy BB, *et al.* Characteristics of assaultive behavior among psychiatric inpatients. *Psychiatr. Serv.* 2003; **54**(7): 1012–1016.

7. Dodge KA, Lochman JE, Harnish JD, Bates JE, Pettit GS. Reactive and proactive aggression in school children and psychiatrically impaired chronically assaultive youth. *J. Abnorm. Psychol.* 1997; **106**(1): 37–51.

8. McDermott BE, Holoyda BJ. Assessment of aggression in inpatient settings. *CNS Spectr.* 2014; **19**(05): 425–431.

9. Nolan KA, Volavka J, Mohr P, Czobor P. Psychopathy and violent behavior among patients with schizophrenia or schizoaffective disorder. *Psychiatr. Serv.* 1999; **50**(6): 787.

10. Patton JH, Stanford MS, Barratt ES. Factor structure of the Barratt impulsiveness scale. *J. Clin. Psychol.* 1995; **51**(6): 768–774.

11. Nolan KA, D'Angelo D, Hoptman MJ. Self-report and laboratory measures of impulsivity in patients with schizophrenia or schizoaffective disorder and healthy controls. *Psychiatry Res.* 2011; **187**(1–2): 301–303.

12. Barratt ES. Impulsivity: integrating cognitive, behavioral, biological, and environmental data. In: McCowan W, Johnson J, Shure M, eds. *The Impulsive Client: Theory, Research, and Treatment.* American Psychological Association; 1993: 39–56.

13. Lipszyc J, Schachar R. Inhibitory control and psychopathology: a meta-analysis of studies using the stop signal task. *J. Int.*

Neuropsychol. Soc. 2010; **16**(6): 1064–1076.

14. Chambers CD, Garavan H, Bellgrove MA. Insights into the neural basis of response inhibition from cognitive and clinical neuroscience. *Neurosci. Biobehav. Rev.* 2009; **33**(5): 631–646.

15. Enticott PG, Ogloff JRP, Bradshaw JL, Daffern M. Contrary to popular belief, a lack of behavioural inhibitory control may not be associated with aggression. *Crim. Behav. Ment. Health.* 2007; **17**(3): 179–183.

16. Whiteside SP, Lynam DR. The five factor model and impulsivity: using a structural model of personality to understand impulsivity. *Personality and Individual Differences.* 2001; **30** (4): 669–689.

17. Cyders MA, Smith GT. Mood-based rash action and its components: positive and negative urgency. *Personality and Individual Differences.* 2007; **43** (4): 839–850.

18. Hoptman MJ, Antonius D, Mauro CJ, Parker EM, Javitt DC. Cortical thinning, functional connectivity, and mood-related impulsivity in schizophrenia: relationship to aggressive attitudes and behavior. *Am. J. Psychiatry.* 2014; **171**(9): 943–948.

19. Cyders MA, Smith GT. Emotion-based dispositions to rash action: positive and negative urgency. *Psychol. Bull.* 2008; **134**(6): 807–828.

20. Cyders MA, Dzemidzic M, Eiler WJ, *et al.* Negative urgency mediates the relationship between amygdala and orbitofrontal cortex activation to negative emotional stimuli and general risk-taking. *Cereb Cortex.* doi:10.1093/cercor/bhu123.

21. Enticott PG, Ogloff JR, Bradshaw JL. Response inhibition and impulsivity in schizophrenia. *Psychiatry Res.* 2008; **157**(1): 251–254.

22. Enticott PG, Ogloff JR, Bradshaw JL. Associations between laboratory measures of executive inhibitory control and self-reported impulsivity. *Personality and Individual Differences.* 2006; **41**(2): 285–294.

23. Pawliczek CM, Derntl B, Kellermann T, *et al.* Inhibitory control and trait aggression: neural and behavioral insights using the emotional stop signal task. *Neuroimage.* 2013; **79**: 264–274.

24. Green MF, Lee J. Neural bases of emotional experience versus perception in schizophrenia. *Biol. Psychiatry.* 2012; **71**(2): 96–97.

25. Insel TR, Cuthbert BN, Garvey MA, *et al.* Research domain criteria (RDoC): toward a new classification framework for research on mental disorders. *Am. J. Psychiatry.* 2010; **167**(7): 748–751.

26. Yudofsky SC, Silver JM, Jackson W, Endicott J, Williams D. The Overt Aggression Scale for the objective rating of verbal and physical aggression. *Am. J. Psychiatry.* 1986; **143**(1): 35–39.

27. Buss AH, Perry M. The aggression questionnaire. *J. Pers. Soc. Psychol.* 1992; **63**(3): 452–459.

28. Taylor SP. Aggressive behavior and physiological arousal as a function of provocation and the tendency to inhibit aggression. *J. Pers.* 1967; **35**(2): 297–310.

29. Cherek DR, Moeller FG, Dougherty DM, Rhoades H. Studies of violent and nonviolent male parolees: II. Laboratory and psychometric measurements of impulsivity. *Biol. Psychiatry.* 1997; **41**(5): 523–529.

30. Soyka M. Neurobiology of aggression and violence in schizophrenia. *Schizophr. Bull.* 2011; **37**(5): 913–920.

31. Hoptman MJ, Antonius D. Neuroimaging correlates of aggression in schizophrenia: an update. *Curr. Opin. Psychiatry.* 2011; **24**(2): 100–106.

32. Weiss EM. Neuroimaging and neurocognitive correlates of aggression and violence in schizophrenia. *Scientifica.* 2012; **2012**: 158646.

33. Volavka J. *Neurobiology of Violence*, 2nd edn. Washington, DC: American Psychiatric Association; 2001.

34. Hoptman MJ, Volavka J, Czobor P, *et al.* Aggression and quantitative MRI measures of caudate in patients with chronic schizophrenia or schizoaffective disorder. *J. Neuropsychiatry Clin. Neurosci.* 2006; **18**(4): 509–515.

35. Hoptman MJ, Volavka J, Weiss EM, *et al.* Quantitative MRI measures of orbitofrontal cortex in patients with chronic schizophrenia or schizoaffective disorder. *Psychiatry Res.* 2005; **140** (2): 133–145.

36. Chakos MH, Lieberman JA, Bilder RM, *et al.* Increase in caudate nuclei volumes of first-episode schizophrenic patients taking antipsychotic drugs. *Am. J. Psychiatry.* 1994; **151**(10): 1430–1436.

37. Rüsch N, Spoletini I, Wilke M, *et al.* Inferior frontal white matter volume and suicidality in schizophrenia. *Psychiatry Res.* 2008; **164**(3): 206–214.

38. Narayan VM, Narr KL, Kumari V, *et al.* Regional cortical thinning in subjects with violent antisocial personality disorder or schizophrenia. *Am. J. Psychiatry.* 2007; **164**(9): 1418–1427.

39. Hoptman MJ, Volavka J, Johnson G, *et al.* Frontal white matter microstructure, aggression, and impulsivity in men with schizophrenia: a preliminary study. *Biol. Psychiatry.* 2002; **52** (1): 9–14.

40. Raine A, Buchsbaum MS, Stanley J, *et al.* Selective reductions in

prefrontal glucose metabolism in murderers. *Biol. Psychiatry*. 1994; **36**(6): 365–373.

41. Volkow ND, Tancredi LR, Grant C, *et al.* Brain glucose metabolism in violent psychiatric patients: a preliminary study. *Psychiatry Res*. 1995; **61**(4): 243–253.

42. Wong MTH, Fenwick PBC, Lumsden J, *et al.* Positron emission tomography in male violent offenders with schizophrenia. *Psychiatry Res*. 1997; **68**(2): 111–123.

43. Joyal C, Putkonen A, Mancini-Marie A, *et al.* Violent persons with schizophrenia and comorbid disorders: a functional magnetic resonance imaging study. *Schizophr. Res*. 2007; **91**(1): 97–102.

44. Kumari V, Das M, Taylor PJ, *et al.* Neural and behavioural responses to threat in men with a history of serious violence and schizophrenia or antisocial personality disorder. *Schizophr. Res*. 2009; **110**(1): 47–58.

45. Dolan MC, Fullam RS. Psychopathy and functional magnetic resonance imaging blood oxygenation level-dependent responses to emotional faces in violent patients with schizophrenia. *Biol. Psychiatry*. 2009; **66**(6): 570–577.

46. Hoptman MJ, D'Angelo D, Catalano D, *et al.* Amygdalofrontal functional disconnectivity and aggression in schizophrenia. *Schizophr. Bull*. 2010; **36**(5): 1020–1028.

47. Szeszko PR. Aggression in schizophrenia and its relationship to neural circuitry of urgency. *Am. J. Psychiatry*. 2014; **171**(9): 897–900.

48. Davidson RJ, Putnam KM, Larson CL. Dysfunction in the neural circuitry of emotion regulation—a possible prelude to violence. *Science*. 2000; **289**(5479): 591–594.

49. Kring AM, Werner KH. Emotion regulation and psychopathology.

In: Philippot P, Feldman RS, eds. *The Regulation of Emotion*. Mahwah, NJ: Lawrence Erlbaum Associates; 2004: 359–385.

50. Gross JJ, Jazaieri H. Emotion, emotion regulation, and psychopathology: an affective science perspective. *Clinical Psychological Science*. 2014; **2**(4): 387–401.

51. Perry Y, Henry JD, Nangle MR, Grisham JR. Regulation of negative affect in schizophrenia: the effectiveness of acceptance versus reappraisal and suppression. *J. Clin. Exp. Neuropsychol*. 2012; **34**(5): 497–508.

52. Krakowski MI, Czobor P, Citrome L, Bark N, Cooper TB. Atypical antipsychotic agents in the treatment of violent patients with schizophrenia and schizoaffective disorder. *Arch. Gen. Psychiatry*. 2006; **63**(6): 622–629.

53. Volavka J, Czobor P, Nolan K, *et al.* Overt aggression and psychotic symptoms in patients with schizophrenia treated with clozapine, olanzapine, risperidone, or haloperidol. *J. Clin. Psychopharmacol*. 2004; **24** (2): 225–228.

54. Arango V, Underwood MD, Mann JJ. Serotonin brain circuits involved in major depression and suicide. *Prog. Brain Res*. 2002; **136**: 443–453.

55. Citrome L, Volavka J. The psychopharmacology of violence: making sensible decisions. *CNS Spectr*. 2014; **19**(5): 411–418.

56. Biswal BB, Mennes M, Zuo XN, *et al.* Toward discovery science of human brain function. *Proc. Natl Acad. Sci. U S A*. 2010; **107**(10): 4734–4739.

57. Bersani F, Minichino A, Enticott P, *et al.* Deep transcranial magnetic stimulation as a treatment for psychiatric disorders: a comprehensive review. *Eur. Psychiatry*. 2013; **28** (1): 30–39.

58. LaConte SM, Peltier SJ, Hu XP. Real-time fMRI using brain-state classification. *Hum. Brain Mapp*. 2007; **28**(10): 1033–1044.

59. Raichle ME, MacLeod AM, Snyder AZ, *et al.* A default mode of brain function. *Proc. Natl Acad. Sci. U S A*. 2001; **98**(2): 676–682.

60. Gusnard DA, Akbudak E, Shulman GL, Raichle ME. Medial prefrontal cortex and self-referential mental activity: relation to a default mode of brain function. *Proc. Natl Acad. Sci. U S A*. 2001; **98**(7): 4259–4264.

61. Ruiz S, Lee S, Soekadar SR, *et al.* Acquired self-control of insula cortex modulates emotion recognition and brain network connectivity in schizophrenia. *Hum. Brain Mapp*. 2013; **34**(1): 200–212.

62. Hampson M, Stoica T, Saksa J, *et al.* Real-time fMRI biofeedback targeting the orbitofrontal cortex for contamination anxiety. *J. Vis. Exp*. 2012; (59): 3535.

63. Sitaram R, Caria A, Veit R, *et al.* Volitional control of the anterior insula in criminal psychopaths using realtime fMRI neurofeedback: a pilot study. *Front. Behav. Neurosci*. 2014; **8**: 344.

64. Keers R, Ullrich S, DeStavola BL, Coid JW. Association of violence with emergence of persecutory delusions in untreated schizophrenia. *Am. J. Psychiatry*. 2014; **171**(3): 332–339.

65. Coid JW, Ullrich S, Kallis C, *et al.* The relationship between delusions and violence: findings from the East London first episode psychosis study. *JAMA Psychiatry*. 2013; **70**(5): 465–471.

66. Johnson SL, Carver CS, Joormann J. Impulsive responses to emotion as a transdiagnostic vulnerability to internalizing and externalizing symptoms. *J. Affect. Disord*. 2013; **150**(3): 872–878.

67. Dambacher F, Sack AT, Lobbestael J, *et al.* Out of control evidence for anterior insula involvement in motor impulsivity and reactive aggression. *Soc. Cogn. Affect. Neurosci.* doi:10.1093/scan/nsu077.

68. Dambacher F, Sack AT, Lobbestael J, *et al.* The role of right prefrontal and medial cortex in response inhibition: Interfering with action restraint and action cancellation using transcranial magnetic brain stimulation. *J. Cogn. Neurosci.* 2014; **26**(8): 1775–1784.

69. Warburton K. The new mission of forensic mental health services: managing violence as a medical syndrome in an environment that balances treatment and safety. *CNS Spectr.* 2014; **19**(5): 368–373.

70. Stahl SM, Morrissette DA, Cummings M, *et al.* California State Hospital Violence Assessment and Treatment (Cal-VAT). *CNS Spectr.* 2014; **19**(5): 449–465.

Chapter 15

Serotonin and impulsive aggression

Emil F. Coccaro, Jennifer R. Fanning, K. Luan Phan, and Royce Lee

Introduction

Aggression has been studied from a variety of perspectives, including the political, social, psychological, and neurobiological. Aggressive behavior serves an adaptive function to enable the organism to defend itself, or its offspring, against attack and/or to secure access to the resources it needs to survive. The fact that aggressive behavior has been preserved over time and across species speaks to its adaptive value. In humans, however, aggression is often not advantageous, especially as our species has become more civilized and, in today's society, there are limited circumstances in which aggressive behavior is acceptable (e.g., in the case of "self-defense").

Typically, we distinguish at least two forms of aggression: instrumental and impulsive (also called proactive or reactive [1]). Instrumental aggression is carried out with the primary goal of obtaining some benefit or reward. This type of aggression is most closely associated with psychopathy and/or antisocial personality disorder. In contrast, aggression that is carried out impulsively or in anger is termed impulsive or reactive aggression. Impulsive aggression characteristically occurs in response to a provocation (which is often social), threat, or frustration. This type of aggression, when it is sufficiently frequent and severe, is exemplified by the diagnosis of intermittent explosive disorder (IED) [2]. However impulsive aggression is also commonly associated with Cluster B personality disorders, in particular borderline personality disorder and antisocial personality disorder [3]. In IED, aggression is not due primarily to a neurological lesion or condition, substance intoxication, mood disorder, or psychotic disorder. The fact that between 5% and 7% of the general population will meet criteria for IED at some point during their lifetime highlights the importance of understanding and addressing aggressive behavior [4].

The most extensively studied neurotransmitter with respect to impulsive aggression has been serotonin [5] (5-hydroxytryptamine; 5-HT), with a large literature strongly suggesting the involvement of 5-HT in impulsive aggressive behavior in humans (Table 15.1). While other neurotransmitters [6–9] and modulators [10] have been shown to have a possible role in aggression, this article will focus on the previous, decades-long study of serotonin function and aggression, and then will conclude with the clinical implications of this research.

Serotonin and Suicidality: Precursor Studies to Those Involving Aggression

Early human studies on 5-HT focused on its role in suicidal behavior [11]. This early work revealed that individuals who had committed suicide had lower post-mortem concentrations of 5-HT and the 5-HT metabolite, 5-hydroxyindoleacetic acid (5-HIAA), compared to those who died by other causes [12–14]. The work was followed by studies of cerebrospinal fluid (CSF) levels of 5-HIAA (CSF 5-HIAA), the major, stable metabolite of serotonin in the CSF which is thought to reflect serotonin turnover via the degradation of serotonin following release into the synapse. Since CSF 5-HIAA levels correlate with brain 5-HIAA levels, CSF 5-HIAA has been utilized as a marker of central 5-HT activity [15]. In one of the earliest human studies in depression, Asberg et al. [16] found a bimodal distribution of CSF 5-HIAA with 29% of depressed subjects comprising a "low 5-HIAA" group. Subjects who attempted suicide using violent methods were significantly more likely to belong to the low 5-HIAA group. Other studies have

Table 15.1 Relationship between measures of aggression and indices of 5-HT in living human subjects

Study type	Brain imaging	CSF	Peripheral (pituitary or platelet)
Neurochemical:			
5-HIAA	—	Inverse correlation in several [12,13], but not all studies [45]	—
Tryptophan	Reduced "trapping" correlates with impulsivity [56]	—	Positive correlation in females but not males [23]
5-HT	—	—	Inverse correlation [24]
Pharmaco-challenge with non-selective 5-HT agents:			
Fenfluramine	Reduction in response in OFC [53]	—	Inverse correlation with PRL[FEN] [21,22]
m-CPP	Reduction in response in ACC [54]	—	Inverse correlation with PRL[m-CPP] [17,33]
5-HT receptors:			
5-HT Transporters	Reduced "ACC" binding in aggressive subjects [57]	—	Inverse correlation [25,26]
5-HT1a (pre-)	—	—	Reduced [32] or same [47] thermal response to ipsapirone
5-HT1a (post-)	—	—	Cortisol response to ipsapirone: inverse correlation in personality disordered subjects [47]
5-HT2a	Increased in frontal areas of aggressive subjects [52]	—	—

also observed lower CSF 5-HIAA levels in those who have attempted suicide compared to healthy individuals [17–19]. In addition, a meta-analysis found clear support for the relationship between suicidal behavior and low CSF 5-HIAA levels [20], while these authors found mixed support for the notion that lower CSF 5-HIAA levels are associated with violent (as opposed to nonviolent) suicide attempts.

Serotonin and Impulsive Aggression: Neurochemical Studies

The earliest study to explore the 5-HT/aggression relationship in humans reported a significant and inverse correlation between CSF 5-HIAA levels and life history of aggressive behavior ($r = -0.78$) in adult Navy recruits being evaluated for "fitness of duty" due to either aggressive or passive aggressive behavior [17]. Moreover, subjects with a history of suicide attempt ($n = 11$) had a higher life history of aggression scores and lower 5-HIAA levels compared to subjects with no such history. This correlation between CSF 5-HIAA level and life history of aggression was replicated in a subsequent sample of men with borderline personality disorder [18]. Several studies of impulsive violent offenders also report lower CSF 5-HIAA levels [19], though not all studies, especially those in subjects not drawn from a criminal justice system, have reported this finding [21–23]. For example, Coccaro et al. [21,22] found no relationship between CSF 5-HIAA levels and life history of aggression in two separate samples of personality disorder subjects. Simeon et al. [24] found no relation between several indices of 5-HT functioning and life history of aggression or impulsivity in a sample of personality disordered individuals with a history of self-harm. In contrast, a more recent study found that when both CSF 5-HIAA and CSF HVA levels are placed in the same statistical model, CSF 5-HIAA demonstrates a significant, and positive, correlation with aggression [25]. This is consistent with reduced 5-HT receptor responsiveness as demonstrated in pharmaco-challenge studies [26,27]. While it is far easier to assess 5-HT–related measures in the periphery, there are limited studies of peripheral levels of tryptophan or of 5-HT and aggression. One study reports a positive relationship of plasma tryptophan with aggression in healthy female, but not male, subjects [28], while another reports an inverse relationship between platelet 5-HT and aggression in personality disordered subjects [29].

Serotonin and Impulsive Aggression: Receptor Studies

Receptor markers on circulating blood platelets have long been used as a model of 5-HT receptors in the central nervous system. Despite considerable platelet receptor work in other psychiatric populations, relatively little research in this area has been published in impulsively aggressive subjects. Simeon et al. [24] reported an inverse correlation between the number of platelet ^{3}H-impiramine (5-HT transporter) binding sites and self-mutilation and impulsivity in personality disordered subjects with, but not without, a history of self-mutilation. Coccaro et al. [30] first reported that the number of platelet ^{3}H-paroxetine (5-HT transporter) binding sites was inversely correlated with life history of aggression in personality disordered subjects. In a study of overlapping subjects, the same authors noted a positive relationship between platelet 5-HT2$_a$ receptors and aggression [31]. However, while a larger study confirmed the relationship between aggression and platelet ^{3}H-paroxetine binding sites [32], this was not true for platelet 5-HT2$_a$ binding sites [33].

Serotonin and Impulsive Aggression: Pharmaco-Challenge Studies

Pharmaco-challenge studies have also provided evidence of a relationship between central 5-HT function and aggression. Coccaro et al. [26] reported a relationship between the prolactin response to d,l-fenfluramine (PRL [d,l-FEN]) challenge and both life history of aggression ($r = -0.57$) as well as the tendency to be aggressive as a personality trait ($r = -0.52$) in subjects with personality disorders. A subsequent study, with a much larger sample, also reported a significant relationship between PRL[d-FEN] and life history of aggression in personality disordered (PD) subjects, though the inverse correlation was smaller in magnitude [27]. Similar associations were observed by New et al. [34] in a large sample of PD subjects between PRL[d,l-FEN] and tendency to be aggressive as a personality trait in PD men ($r = -0.21$). Other studies have also found a relationship between blunted hormonal response to 5-HT challenge in patients with borderline personality disorder [35], antisocial personality disorder [36], and substance use disorder [37,38].

Serotonin and Impulsive Aggression: Behavioral Challenge Studies

In laboratory studies utilizing behavioral measures that provoke anger in the laboratory (e.g., Taylor Aggression Paradigm or the Point Subtraction Aggression Paradigm), aggressiveness has been correlated with blunted PRL response to d-FEN challenge [39] and blunted thermal response to ipsapirone challenge [40]. Laboratory manipulations of central 5-HT using tryptophan depletion [41] or supplementation [42] have also demonstrated an inverse relationship between provoked aggressive responding and 5-HT activity, particularly in subjects with high trait levels of aggression [43].

Serotonin and Impulsive Aggression: Commentary on Extant Empiric Data

Overall, there is considerable data to support the hypothesis that 5-HT is involved in behaviors described as "impulsive" rather than "premeditated." Linnoila et al. [44] reported lower CSF 5-HIAA levels among murderers and attempted murderers who had committed impulsive crimes compared to those who committed premeditated crimes, and several hypotheses have been offered to explain the role of 5-HT in modulating behavior. Spoont [45] proposed that 5-HT stabilizes information flow by supporting phase coherence in neural activity, and thereby modulates reactivity to stimuli both internal and external. In this model, high central 5-HT levels are associated with behavioral constraint, while low 5-HT levels are associated with impulsivity and stimulus activity [45]. Similarly, Linnoila and Virkkunen [46] postulated that a "low 5-HT syndrome" characterizes many individuals who engage in violent, impulsive, and antisocial behavior. This hypothesis was largely derived from studies of CSF 5-HIAA. These authors posit that 5-HT serves to constrain behavior, so a 5-HT deficit is associated with increased impulsivity [46]. Another model, the "irritable aggression model" by Coccaro et al. [47], suggests that a net hypo-serotonergic state is associated with greater irritability, which is conceptualized as a lower threshold for responding to noxious stimuli with aggressive behavior. This is consistent with findings of an inverse correlation between irritability and PRL[d,l-FEN] [26], as well as other reports which have suggested that impulsivity may not correlate with measures of 5-HT independently

of aggression [27,32]. Furthermore, research in both animals and humans suggests that noxious, threatening, or provocative stimuli are necessary to elicit aggressive behavior in an organism in a hypo-serotonergic state [48,49].

While early studies in this area produced large effect sizes, a recent meta-analysis reports a more modest estimate of relationship between 5-HT and aggression in human subjects. Duke et al. [50] analyzed 171 studies on the serotonin–aggression relationship that examined (a) CSF 5-HIAA levels, (b) acute tryptophan depletion (ATD), (c) pharmaco-challenge, and (d) endocrine challenge. These authors found a small ($r = -0.12$), but significant, inverse relation between measures of 5HT functioning and aggression. Pharmaco-challenge studies yielded the largest ($r = -0.21$), while CSF 5-HIAA studies yielded the smallest, and a nonsignificant, effect size ($r = -0.06$, ns). Small, significant, mean effects were also found for ATD ($r = -0.10$) and endocrine challenge ($r = -0.14$); cortisol response variables were not significantly related to aggression ($r = -0.02$). Neither phenomenological nor drug type characteristics of the subjects moderated the relationships between indices of 5-HT functioning and aggression. These results, as well as other conflicting findings in the literature, suggest that the relationship between 5-HT and behavior is more complex than previously thought.

Serotonin and Impulsive Aggression: 5-HT Receptors and Brain Circuitry

Serotonergic neurons project throughout the brain, with particularly dense projections in the cerebral cortex, limbic structures, basal ganglia, and brainstem. In addition, the 5-HT system comprises at least 14 types of receptors. Certain receptor subtypes (5-HT$_{1a}$ and 5-HT$_{1b}$) are expressed at both pre- and post-synaptic locations, and 5-HT receptor subtypes appear to exert unique, and perhaps opposing, effects on aggression. For example, aggressive individuals have been shown to have blunted response to 5-HT$_{1a}$ receptor agonists [51,52], and suicidal subjects have demonstrated unique patterns of 5-HT1$_a$ receptor binding, although the results have been mixed [53]. 5-HT1$_b$ agonists may also reduce aggression through effects on impulsivity and 5-HT1$_b$ hetero-receptors (located at post-synaptic sites on non-5-HT neurons) in the hypothalamus may be involved in regulating offensive, rather than reactive [54], aggression. The relationship between the 5-HT2_a receptor and impulsive aggression has been mixed, with some studies reporting inverse associations with 5-HT2_a indices [55,56], while other studies have reported positive associations [57] in areas of the prefrontal cortex. For example, Rosell *et al.* [57] saw increased 5-HT2_a availability associated with current, but not past, impulsive aggression in PD subjects, which suggests that dynamic changes in this index may reflect state changes in aggressive behavior. Finally, the 5-HT2_c receptor has been of interest because of its possible anti-aggressive effects when stimulated [53], and because the PRL[d-FEN] response appears, in part, to reflect 5-HT2_c stimulation [27].

Neuroimaging methodologies represent a significant advance in the area of psychiatry research. In one of the earliest Positron Emission Tomography (PET) studies in personality disorder subjects, Siever *et al.* [58] imaged glucose metabolism in impulsively aggressive subjects ($n = 6$) with personality disorder and healthy control ($n = 5$) subjects following a single acute challenge dose of d,l-FEN or placebo. In healthy subjects, the d,l-FEN challenge was associated with increased glucose utilization in the left orbitofrontal (OFC) and anterior cingulate cortex (ACC), while impulsively aggressive subjects had reduced glucose utilization in these areas. Only the inferior parietal lobe showed increased metabolism in response to d,l-FEN in PD subjects. PRL[d,l-FEN] (placebo-corrected) responses did not differ between the aggressive subjects and healthy controls. PRL[d,l-FEN] correlated in the medial frontal cortex ($r = 0.58$) and right middle cingulate ($r = 0.63$). These correlations were not significant due to the small sample size. A similar finding was obtained in a larger follow-up study. New *et al.* [59] studied similarly impulsively aggressive PD ($n = 13$) and healthy ($n = 13$) subjects with a meta-chlorophenylpiperazine (m-CPP) challenge. Healthy, but not aggressive, subjects showed increased glucose utilization in OFC and anterior cingulate (i.e., areas involved in inhibiting aggressive behavior) following m-CPP challenge relative to placebo. Furthermore, these investigators reported that three months of fluoxetine treatment appeared to normalize OFC function in impulsively aggressive subjects, which supports the hypothesis that deficits in OFC function are, partially, supported by abnormalities in serotonin function [60].

Other studies suggest that impulsively aggressive subjects have abnormal 5-HT synthesis. In one study, males with borderline personality disorder displayed reduced trapping of a 5-HT precursor analog (i.e., reduced 5-HT synthesis capacity) in the medial frontal gyrus, anterior cingulate gyrus (ACG), superior temporal gyrus (STG), and corpus striatum compared to healthy controls, while similar women had lower trapping in the right ACT and superior temporal gyrus [61]. Another study using PET radiotracer for the serotonin transporter (5-HTT) also showed reduced 5-HTT availability in ACG in impulsively aggressive subjects [62]. Finally, a study by Koch *et al.* [63] using single-photon emission computed tomography (SPECT) examined binding of $[I^{123}]$ ADAM to the serotonin transporter, and found increased binding in impulsively aggressive subjects in both the hypothalamus and brainstem. ADAM binding correlated significantly with impulsivity but not with depression.

Serotonin and Impulsive Aggression: Treatment Correlates

Treatment with selective serotonin reuptake inhibitors (SSRIs; e.g., fluoxetine) has been shown to reduce impulsive aggression in human subjects with prominent histories of impulsive aggressive behavior. In addition to several open-label studies, five double-blind, placebo-controlled studies [64–68] have reported significant reduction in impulsive aggressive behavior in nonbipolar/ nonpsychotic psychiatric patients treated with SSRIs. While such treatment brings about full remission of impulsive aggressive behaviors in less than one-third of subjects, up to nearly 50% achieve either full or partial remission [64].

Further, in small, preliminary studies, we have found that anti-aggressive responses to SSRIs appear to be directly related to the intactness of 5-HT synaptic function and to the degree to which cortico-limbic circuits are impacted by treatment. The first work in this area found a positive relationship between the PRL response to d-FEN and improvement in OAS-M Aggression scores. In other words, the lower the PRL[d-FEN] value pre-treatment, the lower the anti-aggressive response to the SSRI [69]. While seemingly counterintuitive, these data suggest that in order for SSRIs to have anti-aggressive efficacy, 5-HT synaptic function must be somewhat functional, at the least. This is because SSRIs work by attaching to 5-HT

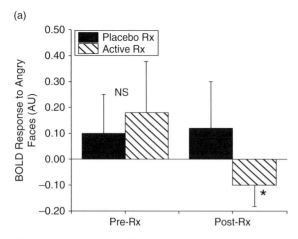

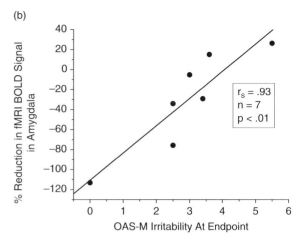

Figure 15.1a Amygdala BOLD responses to social threat (angry faces) before and after 12 weeks of treatment with placebo ($n = 10$) vs. fluoxetine ($n = 3$) or divalproex ($n = 4$); *$p <0.05$.

Figure 15.1b Endpoint Overt Aggression Scale–Modified (OAS-M) Irritability Score correlates (Spearman) directly with percent suppression of amygdala BOLD responses to social threat (angry faces) after 12 weeks of fluoxetine ($n = 3$) or divalproex ($n = 4$) in subjects currently meeting DSM-5 criteria for IED.

transporters, which leads to an increase in synaptic 5-HT. However, if 5-HT transporters are inversely related to aggression, then there would be fewer for the SSRI to bind to, and therefore would work to block 5-HT uptake. This would lead to less of an increase in synaptic 5-HT as a function of aggression. This is also consistent with data showing that aggressive individuals with the "s" allele (which is associated with less production of the transporter protein) have a poorer anti-aggressive response to SSRIs [66]. More recent preliminary work suggests that effective anti-aggressive treatment, by either SSRIs (fluoxetine) or mood stabilizers (divalproex), is associated with a reduction in the amygdala response to social threat ("anger faces"; see Figure 15.1a) and a possible normalization of heightened amygdala, and blunted orbito-frontal, response to social threat. Specifically, placebo had no effect on functional magnetic resonance imaging (fMRI) Blood Oxygenation Level Dependent (BOLD) responses in amygdala, but active drug treatment reduced fMRI BOLD signal activity responses to anger faces ($p<0.05$; 181% reduction in signal from 122% to –0.099%). In addition, percent reduction in amygdala signal activity to anger faces correlated highly with post-treatment endpoint scores on aggression variables in drug-treated subjects (irritability score on the Overt Aggression Scale: $r_s = 0.93$, $p<0.01$; see Figure 15.1b). Conversely, a trend was seen for an increase in fMRI BOLD signal activity to anger faces in OMPFC ($p<0.10$; a 75% increase in signal from –0.173% to –0.043%). In addition, percent

increase in Orbitomedial Prefrontal Cortex (OMPFC) fMRI BOLD activity to anger faces was inversely (though not significantly) correlated with post-treatment scores of OAS-M Irritability ($r_s = -0.60$). This suggests that such agents not only affect central 5-HT function, but also alter cortico-limbic circuitry, as expected by our current understanding of clinical neuroscience [70].

Clinical Implications

If central 5-HT function plays an important role in the regulation of impulsive aggression, how can clinicians utilize these research data to improve the care of their own patients? First, it is critical that clinicians know that 5-HT is not a unitary system. However, while the various components of the system (receptors and their location in the brain) may have different effects on behavior, a direct relationship between 5-HT and behavioral inhibition is the most parsimonious way to conceptualize the role of 5-HT and impulsive aggression. Thus, the greater the 5-HT system activity, the greater behavioral inhibition the individual will have when confronted with threat or frustration.

As we have discussed above, agents that increase 5-HT activity, such as SSRIs, have efficacy to reduce impulsive aggressive behavior up to a point. If so, other ways to stimulate the central 5-HT system will be needed. For example, one could attempt to increase 5-HT receptor activation by giving a direct

5-HT agonist. Recently, a direct 5-HT2c agonist (lorcaserin) has come onto the market for weight loss and may be studied for its effects on impulsive aggression. Since the PRL response to fenfluramine appears to be mediated by activation of 5-HT2c receptors, it is possible that this agent could reduce impulsive aggression on its own or provide added efficacy to SSRI treatment. Other agents that may or may not have an effect on the central 5-HT system may also be efficacious in reducing aggression include mood stabilizers and some atypical antipsychotic agents. Randomized controlled trial data for SSRIs and for mood stabilizer/antipsychotic agents is not extensive, but studies suggest anti-aggressive doses that are similar to those for treating mood disorders.

Behavioral interventions may also reduce impulsive aggressive behavior, but we do not know yet if these interventions are mediated by changes in brain 5-HT function. We also do not know if the combination of pharmacologic and behavioral treatment will produce better efficacy than either modality alone because such studies have not been performed. Knowing that either modality produces similar results, likely through different pathways, we expect that the combination will result in an improved outcome for combined versus single treatment.

Other gaps in our knowledge include the possibility of gender or age differences in treatment response, as well as when to treat and exactly how to treat. We suggest that treatment is warranted when the frequency and severity of impulsive aggressive outbursts has reached the threshold for meeting *Diagnostic and Statistical Manual of Mental Disorders*, Fifth Edition (DSM-5) criteria for intermittent explosive disorder because these criteria define the presence of a disorder of impulsive aggression. The type of treatment should include both pharmacologic and behavioral

interventions. There is no empiric data to inform us as to which should be tried first, but our recommendation is that behavioral intervention may be tried first when the severity of IED is moderate, but the reverse may be true when IED is more severe.

Conclusion

In summary, an extensive literature supports a role for serotonin in impulsive aggression (and suicidality). Evidence suggests that serotonin modulates activity in areas of the prefrontal cortex, including the orbitofrontal cortex and anterior cingulate, which are implicated in "top-down" control of limbic response to stimuli. Individuals with personality disorder display impaired serotonergic functioning in these brain regions, which may account for the aggressive and, perhaps, impulsive behaviors seen in these disorders. Treatment of impulsive aggressive behaviors with serotonergic agents may be a good strategy, but this may be less effective in those with severely impaired 5-HT system function. As serotonin is not the only relevant neurotransmitter underlying aggressive behavior [5], more work needs to be done to examine the role of other neurotransmitter systems in order to more comprehensively treat these behaviors. In addition, neuroimaging methods have the great potential to enhance our understanding of both neurotransmitter and neurocircuitry function in human aggression [70].

Disclosures

Emil Coccaro has the following disclosure: Azevan, Inc., consultant, consulting fees. Royce Lee has the following disclosure: Azevan, Inc., principal investigator, research support. Jennifer Fanning and K. Luan Phan do not have anything to disclose.

References

1. Dodge KA. The structure and function of reactive and proactive aggression. In: Peppler D, Rubin K eds. *The Development and Treatment of Childhood Aggression*. Hillsdale, NJ: Erlbaum; 1991: 201–218.

2. Coccaro EF. Intermittent explosive disorder as a disorder of impulsive aggression for DSM-5.

Am. J. Psychiatry. 2012; **169**(6): 577–588.

3. Berman ME, Fallon AE, Coccaro EF. The relationship between personality psychopathology and aggressive behavior in research volunteers. *J. Abnorm. Psychol.* 1998; **107**(4): 651–658.

4. Kessler RC, Coccaro EF, Fava M, *et al.* The prevalence and correlates of DSM-IV intermittent explosive disorder in the National

Comorbidity Survey Replication. *Arch. Gen. Psychiatry.* 2006; **63**(6): 669–678.

5. Yanowitch R, Coccaro EF. The neurochemistry of human aggression. *Adv. Genet.* 2011; **75**: 151–169.

6. Coccaro EF, Kavoussi RJ, Hauger RL, Cooper TB, Ferris CF. Cerebrospinal fluid vasopressin levels: correlates with aggression and serotonin function in

personality-disordered subjects. *Arch. Gen. Psychiatry.* 1998; **55**(8): 708–714.

7. Coccaro EF, Lee R, Liu T, Mathé AA. CSF NPY correlates with aggression in human subjects. *Biol. Psychiatry.* 2012; **72**(12): 997–1003.

8. Coccaro EF, Lee R, Owens MJ, Kinkead B, Nemeroff CB. Cerebrospinal fluid substance P-like immunoreactivity correlates with aggression in personality disordered subjects. *Biol. Psychiatry.* 2012; **72**(3): 238–243.

9. Coccaro EF, Lee R, Vezina P. Cerebrospinal fluid glutamate concentration correlates with impulsive aggression in human subjects. *J. Psychiatr. Res.* 2013; **47**(9): 1247–1253.

10. Coccaro EF, Lee R, Coussons-Read M. Elevated plasma inflammatory markers in individuals with intermittent explosive disorder and correlation with aggression in humans. *JAMA Psychiatry.* 2014; **71**(2): 158–165.

11. Asberg M, Schalling D, Traskman-Bendz L, Wagner A. Psychobiology of suicide, impulsivity, and related phenomena. In Davis K ed. *Psychopharmacology: The Third Generation of Progress.* New York: Raven Press; 1987: 665–668.

12. Bourne HR, Bunney WE, Colburn RW, *et al.* Noradrenaline, 5-hydroxytryptamine, and 5-hydroxyindoleacetic acid hindbrains of suicidal patients. *Lancet.* 1968; **2**(7572): 805–808.

13. Pare CMB, Yeung DPH, Price K, Stacey RS. 5-Hydroxytryptamine, noradrenaline, and dopamine in brainstem, hypothalamus, and caudate nucleus of controls and of patients committing suicide by coal-gas poisoning. *Lancet.* 1969; **2**(7612): 133–135.

14. Shaw DM, Eccleston EG, Camps FE. 5-Hydroxytryptamine in the hind-brain of depressive suicides.

Br. J. Psychiatry. 1967; **113**(505): 1407–1411.

15. Stanley M, Traskman-Bendz L, Dorovini-Zis K. Correlations between aminergic metabolites simultaneously obtained from human CSF and brain. *Life Sci.* 1985; **37**(14): 1279–1286.

16. Asberg M, Träskman L, Thorén P. 5-HIAA in the cerebrospinal fluid: a biochemical suicide predictor? *Arch. Gen. Psychiatry.* 1976; **33**(10): 1193–1197.

17. Brown GL, Goodwin FK, Ballenger JC, Goyer PF, Major LF. Aggression in humans correlates with cerebrospinal fluid amine metabolites. *Psychiatry Res.* 1979; **1**(2): 131–139.

18. Brown GL, Ebert MH, Goyer PF, *et al.* Aggression, suicide, and serotonin: relationships to CSF aminemetabolites. *Am. J. Psychiatry.* 1982; **139**(6): 741–746.

19. Lidberg L, Tuck JR, Asberg M, Scalia-Tomba GP, Bertilsson L. Homicide, suicide, and CSF 5-HIAA. *Acta Psychiatr. Scand.* 1985; **71**(3): 230–236.

20. Lester D. The concentration of neurotransmitter metabolites in cerebrospinal fluid of suicidal individuals: a meta-analysis. *Pharmacopsychiatry.* 1995; **28**(2): 45–50.

21. Coccaro EF, Kavoussi RJ, Cooper TB, Hauger RL. Central serotonin activity and aggression: inverse relationship with prolactin response to d-fenfluramine, but not CSF 5-HIAA concentration, in human subjects. *Am. J. Psychiatry.* 1997; **154**(10): 1430–1435.

22. Coccaro EF, Kavoussi RJ, Trestman RL, *et al.* Serotonin function in human subjects: intercorrelations among central 5-HT indices and aggressiveness. *Psychiatry Res.* 1997; **73**(1–2): 1–14.

23. Hibbeln JR, Umhau JC, George DT, *et al.* Plasma total cholesterol

concentrations do not predict cerebrospinal fluid neurotransmitter metabolites: implications for the biophysical role of highly unsaturated fatty acids. *Am. J. Clin. Nutr.* 2000; **71**(1 Suppl): 331S–338S.

24. Simeon D, Stanley B, Frances A, *et al.* Self-mutilation in personality disorders: psychological and biological correlates. *Am. J. Psychiatry.* 1992; **149**(2): 221–226.

25. Coccaro EF, Lee R. Cerebrospinal fluid 5-hydroxyindolacetic acid and homovanillic acid: reciprocal relationships with impulsive aggression in human subjects. *J. Neural. Transm.* 2010; **117**(2): 241–248.

26. Coccaro EF, Siever LJ, Klar HM, *et al.* Serotonergic studies in patients with affective and personality disorders: correlates with suicidal and impulsive aggressive behavior. *Arch. Gen. Psychiatry.* 1989; **46**(7): 587–599.

27. Coccaro EF, Lee R, Kavoussi RJ. Aggression, suicidality, and intermittent explosive disorder: serotonergic correlates in personality disorder and healthy control subjects. *Neuropsychopharmacology.* 2010; **35**(2): 435–444.

28. Suarez EC, Krishnan KR. The relation of free plasma tryptophan to anger, hostility, and aggression in a nonpatient sample of adult men and women. *Ann. Behav. Med.* 2006; **31**(3): 254–260.

29. Goveas JS, Csernansky JG, Coccaro EF. Platelet serotonin content correlates inversely with life history of aggression in personality-disordered subjects. *Psychiatry Res.* 2004; **126**(1): 23–32.

30. Coccaro E, Kavoussi R, Sheline Y, Lish J, Csernansky J. Impulsive aggression in personality disorder correlates with tritiated paroxetine

binding in the platelet. *Arch. Gen. Psychiatry*. 1996; **53**(6): 531–536.

31. Coccaro EF, Kavoussi RJ, Sheline YI, Berman ME, Csernansky JG. Impulsive aggression in personality disorder correlates with platelet 5-HT2A receptor binding. *Neuropsychopharmacology*. 1997; **16**(3): 211–216.

32. Coccaro EF, Lee R, Kavoussi RJ. Inverse relationship between numbers of 5-HT transporter binding sites and life history of aggression and intermittent explosive disorder. *J. Psychiatr. Res*. 2009; **44**(3): 137–142.

33. Marseille R, Lee R, Coccaro EF. Inter-relationship between different platelet measures of 5-HT and their relationship to aggression in human subjects. *Prog. Neuropsychopharmacol. Biol. Psychiatry*. 2012; **36**(2): 277–281.

34. New AS, Trestman RL, Mitropoulou V, *et al*. Serotonergic function and self-injurious behavior in personality disorder patients. *Psychiatry Res*. 1997; **69**(1): 17–26.

35. Paris J, Zweig-Frank H, Kin NM, *et al*. Neurobiological correlates of diagnosis and underlying traits in patients with borderline personality disorder compared with normal controls. *Psychiatry Res*. 2004; **121**(3): 239–252.

36. O'Keane V, Moloney E, O'Neill H, *et al*. Blunted prolactin responses to d-fenfluramine in sociopathy: evidence for subsensitivity of central serotonergic function. *Br. J. Psychiatry*. 1992; **160**(5): 643–646.

37. Moeller FG, Steinberg JL, Petty F, *et al*. Serotonin and impulsive/aggressive behavior in cocaine dependent subjects. *Prog. Neuropsychopharmacol. Biol. Psychiatry*. 1994; **18**(6): 1027–1035.

38. Moss HB, Yao JK, Panzak GL. Serotonergic responsivity and behavioral dimensions in antisocial personality disorder with substance abuse. *Biol. Psychiatry*. 1990; **28**(4): 325–338.

39. Coccaro EF, Berman ME, Kavoussi RJ, Hauger RL. Relationship of prolactin response to d-fenfluramine to behavioral and questionnaire assessments of aggression in personality-disordered men. *Biol. Psychiatry*. 1996; **40**(3): 157–164.

40. Moeller FG, Allen T, Cherek DR, *et al*. Ipsapirone neuroendocrine challenge: relationship to aggression as measured in the human laboratory. *Psychiatry Res*. 1998; **81**(1): 31–38.

41. Pihl RO, Young SN, Harden P, *et al*. Acute effect of altered tryptophan levels and alcohol on aggression in normal human males. *Psychopharmacology (Berl.)*. 1995; **119**(4): 353–360.

42. Cleare AJ, Bond AJ. The effect of tryptophan depletion and enhancement on subjective and behavioural aggression in normal male subjects. *Psychopharmacology (Berl.)*. 1995; **118**(1): 72–81.

43. Dougherty DM, Bjork JM, Marsh D, Moeller FG. Influence of trait hostility on tryptophan depletion-induced laboratory aggression. *Psychiatry Res*. 1999; **88**(3): 227–232.

44. Linnoila M, Virkkunen M, Scheinin M, *et al*. Low cerebrospinal fluid 5-hydroxyindoleacetic acid concentration differentiates impulsive from nonimpulsive violent behavior. *Life Sci*. 1983; **33**(26): 2609–2614.

45. Spoont MR. Modulatory role of serotonin in neural information processing: implications for human psychopathology. *Psychol. Bull*. 1992; **112**(2): 330–350.

46. Linnoila VM, Virkkunen M. Aggression, suicidality, and serotonin. *J. Clin. Psychiatry*. 1992; **53**(Suppl): 46–51.

47. Coccaro EF, Kavoussi RJ, Lesser JC. Self- and other-directed human aggression: the role of the central serotonergic system. *Int. Clin. Psychopharmacol*. 1992; **6** (Suppl 6): 70–83.

48. Berman ME, McCloskey MS, Fanning JR, Schumacher JA, Coccaro EF. Serotonin augmentation reduces response to attack in aggressive individuals. *Psychol. Sci*. 2009; **20**(6): 714–720.

49. Marks DJ, Miller SR, Schulz KP, Newcorn JH, Halperin JM. The interaction of psychosocial adversity and biological risk in childhood aggression. *Psychiatry Res*. 2007; **151**(3): 221–230.

50. Duke AA, Bègue L, Bell R, Eisenlohr-Moul T. Revisiting the serotonin-aggression relation in humans: a meta-analysis. *Psychol. Bull*. 2013; **139**(5): 1148–1172.

51. Cleare AJ, Bond AJ. Ipsapirone challenge in aggressive men shows an inverse correlation between 5-HT1A receptor function and aggression. *Psychopharmacology (Berl.)*. 2000; **148**(4): 344–349.

52. Almeida M, Lee R, Coccaro EF. Cortisol responses to ipsapirone challenge correlate with aggression, while basal cortisol levels correlate with impulsivity, in personality disorder and healthy volunteer subjects. *J. Psychiatr. Res*. 2010; **44**(14): 874–880.

53. Bortolato M, Pivac N, Muck Seler D, *et al*. The role of the serotonergic system at the interface of aggression and suicide. *Neuroscience*. 2013; **236**: 160–185.

54. Olivier B, van Oorschot R. 5-HT1B receptors and aggression: a review. *Eur. J. Pharmacol*. 2005; **526**(1–3): 207–217.

55. Meyer JH, Wilson AA, Rusjan P, *et al*. Serotonin2A receptor binding potential in people with aggressive and violent behaviour.

J. Psychiatry Neurosci. 2008; **33**(6): 499–508.

56. Soloff PH, Price JC, Mason NS, Becker C, Meltzer CC. Gender, personality, and serotonin-2A receptor binding in healthy subjects. *Psychiatry Research: Neuroimaging.* 2010; **181**(1): 77–84.

57. Rosell DR, Thompson JL, Slifstein M, *et al.* Increased serotonin 2A receptor availability in the orbitofrontal cortex of physically aggressive personality disordered patients. *Biol. Psychiatry.* 2010; **67** (12): 1154–1162.

58. Siever LJ, Buchsbaum MS, New AS, *et al.* d,l-fenfluramine response in impulsive personality disorder assessed with [18F] fluorodeoxyglucose positron emission tomography. *Neuropsychopharmacology.* 1999; **20**(5): 413–423.

59. New AS, Hazlett EA, Buchsbaum MS, *et al.* Blunted prefrontal cortical 18fluorodeoxyglucose positron emission tomography response to meta-chlorophenylpiperazine in impulsive aggression. *Arch. Gen. Psychiatry.* 2002; **59**(7): 621–629.

60. New AS, Buchsbaum MS, Hazlett EA, *et al.* Fluoxetine increases relative metabolic rate in prefrontal cortex in impulsive aggression. *Psychopharmacology (Berl.).* 2004; **176**(3–4): 451–458.

61. Leyton M, Okazawa H, Diksic M, *et al.* Brain regional alpha-[11C] methyl-L-tryptophan trapping in impulsive subjects with borderline personality disorder. *Am. J. Psychiatry.* 2001; **158**(5): 775–782.

62. Frankle WG, Lombardo I, New AS, *et al.* Brain serotonin transporter distribution in subjects with impulsive aggressivity: a positron emission study with [11C]McN 5652. *Am. J. Psychiatry.* 2005; **162**(5): 915–923.

63. Koch W, Schaaff N, Pöpperl G, *et al.* [I-123] ADAM and SPECT in patients with borderline personality disorder and healthy control subjects. *J. Psychiatry Neurosci.* 2007; **32**(4): 234–240.

64. Coccaro EF, Lee R, Kavoussi RJ. A double-blind, randomized, placebo-controlled trial of fluoxetine in patients with intermittent explosive disorder. *J. Clin. Psychiatry.* 2009; **70**(5): 653–662.

65. George DT, Phillips MJ, Lifshitz M, *et al.* Fluoxetine treatment of alcoholic perpetrators of domestic violence: a 12-week, double-blind, randomized, placebo-controlled intervention study. *J. Clin. Psychiatry.* 2011; **72**(1): 60–65.

66. Silva H, Iturra P, Solari A, *et al.* Fluoxetine response in impulsive-aggressive behavior and serotonin transporter polymorphism in personality disorder. *Psychiatr. Genet.* 2010; **20**(1): 25–30.

67. Heiligenstein JH, Coccaro EJ, Potvin JH, *et al.* Fluoxetine not associated with increased violence or aggression in controlled clinical trials. *Ann. Clin. Psychiatry.* 1992; **4**(4): 285–295.

68. Salzman C, Wolfson AN, Schatzberg A, *et al.* Effect of fluoxetine on anger in symptomatic volunteers with borderline personality disorder. *J. Clin. Psychopharmacol.* 1995; **15** (1): 23–29.

69. Coccaro EF, Kavoussi RJ, Hauger RL. Serotonin function and antiaggressive response to fluoxetine: a pilot study. *Biol. Psychiatry.* 1997; **42**(7): 546–552.

70. Coccaro EF, Sripada CS, Yanowitch RN, Phan KL. Corticolimbic function in impulsive aggressive behavior. *Biol. Psychiatry.* 2011; **69**(12): 1153–1159.

Chapter

16

California State Hospital Violence Assessment and Treatment (Cal-VAT) guidelines

Stephen M. Stahl, Debbi A. Morrissette, Michael A. Cummings, Allen Azizian, Shannon M. Bader, Charles Broderick, Laura J. Dardashti, Darci Delgado, Jonathan M. Meyer, Jennifer A. O'Day, George J. Proctor, Benjamin Rose, Marie Schur, Eric H. Schwartz, Susan Velasquez, and Katherine D. Warburton

Introduction

Violence and aggression arise from a complex inter-action of personal and environmental factors; however, treatment of the violent or aggressive individual often proceeds without an adequate consideration of the sources of the patient's threatening or violent behavior. Furthermore, there are no recent published guidelines about how to assess and treat violence in an inpatient forensic or state hospital system, where most of the patients have diagnoses of psychosis, especially schizophrenia. That is, most published guidelines that discuss the treatment of violence or aggression are focused on one particular diagnosis, such as dementia, attention deficit hyperactivity disorder (ADHD), post-traumatic stress disorder (PTSD), traumatic brain injury (TBI), borderline personality disorder, or intellectual disability [1–12]. The published guidelines that do address treatment of violent or aggressive behaviors in a more general sense and across a variety of diagnostic categories were all published nearly a decade or more ago, the most recent being published in 2007 [13–17]. Since the publication of these guidelines, many advances in psychopharmacology have occurred, not the least of which is the introduction of several additional antipsychotic agents.

Recent research has also suggested that among psychiatric inpatients, personal factors leading to aggression and violence commonly fall into several broad categories, including psychotic persecutory distortions of reality, increased impulsivity, and antisocial (predatory) personality features, with substance abuse and cognitive impairment frequently playing aggravating comorbid roles with the other domains [18].

Environmental factors may also exert significant influences on the risk of aggressive or violent behavior. While it is recognized that, in many patients, more than one personal or environmental factor may be operative, it is the aim of these guidelines to ask the clinician to generate a data-driven hypothesis regarding the principal or proximate factors that promote the individual's aggression or violence, and then to provide a roadmap for the further evaluation and treatment of the patient. These guidelines make the assumption that a logical, step-wise process of data collection, data analysis, and evidence-based treatment will maximize the probability of resolving or ameliorating the treated person's risk of violent behavior [19].

These guidelines were written for a presumed clinical environment in which, based on level of risk and probable resistance to treatment, the patient may be moved to higher or lower levels of secure care, from a regular hospital unit to an enhanced treatment unit and then to less secure treatment settings as the danger of violence and aggression declines [20]. In order to ease the use of these guidelines in clinical practice, they are presented in a bulleted format with numerous tables and treatment algorithms (many available in the online Supplemental Material).

Overview and Key Points

- Determine type of aggression (psychotic, impulsive, predatory) as well as environmental factors that may exacerbate aggressive behaviors
- Actively monitor for and treat comorbid conditions that may contribute to aggressive behavior, including substance abuse

- Continually evaluate patients using violence risk assessment tools
- Integrate psychosocial therapies into the treatment plan for patients who are chronically aggressive
- Actively monitor therapeutic drug levels during treatment
- Strongly consider using high-dose antipsychotic monotherapy or antipsychotic polypharmacy in patients who are aggressive and violent
- Strongly consider clozapine for patients with persistent aggression

Assessment
Determine etiology of aggressive behavior

- Evaluate patient for causes of aggression [21]
  - Aggression type [22–24]
    - Psychotic [25]
      - Patient misunderstands or misinterprets environmental stimuli
      - Attributable to positive symptoms of psychosis
        - Paranoid delusions of threat or persecution
        - Command hallucinations
        - Grandiosity
      - Accompanied by autonomic arousal
    - Impulsive
      - Hyper-reactivity to stimuli
      - Emotional hypersensitivity
      - Exaggerated threat perception
      - Involves no planning
      - Accompanied by autonomic arousal
    - Predatory [26]
      - Planned assaults
      - Goal-directed
      - Lack of remorse
      - Autonomic arousal absent
- Physical conditions that may contribute to violence risk [27]
  - Psychomotor agitation
  - Akathisia
  - Pain or physical discomfort
  - Delirium
  - Intoxication or withdrawal

- Complex partial seizures
- Sleep issues
- Abnormal laboratory results that may contribute to violence risk [28]
  - Plasma glucose
  - Plasma calcium
  - White blood cell count to rule out sepsis
  - Infectious disease screens as clinically indicated
  - Plasma sodium to rule out hyponatremia or hypernatremia
  - Oxygen saturation as clinically indicated
  - Serum ammonia as clinically indicated
  - Thyroid status
  - Sedimentation rate if history of inflammatory disease
- Adverse medication effects
  - Extrapyramidal symptoms (EPS)
    - Akathisia
    - Dystonia
    - Parkinsonism
  - Sedation
  - Orthostasis
  - Adverse anticonvulsant effects
    - Ataxia
    - Tremor
    - Cognitive impairment
  - Adverse lithium effects
    - Polyuria
    - Tremor
    - Cognitive impairment
  - Adverse beta blocker effects
    - Hypotension
    - Bronchospasm
    - Bradycardia
- Environmental factors that may contribute to violence risk [29]
  - Physical environment [30–32]
    - Regulation of daily life/activities
      - Meals, medication, showers, etc., on a fixed schedule
      - Personal choices about attire, food, and leisure time are limited

- • All actions supervised
  - ▪ Waiting in line required
  - ▪ Limited privacy
    - • Shared bedrooms/bathrooms
  - ▪ Crowded communal areas
  - ▪ Conversely, constant monitoring and structured activities may be beneficial for decreasing violence

- ○ Treatment unit factors

  - ▪ Younger age of unit population [33,34]
  - ▪ Unsafe population mix [35]
    - • Unit population is unadjusted according to violence risk, age, and diagnoses of patients
  - ▪ Crowding [30,36-38]
  - ▪ Poor unit management [39–44]
    - • Unreliable schedules and routines
    - • Staff roles not clearly defined
    - • Poor teamwork among staff
    - • Absence of a committed and active psychiatrist/leader
    - • Poor therapeutic alliance between patient and staff
    - • Lack of therapeutic activities
    - • Sensory overload from excessive noise
  - ▪ Lack of a sense of community/therapeutic community [45]

- ○ Staff factors [35,43,44,46-49]

  - ▪ Inexperienced staff
  - ▪ Shift and unit staff assignments are unadjusted for experience levels of staff
  - ▪ Understaffing
  - ▪ High turnover of staff
  - ▪ Inadequate or improper staff training [50,51]
  - ▪ Noncompliance with risk-reducing policies and procedures
  - ▪ Overtime shifts
  - ▪ Lack of discipline for staff who show a repetitive pattern of poor-quality relationships with patients
  - ▪ Staff burnout (Supplemental Table 4)

- ○ Institutional factors [35]

  - ▪ Limited ability of staff to quickly access risk-relevant patient information

- ▪ Lack of an effective crisis management plan
- ▪ Poor management [52]
  - • Failure to resolve conflicts among staff members
  - • Senior management absent from treatment units
  - • Absence of a designated person in charge of violence management
  - • Incomplete or inaccurate written policies related to aggression [45,53]
  - • Acceptance of risky current practices
- ▪ Lack of transfer options for patients who are too dangerous to be housed in current facility

- ○ Schedule factors [54–60]

  - ▪ Unstructured activities
  - ▪ Periods of transition, patient movement, patient lines, high-volume patient–staff interactions

Violence risk assessment

- • Areas of elevated social interaction and physical proximity (e.g., hallways) [56,58,61]
- • Violence risk assessment should include a systematic collection of patient information and documenting of violence risk factors [62,63]
- • Violence risk assessment should include both

  - ○ Validated violence risk assessments
  - ○ Structured clinical judgment processes

- • Violence risk assessment should be conducted by a credentialed mental health professional

  - ○ With specialized education and supervised training in the use and limitations of psychological assessment instruments and structured clinical judgment processes
  - ○ Who completes ongoing training to maintain expertise in the use of violence risk assessments

- • Review prior history and assessments

  - ○ Frequency of violence
  - ○ Severity of violence
  - ○ Patient factors associated with violence
  - ○ Environmental factors associated with violence

- Cause of latest decompensation
- Comorbid factors associated with violence

  - Psychosis
  - Substance abuse
  - Criminal thinking/psychopathy
  - Emotional instability
  - Borderline personality disorder
  - Intellectual disability
  - Traumatic brain injury

- Evaluate previous treatments and treatment efficacy [64]
- Review all incident reports, progress notes, laboratory reports, prior psychological and neuropsychological testing results, treatment team documents, and court records
- Include collateral reports of previous violence incidents, if available
- Interview treatment team members and level-of-care staff
- Conduct a clinical interview with the patient including a full mental status examination

- Supplementary assessment tools (Supplemental Tables 1 and 2)

  - Structured professional judgment violence risk assessment instruments

    - Historical Clinical Risk Management-20 (HCR-20) [65]
    - Short-Term Assessment of Risk and Treatability (START) [66]
    - Violence Risk Screening-10 (V-RISK-10) [67]

  - Psychopathy

    - Psychopathy Checklist-Revised (PCL-R) [68]
    - Psychopathy Checklist-Short Version (PCL-SV)

  - Actuarial violence risk assessment instruments

    - Classification of Violence Risk (COVR) [69]
    - Violence Risk Appraisal Guide (VRAG) [70,71]
    - Violence Risk Scale (VRS) [72]

  - Observational rating scales and checklists

    - Dynamic Appraisal of Situational Aggression (DASA) [21,73]

- Staff Observation Aggression Scale-Revised (SOAS-R) [74]
- Buss–Perry Aggression Questionnaire
- Brief Psychiatric Rating Scale (BPRS)
- Cohen–Mansfield Agitation Inventory (CMAI)

- If patient poses an immediate threat

  - Evaluate need for seclusion or restraint

    - Clinical observation
    - Clinical interview
    - Use of rating scales (e.g., DASA)

Treatment

- Treatment of acute agitation (Figure 16.1) [75,76]

  - When possible, choose an antipsychotic that is also being used as part of the primary treatment. Available dose forms may limit this option
  - Recent studies have suggested that additional agents, such as midazolam and promethazine, may play adjunctive roles in controlling acute aggression and violence [77–80]

- Long-term treatment

  - Note that absence of any adverse effects despite adequate plasma concentrations of antipsychotics may reflect a need for higher-than-standard doses to achieve adequate receptor occupancy (Tables 16.1 and 16.2)
  - A partial response ($<20\%$–30% on the Positive and Negative Syndrome Scale [PANSS] or BPRS) with minimal or no adverse effects argues for a higher-dose trial of the present antipsychotic
  - Failure of two or more adequate trials of antipsychotics, with at least one being an atypical antipsychotic, argues for a trial of clozapine
  - Tailor treatments to target specific symptoms that may contribute to violence risk (Table 16.3 and Figure 16.2)
  - There are a variety of pharmacokinetic and drug–drug interaction effects of the anticonvulsants, lithium, and beta blockers that should be considered [81]

    - e.g., phenytoin with zero-order kinetics
    - e.g., carbamazepine induces CYP450

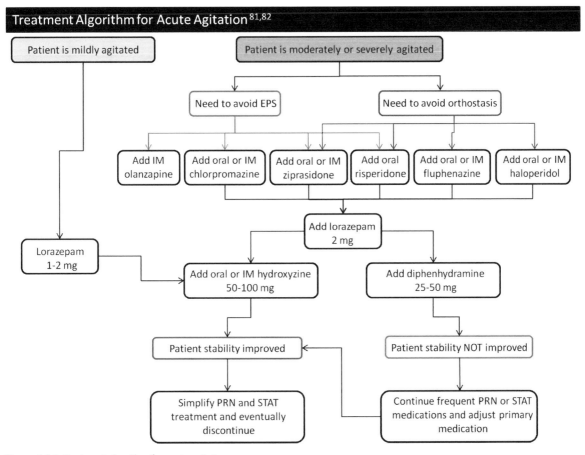

Figure 16.1 Treatment algorithm for acute agitation.

- e.g., angiotensin-converting enzyme inhibitors and nonsteroidal anti-inflammatory drugs (NSAIDS) raise lithium levels
- e.g., nonselective beta blockers are contraindicated in asthma
  - A partial response (small decline in Barratt Impulsiveness Scale [BIS-11]) with adequate anticonvulsant plasma concentrations argues for the addition of an anticonvulsant or other medication with a mechanism of action distinct from that of the primary treatment [82,83]

Psychotic aggression

- Confirm that the patient's violent and aggressive behaviors arise primarily from psychosis

- Associated with a primary psychotic disorder (Figure 16.3) [2,3]
  - Schizophrenia spectrum disorders
  - Bipolar spectrum disorders
- Associated with a major cognitive disorder (Supplemental Figure 1) [4,7,10,11]
  - Alzheimer's disease [84]
  - Vascular dementia
  - Major cognitive disorder with Lewy bodies
  - Traumatic brain injury [12]
    - Antipsychotics increase the risk of mortality by 1.5- to 2-fold in elderly demented patients but may be worthwhile if alternative choices to control agitation and violence are ineffective [85,86]
- Periodically test whether antipsychotic dose is required to maintain stability

Table 16.1 Dosing recommendations: conventional antipsychotics

Medication (*brand*)	Recommended dose range	High-dosing recommendations	Recommended plasma concentration	Long-acting depot recommendations
Chlorpromazine (*Thorazine*)	300–1000 mg/day			
Fluphenazine (*Prolixin*)	6–20 mg/day	20–60 mg/day	0.8–2.0 ng/ml Up to 4.0 ng/ml may be required	2–3 week depot available. 25–100 mg/14 days
Haloperidol (*Haldol, Serenace*)	6–40 mg/day	20–80 mg/day Higher doses especially when failing to respond to doses up to 20 mg/day	5–20 ng/ml Up to 30 ng/ml may be required	4-week depot available. 200–300 mg/28 days after loading with 200–300 mg/weekly times 3
Loxapine (*Loxitane*)	30–100 mg/day			
Perphenazine (*Trilafon*)	12–64 mg/day			
Thiothixene (*Navane*)	15–50 mg/day			
Trifluoperazine (*Stelazine*)	15–50 mg/day			

See full prescribing information for details.

- It is recommended that antipsychotics be tapered and discontinued after major cognitive disorders have stabilized or progressed
  - Note that, although no response by weeks 4–6 of adequate to high-dose antipsychotic treatment portends a poor outcome, many patients show ongoing improvement for many weeks to months following a favorable, albeit partial, response to early treatment [87]
- Some patients may require higher than cited antipsychotic plasma concentrations to achieve stabilization (Tables 16.1 and 16.2)

Impulsive aggression

- Confirm that patient's violent and aggressive behaviors result primarily from impulsive aggression
  - Characterized by reactive or emotionally charged response that has a loss of behavioral control and failure to consider consequences
  - Associated with
    - Schizophrenia spectrum disorders
    - Cognitive disorders [88]
    - ADHD (Supplemental Figure 2) [5,89]
    - Bipolar disorder (Supplemental Figure 3) [90–100]
    - Depressive disorders (Supplemental Figure 4) [101–114]
    - Cluster B personality disorders (Supplemental Figure 5) [115,116]
    - Intermittent explosive disorder (Supplemental Figure 6) [82]
    - PTSD (Supplemental Figure 7) [8]
    - TBI (Supplemental Figure 8) [12]
    - Unknown origin (Supplemental Figure 9) [81,82,117–120]
  - Strongly associated with substance use disorders
  - Past history of psychological trauma increases risk of impulsive aggression and is often comorbid with substance use disorders and personality disorders

Table 16.2 Dosing recommendations: atypical antipsychotics

Medication (*brand*)	Recommended dose range	High-dosing recommendations	Recommended plasma concentration	Long-acting depot recommendations
Aripiprazole (*Abilify*)	10–30 mg/day	Higher doses usually not more effective and possibly less effective		4-week depot available
Asenapine (*Saphris*)	10–20 mg/day	High-dosing not well-studied		No depot available
Clozapine (*Clozaril*)	150–450 mg/day	FDA max 900 mg/day Doses >550 mg/day may require concomitant anticonvulsant administration to reduce seizure risk		No depot available
Iloperidone (*Fanapt*)	12–24 mg/day	High-dosing not well-studied		No depot available
Lurasidone (*Latuda*)	40–160 mg/day Must be taken with food. Nightly administration may improve tolerability	Efficacy of high-dosing (>160 mg/day) not well-studied		No depot available
Olanzapine (*Zyprexa*)	10–30 mg/day	40–60 mg/day. Up to 90 mg/day for more difficult cases	80–120 ng/ml	2- and 4-week depots available
Paliperidone ER (*Invega*)	3–12 mg/day	Max dose is generally 12 mg/day		4-week depot available 234 mg followed after 1 week by 156 mg then continuing at 117–234 mg/28 days
Quetiapine (*Seroquel, SeroquelXR*)	300–750 mg/day	Up to 1800 mg /day or more for difficult cases		No depot available
Risperidone (*Risperdal*)	2–8 mg/day	FDA-approved up to 16 mg/day. Very high doses are usually not well-tolerated		2-week depot available
Ziprasidone (*Geodon*)	80–160 mg/day Must be taken with food	Up to 360 mg/day for difficult cases		No depot available

See full prescribing information for details.

○ For mood disorders, the goal of treatment is resolution of the mood symptoms, or improvement to the point that only one or two symptoms of mild intensity persist

- Resolution of psychosis is required for remission

○ For patients with mood disorders who do not achieve remission, a reasonable goal is response that entails stabilization of the patient's safety and substantial improvement in the number, intensity, and frequency of mood (and psychotic) symptoms [121]

Table 16.3 Dosing recommendations: other medications

Medication (*brand*)	Recommended dose range	Dosing considerations
Bupropion (*Wellbutrin*)	150–450 mg/day	High risk of abuse in forensic settings
Benzodiazepines	Various	Dose clonazepam at 0.5–2.0 mg TID and then taper as patient stabilizes. High risk of abuse in forensic settings
Beta blockers	Various	
Carbamazepine (*Tegretol, generic*)	400–1200 mg/day	Target plasma concentration of 8–12 ng/ml. Recheck plasma concentration for decrease due to autoinduction 4–6 weeks after initiating. May lower plasma levels of other medications
Diphenhydramine (*Benadryl*)	25–300 mg/day	
Divalproex (*Depakote, DepakoteER, generic*)	750 mg/day up to 60 mg/kg/day BID or TID	May be loaded at 20–30 mg/kg, reaching steady state at around 3 days with plasma concentrations of 80–120 mcg/ml
Lamotrigine (*Lamictal, generic*)	Various	
Lithium (*Eskalith, generic*)	900–2400 mg/day	May be initiated at 600 mg/day and titrated by 300 mg every other day to 900–1800 mg/day. Once per day dosing spares renal function. Plasma concentrations should be 0.6–1.2 mEq/l (up to 1.4 mEq/l in acute mania). Lower doses for unipolar depression (900 mg/day with serum levels of 0.6–0.9 mEq/l)
Oxcarbazepine (*Trileptal, generic*)	1200–2400 mg/day	Less potent induction than carbamazepine, but may lower plasma levels of other medications.
Phenytoin (*Dilantin, generic*)	300–900 mg/day	Zero-order kinetics make dosage increases result in dramatic increases in plasma concentration. Desired range is 10–20 mcg/ml. May lower plasma levels of other medications
SNRIs	Various	
SSRIs	Various	
TCAs	Various	Desipramine (150–300 ng/ml) and nortriptyline (50–150 ng/ml) are first-line TCAs for impulsive aggression associated with ADHD.
Topiramate (*Topamax*)	200–400 mg/day	
Trazodone (*Oleptro, Desyrel, generic*)	25–600 mg /day	
Zolpidem (*Ambien*)	5–10 mg/day	

See full prescribing information for details.

Predatory aggression

- Confirm that patient's violent and aggressive behaviors result primarily from predatory aggression
  - ○ Purposeful, planned behavior that is associated with attainment of a goal
  - ○ Some patients who engage in predatory acts may have the constellation of personality traits commonly known as psychopathy
- Avoid countertransference reactions (Supplemental Table 3)

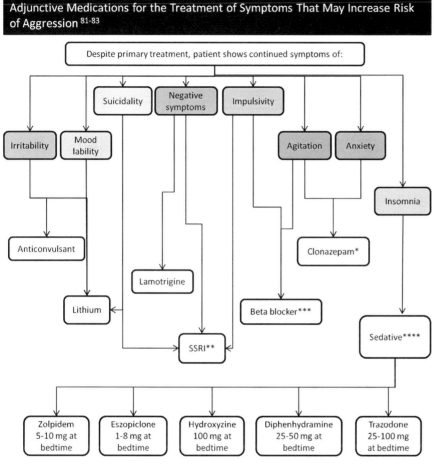

Figure 16.2 Adjunctive medications for the treatment of symptoms that may increase risk of aggression.

- Determine potential reasons for predatory aggression (Supplemental Table 4) [65,68,70,122]
- Provide opportunities to attain acceptable goals using social learning principles, differential reinforcement, and cognitive restructuring (Figure 16.4) [123]
- Utilize the Risk–Need–Responsivity principles to determine risk level, treatment needs, and the best way to deliver and optimize treatment (Supplemental Tables 5 and 6)

- Regularly evaluate the progress of predatory aggression treatment (Supplemental Table 7) [124]
- Consider using mood stabilizers, SSRIs, or other antidepressants for persistent tension, explosive anger, mood swings, and impulsivity
- While level of security and psychosocial interventions remain the mainstays of addressing predatory violence, preliminary

163

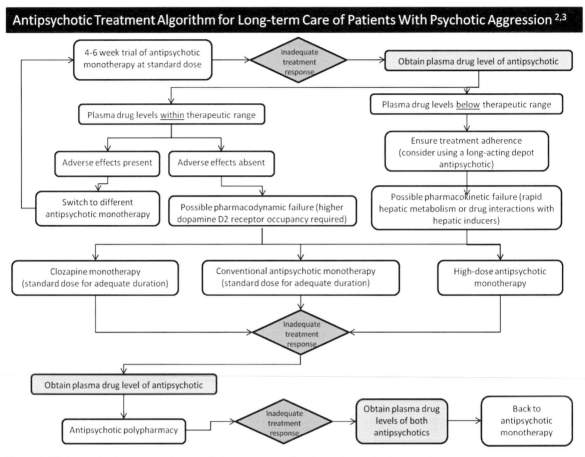

Antipsychotic Treatment Algorithm for Long-term Care of Patients With Psychotic Aggression [2,3]

Figure 16.3 Antipsychotic treatment algorithm for long-term care of patients with psychotic aggression.

data have suggested that clozapine also may reduce such aggression and violence [125]

Psychosocial Interventions

- It is often the case that when treating the violently mentally ill, both medications and therapeutic interventions are needed in order to impact change
- Pairing medication with appropriate psychosocial interventions can impart new coping strategies and increase medication adherence
- Psychosocial interventions should also give weight to the etiology of the aggression
  - Once an etiology has been identified, a behavioral treatment must be further

individualized based on the patient's needs, capabilities, and other logistical limitations

- Utilize the Risk–Need–Responsivity Model (Supplemental Table 6) [126–128]
  - Risk principle
    - Assessment of patient's level of risk and contributing factors to his or her aggressive behavior
  - Need principle
    - Assessment of criminogenic needs
      - In this context, criminogenic needs refer to dynamic (treatable) risk factors that are correlated with criminal behavior, and when treated, reduce recidivism

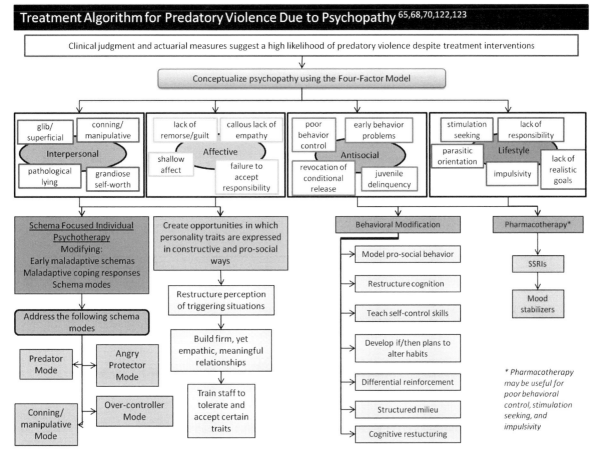

Figure 16.4 Treatment algorithm for predatory aggression.

- Provides specific targets for treatment to reduce violence
  - Early antisocial behavior
  - Impulsive personality patterns
  - Negative criminal attitudes and values
  - Delinquent or criminal associates
  - Dysfunctional family relationships
  - Poor investment in school or work
  - Little involvement in legitimate leisure pursuits
  - Substance abuse
  - Responsivity principle
    - Individually tailor treatments to maximize the patient's ability to learn from the interventions

- Intervention is tailored toward the patient's
  - Learning style
  - Motivation
  - Abilities
  - Strengths
- Offer high-standard training on de-escalation and prevention strategies such as awareness of one's presence (body posture), content of speech, reflective listening skills, negotiation, positive affirmation, and offering an alternative solution
- Provide supportive and nonjudgmental briefing sessions to staff who are involved in incidents to discuss their subjective experience

Psychosocial interventions for psychotic aggression

- General factors [129]

    ◦ Good communication is essential
    ◦ Multiple and coordinated treatment approaches should be used, including administrative, psychosocial, and psychotropic approaches
    ◦ A sufficient dose of the selected treatment should be administered
    ◦ Treatment integrity, including well-trained staff, supportive administration, and well-coordinated evaluation efforts, is vital
    ◦ Treatment should be tailored to the individual
    ◦ There should be a clear connection between risk assessment and treatment

- Specific interventions have some evidence for efficacy in reducing violence associated with mental illness

    ◦ Using cognitive behavioral methods

        ▪ Behavioral modification–reinforcement
            • Unit and individual reinforcement
        ▪ Group therapy
            • Cognitive therapy for psychotic symptoms
            • Anger management
            • Teaching cognitive and problem solving skills

    ◦ Individual therapy

        ▪ Can use various approaches
        ▪ Focus on reality testing
        ▪ Building alliance

    ◦ Social learning [130]

        ▪ Modeling by staff
        ▪ Teaching cognitive and problem solving skills
        ▪ Using behavioral methods

    ◦ Anger management [131,132]
    ◦ Dialectical behavior therapy (DBT) [133]

        ▪ Associated with reduction in severity but not in frequency of violence in the mentally ill population

    ◦ Seclusion

        ▪ For up to 48 hours but not less than 4 hours
        ▪ It is worth noting that anecdotal evidence suggests that some patients may respond to preventative interventions, such as time-outs, or to shorter periods of seclusion
        ▪ Most experts caution against using methods that may seem punitive

    ◦ Institutional approaches

        ▪ Total quality management [60]
            • Including rewarding good behavior and changing the environment
        ▪ Identifying the most aggressive individuals and targeting them for intense treatment [134]
        ▪ Social structures that provide strong clinical leadership [41]
        ▪ A predictable, competent, interactive, trusting environment
        ▪ Intrapsychic humanism [135]

Psychosocial interventions for impulsive aggression

- The goal of treatment is to increase behavioral control and decrease emotional dysregulation [136]

    ◦ DBT [137,138]

        ▪ Established as a validated treatment for borderline personality disorder and self-injurious behavior

    ◦ Reinforcement/behavioral interventions
    ◦ Positive coping
    ◦ Individual therapy: exploration of impulsive episodes, coping, and triggers
    ◦ Group therapy: anger management and social skills

- Psychosocial interventions for impulsive aggression with a trauma component:

    ◦ Past history of psychological trauma increases risk of impulsive aggression and is often comorbid with substance use disorders and personality disorders
    ◦ Treatments that incorporate trauma-informed strategies may be effective for impulsive aggression that is not responsive to other interventions [139–148]

- o Previous experiences of victimization often lead to difficulties in forming close relationships and ineffective coping strategies
- o Special emphasis on safety and therapeutic alliance
- o May be incorporated into many existing treatments, especially treatments for ongoing mood disorders or substance use disorders
- o In the case of trauma, be mindful of restraint conditions, which may re-traumatize
- o Exposure therapy may be useful for aggression stemming from PTSD or other traumatic experiences
- More intensive and specialized treatment may be required for severely ill patients or those with chronic coping deficits or personality disorders

Psychosocial interventions for aggression due to cognitive impairment

- Psychosocial interventions for aggression due to cognitive impairment
  - o Cognitive impairment is found consistently in serious mental illness, especially schizophrenia [149–151]
  - o Addressing complex aggressive behavior and cognitive issues should be the target of treatment
  - o Recovery Inspired Skills Enhancement (RISE)
    - Multifaceted neurocognitive and social cognition training program for individuals with psychiatric disorders and severe cognitive needs and challenges
    - Goal of RISE is to eliminate maladaptive behaviors that interfere with an individual's recovery process and acquisition of skills necessary for adaptive functioning

Psychosocial interventions for predatory aggression

- Interventions that are tailored to the individual and provided for a sufficient amount of time can result in treatment gains [152–155]
  - o Keeping in mind, treatment gains may be modest or non-existent
- Treatments that address patients' dynamic risk factors through psychotherapy and structured milieu interventions are most effective

- Interventions to address maladaptive patterns of thinking and behavior [156]
  - o Reasoning and Rehabilitation (R&R) [157,158]
  - o Enhanced Thinking Skills (ETS) [159]
  - o Think First (TF)
- Psychotherapy [160–162]
  - o May include theme-centered psychoeducation and process components
  - o Modify antisocial attitudes
  - o Improve problem solving abilities and self-regulation
  - o Reduce resistance and impulsive lifestyles
  - o Focus on early maladaptive schemas, schema modes, and coping responses
  - o Seek to increase the patient's awareness of how hostile thoughts, biases, and worldviews have contributed to his or her maladaptive behavior
  - o If the patient is particularly psychopathic, individual therapy may be contraindicated
- Milieu
  - o Highly structured environment
  - o Lack of access to dangerous materials
  - o Staff having strong boundaries is crucial
  - o Increased monitoring/externally imposed supervision
    - Cameras
    - Hospital security officers
  - o Consider a rotation
- Every interaction between the patients and a staff member should be considered an opportunity to reinforce prosocial behaviors and practice learned skills
- Reinforce and model prosocial ways to achieve one's goals

Setting and Housing

- Make all efforts to preserve patients' self-determination, autonomy, and dignity within the treatment environment [163]
- Avoid seclusion, physical restraint, and sedation when possible
  - o Finding the right balance is key
    - For instance, staff should not avoid the use of restraint and seclusion to the point where the patient does not have to follow unit rules

- Hospitalize patients in an enhanced treatment unit (ETU) who have [164]
  - Recently committed/threatened acts of violence or aggression that put others at risk of physical injury and cannot be managed in a standard treatment setting
  - Recurrent violent or aggressive behaviors that are unresponsive to all therapeutic interventions available in a standard treatment setting

    - Review attempted interventions to ensure that standard of care has been met
      - Communicate with treating clinicians to discuss past treatment plans
      - Review medications to determine if pharmacotherapy meets standard of care for the identified disorders
      - Review psychological assessments to determine if the relevant assessments have been attempted
      - Review past psychological interventions, including behavioral plans, group treatment enrollment, and individual therapy progress

  - A high risk of violence that cannot be contained in a standard treatment environment determined by a violence risk assessment process in conjunction with clinical judgment

    - The patient shows continued symptoms that increase risk for violence despite standard care
    - The patient refuses to engage in treatment activities
    - The patient refuses medication
    - The patient possesses prominent risk factors for violence

  - Examples of violence or aggression that meet criteria for ETU admission

    - One severe act of violence to staff or peers that causes bodily injury
    - Multiple acts of moderate physical violence with the potential to cause injury
    - A threat of significant violence (e.g., "I'm going to kill you!") with a history of past violence
    - Threatening gestures or words (e.g., raised fist, slicing hand across throat) or words constituting a threat of violence

    - Intentional destruction of property to cause intimidation, discomfort, pain, or humiliation
    - Acts of sexualized violence or attempted sexual violence

  - Examples of behaviors that DO NOT meet criteria for ETU admission

    - Nuisance behavior that is disruptive but does not cause injury to peers or staff, or has little foreseeable likelihood to result in injury
    - Minor forms of injurious behavior unlikely to cause substantial injury or permanent damage
    - Sexual behavior that is consensual and does not include an aggressive or violent component
    - Destruction of property lacking intent or risk of personal or interpersonal harm
    - Inappropriate masturbation

- Discharge patients from ETU who meet all of these criteria
  - No evident risk of aggressive or violent behavior as demonstrated by absence of

    - Serious rule violations
    - Heightened risk factors for assaultive or aggressive acts as determined by the violence risk assessment process
    - Threatening acts (e.g., spitting, leering, posturing to fight)
    - Assaultive acts
    - Intimidating acts

  - Reasonable probability that the patient will be able to maintain psychiatric stability in a less structured environment and will continue to participate in ongoing treatment activities designed to reduce violence risk

    - Based on documented treatment records including notes, treatment plans, and consultations

  - Risk assessment indicates that the patient's current risk for aggression on a standard treatment unit or in a less structured environment is no longer elevated

    - The risk assessment process should include objective inpatient violence risk factors

- Underlying risk factors that contributed to elevated violence risk and placement in the ETU have been mitigated

Conclusion

In conclusion, the task before clinicians who treat violent mentally ill patients is great. We are challenged to help these individuals by whatever means necessary, while at the same time working within the practical restrictions of a hospital setting. The above guidelines will hopefully provide assistance with this task, and can be used as a reference. It is important to remember that many of our patients do not wish to harm others; they are simply struggling to hold themselves together, day in and day out, and it is our duty to help them achieve their highest potential. We must make every attempt to keep all those at our hospitals safe – patients and staff alike. Our concluding thought is to remember that our efforts matter; that by using science, and the best tools available, we can change the course of a life.

Supplementary Material

To view supplementary material for this article, please visit http://dx.doi.org/10.1017/S1092852914000376.

Disclosures

Debbi Ann Morrissette has nothing to disclose.
Marie Cugini Schur has nothing to disclose.
Jonathan Meyer has the following disclosures:

- BMS, Speaker, Speaker's fee
- Genentech, Speaker, Speaker's fee
- Genentech, Advisor, Honoraria
- Otsuka, Speaker, Speaker's fee
- Sunovion, Speaker, Speaker's fee

Eric Schwartz has nothing to disclose.
Susan Velasquez has nothing to disclose.
Darci Delgado has nothing to disclose.
Laura Dardashti has nothing to disclose.
Katherine Warburton has nothing to disclose.
George Proctor has nothing to disclose.
Michael Cummings has nothing to disclose.
Jennifer O'Day has nothing to disclose.
Charles Broderick has nothing to disclose.
Allen Azizian has nothing to disclose.
Benjamin Rose has nothing to disclose.
Shannon Bader has nothing to disclose.

Stephen M. Stahl,MD, PhD is an Adjunct Professor of Psychiatry at the University of California, San Diego School of Medicine, Honorary Visiting Senior Fellow at the University of Cambridge, UK and Director of Psychopharmacology for California Department of State Hospitals. Dr. Stahl has served as a Consultant for Astra Zeneca, Avanir, Biomarin, Envivo, Forest, Jazz, Lundbeck, Neuronetics, Noveida, Orexigen, Otsuka, PamLabs, Servier, Shire, Sunovion, Taisho, Takeda and Trius; he is a board member of RCT Logic and GenoMind; on the Speakers Bureau for Astra Zeneca, Janssen, Otsuka, Sunovion and Takeda and he has received research and/or grant support from AssureX, Eli Lilly, EnVivo, Janssen, JayMac, Jazz, Lundbeck, Mylan, Neuronetics, Novartis, Otsuka, Pamlabs, Pfizer, Roche, Shire, Sunovion, Takeda, Teva and Valeant.

References

1. Diaz-Marsa M, Gonzalez Bardanca S, Tajima K, *et al.* Psychopharmacological treatment in borderline personality disorder. *Actas Esp. Psiquiatr.* 2008; **36**(1): 39–49.

2. Buscema CA, Abbasi QA, Barry DJ, Lauve TH. An algorithm for the treatment of schizophrenia in the correctional setting: the Forensic Algorithm Project. *J. Clin. Psychiatry.* 2000; **61**(10): 767–783.

3. Castle D, Daniel J, Knott J, *et al.* Development of clinical guidelines for the pharmacological management of behavioural disturbance and aggression in people with psychosis. *Australas. Psychiatry.* 2005; **13**(3): 247–252.

4. Herrmann N, Lanctôt KL, Hogan DB. Pharmacological recommendations for the symptomatic treatment of dementia: the Canadian Consensus Conference on the Diagnosis and Treatment of Dementia 2012. *Alzheimers Res. Ther.* 2013; **5**(Suppl 1): S5.

5. List BA, Barzman DH. Evidence-based recommendations for the treatment of aggression in pediatric patients with attention deficit hyperactivity disorder. *Psychiatr. Q.* 2011; **82**(1): 33–42.

6. Morana HC, Camara FP. International guidelines for the management of personality disorders. *Curr. Opin. Psychiatry.* 2006; **19**(5): 539–543.

7. Oliver-Africano P, Murphy D, Tyrer P. Aggressive behaviour in

adults with intellectual disability: defining the role of drug treatment. *CNS Drugs.* 2009; **23**(11): 903–913.

8. Taft CT, Creech SK, Kachadourian L. Assessment and treatment of posttraumatic anger and aggression: a review. *J. Rehabil. Res. Dev.* 2012; **49**(5): 777–788.

9. Tyrer P, Seivewright N. Pharmacological treatment of personality disorders. *Clin. Neuropharmacol.* 1988; **11**(6): 493–499.

10. Vickland V, Chilko N, Draper B, *et al.* Individualized guidelines for the management of aggression in dementia— Part 2: appraisal of current guidelines. *Int. Psychogeriatr.* 2012; **24**(7): 1125–1132.

11. Vickland V, Chilko N, Draper B, *et al.* Individualized guidelines for the management of aggression in dementia— Part 1: key concepts. *Int. Psychogeriatr.* 2012; **24**(7): 1112–1124.

12. Warden DL, Gordon B, McAllister TW, *et al.* Guidelines for the pharmacologic treatment of neurobehavioral sequelae of traumatic brain injury. *J. Neurotrauma.* 2006; **23**(10): 1468–1501.

13. Allen MH. Currier GW, Hughes DH, *et al.* Treatment of behavioral emergencies: a summary of the expert consensus guidelines. *J. Psychiatr. Pract.* 2003; **9**(1): 16–38.

14. Fava M. Psychopharmacologic treatment of pathologic aggression. *Psychiatr. Clin. North Am.* 1997; **20**(2): 427–451.

15. Sheard MH. Clinical pharmacology of aggressive behavior. *Clin. Neuropharmacol.* 1988; **11**(6): 483–492.

16. Tardiff K. The current state of psychiatry in the treatment of violent patients. *Arch. Gen. Psychiatry.* 1992; **49**(6): 493–499.

17. Wong SC, Gordon A, Gu D. Assessment and treatment of violence-prone forensic clients: an integrated approach. *Br. J. Psychiatry Suppl.* 2007; **49**: s66–s74.

18. Dack C, Ross J, Papadopoulos C, Stewart D, Bowers L. A review and meta-analysis of the patient factors associated with psychiatric in-patient aggression. *Acta Psychiatr. Scand.* 2013; **127**(4): 255–268.

19. Howland RH. Limitations of evidence in the practice of evidence-based medicine. *J. Psychosoc. Nurs. Ment. Health Serv.* 2007; **45**(11): 13–16.

20. Kennedy HG. Therapeutic uses of security: mapping forensic mental health services by stratifying risk. *Advances in Psychiatric Treatment.* 2002; **8**(6): 433–443.

21. Vaaler AE, Iversen VC, Morken G, *et al.* Short-term prediction of threatening and violent behaviour in an acute psychiatric intensive care unit based on patient and environment characteristics. *BMC Psychiatry.* 2011; **11**: 44.

22. Bandura A. Psychological mechanisms of aggression. In: Geen RG, Donnerstein EI, eds. *Aggression: Theoretical and Empirical Reviews—Vol 1, Theoretical and Methodological Issues.* New York: Academic Press; 1983: 1–40.

23. Berkowitz L. *Aggression: Its Causes, Consequences, and Control.* New York: McGraw-Hill Higher Education; 1993.

24. Hemphill JF, Hare RD, Wong S. Psychopathy and recidivism: a review. *Legal Criminol. Psych.* 1998; **3**(1): 139–170.

25. Volavka J, Citrome L. Pathways to aggression in schizophrenia affect results of treatment. *Schizophr. Bull.* 2011; **37**(5): 921–929.

26. Hare RD, Neumann CS. Psychopathy as a clinical and empirical construct. *Annu. Rev. Clin. Psychol.* 2008; **4**: 217–246.

27. Hankin CS, Bronstone A, Koran LM. Agitation in the inpatient psychiatric setting: a review of clinical presentation, burden, and treatment. *J. Psychiatr. Pract.* 2011; **17**(3): 170–185.

28. Joshi A, Krishnamurthy VB, Purichia H, *et al.* "What's in a name?" Delirium by any other name would be as deadly: a review of the nature of delirium consultations. *J. Psychiatr. Pract.* 2012; **18**(6): 413–418.

29. Wortley R. *Situational Prison Control: Crime Prevention in Correctional Institutions.* Cambridge, UK: Cambridge University Press; 2002.

30. Gadon L, Johnstone L, Cooke D. Situational variables and institutional violence: a systematic review of the literature. *Clin. Psychol. Rev.* 2006; **26**(5): 515–534.

31. Baldwin S. Effects of furniture rearrangement on the atmosphere of wards in a maximum-security hospital. *Hosp. Community Psychiatry.* 1985; **36**(5): 525–528.

32. Zaslove MO, Beal M, McKinney RE. Changes in behaviors of inpatients after a ban on the sale of caffeinated drinks. *Hosp. Community Psychiatry.* 1991; **42**(1): 84–85.

33. Ekland-Olson S, Barrick DM, Cohen LE. Prison overcrowding and disciplinary problems: an analysis of the Texas prison system. *J. Appl. Behavioral Science.* 1983; **19**(2): 163–192.

34. Mabli J, Holley C, Patrick J, Walls J. Age and prison violence: increasing age heterogeneity as a violence-reducing strategy in prisons. *Crim. Justice Behav.* 1979; **6**(2): 175–186.

35. Cooke DJ, Wozniak E. PRISM applied to a critical incident review: a case study of the Glendairy prison riot and its aftermath in Barbados. *Int. J. Forensic Ment. Health.* 2010; **9**(3): 159–172.

36. Ekland-Olson S. Crowding, social control, and prison violence: evidence from the post-Ruiz years in Texas. *Law & Society Review.* 1986; **20**(3): 389–421.

37. Lester D. Overcrowding in prisons and rates of suicide and homicide. *Percept. Mot. Skills.* 1990; **71**(1): 274.

38. Palmstierna T, Huitfeldt B, Wistedt B. The relationship of crowding and aggressive behavior on a psychiatric intensive care unit. *Hosp. Community Psychiatry.* 1991; **42**(12): 1237–1240.

39. Flannery RB Jr, Hanson MA, Penk WE, Flannery GJ. Violence and the lax milieu? *Preliminary data.. Psychiatr. Q.* 1996; **67**(1): 47–50.

40. Morrison E, Morman G, Bonner G, *et al.* Reducing staff injuries and violence in a forensic psychiatric setting. *Arch. Psychiatr. Nurs.* 2002; **16**(3): 108–117.

41. Katz P, Kirkland FR. Violence and social structure on mental hospital wards. *Psychiatry.* 1990; **53**(3): 262–277.

42. Flannery RB Jr. Precipitants to psychiatric patient assaults on staff: review of empirical findings, 1990–2003, and risk management implications. *Psychiatr. Q.* 2005; **76**(4): 317–326.

43. Flannery RB Jr, Hanson MA, Penk WE. Risk factors for psychiatric inpatient assaults on staff. *J. Ment. Health Admin.* 1994; **21**(1): 24–31.

44. Flannery RB, Staffieri A, Hildum S, Walker AP. The violence triad and common single precipitants to psychiatric patient assaults on staff: 16-year analysis of the Assaulted Staff Action Program. *Psychiatr. Q.* 2011; **82**(2): 85–93.

45. Mistral W, Hall A, McKee P. Using therapeutic community principles to improve the functioning of a high care psychiatric ward in the UK. *Int. J. Ment. Health Nurs.* 2002; **11**(1): 10–17.

46. Flannery RB Jr, White DL, Flannery GJ, Walker AP. Time of psychiatric patient assaults: fifteen-year analysis of the Assaulted Staff Action Program (ASAP). *Int. J. Emerg. Ment. Health.* 2007; **9**(2): 89–95.

47. Davies W, Burgess PW. Prison officers' experience as a predictor of risk of attack: an analysis within the British prison system. *Med. Sci. Law.* 1988; **28**(2): 135–138.

48. Hamadeh RR, Al Alaiwat B, Al Ansari A. Assaults and nonpatient-induced injuries among psychiatric nursing staff in Bahrain. *Issues Ment. Health Nurs.* 2003; **24**(4): 409–417.

49. Webster CD, Nicholls TD, Martin ML, Desmarais SL, Brink J. Short-Term Assessment of Risk and Treatability (START): the case for a new structured professional judgment scheme. *Behav. Sci. Law.* 2006; **24**(6): 747–766.

50. Stewart D, Van der Merwe M, Bowers L, Simpson A, Jones J. A review of interventions to reduce mechanical restraint and seclusion among adult psychiatric inpatients. *Issues Ment. Health Nurs.* 2010; **31**(6): 413–424.

51. Bowers L, Stewart D, Papadopoulos C, *et al. Inpatient Violence and Aggression: A Literature Review.* Report from the Conflict and Containment Reduction Research Programme London: Institute of Psychiatry, King's College London; 2011.

52. Reisig MD. Administrative control and inmate homicide. *Homicide Studies.* 2002; **6**(1): 84–103.

53. Templeton L, Gray S, Topping J. Seclusion: changes in policy and practice on an acute psychiatric unit. *J. Ment. Health.* 1998; **7**(2): 199–202.

54. Jayewardene CH, Doherty P. Individual violence in Canadian penitentiaries. *Can. J. Criminol.* 1985; **27**(4): 429–439.

55. Porporino FJ, Doherty PD, Sawatsky T. Characteristics of homicide victims and victimizations in prisons: a Canadian historical perspective. *Int. J. Offender Therapy Comp. Criminol.* 1987; **31**(2): 125–136.

56. Bader S, Evans SE, Welsh E. Aggression among psychiatric inpatients: the relationship between time, place, victims, and severity ratings. *J. Am. Psychiatr. Nurses Assoc.* 2014; **20**(3): 179–186.

57. Grainger C, Whiteford H. Assault on staff in psychiatric hospitals: a safety issue. *Aust. N. Z. J. Psychiatry.* 1993; **27**(2): 324–328.

58. Hodgkinson PE, McIvor L, Phillips M. Patient assaults on staff in a psychiatric hospital: a two-year retrospective study. *Med. Sci. Law.* 1985; **25**(4): 288–294.

59. Weizmann-Henelius G. Suutala HJO. Violence in a Finnish forensic psychiatric hospital. *Nord. J. Psychiatry.* 2000; **54**(4): 269–273.

60. Hunter ME, Love CC. Total quality management and the reduction of inpatient violence

and costs in a forensic psychiatric hospital. *Psychiatr. Serv.* 1996; **47**(7): 751–754.

61. Harris GT, Varney G. A ten-year study of assaults and assaulters on a maximum security psychiatric unit. *Journal of Interpersonal Violence.* 1986; **1**(2): 173–191.

62. Heilbrun K, Lander T. Forensic mental health assessment. In: Spielberger C, ed. *Encyclopedia of Applied Psychology*, Vol 2. New York: Elsevier Academic Press; 2004: 29–42.

63. Maden A. *Treating Violence: A Guide to Risk Management in Mental Health.* New York: Oxford University Press; 2007.

64. Lopez LV, Kane JM. Plasma levels of second-generation antipsychotics and clinical response in acute psychosis: a review of the literature. *Schizophr. Res.* 2013; **147**(2–3): 368–374.

65. Douglas KS, Hart SD, Webster CD, Belfrage H. *HCR-20V3: Assessing Risk of Violence—User Guide.* Burnaby, Canada: Mental Health, Law, and Policy Institute, Simon Fraser University; 2013.

66. Webster CD, Martin ML, Brink J, Nicholls TD, Desmarais SL. *Manual for the Short-Term Assessment of Risk and Treatability (START) (Version 1.1).* Port Coquitlam, BC, Canada: Forensic Psychiatric Services Commission and St. Joseph's Healthcare; 2009.

67. Bjørkly S, Hartvig P, Heggen FA, Brauer H, Moger TA. Development of a brief screen for violence risk (V-RISK-10) in acute and general psychiatry: an introduction with emphasis on findings from a naturalistic test of interrater reliability. *Eur. Psychiatry.* 2009; **24**(6): 388–394.

68. Hare RD. *Manual for the Revised Psychopathy Checklist*, 2nd edn. Toronto: Multi-Health Systems; 2003.

69. Monahan J, Steadman HJ, Robbins PC, *et al.* An actuarial model of violence risk assessment for persons with mental disorders. *Psychiatr. Serv.* 2005; **56**(7): 810–815.

70. Dolan M, Fullam R, Logan C, Davies G. The Violence Risk Scale Second Edition (VRS-2) as a predictor of institutional violence in a British forensic inpatient sample. *Psychiatry Res.* 2008; **158**(1): 55–65.

71. Quinsey VL, Harris GT, Rice ME, Cormier CA. *Violent Offenders: Appraising and Managing Risk.* Washington, DC: American Psychological Association; 1998.

72. Wong S, Gordon A. *The Violence Risk Scale.* Saskatchewan, Canada: Research Unit, Regional Psychiatric Centre, Saskatoon; 2000.

73. Ogloff JRP, Daffern M. The Dynamic Appraisal of Situational Aggression: an instrument to assess risk for imminent aggression in psychiatric inpatients. *Behav. Sci. Law.* 2006; **24**(6): 799–813.

74. Nijman HLI, Muris P, Merckelbach HLGJ, *et al.* The staff observation aggression scale–revised (SOAS-R). *Aggressive Behavior.* 1999; **25**(3): 197–209.

75. Marder SR. A review of agitation in mental illness: treatment guidelines and current therapies. *J. Clin. Psychiatry.* 2006; **67**(Suppl 10): 13–21.

76. National Institute for Health and Clinical Excellence. *Violence: The Short-Term Management of Disturbed/Violent Behaviour in In-Patient Psychiatric Settings and Emergency Departments.* London: Royal College of Nursing; 2005.

77. Huf G, Alexander J, Allen MH, Raveendran NS. Haloperidol plus promethazine for psychosis-induced aggression. *Cochrane Database Syst Rev.* 2009; (3): CD005146.

78. Huf G, Coutinho ES, Adams CE. Rapid tranquillisation in psychiatric emergency settings in Brazil: pragmatic randomised controlled trial of intramuscular haloperidol versus intramuscular haloperidol plus promethazine. *BMJ.* 2007; **335**(7625): 869.

79. Raveendran NS, Tharyan P, Alexander J, Adams CE. Rapid tranquillisation in psychiatric emergency settings in India: pragmatic randomised controlled trial of intramuscular olanzapine versus intramuscular haloperidol plus promethazine. *BMJ.* 2007; 335(7625): 865.

80. Nobay F, Simon BC, Levitt MA, Dresden GM. A prospective, doubleblind, randomized trial of midazolam versus haloperidol versus lorazepam in the chemical restraint of violent and severely agitated patients. *Acad. Emerg. Med.* 2004; **11**(7): 744–749.

81. Silver JM, Yudofsky SC, Slater JA, *et al.* Propranolol treatment of chronically hospitalized aggressive patients. *J. Neuropsychiatry Clin. Neurosci.* 1999; **11**(3): 328–335.

82. Stanford MS, Anderson NE, Lake SL, Baldridge RM. Pharmacologic treatment of impulsive aggression with antiepileptic drugs. *Curr. Treat. Options Neurol.* 2009; **11**(5): 383–390.

83. Stanford MS, Mathias CW, Dougherty DM, *et al.* Fifty years of the Barratt Impulsiveness Scale: an update and review. *Personality and Individual Differences.* 2009; **47**(5): 385–395.

84. Azermai M, Petrovic M, Elseviers MM, *et al.* Systematic appraisal of dementia guidelines for the management of behavioural and psychological symptoms. *Ageing Res. Rev.* 2012; **11**(1): 78–86.

85. Langballe EM, Engdahl B, Nordeng H, *et al.* Short- and long-

term mortality risk associated with the use of antipsychotics among 26,940 dementia outpatients: a population-based study. *Am. J. Geriatr. Psychiatry.* 2014; **22**(4): 321–331.

86. Ballard C, Corbett A. Agitation and aggression in people with Alzheimer's disease. *Curr. Opin. Psychiatry.* 2013; **26**(3): 252–259.

87. Ruberg SJ, Chen L, Stauffer V, *et al.* Identification of early changes in specific symptoms that predict longer-term response to atypical antipsychotics in the treatment of patients with schizophrenia. *BMC Psychiatry.* 2011; **11**: 23.

88. Tombaugh TN. Trail Making Test A and B: normative data stratified by age and education. *Arch. Clin. Neuropsychol.* 2004; **19**(2): 203–214.

89. Erhardt D, Epstein JN, Conners CK, Parker JDA, Sitarenios G. Self-ratings of ADHD symptoms in adults II: reliability, validity, and diagnostic sensitivity. *Journal of Attention Disorders.* 1999; **3**(3): 153–158.

90. Ketter TA. Monotherapy versus combined treatment with second-generation antipsychotics in bipolar disorder. *J. Clin. Psychiatry.* 2008; **69**(Suppl 5): 9–15.

91. Yatham LN, Grossman F, Augustyns I, Vieta E, Ravindran A. Mood stabilisers plus risperidone or placebo in the treatment of acute mania: international, double-blind, randomised controlled trial. [Erratum appears in *Br. J. Psychiatry.* 2003;182:369]. *Br. J. Psychiatry.* 2003; **182**(2): 141–147.

92. Keck PE Jr. The role of second-generation antipsychotic monotherapy in the rapid control of acute bipolar mania. *J. Clin. Psychiatry.* 2005; **66**(Suppl 3): 5–11.

93. Swann AC, Bowden CL, Calabrese JR, Dilsaver SC, Morris DD. Differential effect of number of previous episodes of affective disorder on response to lithium or divalproex in acute mania. *Am. J. Psychiatry.* 1999; **156**(8): 1264–1266.

94. Bauer M, Berghofer A, Bschor T, *et al.* Supraphysiological doses of L-thyroxine in the maintenance treatment of prophylaxis-resistant affective disorders. *Neuropsychopharmacology.* 2002; **27**(4): 620–628.

95. Kupka RW. Treatment options for rapid cycling bipolar disorder. *Clinical Approaches in Bipolar Disorders.* 2006; **5**(1): 22–29.

96. Calabrese JR, Kimmel SE, Woyshville MJ, *et al.* Clozapine for treatment-refractory mania. *Am. J. Psychiatry.* 1996; **153**(6): 759–764.

97. Green AI, Tohen M, Patel JK, *et al.* Clozapine in the treatment of refractory psychotic mania. *Am. J. Psychiatry.* 2000; **157**(6): 982–986.

98. Suppes T, Ozcan ME, Carmody T. Response to clozapine of rapid cycling versus non-cycling patients with a history of mania. *Bipolar Disord.* 2004; **6**(4): 329–332.

99. Suppes T, Webb A, Paul B, *et al.* Clinical outcome in a randomized 1-year trial of clozapine versus treatment as usual for patients with treatment-resistant illness and a history of mania. *Am. J. Psychiatry.* 1999; **156**(8): 1164–1169.

100. Grunze H, Vieta E, Goodwin GM, *et al.* The World Federation of Societies of Biological Psychiatry (WFSBP) guidelines for the biological treatment of bipolar disorders: update 2009 on the treatment of acute mania. [Erratum appears in *World J. Biol. Psychiatry.* 2009;10(3):255. Note: Dosage error in article text].

World J. Biol. Psychiatry. 2009; **10**(2): 85–116.

101. Osterberg L, Blaschke T. Adherence to medication. *N. Engl. J. Med.* 2005; **353**(5): 487–497.

102. Bauer M, Adli M, Bschor T, *et al.* Lithium's emerging role in the treatment of refractory major depressive episodes: augmentation of antidepressants. *Neuropsychobiology.* 2010; **62**(1): 36–42.

103. Bauer M, Forsthoff A, Baethge C, *et al.* Lithium augmentation therapy in refractory depression—update 2002. *Eur. Arch. Psychiatry Clin. Neurosci.* 2003; **253**(3): 132–139.

104. Crossley NA, Bauer M. Acceleration and augmentation of antidepressants with lithium for depressive disorders: two meta-analyses of randomized, placebo-controlled trials. *J. Clin. Psychiatry.* 2007; **68**(6): 935–940.

105. Joffe RT, Singer W, Levitt AJ, MacDonald C. A placebo-controlled comparison of lithium and triiodothyronine augmentation of tricyclic antidepressants in unipolar refractory depression. *Arch. Gen. Psychiatry.* 1993; **50**(5): 387–393.

106. Nierenberg AA, Fava M, Trivedi MH, *et al.* A comparison of lithium and T(3) augmentation following two failed medication treatments for depression: a STAR*D report. *Am. J. Psychiatry.* 2006; **163**(9): 1519–1530; quiz 1665.

107. Komossa K, Depping AM, Gaudchau A, Kissling W, Leucht S. Second-generation antipsychotics for major depressive disorder and dysthymia. *Cochrane Database Syst. Rev.* 2010: **12**, CD008121.

108. Nelson JC, Papakostas GI. Atypical antipsychotic augmentation in major depressive disorder: a meta-analysis of placebo-controlled randomized

trials. *Am. J. Psychiatry.* 2009; **166**(9): 980–991.

109. Lam RW, Kennedy SH, Grigoriadis S, *et al.* Canadian Network for Mood and Anxiety Treatments (CANMAT) clinical guidelines for the management of major depressive disorder in adults. *III. Pharmacotherapy. J. Affect. Disord.* 2009; **117**(Suppl 1): S26–S43.

110. Kho KH, van Vreeswijk MF, Simpson S, Zwinderman AH. A metaanalysis of electroconvulsive therapy efficacy in depression. *J ECT.* 2003; **19**(3): 139–147.

111. National Collaborating Centre for Mental Health. *The Treatment and Management of Depression in Adults.* Updated edn. London: The British Psychological Society and The Royal College of Psychiatrists; 2010.

112. Pagnin D, de Queiroz V, Pini S, Cassano GB. Efficacy of ECT in depression: a meta-analytic review. *J ECT.* 2004; **20**(1): 13–20.

113. Spijker J, Nolen WA. An algorithm for the pharmacological treatment of depression. *Acta Psychiatr. Scand.* 2010; **121**(3): 180–189.

114. UK ECT Review Group. Efficacy and safety of electroconvulsive therapy in depressive disorders: a systematic review and meta-analysis. *Lancet.* 2003; **361**(9360): 799–808.

115. Jones RM, Arlidge J, Gillham R, *et al.* Efficacy of mood stabilisers in the treatment of impulsive or repetitive aggression: systematic review and meta-analysis. *Br. J. Psychiatry.* 2011; **198**(2): 93–98.

116. Frogley C, Anagnostakis K, Mitchell S, *et al.* A case series of clozapine for borderline personality disorder. *Ann. Clin. Psychiatry.* 2013; **25**(2): 125–134.

117. Butler T, Schofield PW, Greenberg D, *et al.* Reducing impulsivity in repeat violent offenders: an open label trial of a selective serotonin reuptake inhibitor. *Aust. N. Z. J. Psychiatry.* 2010; **44**(12): 1137–1143.

118. Huband N, Ferriter M, Nathan R, Jones H. Antiepileptics for aggression and associated impulsivity. *Cochrane Database Syst. Rev.* 2010; **17**(2): CD003499.

119. Mattes JA. Medications for aggressiveness in prison: focus on oxcarbazepine. *J. Am. Acad. Psychiatry Law.* 2012; **40**(2): 234–238.

120. Takahashi A, Quadros IM, de Almeida RM, Miczek KA. Brain serotonin receptors and transporters: initiation vs. termination of escalated aggression. *Psychopharmacology (Berl.).* 2011; **213**(2–3): 183–212.

121. Young RC, Biggs JT, Ziegler VE, Meyer DA. A rating scale for mania: reliability, validity and sensitivity. *Br. J. Psychiatry.* 1978; **133**(5): 429–435.

122. Hart SD, Cox DN, Hare RD. *The Hare Psychopathy Checklist: Screening Version.* Toronto: Multi-Health Systems; 1995.

123. Hare RD. Psychopathy: a clinical and forensic overview. *Psychiatr. Clin. North Am.* 2006; **29**(3): 709–724.

124. Ross RR, Ross RD. Programme development through research. In: Ross RR, Ross RD, eds. *Thinking Straight: The Reasoning and Rehabilitation Program for Delinquency Prevention and Offender Rehabilitation.* Ottawa: Air Training and Publications; 1995.

125. Brown D, Larkin F, Sengupta S, *et al.* Clozapine: an effective treatment for seriously violent and psychopathic men with antisocial personality disorder in a UK high-security hospital. *CNS Spectr.* 2014; **19**(5): 391–402. DOI: 10.1017/S1092852914000157.

126. Bonta J, Andrews DA. *Risk–Need–Responsivity Model for Offender Assessment and Rehabilitation 2007–06.* Ottawa: Her Majesty the Queen in Right of Canada; 2007.

127. Dvoskin JA, Skeem JL, Novaco RW, Douglas KS, eds. *Using Social Science to Reduce Violent Offending.* New York: Oxford University Press; 2012.

128. Hanson RK, Bourgon G, Helmus L, Hodgson S. The principles of effective correctional treatment also apply to sexual offenders: a meta-analysis. *Criminal Justice and Behavior.* 2009; **36**(9): 865–891.

129. Douglas KS, Nicholls TD, Brink J. Reducing the risk of violence among people with serious mental illness: a critical analysis of treatment approaches. In: Kleespies PM, ed. *Behavioral Emergencies: An Evidence-Based Resource for Evaluating and Managing Risk of Suicide, Violence, and Victimization.* Washington, DC: American Psychological Association; 2009: 351–376.

130. Beck NC, Menditto AA, Baldwin L, Angelone E, Maddox M. Reduced frequency of aggressive behavior in forensic patients in a social learning program. *Hosp. Community Psychiatry.* 1991; **42**(7): 750–752.

131. Becker M, Love CC, Hunter ME. Intractability is relative: behaviour therapy in the elimination of violence in psychotic forensic patients. *Legal and Criminological Psychology.* 1997; **2**(1): 89–101.

132. Stermac LE. Anger control treatment for forensic patients. *Journal of Interpersonal Violence.* 1986; **1**(4): 446–457.

133. Evershed S, Tennant A, Boomer D, *et al.* Practice-based outcomes of dialectical behaviour therapy (DBT) targeting anger and violence, with male forensic

patients: a pragmatic and non-contemporaneous comparison. *Crim. Behav. Ment. Health.* 2003; **13**(3): 198–213.

134. Drummond DJ, Sparr LF, Gordon GH. Hospital violence reduction among high-risk patients. *JAMA.* 1989; **261**(17): 2531–2534.

135. Carroll E, Tyson K. Therapeutic management of violence in residential care for severely mentally ill clients: an application for intrapsychic humanism. *Smith College Studies in Social Work.* 2004; **74**(3): 539–561.

136. Shelton D, Sampl S, Kesten KL, Zhang W, Trestman RL. Treatment of impulsive aggression in correctional settings. *Behav. Sci. Law.* 2009; **27**(5): 787–800.

137. Rizvi SL, Linehan MM. Dialectical behavior therapy for personality disorders. *Curr. Psychiatry Rep.* 2001; **3**(1): 64–69.

138. Berzins LG, Trestman RL. The development and implementation of dialectical behavior therapy in forensic settings. *International Journal of Forensic Mental Health.* 2004; **3**(1): 93–103.

139. Flannery DJ, Singer MI, Van Dulmen M, Kretschmar J, Belliston L. Exposure to violence, mental health and violent behavior. In: Flannery DJ, Vazsonyi AT, Waldman I, eds. *The Cambridge Handbook of Violent Behavior.* Cambridge, UK: Cambridge University Press; 2007: 306–319.

140. Sullivan CP, Elbogen EB. PTSD symptoms and family versus stranger violence in Iraq and Afghanistan veterans. *Law Hum. Behav.* 2014; **38**(1): 1–9.

141. Management of Post-Traumatic Stress Working Group. *VA/DoD Clinical Practice Guideline for Management of Post-Traumatic Stress.* Washington, DC: Department of Defense; 2010.

142. Cauffman E, Feldman SS, Waterman J, Steiner H. Posttraumatic stress disorder among female juvenile offenders. *J. Am. Acad. Child Adolesc. Psychiatry.* 1998; **37**(11): 1209–1216.

143. Steiner H, Garcia IG, Matthews Z. Posttraumatic stress disorder in incarcerated juvenile delinquents. *J. Am. Acad. Child Adolesc. Psychiatry.* 1997; **36**(3): 357–365.

144. Ford JD, Chapman J, Connor DF, Cruise KR. Complex trauma and aggression in secure juvenile justice settings. *Criminal Justice and Behavior.* 2012; **39**(6): 694–724.

145. Physicians for Human Rights— Health and Justice for Youth Campaign. *Unique Needs of Girls in the Juvenile Justice System.* http://createapath.org/wp-content/uploads/2012/08/PHR-Factsheet.pdf, 2009. Accessed January 13, 2014.

146. Flannery DJ, Singer MI, Wester KL. Violence exposure, psychological trauma, and suicide risk in a community sample of dangerously violent adolescents. *J. Am. Acad. Child Adolesc. Psychiatry.* 2001; **40**(4): 435–442.

147. Najavits LM, Schmitz M, Gotthardt S, Weiss RD. Seeking safety plus exposure therapy: an outcome study on dual diagnosis men. *J. Psychoactive Drugs.* 2005; **37**(4): 425–435.

148. Zlotnick C, Najavits LM, Rohsenow DJ, Johnson DM. A cognitive-behavioral treatment for incarcerated women with substance abuse disorder and posttraumatic stress disorder: findings from a pilot study. *J. Subst. Abuse Treat.* 2003; **25**(2): 99–105.

149. Heinrichs RW, Zakzanis KK. Neurocognitive deficit in schizophrenia: a quantitative review of the evidence. *Neuropsychology.* 1998; **12**(3): 426–445.

150. Keefe RS, Bilder RM, Harvey PD, *et al.* Baseline neurocognitive deficits in the CATIE schizophrenia trial. *Neuropsychopharmacology.* 2006; **31**(9): 2033–2046.

151. Keefe RS, Fenton WS. How should DSM-V criteria for schizophrenia include cognitive impairment? *Schizophr. Bull.* 2007; **33**(4): 912–920.

152. Harris GT, Rice ME, Quinsey VL. Violent recidivism of mentally disordered offenders: the development of a statistical prediction instrument. *Criminal Justice and Behavior.* 1993; **20**(4): 315–335.

153. D'Silva K, Duggan C, McCarthy L. Does treatment really make psychopaths worse? A review of the evidence. *J. Personal Disord.* 2004; **18**(2): 163–177.

154. Polaschek DLL, Daly TE. Treatment and psychopathy in forensic settings. *Aggression and Violent Behavior.* 2013; **18**(5): 592–603.

155. Salekin RT. Psychopathy and therapeutic pessimism: clinical lore or clinical reality? *Clin. Psychol. Rev.* 2002; **22**(1): 79–112.

156. McGuire J. General offending behaviour programmes: concept, theory, and practice. In: Hollin CR, Palmer EJ, eds. *Offending Behaviour Programmes: Development, Application, and Controversies.* Chichester, UK: John Wiley & Sons, Ltd; 2008; 69–111.

157. Ross R, Fabiano E. *Reasoning and Rehabilitation: Manual.* Ottawa: Air Training and Publications; 1985.

158. Tong LSJ, Farrington DP. How effective is the "Reasoning and Rehabilitation" programme in reducing reoffending? A metaanalysis of evaluations in four countries. *Psychology, Crime & Law.* 2006; **12**(1): 3–24.

159. Clarke DA. *Theory Manual for Enhanced Thinking Skills—Prepared for the Joint Prison Accreditation Panel.* London: Home Office; 2000.

160. Renner F, van Goor M, Huibers M, *et al.* Short-term group schema cognitive-behavioral therapy for young adults with personality disorders and personality disorder features: associations with changes in symptomatic distress, schemas, schema modes and coping styles. *Behav. Res. Ther.* 2013; **51**(8): 487–492.

161. Bernstein DP, Arntz A. Vos M. Schema focused therapy in forensic settings: theoretical model and recommendations for best clinical practice. *International Journal of Forensic Mental Health.* 2007; **6**(2): 169–183.

162. Livesley WJ. *Practical Management of Personality Disorder.* New York: Guilford Press; 2003.

163. The President's Commission on Mental Health. *Report to the President from The President's Commission on Mental Health.* Vol 1. Washington, DC: U.S. Government Printing Office; 1978.

164. Coombs T, Taylor M, Pirkis J. Benchmarking forensic mental health organizations. *Australas. Psychiatry.* 2011; **19**(2): 133–142.

Chapter

17

Effectiveness of antipsychotic drugs against hostility in patients with schizophrenia in the Clinical Antipsychotic Trials of Intervention Effectiveness (CATIE) study

Jan Volavka, Pál Czobor, Leslie Citrome, and Richard A. Van Dorn

Introduction

Aggressive behavior can be a dangerous complication of schizophrenia. Aggression is overt action intended to harm. This term describes animal and human behavior. The term *aggression* tends to be used in biomedical and psychological contexts. Aggressive behavior has been classified into two subtypes: impulsive or premeditated. Impulsive aggression is a hair-trigger aggressive response to provocation with loss of behavioral control. Premeditated aggression is a planned aggressive act that is neither spontaneous, nor committed in an agitated state.

Violence denotes aggression among humans. The term is more commonly used in sociology and criminology (e.g., violent crime). The terms violence and aggression are used interchangeably, depending on context.

Hostility denotes unfriendly attitudes. Overt irritability, anger, resentment, or aggression are behavioral manifestations of hostility. Hostility is defined operationally by rating scales. The clinical importance of hostility is in its close association with violence and nonadherence to treatment. A detailed discussion of the definitions of aggression, violence, and hostility can be found elsewhere [1].

The Clinical Antipsychotic Trials of Intervention Effectiveness (CATIE) study [2,3] found that at baseline, 18% of subjects had engaged in violent behavior in the previous six months; of these, 4% had committed serious acts of violence involving weapons or causing injury to another person [4]. A Swedish study found that among 8003 schizophrenia patients, 1054 (13.2%) were convicted at least once for violent crime, compared with 5.3% of general population controls [5].

Hostility, as defined by the Positive and Negative Syndrome Scale (PANSS) [6] item, may include overt aggressive behavior among its manifestations. In the CATIE study, for each unit of increase on the rating of PANSS Hostility at baseline, the odds of serious violence during the preceding six months increased by a factor of 1.65 ($P < 0.001$) [4]. A recent meta-analysis of risk factors for violence in individuals diagnosed with psychosis has estimated that hostility during the study period as well as higher hostility scores significantly elevate violence risk [respective odds ratios 2.8 (95% CI 1.8–4.2) and 1.5 (95% CI 1.0–2.1)] [7].

The PANSS Hostility item has been used as a proxy measure for aggression in psychopharmacological studies [1]. Recently, the efficacy of antipsychotics against hostility was examined by post-hoc analyses of the European First-Episode Schizophrenia Trial (EUFEST) [8]. In that randomized, open trial, haloperidol, amisulpride, olanzapine, quetiapine, and ziprasidone were compared regarding their effects on hostility. The scores on the hostility item of the PANSS were analyzed in a subset of 302 patients who showed at least minimal hostility (a score ≥ 2) at baseline. The results indicated significant differences between treatments. Olanzapine was significantly superior to haloperidol, quetiapine, and amisulpride in reducing hostility in the first three months of treatment.

Here we present analogous post-hoc analyses of the hostility item implemented in Phase 1 of the

Violence in Psychiatry, ed. Katherine D. Warburton and Stephen M. Stahl. Published by Cambridge University Press.
© Cambridge University Press 2016.

CATIE. We hypothesized that the medications would differ in their effects on hostility, and that olanzapine's effects on hostility would be superior to those of the other antipsychotics.

Methods
Study population and interventions

Phase 1 of the multicenter CATIE study enrolled 1493 patients with schizophrenia who were recruited at 57 clinical sites in the United States (16 university clinics, 10 state mental health agencies, 7 Veterans Affairs medical centers, 6 private nonprofit agencies, 4 private-practice sites, and 14 mixed-system sites). The study used broad inclusion and minimal exclusion criteria and allowed the enrollment of patients with coexisting conditions and those who were taking other medications. These features of the study make the results widely applicable.

The participants were randomly assigned to receive olanzapine (olanzapine (7.5 to 30 mg per day), perphenazine (8 to 32 mg per day), quetiapine (200 to 800 mg per day), risperidone (1.5 to 6.0 mg per day), or ziprasidone (40 to 160 mg per day) for up to 18 months in a double-blind trial [3]. The ziprasidone treatment arm was added 1 year after the study began, once ziprasidone was approved for use by the US Food and Drug Administration. Patients with current tardive dyskinesia were not assigned to perphenazine.

The participants were followed for up to 18 months as outpatients. Psychopathology was assessed with the PANSS at baseline and at months 1, 3, 6, 9, 12, 15, and 18. Hostility is one of the PANSS items. The hostility item score range is 0–7. A Hostility item score of 1 means "no hostility," whereas 2 is a rating of "minimal" hostility, with the criterion being "questionable pathology; the patient may be at the upper extreme of normal limits" [9]. A rating of 3, "mild," has the descriptor "the patient shows indirect or restrained communication of anger, such as sarcasm, disrespect, hostile expressions and occasional irritability." Ratings of 4 ("moderate") and 5 ("moderate severe") also do not require the presence of physically assaultive behaviors. The highest ratings of 6 ("severe") and 7 ("extreme") are more likely related to aggressive behaviors that would be considered serious, with the respective criteria of "uncooperativeness and verbal abuse or threats notably influence the interview and seriously impact upon

the patient's social relations; the patient may be violent and destructive but is not physically assaultive toward others" and "marked anger by the patient results in extreme uncooperativeness, precluding other interactions, or in a physical assault episode directed toward others." Hostility is one of the positive items on the PANSS scale. The other positive items are delusions, conceptual disorganization, hallucinatory behavior, excitement, grandiosity, and suspiciousness/persecution.

The time to the discontinuation of treatment for any cause was the primary outcome variable to assess effectiveness [3]. The study was approved by the institutional [1] review board at each site, and written informed consent [1] was obtained from the patients or their legal guardians.

Statistical procedures

Similar to the analyses of the hostility change in the EUFEST study, all analyses were based on the subsample of the modified intent-to-treat population from the parent study who displayed a baseline hostility score of at least 2 ("minimal hostility"). This criterion was needed for the exclusion of patients who did not have sufficient initial severity of hostility (i.e., were rated 1, meaning "no hostility"), and therefore had no room for improvement as a result of treatment.

Two statistical approaches were adopted to analyze all available data: (1) the random regression hierarchical linear modeling (HLM), which allows the use of observations with incomplete data; and (2) the traditional analysis of covariance (ANCOVA) analysis of change over time [endpoint, or last observation carried forward analysis (LOCF) for observed change at study endpoint for each subject].

Random regression hierarchical linear modeling (HLM), a longitudinal data-analytic approach that permits the use of observations with incomplete repeated measures data (e.g., patients who discontinue before completing the study), was adopted as the primary statistical model for the study. In the HLM analysis, change in PANSS Hostility over time across study visits served as the dependent variable. The independent factors included "treatment group" and "time." Regarding treatment group, the five different treatments were applied as between-subject factors. Time (in months) from baseline served as a within-subject, random-effect factor. Interactions between the two independent factors were also included in the model. An unstructured covariance matrix was specified in the analyses in order to account for the time-structured nature of the data (serial correlations across time among assessments of efficacy).

Gender, age, and change in the PANSS positive scale were used as covariates in the HLM analyses. The latter variable was applied as a time-varying covariate to ensure that group differences among treatment groups in change over time identified in the study were specific with respect to hostility (i.e., were independent of change in severity of positive symptoms over time). Change in positive symptoms was defined as the sum of changes on the items of the PANSS positive scale, excluding hostility. Accordingly, the following items were included: delusions, conceptual disorganization, hallucinatory behavior, excitement, grandiosity, and suspiciousness/persecution.

The model effects were tested by the F-statistic. The estimation of the degrees of freedom was based on the Satterthwaite approximation [10]. If a significant main effect or interaction involving treatment group and time was detected, post-hoc analyses were performed to examine the direction of changes (time effect) or the differences in change over time among the treatment groups (interaction effect). An α-level of 0.05 (2-sided) was adopted for all analyses of statistical significance. The Tukey–Kramer method was used for adjustment for Type I error inflation due to the multiple comparisons.

ANCOVA using the LOCF approach was used for sensitivity analyses. Furthermore, similar to the approach used previously in this data set [11], we implemented analyses using statistical models that included covariates for whether the participant was recruited before or after the introduction of ziprasidone, whether the participant had tardive dyskinesia at baseline, and for site effects.

Change from baseline at the study endpoint for each individual patient was applied as a dependent variable, whereas treatment group was used as the principal independent variable of interest in the ANCOVA model. Similar to the primary HLM analyses, gender, age, and change in positive symptoms were included as covariates in the ANCOVA analyses. If a significant overall effect of treatment group was detected, post-hoc analyses with the Tukey–Kramer method for correction against alpha-inflation were

performed to investigate the pairwise group differences in change over time among the treatment groups.

The Statistical Analysis System for Windows (version 9.2; SAS Institute, Cary, NC, USA) was used for the implementation of all statistical analyses, including the HLM (Proc Mixed) and ANCOVA (Proc GLM) analyses.

Findings
Descriptive statistics

Demographic and clinical characteristics of the patients who were included in the current study because they had a hostility score ≥ 2 at baseline ($N = 614$) are listed in Table 17.1. At baseline, there were no statistically significant differences between treatment groups in hostility scores. The other baseline characteristics were similar between the treatment groups. They were also similar to the parent population. Patient disposition is shown in Figure 17.1.

Primary analysis of hostility change (HLM)

The results of our primary analysis of hostility change from baseline showed a statistically significant effect of treatment group ($F_{4,1487} = 7.78$, $P < 0.0001$), indicating differential treatment effects on hostility.

Post-hoc treatment group contrasts for change from baseline were computed for each subsequent time point and for overall change. Olanzapine was significantly superior to perphenazine and quetiapine at months 1, 3, 6, and 9. It was also significantly superior to ziprasidone at months 1, 3, and 6, and to risperidone at months 3 and 6. Corrected P values are shown in Figure 17.2. All medications produced statistically significant improvements in comparison with baseline at all time points, except for ziprasidone, which was not significant starting from month 9, and perphenazine at month 18.

We also present the results that were not adjusted for change in positive symptoms. These results showed a statistically significant effect of treatment group ($F_{4,1498} = 7.40$, $P < 0.0001$). Olanzapine was significantly superior to perphenazine at months 1, 3, 6, and 9 ($P \leq 0.0161$). It was also superior to quetiapine at months 1, 3, 6, 9, and 12 ($P \leq 0.0245$); risperidone at months 3 and 6 ($P \leq 0.0319$); and ziprasidone at months 1, 3, and 6 ($P \leq 0.0046$).

The introduction of covariates for whether the participant was recruited before or after the introduction of ziprasidone, whether s/he had tardive

Table 17.1 Sociodemographic and psychopathological characteristics at baseline

	Olanzapine (N = 136)	Perphenazine (N = 113)	Quetiapine (N = 147)	Risperidone (N = 144)	Ziprasidone (N = 74)	Total (N = 614)
Sociodemographic characteristics						
Age (years)[a]	40.3 (10.4)	38.7 (11.1)	40.4 (11.6)	39.9 (11.8)	39.8 (11.1)	39.9 (11.2)
Women	41/136 (30%)	24/113 (21%)	41/147 (28%)	36/144 (25%)	25/74 (34%)	167/614 (27%)
White	85/136 (63%)	64/113 (57%)	102/147 (69%)	99/144 (69%)	42/74 (57%)	392/614 (64%)
Psychopathology score (PANSS)[b]						
Total	82.2 (17.4)	81.9 (17.5)	81.3 (16.1)	82.9 (15.9)	85.5 (18.1)	82.5 (16.8)
Positive	20.2 (5.2)	20.5 (5.5)	21.4 (5.0)	20.8 (4.9)	21.9 (5.5)	20.9 (5.2)
Negative	21.6 (6.1)	22.0 (6.0)	20.0 (6.3)	21.3 (6.4)	22.0 (6.3)	21.3 (6.2)
General	40.4 (9.8)	39.4 (9.7)	39.9 (9.0)	40.9 (8.5)	40.6 (9.8)	40.3 (9.3)
Hostility	2.7 (0.8)	2.6 (0.7)	2.7 (0.9)	2.6 (0.7)	2.7 (0.9)	2.7 (0.8)

[a] Data are n/N (%) or mean (SD), unless otherwise indicated. Denominators change because of incomplete data.
[b] PANSS = positive and negative syndrome scale. For PANSS, theoretical scores range from 30–210 (total scale), 7–49 (positive scale), 7–49 (negative scale), 16–112 (general psychopathology scale), 1–7 (hostility). Higher scores indicate more severe psychopathology.

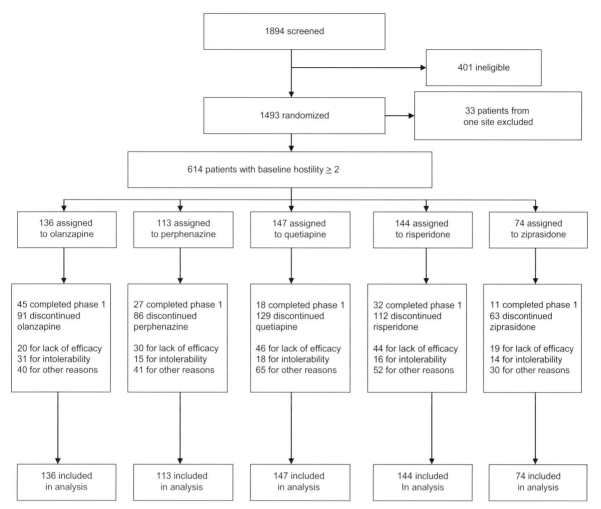

Figure 17.1 Flowchart of patient disposition. The exclusion of data for all 33 patients from one site was caused by concern about the integrity of data from that site. Patients who showed no hostility at baseline (hostility score = 1; *N* = 790) were also excluded (see text).

dyskinesia at baseline, and for site effect had no substantial influence on principal results.

Sensitivity analysis (LOCF)

There was a statistically significant effect of treatment group ($F = 5.48$, $P = 0.0002$). Olanzapine was significantly superior to quetiapine ($P = 0.0002$) and to ziprasidone ($P = 0.0048$). Olanzapine's superiority to risperidone was marginal ($P = 0.0543$).

The results of LOCF analysis not adjusted for change in positive symptoms showed a statistically significant effect of treatment group ($F = 6.87$, $P > 0.0001$). Olanzapine was significantly superior to quetiapine ($P < 0.0001$), risperidone ($P = 0.0143$), and ziprasidone ($P = 0.0007$).

Discussion

The results supported our hypothesis that the medications would differ in their effects on hostility, and that olanzapine's effects would be superior to those of other antipsychotics. Advantages were found for olanzapine compared with perphenazine, quetiapine, risperidone, and ziprasidone for a specific antihostility effect, independent of reduction of other positive symptoms of schizophrenia. Sensitivity analysis using LOCF was generally consistent with our primary HLM analysis.

The trajectory of response for olanzapine, as measured by a decrease in PANSS Hostility over time (Figure 17.2), is consistent with the trajectories of PANSS total score and of Clinical Global Impressions–Severity score as reported for the entire sample in

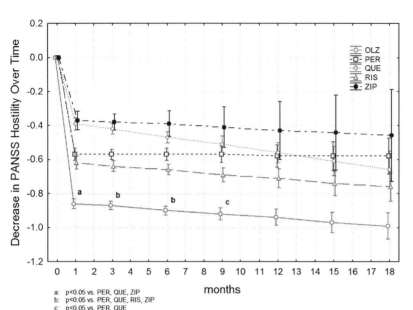

Figure 17.2 Decrease in PANSS Hostility rating over time in CATIE study. Corrected *P* values are shown.

a: p<0.05 vs. PER, QUE, ZIP
b: p<0.05 vs. PER, QUE, RIS, ZIP
c: p<0.05 vs. PER, QUE

the primary CATIE report [3]. Our results are also consistent with those of a similar post-hoc analysis of hostility in first-episode subjects with schizophrenia who were enrolled in the EUFEST trial [8], where olanzapine demonstrated advantages compared with haloperidol, quetiapine, and amisulpride. Our results are also consistent with those reported in a 12-week randomized double-blind clinical trial that was specifically designed to test specific antiaggressive effects of clozapine, olanzapine, and haloperidol [12]. In that study, subjects who were assigned to clozapine had statistically significant lower endpoint aggression scores than patients assigned to either olanzapine or haloperidol. Patients in the olanzapine group had statistically significant lower endpoint aggression scores than patients in the haloperidol group. However, no differences were seen among the three groups in terms of reduction of psychopathology as measured by the PANSS total score, suggesting that clozapine's and olanzapine's advantages were related to a specific antiaggressive effect.

In addition to this report and that from EUFEST, our methods of assessing specific antihostility effects of second-generation antipsychotics have been previously used a priori [13], as well as in a number of other post-hoc analyses [14–16]. Similar techniques have been used post-hoc by others [17–19]. Results

have varied from superiority to haloperidol (compared to risperidone, olanzapine, quetiapine, and ziprasidone) to no difference from haloperidol (for aripiprazole) in terms of antihostility or antiaggressive effect. Compared with haloperidol, the second-generation antipsychotics were associated with fewer extrapyramidal effects and thus were considered more tolerable and overall more effective. Methodologies varied, however, and specific antihostility or antiaggressive effect was not always determined (for olanzapine [17]) or was inconsistently demonstrated (for quetiapine [18,19]).

The correlation of PANSS Hostility item scores and violent outcomes may not be consistent. Although we found that medications differed in their effects on hostility during Phase 1 of CATIE, there were no differences among treatments in their effects on violence during the same Phase [11]. There are several potential explanations of this apparent discrepancy.

First, hostility and violence are different constructs that are assessed using different instruments. A detailed description of the PANSS Hostility item is presented in a preceding section ("Study Populations and Interventions").

In the study by Swanson *et al.* [11], the MacArthur Community Violence Interview was used to measure

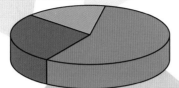

Organized - 29%

Planned behavior not typically associated with frustration or response to immediate threat

Might not be accompanied by autonomic arousal

Planned with clear goals in mind

Also called predatory, instrumental, proactive, or premeditated aggression

Psychotic - 17%

Associated with positive symptoms of psychosis
– typically command hallucinations and/or delusions

Impulsive - 54%

Characterized by high levels of autonomic arousal

Precipitated by provocation

Associated with negative emotions, such as anger or fear

Usually represents response to perceived stress
Also called reactive, affective, or hostile aggression

Figure 9.1 Heterogeneity of aggression. Identifying the type of aggression a patient is displaying may help guide the selection of appropriate treatments that target the underlying dysfunctional circuits. However, violence and aggression arise from a complex combination of neurobiological, genetic, and environmental factors, and are often presented in the context of comorbid conditions.

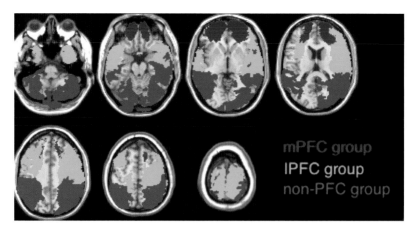

Figure 10.1 Subtraction lesions maps for the mPFC group (red), lPFC group (green), and non-PFC group (blue). For each group, the subtraction lesion map shows those brain areas that were more lesioned in 1 group compared to the other groups. Note that each subject was only included in 1 group.

Maladaptations of the Reward Pathway Can Shift Behavior From Normal to Impulsive to Compulsive

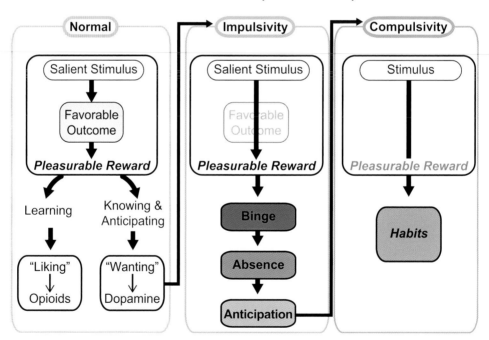

Figure 11.1 Maladaptations of the reward pathway can shift behavior from normal to impulsive to compulsive. Under normal conditions, if a salient stimulus causes a favorable outcome, this behavior will be encoded as a pleasurable reward. The learning of this pleasurable reward is called "liking," and is an opioid-dependent process. The knowledge and anticipation of this pleasurable reward is called "wanting," and is a dopamine-dependent process. An increase in "wanting" is said to underlie impulsivity, such that the drive for the pleasurable reward outweighs the outcome and the behavior is repeated without forethought. In some individuals, there is a higher probability that "wanting" behavior will develop into impulsive behavior due to an underlying environmental or genetic risk. This increased risk is deemed an "impulsivity trait" and can lead to the development of impulsive disorders such as binge eating, drug addiction, and, perhaps, impulsive violence. Repetition of the impulsive behavior, or binging, does not happen all the time; the absence of behavior, however, can lead to a stronger desire, or anticipation, for the reward. It is this cycle of binge–abstinence–anticipation that can lead to compulsivity. When a behavior becomes compulsive, the reward no longer matters and the behavior is strictly driven by stimulus. It is through this mechanism that habits develop.

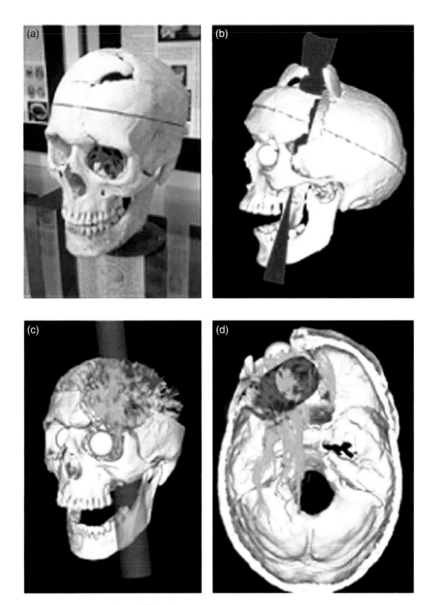

Figure 12.1 Phineas Gage – post-injury analysis of frontal connectivity.

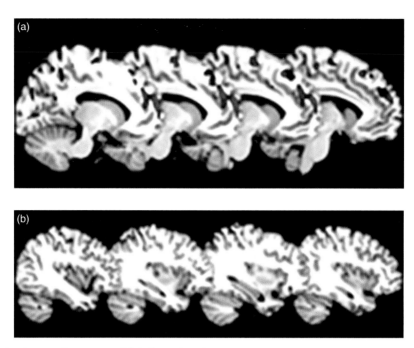

Figure 12.2 Frontal and temporal gray matter deficits in psychopathy.

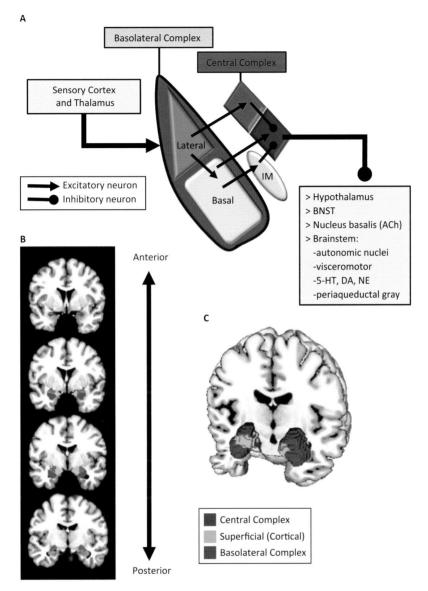

Figure 13.1 Amygdala: functional subdivisions and basic organization of flow of information. The amygdala is not a unitary structure, and consideration of its anatomical subdivisions and circuitry is essential. (A) One of the best characterized models of information flow and intra-amygdala circuitry involves the basolateral nuclear complex (which subsumes lateral and basal nuclei) and the central nuclear complex (which consists of a lateral [light red] and medial component [dark red]); these two complexes are considered the primary input and output components of this circuit, respectively. The basolateral complex receives cortical and thalamic sensory input. The lateral nucleus projects to the basal and central nuclei (lateral component); the basal nucleus projects to the central nucleus (medial component), as well as the intercalated masses (IM). The IMs are clusters of GABAergic inhibitory neurons, nestled between basolateral and central nuclei, which play a critical role in regulating central nucleus activity. The central nucleus projects to various subcortical regions, such as the hypothalamus, bed nucleus of the stria terminalis (BNST), nucleus basalis (major site of acetylcholine [ACh] ascending projection neurons), and various brainstem regions that regulate neurotransmitter systems, autonomic function, innate psychomotor and visceromotor responses, and descending pain-regulation pathways. Central nucleus efferents are believed to consist of tonically active inhibitory projection neurons that activate their downstream targets when their activity is inhibited [30,31]. (B)–(C) Studies of the amygdala in humans have typically considered it as a single functional unit, mainly due to its amorphous shape and relatively small size. Recent imaging studies have demonstrated the ability to differentiate the human amygdala in vivo into the three main nuclear complexes: basolateral, central (centromedial), and superficial (cortical) [32].

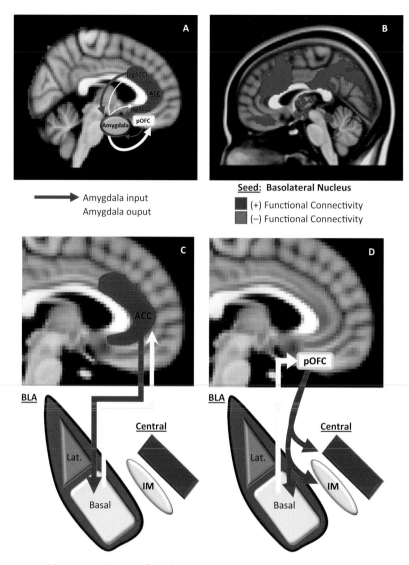

Seed: Basolateral Nucleus

(+) Functional Connectivity
(−) Functional Connectivity

Amygdala input
Amygdala ouput

Figure 13.2 Prefrontal–amygdala circuitry. Altered prefrontal amygdala circuitry has been implicated in the neurobiology of aggression. (A) Preclinical studies in primates and rodents have demonstrated that the portions of the prefrontal cortex most robustly interconnected, anatomically, with the amygdala include two basic regions: the posterior extent of the orbitofrontal cortex (pOFC) and the caudal portions of the anterior cingulate cortex (ACC), roughly corresponding to the subgenual (sg)ACC and pregenual (pg)ACC. Anatomical connectivity between the amygdala and PFC, in general, decreases as it moves toward the dorsal and lateral aspects of the PFC (not depicted in this figure). Although there is significant bilateral anatomical connectivity between the amygdala and both the ACC and pOFC, studies in primates have also demonstrated relatively greater ACC-to-amygdala projections than amygdala-to-ACC projections; the pOFC, on the other hand, receives a greater number of projections from the amygdala compared to projections the pOFC sends to the amygdala. This has been considered to signify that the ACC is more of a sender of amygdala-PFC projections, whereas, the pOFC is more of a receiver [49,50]. (B) These structural data in primates are broadly consistent with intrinsic functional connectivity studies of the amygdala complex in humans, although the latter provides, of course, relatively less anatomical resolution. As illustrated in (B), the subgenual/orbital portion of the medial PFC exhibits positive functional connectivity (red) with the basolateral amygdala complex, which suggests a predominantly feed-forward relationship. The pregenual medial PFC, on the other hand, exhibits negative functional connectivity with the basolateral amygdala complex (blue), which indicates a feed-back role [52]. There is a general absence of functional connectivity with the more dorsal and lateral (not shown) PFC, which is similar to primate structural findings. (C)–(D) There are important anatomical differences in the termination patterns of projections from the OFC and ACC to the amygdala in the primate [51]. Projection neurons from the ACC terminate broadly throughout the basal nucleus (as well as other amygdala nuclei), whereas OFC efferents are relatively unique in that they terminate among the intercalated masses or IMs (clusters of GABAergic inhibitory neurons that regulate central nucleus activity), as well as the central nucleus itself. Therefore, the pOFC may act as a direct arbiter of central nucleus activity, and therefore, determine the extent to which a stimulus representation is infused with a visceral/autonomic or "somatic" component. The ACC, on the other hand, may influence more broadly how sensory inputs to the amygdala are processed. It remains unclear how pregenual and subgenual portions of the ACC may differ in this respect, however.

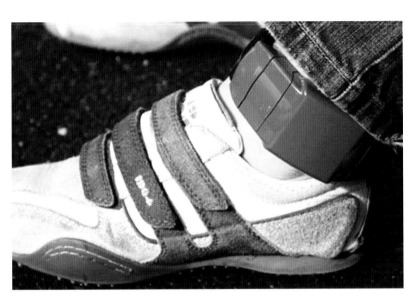

Figure 31.1 The "Buddi" GPS tracker.

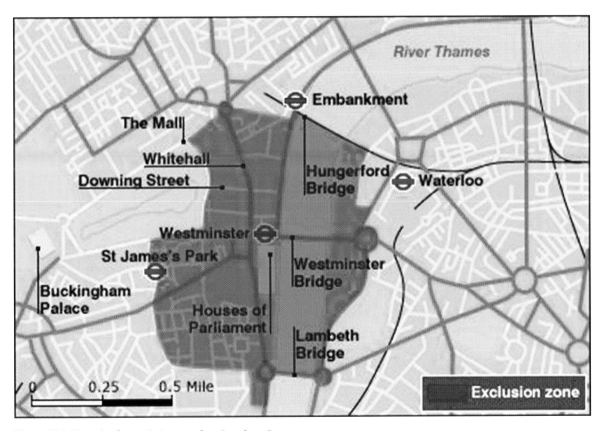

Figure 31.2 Example of an exclusion zone for a "geo-fence."

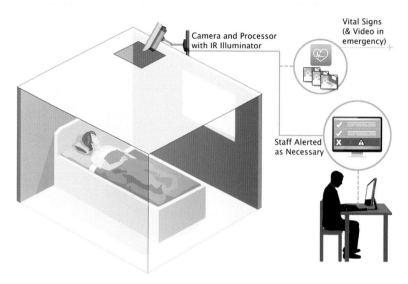

Figure 31.4 Oxecam system.

violent behavior and included minor violence, corresponding to battery without injury or weapon use; and serious violence, corresponding to any battery using a weapon or resulting in injury, any threat with a lethal weapon in hand, or any sexual assault. This level of violence differs qualitatively and quantitatively from the psychopathological symptom of hostility as measured by the PANSS.

Second, the time scale of the assessments of hostility in our study differed from that used in the Swanson study [11] to assess violence. We used multiple PANSS ratings that were based partly on the patient's behavior during the rating interview and partly on the information covering the behavior in the preceding week [9]. Swanson *et al.* conducted two interviews: one at baseline and another at 6 months. Finally, the two studies used different subsets of CATIE patients.

Although hostility is different from violence, it can be a significant barrier to discharge from a hospital and reintegration into the community [20]; in the clinical experience of the authors, hostility is a common treatment target that is identified in individual care plans. The principal concern about hostility as a symptom is the potential for escalation of aggressive behaviors. Hostile behavior is a dynamic risk factor that is strongly associated with increased violence risk in persons who are psychotic, as demonstrated in a meta-analysis of 110 studies that reported on 45,533 individuals [7].

There are several limitations to our study. First, patients recruited for the CATIE study were not necessarily hostile, and those who were tended to display low levels of hostility. However, we note that the effect of olanzapine that was observed in the EUFEST study was very similar to the current results, although the EUFEST patients had higher baseline levels of hostility [8].

Second, with 74% of subjects discontinuing Phase 1, the attrition rate was high, although this rate is generally consistent with those previously observed [21]. The high discontinuation rate was partly due to study design, as subjects were eligible to discontinue Phase 1 and be re-randomized because of perceived lack of efficacy or tolerability with the original randomized medication.

Third, the CATIE was criticized because patients with tardive dyskinesia were not allowed to be randomized to perphenazine; because the maximal dose of olanzapine used was 30 mg per day (instead of the 20 mg per day recommended by the manufacturer), resulting in the average dose of 20 mg per day actually used; and for various other methodological problems [22].

The problem with the olanzapine dose has been somewhat mitigated by a subsequent 8-week study that compared the efficacy of olanzapine 10, 20, and 40 mg per day [23]. All dose groups showed improvement in PANSS total scores from baseline to endpoint without significant dose–response relationship. Thus, the higher dosing of olanzapine used in the CATIE is an unlikely explanation of its superior efficacy against hostility. It should be noted that similar effects of olanzapine against hostility were observed in the EUFEST study that used the recommended dose range of 5–20 mg per day.

Conclusion

Olanzapine demonstrated advantages in terms of a specific antihostility effect over the other antipsychotics tested in Phase 1 of the CATIE trial. This effect replicates, in long-term schizophrenia patients, the findings reported in patients in their first episode [8]. In general, the present findings are consistent with what is already known about olanzapine.

The use of olanzapine in these circumstances needs to be considered within the context of the multiple causes of the hostile behavior and olanzapine's potential for weight gain and changes in metabolic variables [24].

Hostile and aggressive behavior in schizophrenia is etiologically heterogeneous [25]. Violence among adults with schizophrenia may follow at least two distinct pathways: one associated with premorbid conditions, including antisocial conduct, and another associated with the acute psychopathology of schizophrenia [26]. Schizophrenia patients who are violent may show comorbid psychopathic traits [27,28]. The effectiveness of antipsychotics in such cases merits further study.

Disclosures

Jan Volavka does not have anything to disclose. Leslie Citrome has the following disclosures: Alexza, consultant, consulting fees; Alkermes, consultant, consulting fees; Bristol-Myers Squibb, consulting, consultant fees; Bristol-Myers Squibb, speaker, speaker fees; Eli Lilly, consultant, consulting fees; Eli Lilly, speaker, speaker fees; Envivo, consultant, consulting fees; Forest, consultant, consulting fees; Genentech, consultant, consulting fees; Janssen, consultant, consulting fees;

Lundbeck, consultant, consulting fees; Lundbeck, speaker, speaker fees; Merck, consultant, consulting fees; Merck, speaker, speaker fees; Mylan, consultant, consulting fees; Novartis, consultant, consulting fees; Novartis, speaker, speaker fees; Noven, consultant, consulting fees; Otsuka, consultant, consulting fees; Otsuka, speaker, speaker fees; Pfizer, consultant, consulting fees; Pfizer, speaker, speaker fees; Reckitt Benckiser, consultant, consulting fees; Sunovion, consultant, consulting fees; Sunovion, speaker, speaker fees; J & J, small number of shares and common stock; AstraZeneca, speaker, speaker fees. Pál Czobor does not have anything to disclose. Richard A. Van Dorn does not have anything to disclose.

Acknowledgment

Funding for Dr. Van Dorn's time was provided by NIMH Award number 5R01MH093426 to Dr. Van Dorn. The content is solely the responsibility of the authors and does not necessarily represent the official views of the NIMH or the NIH.

Appendix

The CATIE Study Investigators Group included the following: L. Adler, Clinical Insights, Glen Burnie, MD; M. Bari, Synergy Clinical Research, Chula Vista, CA; I. Belz, Tri-County/Mental Health and Mental Retardation Services, Conroe, TX; R. Bland, Southern Illinois University School of Medicine, Springfield, IL; T. Blocher, Mental Health and Mental Retardation Authority of Harris County, Houston, TX; B. Bolyard, Cox North Hospital, Springfield, MO; A. Buffenstein, Queen's Medical Center, Honolulu, HI; J. Burruss, Baylor College of Medicine, Houston, TX; M. Byerly, University of Texas Southwestern Medical Center at Dallas, Dallas, TX; J. Canive, Albuquerque Veterans Affairs Medical Center, Albuquerque, NM; S. Caroff, Behavioral Health Service, Philadelphia, PA; C. Casat, Behavioral Health Center, Charlotte, NC; E. Chavez-Rice, El Paso Community Mental Health and Mental Retardation Center, El Paso, TX; J. Csernansky, Washington University School of Medicine, St. Louis, MO; P. Delgado, University Hospitals of Cleveland, Cleveland, OH; R. Douyon, Veterans Affairs Medical Center, Miami, FL; C. D'Souza, Connecticut Mental Health Center, New Haven, CT; I. Glick, Stanford University School of Medicine, Stanford, CA; D. Goff, Massachusetts General Hospital, Boston, MA; S. Gratz, Eastern Pennsylvania Psychiatric Institute, Philadelphia, PA; G. T. Grossberg, Saint Louis University School of Medicine–Wohl Institute, St. Louis, MO; M. Hale, New Britain General Hospital, New Britain, CT; M. Hamner, Medical University of South Carolina and Veterans Affairs Medical Center, Charleston, SC; R. Jaffe, Belmont Center for Comprehensive Treatment, Philadelphia, PA; D. Jeste, University of California, San Diego, Veterans Affairs Medical Center, San Diego, CA; A. Kablinger, Louisiana State University Health Sciences Center, Shreveport, LA; A. Khan, Psychiatric Research Institute, Wichita, KS; S. Lamberti, University of Rochester, Medical Center, Rochester, NY; M. T. Levy, Staten Island University Hospital, Staten Island, NY; J. A. Lieberman, University of North Carolina School of Medicine, Chapel Hill, NC; G. Maguire, University of California–Irvine, Orange, CA; T. Manschreck, Corrigan Mental Health Center, Fall River, MA; J. McEvoy, Duke University Medical Center, Durham, NC; M. McGee, Appalachian Psychiatric Healthcare System, Athens, OH; H. Meltzer, Vanderbilt University Medical Center, Nashville, TN; A. Miller, University of Texas Health Science Center at San Antonio, San Antonio, TX; D. D. Miller, University of Iowa, Iowa City, IA; H. Nasrallah, University of Cincinnati Medical Center, Cincinnati, OH; C. Nemeroff, Emory University School of Medicine, Atlanta, GA; S. Olson, University of Minnesota Medical School, Minneapolis, MN; G. F. Oxenkrug, St. Elizabeth's Medical Center, Boston, MA; J. Patel, University of Massachusetts Health Care, Worcester, MA; F. Reimherr, University of Utah Medical Center, Salt Lake City, UT; S. Riggio, Mount Sinai Medical Center–Bronx Veterans Affairs Medical Center, Bronx, NY; S. Risch, University of California–San Francisco, San Francisco, CA; B. Saltz, Mental Health Advocates, Boca Raton, FL; T. Simpatico, Northwestern University, Chicago, IL; G. Simpson, University of Southern California Medical Center, Los Angeles, CA; M. Smith, Harbor–UCLA Medical Center, Torrance, CA; R. Sommi, University of Missouri, Kansas City, MO; R. M. Steinbook, University of Miami School of Medicine, Miami, FL; M. Stevens, Valley Mental Health, Salt Lake City, UT; A. Tapp, Veterans Affairs Puget Sound Health Care System, Tacoma, WA; R. Torres, University of Mississippi, Jackson, MS; P. Weiden, SUNY Downstate Medical Center, Brooklyn, NY; J. Wolberg, Mount Sinai Medical Center, New York, NY.

References

1. Volavka J. *Neurobiology of Violence*, 2nd edn. Washington, DC: American Psychiatric Publishing, Inc.; 2002.

2. Stroup TS, McEvoy JP, Swartz MS, *et al.* The National Institute of Mental Health Clinical Antipsychotic Trials of Intervention Effectiveness (CATIE) project: schizophrenia trial design and protocol development. *Schizophr. Bull.* 2003; **29**(1): 15–31.

3. Lieberman JA, Stroup TS, McEvoy JP, *et al.* Effectiveness of antipsychotic drugs in patients with chronic schizophrenia. *N. Engl. J. Med.* 2005; **353**(12): 1209–1223.

4. Swanson JW, Swartz MS, Van Dorn RA, *et al.* A national study of violent behavior in persons with schizophrenia. *Arch. Gen. Psychiatry.* 2006; **63**(5): 490–499.

5. Fazel S, Langstrom N, Hjern A, Grann M, Lichtenstein P. Schizophrenia, substance abuse, and violent crime. *JAMA.* 2009; **301**(19): 2016–2023.

6. Kay SR, Opler LA, Lindenmayer JP. The Positive and Negative Syndrome Scale (PANSS): rationale and standardisation. *Br. J. Psychiatry.* 1989; **155**(Suppl 7): 59–65.

7. Witt K, van Dorn R, Fazel S. Risk factors for violence in psychosis: systematic review and meta-regression analysis of 110 studies. *PLoS One.* 2013; **8**(2): e55942.

8. Volavka J, Czobor P, Derks EM, *et al.* Efficacy of antipsychotic drugs against hostility in the European First-Episode Schizophrenia Trial (EUFEST). *J. Clin. Psychiatry.* 2011; **72**(7): 955–961.

9. Kay SR, Opler LA, Fiszbein A. Positive and Negative Syndrome

Scale (PANSS) rating manual. 1986. Unpublished work.

10. Little RC, Milliken GA, Stroup WW, Wolfinger RD, Schabenberger O. *SAS for Mixed Models*, 2nd edn. Cary, NC: SAS Press; 2006.

11. Swanson JW, Swartz MS, Van Dorn RA, *et al.* Comparison of antipsychotic medication effects on reducing violence in people with schizophrenia. *Br. J. Psychiatry.* 2008; **193**(1): 37–43.

12. Krakowski MI, Czobor P, Citrome L, Bark N, Cooper TB. Atypical antipsychotic agents in the treatment of violent patients with schizophrenia and schizoaffective disorder. *Arch. Gen. Psychiatry.* 2006; **63**(6): 622–629.

13. Citrome L, Volavka J, Czobor P, *et al.* Effects of clozapine, olanzapine, risperidone, and haloperidol on hostility in treatment resistant patients with schizophrenia and schizoaffective disorder. *Psychiatr. Serv.* 2001; **52**(11): 1510–1514.

14. Czobor P, Volavka J, Meibach RC. Effect of risperidone on hostility in schizophrenia. *J. Clin. Psychopharmacol.* 1995; **15**(4): 243–249.

15. Volavka J, Czobor P, Citrome L, *et al.* Efficacy of aripiprazole against hostility in schizophrenia and schizoaffective disorder: data from 5 double-blind studies. *J. Clin. Psychiatry.* 2005; **66**(11): 1362–1366.

16. Citrome L, Volavka J, Czobor P, *et al.* Efficacy of ziprasidone against hostility in schizophrenia: post hoc analysis of randomized, openlabel study data. *J. Clin. Psychiatry.* 2006; **67**(4): 638–642.

17. Kinon BJ, Roychowdhury SM, Milton DR, Hill AL. Effective resolution with olanzapine of acute presentation of behavioral

agitation and positive psychotic symptoms in schizophrenia. *J. Clin. Psychiatry.* 2001; **62**(Suppl 2): 17–21.

18. Arango C, Bernardo M. The effect of quetiapine on aggression and hostility in patients with schizophrenia. *Hum. Psychopharmacol.* 2005; **20**(4): 237–241.

19. Chengappa KN, Goldstein JM, Greenwood M, John V, Levine J. A post hoc analysis of the impact on hostility and agitation of quetiapine and haloperidol among patients with schizophrenia. *Clin. Ther.* 2003; **25**(2): 530–541.

20. Volavka J, Swanson JW, Citrome LL. Understanding and managing violence in schizophrenia. In: Lieberman JA, Murray RM, eds. *Comprehensive Care of Schizophrenia: A Textbook of Clinical Management*, 2nd edn. New York: Oxford University Press; 2012: 262–290.

21. Geddes J, Freemantle N, Harrison P, Bebbington P. Atypical antipsychotics in the treatment of schizophrenia: systematic overview and meta-regression analysis. *BMJ.* 2000; **321**(7273): 1371–1376.

22. Moller HJ. Do effectiveness ("real world") studies on antipsychotics tell us the real truth? *Eur. Arch. Psychiatry Clin. Neurosci.* 2008; **258**(5): 257–270.

23. Kinon BJ, Volavka J, Stauffer V, *et al.* Standard and higher dose of olanzapine in patients with schizophrenia or schizoaffective disorder: a randomized, double-blind, fixed-dose study. *J. Clin. Psychopharmacol.* 2008; **28**(4): 392–400.

24. Citrome L, Holt RI, Walker DJ, Hoffmann VP. Weight gain and changes in metabolic variables following olanzapine treatment in schizophrenia and bipolar disorder.

Clin. Drug Investig. 2011; **31**(7): 455–482.

25. Volavka J, Citrome L. Heterogeneity of violence in schizophrenia and implications for long-term treatment. *Int. J. Clin. Pract.* 2008; **62**(8): 1237–1245.

26. Swanson JW, Van Dorn RA, Swartz MS, *et al.* Alternative pathways to violence in persons with schizophrenia: the role of childhood antisocial behavior problems. *Law Hum. Behav.* 2008; **32**(3): 228–240.

27. Laajasalo T, Salenius S, Lindberg N, Repo-Tiihonen E, Hakkanen-Nyholm H. Psychopathic traits in Finnish homicide offenders with schizophrenia. *Int. J. Law Psychiatry.* 2011; **34**(3–4): 324–330.

28. Abushua'leh K, bu-Akel A. Association of psychopathic traits and symptomatology with violence in patients with schizophrenia. *Psychiatry Res.* 2006; **143**(2–3): 205–211.

Chapter

18

Clozapine: an effective treatment for seriously violent and psychopathic men with antisocial personality disorder in a UK high-security hospital

Darcy Brown, Fintan Larkin, Samrat Sengupta, Jose L. Romero-Ureclay, Callum C. Ross, Nitin Gupta, Morris Vinestock, and Mrigendra Das

Introduction

In recent years, the evidence base to support the use of pharmacotherapy in personality disorders has grown. A number of recent systematic reviews examining this issue concluded that, of the available treatments, mood stabilizers and atypical antipsychotics demonstrated the most clinical benefit [1–3].

A number of atypical antipsychotics, including quetiapine [4–6], aripiprazole [7], and paliperidone [8], have been found to be effective in improving the clinical symptoms of borderline personality disorder (BPD) [9]. In addition to displaying a positive effect in BPD [10–14], olanzapine also reduces symptoms of psychosis and depression in schizotypal personality disorder [15]. Similarly, low-dose risperidone reduces the severity of schizotypal [16] and borderline [17] personality disorders.

Of the atypical antipsychotics, clozapine has shown promising results in the treatment of personality disorder. Clozapine, an atypical antipsychotic with a wide-ranging receptor profile [18], is used in the treatment of schizophrenia. Studies have shown that it is of particular benefit in treatment-resistant schizophrenia [19], with response rates between 30% and 60% [20–22]. Clozapine was found to significantly reduce incidents of self-harm and aggression in a case series of seven female patients with severe BPD [23]. Other studies, including a case report [24], two case series [25,26], and a prospective open-label study involving 15 patients [27], replicated similarly positive results.

Clozapine is also widely known for its anti-aggressive effects [28,29], which have most commonly been demonstrated among schizophrenia patients [30–35]. In a randomized control trial comparing clozapine, olanzapine, and haloperidol, all three drugs showed similar antipsychotic effects; however, clozapine showed a significantly better effect in reducing violent incidents, thus indicating its specific anti-aggressive effects [36].

As clozapine has been shown to be of benefit in certain subtypes of personality disorder and also in reducing aggression in schizophrenia, it is reasonable to hypothesize that it may improve the clinical severity and also reduce aggression and violence in patients with antisocial personality disorder. There is currently limited research in this area.

We present a case series of seven men with a primary diagnosis of antisocial personality disorder (ASPD) and who also scored high on psychopathy (as assessed by a validated psychopathy checklist) [37,38]. All patients had a significant history of serious violence and were commenced on clozapine treatment while being cared for in a high-security hospital.

Method

All patients reported in this article were inpatients at Broadmoor Hospital (a high-security hospital). There are three high-security hospitals in England and Wales with 797 beds, caring for a population of 56 million. High-security hospitals treat patients who have committed serious offences, have severe psychiatric conditions, and therefore pose the highest level of risk to others such that they cannot be managed in other security settings. Typically, the most common

Violence in Psychiatry, ed. Katherine D. Warburton and Stephen M. Stahl. Published by Cambridge University Press.
© Cambridge University Press 2016.

diagnosis is schizophrenia, followed by personality disorder. Patients are detained under the Mental Health Act and include patients transferred from less security hospital units or prisons, or those who receive a hospital treatment order at sentencing from court. The hospital has wards that are distinguished by the level of dependency or risk that the patient poses. This ranges from Intensive Care or High Dependency to rehabilitation wards from where patients are discharged. Patients are discharged to less security hospitals or repatriated to prison once their treatment is complete.

At the time of writing of this case series, six ASPD patients were receiving clozapine in the hospital. Through examining pharmacy records, one further patient was noted to have received a previous discontinued trial of clozapine, and he was also included in this case-series study. All the patients were able to provide informed consent for this retrospective case series. Patients were initiated on clozapine as per the hospital's titration protocol while they were inpatients on a high-dependency ward in the hospital. Doses of clozapine for each patient were recorded, and any changes in these doses and any concurrent medications were noted.

The Clinical Global Impression (CGI) Scale was used to assess the clinical severity and post-intervention changes of patient symptoms [39]. CGI is a commonly used scale for measuring the effect of pharmacological intervention in various studies on personality disorders [40,41]. Scores were formulated retrospectively by the authors (MD, DB) using clinical information examining the patients' illness severity before and after commencement of clozapine treatment. Outcome variables (as described by Soloff [42] and Ingenhoven et al. [1]) were also derived, this time by the treating psychiatrist using the following symptom domains: cognitive-perceptual symptoms, impulsive behavioral dyscontrol, and affective dysregulation. The treating psychiatrists were asked to rate patients' response, following clozapine treatment, in these domains as follows: worsened, remained the same, some improvement, or much improvement. The cognitive-perceptual domain included feelings of paranoia, suspiciousness, referential thinking, depersonalization, illusions, and hallucination-like symptoms; impulsive-behavioral dyscontrol described symptoms such as impulsive aggression, self-harm, promiscuity, excessive spending, and substance abuse; the affective dysregulation domain illustrated

abnormal emotional responses such as mood lability, rejection sensitivity, outbursts of temper, low mood, and inappropriateness of intense anger. This final domain had four subdomains: low mood, anxiety, anger, and mood lability.

Psychopathy was assessed by either the Revised Psychopathy Checklist (PCL-R) [37], which is a validated tool assessing psychopathy, or the Psychopathy Checklist–Screening Version (PCL-SV) [38]. Scores of 28 or more out of a possible score of 40 on PCL-R or a score of 16 or more out of a possible score of 24 on PCL-SV were considered indicative of psychopathy.

The case notes were also reviewed for episodes of seclusion, violent incidents, and episodes of self-harm and positive factors such as engagement in occupational therapy (OT), vocational activities, and psychological therapies. Formal risk assessments (HCR-20) [43] and the hospital's own high risk assessment were reviewed to gauge change in risk status. Planned moves to lower or higher dependency wards were also noted. Clinical reports were examined for details of patients' index offences. All of this information was used to measure risk of aggression prior to and after commencement of clozapine.

We examined metabolic parameters, where these were available, using the latest value prior to and after initiation of clozapine, including BMI (body mass index), total cholesterol:high density lipid (HDL) ratio, and blood glucose levels.

Results

None of the patients had a comorbid diagnosis of schizophrenia or schizoaffective disorder. They also did not have any history of learning disability, brain injury, epilepsy, or concurrent substance abuse. Patients had an average age of 33.3 years. All patients were diagnosed by the treating consultant psychiatrist with primary ASPD. They also had other personality disorder traits (see Table 18.1). All clinical diagnoses and exclusions were made by the treating consultant psychiatrist using International Statistical Classification of Diseases and Related Health Problems, 10th revision (ICD-10) [44] and Diagnostic and Statistical Manual of Mental Disorders, 4th edition (DSM-IV) [45] criteria. Patients received a mean clozapine dosage of 171 mg per day (range 100 mg to 325 mg per day) for at least 7 weeks (range 7 to 67 weeks, median 14 weeks).

Table 18.1 Sample clinical characteristics

Patient	Age	Diagnosis	PCL-SV score	Current duration in HSH (months)	Previous time as inpatient (months)	Descriptors of aggression, self-harm, and details of index offense	Previous medications tried
A	25–29	Antisocial personality disorder with paranoid traits	21/24	34	60	Numerous assaults, interpersonal violence, violence toward animals. Cuts on his hands, banging arms and knuckles. Index offense: attempted murder of close relative.	Clozapine, quetiapine, mirtazepine, citalopram, venlafaxine
B	30–34	Antisocial-schizoid personality disorder with borderline, paranoid, and narcissistic traits	21/24	4	0	Numerous assaults, arson, sexual assault, attempted murder. History of overdose and cutting his arms. Index offense: murder of fellow prisoner by strangulation followed by attempt at decapitation.	Amitriptyline, promethzaine
C	30–34	Antisocial personality disorder with borderline traits	19/24	11	0	Numerous assaults, weapon possession, actual bodily harm, and has frequent fantasies about violence. No history of self-harm. Index offense: extremely violent murder.	Olanzapine
D	25–29	Antisocial-paranoid personality disorder	19/24	28	6	Numerous assaults, violence toward animals, strangulation, and stabbing.	Citalopram, fluoxetine, quetiapine, sertraline, mianserin
E	50–54	Antisocial personality disorder with borderline traits	19/24*	18	48	Multiple sexual assaults, violent assaults, theft. Self-neglect, refusal to eat, self-mutilation. Index offense: Three counts of rape.	Diazepam

Table 18.1 (cont.)

Patient	Age	Diagnosis	PCL-SV score	Current duration in HSH (months)	Previous time as inpatient (months)	Descriptors of aggression, self-harm, and details of index offense	Previous medications tried
F	30–34	Antisocial personality disorder with borderline and paranoid traits	19/24	78	72	Numerous assaults to staff and patients, assault on family members, stabbing, use of weapons. History of cutting himself, attempted to hang himself. Index offense: Actual bodily harm, possession of a weapon, and affray.	Aripiprazole, citalopram, clonazapam, diazepam, lithium carbonate, mirtazepine, palperidone, promethazine, risperidone
G	30–34	Antisocial-paranoid personality disorder with borderline traits.	19/24	16	0	Numerous assaults and interpersonal violence. History of creating and using weapons. No history of self-harm. Index offense: burglary and assaulted shop-keeper with a knife.	Aripiprazole, diazepam, zopiclone

PCL-SV: Psychopathy Checklist-Screening Version [38]. A score of 16/24 or greater indicates psychopathy; HSH: High-security hospital.
* This patient had an additional PCL-R (Hare Psychopathy Checklist–Revised) [37]. This patient scored 28/40, which indicates psychopathy.

Symptom improvement

Of the seven patients, one had a CGI score that displayed "vast improvement" (reduced CGI by 4 points), one showed "major improvement" (reduced CGI by 3 points), and all other patients (N = 5) displayed "significant improvement" (reduced CGI by 2 points). The severity of illness decreased significantly for all patients (see Table 18.2).

With regard to improvement in specific symptom domains, six of the seven patients showed improvement in the cognitive-perceptual domain. All of the patients showed improvement in impulsive-behavioral dyscontrol. All patients showed improvement in some aspect of affective dysregulation; specifically, four showed improved symptoms of low mood, five in anxiety, all demonstrated improved anger control, and six of the seven improved mood lability.

Clozapine and nor-clozapine serum levels, concurrent medication

Data were available for clozapine and nor-clozapine levels for six of the seven patients. Levels were not available for one patient (Patient F), as he was on clozapine for 7 weeks only, and subsequently it was discontinued. Serum clozapine level results were as follows: 150, 160, 170, 230, 270, and 350 ng/ml. Concurrent psychotropic medication was recorded (see Table 18.2). None of the patients was started on any antipsychotic or other psychotropic medication concurrently after the initiation of clozapine.

PCL-SV and PCL-R scores

All patients scored highly on psychopathy as assessed by the PCL-SV (all scored 19 or above out of 24; mean: 19.6; range: 19–21). One patient had an

Table 18.2 Treatment details and results

Patient	Duration of clozapine treatment (weeks)	Clozapine dose (mg/day)	Concurrent medication (mg/day)	Clozapine/ norclozapine level (ng/mL)	CGI Pre	CGI Post	AD CP	AD IB	AD Low mood	AD Anxiety	AD Anger	AD Lability
A	12	325	Quetiapine (200 mg tapering dose)	350/140	6	4	↑	↑↑	↔	↑	↑↑	↑
B	14	200	Mirtazapine (30 mg)	270/210	5	3	↔	↑↑	↔	↔	↑	↔
C	12	175	Chlorpromazine (400 mg) Duloxetine (30 mg) Sodium-valproate (1600 mg)	160/70	5	3	↑↑	↑↑	↑↑	↑↑	↑↑	↑
D	38	150	Chlorpromazine (125 mg) Methadone (30 mg) Tropimarate (200 mg) Trihexyphenidyl (6 mg)	230/110	5	3	↑	↑	↑↑	↑	↑	↑↑
E	65	100	Fluoxetine (40 mg)	150/60	7	3	↑↑	↑↑	↑↑	↑↑	↑↑	↑↑
F	7	100	Amisulpride (600 mg) Diazepam (15 mg) Trihexyphenidyl (20 mg) Venlafaxine (300 mg)	N/A	5	3	↑	↑↑	↔	↔	↑	↑
G	67	150	Sertaline (50 mg) Sodium valproate (1200 mg) Pregabalin (300 mg)	170/80	6	3	↑↑	↑↑	↑↑	↑↑	↑	↑

mg: milligrams; ng/ml: nanograms per milliliter; Pre: before clozapine initiation; Post: after clozapine initiation; CGI: Clinical Global Impression Scale.[39] 1 = normal, not at all ill, 2 = borderline mentally ill, 3 = mildly ill, 4 = moderately ill, 5 = markedly ill, 6 = severely ill, 7 = among the most extremely ill, 0 = not assessed.
Symptom domains: CP: cognitive perceptual symptoms; IB: impulsive-behavioral dyscontrol; AD: affective dysregulation; ↓ worse; ↔ no change; ↑ some improvement; ↑↑ much improved.

additional PCL-R assessment and scored 28 out of 40. These tests were administered by a trained psychologist or doctor.

Improvement in aggression and violence

All patients' risk of violence and aggression to others reduced following treatment with clozapine, as quantified by formal risk assessment changes and staff opinions recorded in the weekly records. In all cases, this risk reduction was associated with clinical improvement in symptoms and positive engagement with OT and psychological therapies. In three of the seven patients, their risk reduced sufficiently to merit a move to a lower dependency ward or transfer to a medium-security unit. None of the patients had to be moved to a higher dependency ward following commencement on clozapine.

Incidents of violence logged in the hospital's incident reporting system were assessed in the 90 days before clozapine was initiated and in the most recent 90 days on clozapine at the time of the writing of this report. It will be pertinent to mention here that in cases where clozapine was started less than 90 days after admission to the hospital, potential incidents may have been missed, as we did not have access to other hospitals' or prison service records. Post-clozapine initiation, no incidents were missed for any patient, as all hospital records were available. Incidents were divided into the following subgroups: verbal aggression, aggression toward property, aggression toward others (physical), and self-harm.

Six of the seven patients showed a reduction in their number of total violent incidents, with four of the six demonstrating a 100% reduction (see Table 18.3 and Figure 18.1). The remaining patient (Patient C: see Case Reports) did not have any recorded incidents before or after clozapine was initiated, but reported a diminished preoccupation with violent fantasies.

Metabolic parameters (see Table 18.4) and side effects

Four patients' body mass index (BMI) increased and 3 decreased over the treatment time period. The mean BMI was 30.2 before clozapine was initiated; this increased to 31.6 after treatment. The result was positively skewed by Patient G's significant BMI increase from 31.8 to 37.4. There was a minor increase in fasting blood sugar results (mean 5.0 pre-clozapine and 5.2 post-clozapine). Finally, there was a slight

Table 18.3 Change in levels of aggression 90 days before and after clozapine initiation

| | Total number of violent incidents | | | | | | | | | | |
| | Verbal aggression | | Aggression against property | | Aggression against others | | Self-harm | | % Reduction in total number of incidents | Risk of violence to others* | Dependency level |
Patient	Pre	Post	Pre	Post	Pre	Post	Pre	Post			
A	22	0	–	–	–	–	–	–	100%	↓	↔
B	2	2	1	0	–	–	–	–	33.3%	↓	↓
C	–	–	–	–	–	–	–	–	–	↓	↔
D	6	1	–	–	–	–	–	–	83.3%	↓	↔
E	6	0	–	–	1	0	2	0	100%	↓	↓
F	1	0	3	0	–	–	–	–	100%	↓	↔
G	5	0	1	0	–	–	–	–	100%	↓	↓

Pre: number of incidents in 90 days prior to starting clozapine; Post: number of incidents in most recent 90 days on clozapine; ↓ reduction; ↑ increase; ↔ no change; and – no incidents.
* As assessed by HCR-20 [41,43] and hospital risk assessment.

Table 18.4 Metabolic parameters

	Pre-clozapine			Post-clozapine			
Patient	BMI	Fasting blood glucose	Total cholesterol: HDL ratio	BMI	Fasting blood glucose	Total cholesterol: HDL ratio	Side effects
A	33.9	n/a	3.4:1	32.0	5.4	3.1:1	Drowsy, tachycardia
B	29.1	5.0	8.6:1	32.2	5.7	11.9:1	Hypersalivation, drowsy, slurred speech
C	28.4	5.0	4.6:1	31.8	5.0	n/a	Drowsy, slurred speech, hypersalivation
D	27.1	5.7	9.6:1	24.4	5.6	4.6:1	Drowsy
E	27.5	4.8	4.0:1	31.5	5.6	5.2:1	Drowsy
F	33.7	4.8	2.9:1	31.7	4.1	5.3:1	Various: non-specific, drowsy
G	31.8	4.9	n/a	37.4	4.8	5.5:1	Drowsy, slurred speech, weight gain

BMI: Body Mass Index, HDL: high density lipid, n/a: information not available.

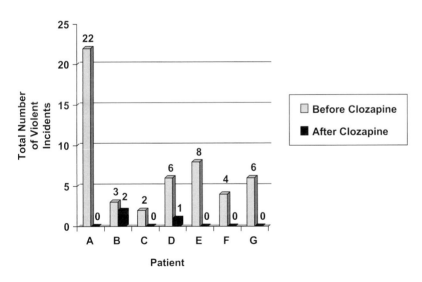

Figure 18.1 Number of violent incidents before and after clozapine treatment. Before clozapine: number of incidents in 90 days prior to starting clozapine; After clozapine: number of incidents in most recent 90 days on clozapine.

increase in total cholesterol:HDL ratios (mean 5.5:1 pre-clozapine, 5.9:1 post-clozapine).

All patients reported a similar profile of side effects. These included drowsiness, hypersalivation, and slurred speech. One patient (Patient F) discontinued clozapine, despite "feeling better," due to various side effects and his subsequent noncompliance.

None of the patients presented with neutropenia or agranulocytosis after initiation of clozapine.

Patient case reports

Patient A has a history of conduct disorder as a child, and presented in his adolescence with violent thoughts, animal abuse, and incidents of interpersonal violence. His index offence involved a serious assault on one of his parents with a knife, and he was convicted of attempted murder. He came to the hospital with symptoms of self-harm, emotional lability, and numerous acts of violence against fellow patients and staff. He has remained an inpatient for the last 7 years. Since 2011, he has had over 88 incidents of verbal aggression and has physically assaulted or attempted to assault fellow patients and staff on 16 accounts. Two years ago, he responded to clozapine for 8 months, but this was stopped due to poor compliance. Since being re-challenged on clozapine, his incidents of aggression have completely ceased, his seclusion hours have more than halved, he is less irritable, and he engages better with staff and fellow patients.

Patient B has a significant history of violence dating back to his early childhood and has over 60 convictions, including assault, arson, criminal damage, sexual assault, attempted murder, and witness intimidation. His index offence was the murder of a fellow prisoner by strangulation and attempted decapitation. He has had several incidents since moving from prison to hospital services, including barricading a door and making serious threats of violence toward staff. Since starting clozapine, he has appeared calmer, violent incidents have reduced, there has been no self-harm, and he has engaged better with staff and other patients. In light of clinical improvement, there are now plans to move him back to prison and prepare him for release on license after he has finished serving his sentence.

Patient C has multiple convictions for assault, actual bodily harm, and the possession of weapons. His index offence was an extremely violent homicide where the victim was hit over the head 30–40 times with a metal bar. He frequently has violent fantasies about killing others and stabbing people with knives. Despite these intense feelings, he has managed to control his impulses while in the hospital and has had no recent incidents of outward aggression toward staff or patients. After the addition of clozapine to his treatment regime, which already included chlorpromazine, Patient C reported feeling better "mentally." Since starting clozapine, his internal aggression and tendency for violence has improved, and he has engaged well with dialectical behavioral therapy and occupational therapies.

Patient D has an index offence of robbery and wounding with intent to cause grievous bodily harm. He has a significant history of assault, robbery, animal cruelty, and substance misuse, and he poses a significant risk of violence to others. Before starting clozapine, the patient was stable but could be verbally abusive toward staff at times. He also refused to engage in any OT or psychological therapies. After commencing treatment on clozapine, his episodes of aggression have reduced, he is now engaging better with staff, and he has been removed from the high-risk register.

Patient E has multiple convictions of rape and sexual violence, and he has displayed significant interpersonal violence toward others while in prison and hospital care. He also has a high risk of self-harm and made serious attempts to self-mutilate while in prison. Before starting clozapine, Patient E could be aggressive and had to be reminded about inappropriate behavior toward female staff. After clozapine was started, it was noted by staff that he appeared calmer. At this point, he also began to engage more frequently in OT and psychological treatment with great success. He has displayed few incidences of violence, engages well, and has been moved to a rehabilitation ward. There is a plan to move him to a medium-security unit.

Patient F has numerous violent convictions, including assault, actual bodily harm, and the possession of weapons. While in the hospital, this violence has continued, and he is at high risk of aggression, assault, and fashioning weapons from sharp objects. During his short trial of clozapine, it was noted by staff that he showed improvement and was more settled. The patient stated that he "felt better," and he continued to engage well with psychological therapies. There were plans for him to be moved to a lower dependency rehabilitation ward. However, clozapine was stopped after only seven weeks due to side effects, including drowsiness, which led to patient noncompliance. In the weeks following discontinuation of clozapine, Patient F did not show any signs of immediate relapse. However, several months later, he had to be moved to a higher dependency ward, as he had begun to destabilize. While writing this report, it was noted that patient F has been restarted on clozapine in the hope he will show a similar response as in his previous trial.

Patient G has various convictions beginning at adolescence. His index offence was robbery with assault, which resulted in grievous bodily harm, and assaults on prison staff on numerous occasions causing serious injuries. Upon admission to the hospital, he had a history of self-harm, failure to comply with medication, and violence toward staff. His aggression toward others seemed to settle after only a few weeks on clozapine, and there was a significant reduction in the frequency of incidents reported. At this time, he has begun engaging well with activities off-ward and was moved to a lower security, rehabilitation ward. He has recently been recommended for transfer to a medium-security unit.

Discussion

We report a case series of seven forensic patients with ASPD and significant histories of violence toward others who were being treated with clozapine in a high-security hospital. Among the robust socio-demographic and clinical predictors for dangerousness in people suffering with mental illnesses, previous history of violence and/or incarceration, aggression at the time of referral, and aggression at the time of hospitalization have been identified [46]. These factors are present in our patients, and hence initiation of clozapine was clinically justified, keeping in perspective the additional facts that clozapine has been shown to be of benefit in certain subtypes of personality disorders [23,27], coupled with reducing aggression in schizophrenia [46].

All of the patients also scored high on psychopathy as determined by PCL-SV and additionally by PCL-R (in one patient). All seven of the patients showed clinical improvement in symptoms with the commencement of clozapine treatment and also a reduction in their risk of violence to others. Specifically, six of the seven patients showed improvement in cognitive-perceptual symptoms, all showed improvement in impulsive-behavioral dyscontrol, four in low mood, five in anxiety, seven in anger, and six in mood lability domains. Overall, clozapine treatment showed exceptional improvement in treating all symptom domains, with maximum benefit in the improvement of the severity of impulsive-behavioral dyscontrol and reducing anger.

Two of the patients who had a presentation of self-harming behavior showed a reduction in this risk. Six of the seven patients displayed a reduction in the total number of violent incidents, with four of the six showing a 100% reduction. The dose of clozapine prescribed was below the therapeutic dose for schizophrenia (350 ng/ml) [47] for five of the six patients whose levels were sampled. All patients showed an improvement in engagement with occupational, vocational, and/or psychological work. Metabolic parameters (where available) were largely unchanged, except for one patient who had a significant increase in BMI from 31.8 to 37.4. Considering this effect, clozapine may have caused minor weight gain in our patient sample. In some cases, there was unexpected improvement in metabolic parameters, which may be due to increased engagement in physical activities such as sports and leisure facilities. Side effects reported by the patients included drowsiness, hypersalivation, and slurred speech, which are all commonly reported side effects. It is relevant to mention here that patients were notified of the potential for these side effects before commencing clozapine. In one patient, various side effects led to the discontinuation of clozapine treatment after only seven weeks. To our knowledge, this is the first report to demonstrate that clozapine treatment may have a beneficial effect on ASPD patients with high psychopathy, especially in reducing the risk of violence to others.

Pharmacodynamic rationale for treatment with clozapine

Clozapine has an extensive range of actions, and has a potent affinity for D_1, D_2, D_4, 5-HT_{2A}, 5-HT_{2C}, 5-HT_3, muscarinic, α-adrenergic, and histamine H_1 receptors; inverse agonist activity at histamine H_2 receptors [48]. The full range of actions induced by clozapine is not yet fully understood [18,19,21,49]. The virtue by which clozapine is particularly efficacious in treatment-resistant schizophrenia, and in reducing violence, may be because of this diverse receptor profile.

Animal studies suggest that dopamine has considerable influence in mediating emotion, stress response, aggression, and impulsivity [50–52]. Additionally several studies have demonstrated the association between abnormal dopamine metabolite (HVA) levels and impulsivity [53,54]. These effects are particularly relevant to borderline and antisocial personality disorders, which are characterized by emotional dysregulation and impulsivity [45]. Dopamine dysfunction has been postulated as an underlying pathology in BPD, and this is supported by evidence that personality disorder symptoms can be treated by neuromodulators that improve dopamine dysfunction, such as the atypical antipsychotic clozapine [55].

Additionally, it has been shown that serotonin (5HT) has a key role in the modulation of aggressive behavior [54–62], and several studies have identified an association between serotonin metabolite (5-HIAA) in human cerebrospinal fluid and antisocial behavior such as violence, homicide, arson, and child abuse [57,58,63]. The extent to which serotoninergic dysfunction influences aggression is dependent on a complex interplay between multiple environmental factors [64].

Through its complex action on both the dopaminergic and serotinergic systems, clozapine induces anti-aggressive properties [28,65], which can be of benefit in the treatment of personality disorders. However, further research is needed to evaluate the pharmacodynamic basis for clozapine's efficacy in this patient group.

Existing literature

It is difficult to compare our results with the current literature due to scarcity of studies reporting on pharmacological treatment in ASPD. However, there are several studies that demonstrate the positive effect of clozapine treatment in BPD [23–27]. While we report seven patients with primary ASPD, it is notable that five of these patients had concurrent borderline personality traits. Hence, one may argue that the improvement in violence may be the effect of clozapine in ameliorating the borderline pathology. Antisocial personality is remarkably similar to borderline type personality, as they share the same core pathology – affective instability and impulsivity [66]. It can therefore be suggested that the benefit of clozapine is not due to the treatment of comorbid borderline traits, but rather that it targets the same spectrum of symptoms that are found in both BPD and ASPD.

However, our patient subgroup is very different to the subgroups in literature that have demonstrated the effectiveness of clozapine in BPD. Our patients' primary difficulties were antisocial behavior, histories of serious violence including homicide, and levels of risk such that they necessitated high-security hospital treatment. Therefore, we suggest that the benefits of clozapine our patients displayed are not merely explained by an amelioration of their borderline pathology.

We have considered the role of concurrent medication, as five of the patients were on antidepressants,

and four were on mood stabilizers. Both can improve symptom domains. However, it is to be noted that these concurrent medications pre-dated the initiation of clozapine, and no changes in dose were made after initiation of clozapine. Also, clozapine treatment was only considered because the concurrent medication (antidepressant or mood stabilizer) in itself was ineffective.

A meta-analysis [1] examined the actions of psychotropic medication on various symptom domains in severe personality disorder and found that antipsychotics rather than mood stabilizers or antidepressants (level of evidence: randomized controlled trials) led to improvement in cognitive perceptual symptoms, whereas improvement in the impulsive-behavioral dyscontrol and in the affective dysregulation domains were found to respond to either antipsychotics, antidepressants, or mood stabilizers. Therefore, the mechanism for improvement in the cognitive perceptual domain may be due to improvement in potential dopamine dysfunction, whereas, impulsive-behavior dyscontrol and affective dysregulation domains are governed in addition by potential serotonin and noradrenergic dysfunction, respectively [67]. Our findings were that clozapine improved functioning in all symptom domains, which may be attributed to the diverse spectrum of receptor actions by clozapine [23].

Our patients were detained in a high-security hospital by virtue of posing the highest levels of risk of violence toward others. Importantly, there was a significant reduction in this risk as demonstrated by reduction in incidents, risk assessments, and movement of patients to lower dependency wards. While this may be due to the specific anti-aggressive property of clozapine, it may be secondary to improvement in cognitive perceptual or impulsive-behavioral dyscontrol domains.

Low dose

The patients in our study achieved clinical response with relatively low doses of clozapine (mean dose: 171 mg, range: 100–325 mg). Five of the six clozapine level samples were below the recommended therapeutic dose level for treatment of schizophrenia (350 ng/ml) [47], and the seventh patient (for whom clozapine levels could not be done) showed clinical benefit with only 100 mg/day of clozapine.

Our findings of low-dose treatment efficacy are similar to that of a previous study that investigated successful low-dose clozapine treatment in BPD [25] and recent reviews on pharmacotherapy of BPD [68,69]. Hence, further research is warranted on treatment dosing and plasma levels of clozapine for the specific treatment of personality disorders, especially ASPD.

We consider that personality disorder treatment may require lower doses of clozapine, as the focus is on improvement in impulsivity and emotion regulation, i.e., symptomatic improvement. Treatment of these symptoms may require lower doses of clozapine compared to the psychotic symptoms displayed in schizophrenia [68]. In fact, in a recent review, it has been pointed out that heterogeneous presentation of BPD lends itself to a symptom-targeted approach based on available research evidence [69]; this issue may operate similarly for patients with ASPD.

Psychopathy

All the patients presented with high psychopathy, with the minimum assessed PCL-SV level falling at the 83rd percentile for forensic psychiatric populations (mean: 19.7; approximately 88th percentile) [38]. The prevalence of psychopathy in the general population is estimated to be 1%, and between 15%–25% of the prison population [70]. Although similar and often comorbid, ASPD and psychopathy are considered separate diagnoses. Research on prisoners found that 50%–80% had ASPD, but only 20% qualified, and therefore were considered to be high psychopathy [71]. High psychopathy in ASPD patients is considered to be clinically relevant because it has proven to be a valid predictor of future violence and risk of reoffending [72].

There is emerging evidence that psychopathy is strongly associated with dopaminergic system abnormalities and possibly serotonin dysregulation [73–75]. Neuroimaging studies support prefrontal structural and functional impairments in this offender subgroup [76–78]. To date there is no literature on the effectiveness of antipsychotics in psychopathic personality disorder. Our findings support the notion that clozapine may provide clinical benefit leading to risk reduction of violence in psychopathic ASPD. We consider this an important area for future research.

Concurrent Axis I diagnosis

Our patients benefited from detailed psychiatric assessments by a range of professionals and treatment in both hospital and prison settings. This detailed evaluation process did not substantiate the presence of an Axis I disorder such as schizophrenia or schizoaffective disorder. The presentation of quasipsychotic symptoms or psychotic-like symptoms in severe personality disorder with borderline/paranoid pathology is not uncommonly encountered [79], and symptoms are known to respond to treatment with atypical antipsychotics [27]. It is unlikely that our patients showed a response due to treatment of a concurrent psychotic illness, but instead benefited from the reduction in the severity of their personality disorder.

Important considerations

The retrospective nature of this case series, lack of objective rating scales, and the small sample size are some of the factors that limit our ability to draw firm conclusions from our data. The data in the medical records as available to the authors may not have been collected similarly across and within subjects. Studies conducted in a high-security hospital typically involve patients who are considered extreme cases in terms of their presentation and associated risks (and accordingly their management), and this may limit the ability of our results to be generalized and be representative of a larger population. This study also did not control for confounding variables such as other medications or psychological therapies and the therapeutic relationship between the patients and their treating team, and this may well have contributed to their improvement. All subjects reported drowsiness as a side effect, which may have confounded behavioral outcomes; however, this may not be the case, as their increased engagement in occupational therapies indicated a genuine behavioral improvement.

However, there are also advantages to our approach. We were able to access large volumes of historical data in a longitudinal perspective for all patients, as participants were inpatients in a high-security setting with stringent and detailed recording of clinical information. Additionally, in such a setting, there are no confounding issues in the form of concurrent substance misuse or irregular/lack of adherence to medications. All patients were fully adherent to the clozapine treatment, and only one patient had to stop treatment due to its side effects. However, this aspect of adherence to a medication such as clozapine merits further consideration, keeping in perspective earlier research that has acknowledged and cautioned regarding the issue of ensuring compliance to oral antipsychotics (including clozapine) after discharge into the community [32].

Cost benefit and future recommendations

All these patients had been transferred to high-security hospital services from medium-security hospitals or from custodial settings due to unmanageable aggression and their need for treatment. High-security hospital care is extremely expensive in comparison to these alternatives, and therefore, if proved beneficial, clozapine would be of immense cost benefit to health services. Effective treatment with clozapine in these patients would reduce the duration of high-security hospital stay and encourage progression to a medium-security hospital or return to prison services, thereby mitigating the overall cost of treatment.

There is a considerable lack of evidence to support pharmacological treatment in ASPD; if available, it is of low impact due to small sample sizes [80]. Additionally, research exploring pharmacotherapy in forensic patients is difficult to conduct, and the subjects that are enrolled in randomized controlled trials are not representative of the most difficult-to-manage patients in security units [81]. Due to the scarcity of evidence, future research is definitely indicated in the field of pharmacotherapy for patients with ASPD and psychopathy.

Conclusion

Clozapine is an atypical antipsychotic that has shown to be of benefit in reducing the risk of violence in schizophrenia. We report our experience of clozapine treatment in violent ASPD patients, with predominantly high psychopathic traits, in the setting of a high-security hospital, where we found that all patients achieved clinical benefit and had reduced risk of violence toward others. To the best our knowledge, this is the first time that clozapine has been shown to be of benefit in patients with ASPD with comorbid high psychopathy. Therefore, there is need for further research to explore the effectiveness of clozapine or other atypical antipsychotics in this subgroup of personality disorder patients.

Disclosures

The authors do not have an affiliation with or financial interest in any organization that might pose a conflict of interest.

References

1. Ingenhoven T, Lafay P, Rinne T, *et al.* Effectiveness of pharmacotherapy for severe personality disorders: meta-analyses of randomized controlled trials. *J. Clin. Psychiatry.* 2010; **71**(1): 14–25.

2. Lieb K, Völlm B, Rücker G, *et al.* Pharmacotherapy for borderline personality disorder: Cochrane systematic review of randomised trials. *Br. J. Psychiatry.* 2010; **196**(1): 4–12.

3. Stoffers JBA, Völlm G, Rücker A, *et al.* Pharmacological interventions for borderline personality disorder. *Cochrane Database Syst Rev.* 2010; (**6**): CD005653.

4. Bellino S, Paradiso E, Bogetto F. Efficacy and tolerability of quetiapine in the treatment of borderline personality disorder: a pilot study. *J. Clin. Psychiatry.* 2006; **67**(7): 1042–1046.

5. Hilger E, Barnas C, Kasper S. Quetiapine in the treatment of borderline personality disorder. *World J. Biol. Psychiatry.* 2003; **4**(1): 42–44.

6. Villeneuve E, Lemelin S. Open-label study of atypical neuroleptic quetiapine for treatment of borderline personality disorder: impulsivity as main target. *J. Clin. Psychiatry.* 2005; **66**(10): 1298–1303.

7. Nickel M, Muehlbacher M, Nickel C, *et al.* Aripiprazole in the treatment of patients with borderline personality disorder: a double-blind, placebo-controlled study. *Am. J. Psychiatry.* 2006; **163** (5): 833–838.

8. Bellino S, Bozzatello P, Rinaldi C, Bogetto F. Paliperidone ER in the treatment of borderline personality disorder: a pilot study of efficacy and tolerability. *Depress. Res. Treat.* 2011; **2011**: 680194.

9. Grootens KP, Verkes RJ. Emerging evidence for the use of atypical antipsychotics in borderline personality disorder. *Pharmacopsychiatry.* 2005; **38**(01): 20–23.

10. Bogenschutz MP, Nurnberg G. Olanzapine versus placebo in the treatment of borderline personality disorder. *J. Clin. Psychiatry.* 2004; **65**(1): 104–109.

11. Linehan MM, McDavid JD, Brown MZ, Sayrs JH, Gallop RJ. Olanzapine plus dialectical behavior therapy for women with high irritability who meet criteria for borderline personality disorder: a double-blind, placebo-

controlled pilot study. *J. Clin. Psychiatry.* 2008; **69**(6): 999–1005.

12. Schulz CS, Camlin KL, Berry SA, Jesberger JA. Olanzapine safety and efficacy in patients with borderline personality disorder and comorbid dysthymia. *Biol. Psychiatry.* 1999; **46**(10): 1429–1435.

13. Zanarini MC, Frankenburg FR, Parachini EA. A preliminary, randomized trial of fluoxetine, olanzapine, and the olanzapine–fluoxetine combination in women with borderline personality disorder. *J. Clin. Psychiatry.* 2004; **65**(7): 903–907.

14. Zanarini MC, Frankenburg FR. Olanzapine treatment of female borderline personality disorder patients: a double-blind, placebo controlled pilot study. *J. Clin. Psychiatry.* 2001; **62**(11): 849–854.

15. Keshavan M, Shad M, Soloff P, Schooler N. Efficacy and tolerability of olanzapine in the treatment of schizotypal personality disorder. *Schizophr. Res.* 2004; **71**(1): 97–101.

16. Koenigsberg HW, Reynolds D, Goodman M, *et al.* Risperidone in the treatment of schizotypal personality disorder. *J. Clin. Psychiatry.* 2003; **64**(6): 628–634.

17. Rocca P, Marchiaro L, Cocuzza E, Bogetto F. Treatment of borderline personality disorder with risperidone. *J. Clin. Psychiatry.* 2002; **63**(3): 241–244.

18. Vauquelin G, Bostoen S, Vanderheyden P, Seeman P. Clozapine, atypical antipsychotics, and the benefits of fast-off D2 dopamine receptor antagonism. *Naunyn Schmiedebergs Arch. Pharmacol.* 2012; **385**(4): 337–372.

19. Fakra E, Azorin J. Clozapine for the treatment of schizophrenia. *Expert Opin. Pharmacother.* 2012; **13**(3): 1923–1935.

20. Chakos M, Lieberman J, Hoffman E, Bradford D, Sheitman B. Effectiveness of second-generation antipsychotics in patients with treatment-resistant schizophrenia: a review and meta-analysis of randomized trials. *Am. J. Psychiatry.* 2001; **158**(4): 518–526.

21. Kane J, Honigfeld G, Singer J, Meltzer H. Clozapine for the treatment-resistant schizophrenic: a double-blind comparison with chlorpromazine. *Arch. Gen. Psychiatry.* 1988; **45**(9): 789–796.

22. Meltzer, Herbert Y. Treatment-resistant schizophrenia-the role of clozapine. *Curr. Med. Res. Opin.* 1997; **14**(1): 1–20.

23. Chengappa KN, Ebeling T, Kang JS, Levine J, Parepally H. Clozapine reduces severe self-mutilation and aggression in psychotic patients with borderline personality disorder. *J. Clin. Psychiatry.* 1999; **60**(7): 477–484.

24. Vohra AK. Treatment of severe borderline personality disorder with clozapine. *Indian J. Psychiatry.* 2010; **52**(3): 267–269.

25. Benedetti F, Sforzini L, Colombo C, Maffei C, Smeraldi E. Low-dose clozapine in acute and continuation treatment of severe borderline personality disorder. *J. Clin. Psychiatry.* 1998; **59**(3): 103–107.

26. Swinton M. Clozapine in severe borderline personality disorder. *The Journal of Forensic Psychiatry.* 2001; **12**(3): 580–591.

27. Frankenburg FR, Zanarini MC. Clozapine treatment of borderline patients: a preliminary study. *Compr. Psychiatry.* 1993; **34**(6): 402–405.

28. Buckley P, Bartell J, Donenwirth K, *et al.* Violence and schizophrenia: clozapine as a specific antiaggressive agent. *Bull. Am. Acad. Psychiatry Law.* 1995; **23**(4): 607–611.

29. Frogley C, Taylor D, Dickens G, Picchioni M. A systematic review of the evidence of clozapine's anti-aggressive effects. *Int. J. Neuropsychopharmacol.* 2012; **15**(9): 1351–1371.

30. Chengappa KNR, Vasile J, Levine J, *et al.* Clozapine: its impact on aggressive behaviour among patients in a state psychiatric hospital. *Schizophr. Res.* 2002; **53**(1–2): 1–6.

31. Citrome L, Volavka J, Czobor P, *et al.* Effects of clozapine, olanzapine, risperidone, and haloperidol on hostility among patients with schizophrenia. *Psychiatr. Serv.* 2001; **52**(11): 1510–1514.

32. Dalal B, Larkin E, Leese M, Taylor PJ. Clozapine treatment of longstanding schizophrenia and serious violence: a two-year follow-up study of the first 50 patients treated with clozapine in Rampton high security hospital. *Crim. Behav. Ment. Health.* 1999; **9**(2): 168–178.

33. Rabinowitz J, Avnon M, Rosenberg V. Effect of clozapine on physical and verbal aggression. *Schizophr. Res.* 1996; **22**(3): 249–255.

34. Ratey JJ, Leveroni C, Kilmer D, Gutheil C. The effects of clozapine on severely aggressive psychiatric inpatients in a state hospital. *J. Clin. Psychiatry.* 1993; **54**(6): 219–223.

35. Volavka J. The effects of clozapine on aggression and substance abuse in schizophrenic patients. *J. Clin. Psychiatry.* 1999; **60**(Suppl 12): 43–46.

36. Krakowski MI, Czobor P, Citrome L, Bark N, Cooper TB. Atypical antipsychotic agents in the treatment of violent patients with schizophrenia and schizoaffective disorder. *Arch. Gen. Psychiatry.* 2006; **63**(6): 622–629.

37. Hare RD. *Manual for the Revised Psychopathy Checklist* (1st edn). 1991. Toronto, ON, Canada: Multi-Health Systems. URL for other refs: http://scholar.google.co.uk/scholar?

hl5en&q5hare1checklist&
btnG5&as_sdt51%2C5&as_sdtp5

38. Hart SD, Cox DN, Hare RD. *The Hare Psychopathy Checklist: Screening Version (PCL: SV)*. Toronto, ON, Canada: Multi-HealthSystems, Inc.; 1995.

39. Guy W. The Clinical Global Impression Scale. In: Guy W, ed. *ECDEU Assessment Manual for Psychopharmacology*. Rev. edn. Rockville, MD: U.S. Department of Health, Education and Welfare, ADAMHA, MIMH Psychopharmacology Research Branch; 1976:218–222.

40. Frankenburg FR, Zanarini MC. Clozapine treatment of borderline patients: a preliminary study. *Compr. Psychiatry*. 1993; **34**(6): 402–405.

41. Binks CA, Fenton M, McCarthy L, *et al*. Psychological therapies for people with borderline personality disorder. *Cochrane Database Syst. Rev.* 2006; (**1**): CD005652.

42. Soloff PH. Algorithms for pharmacological treatment of personality dimensions: symptom-specific treatments for cognitive-perceptual, affective, and impulsive-behavioural dysregulation. *Bull. Menninger Clin.* 1997; **62**(2): 195–214.

43. Webster C, Douglas K, Eaves D, Hart S. *HCR-20: Assessing Risk for Violence*. Version 2; 1992. Burnaby, BC, Canada: Mental Health, Law and Policy Institute, Simon Fraser University.

44. World Health Organization. *The ICD-10 Classification of Mental and Behavioral Disorders: Clinical Descriptions and Diagnostic Guidelines*. Geneva: World Health Organization; 1992; 50.

45. American Psychiatric Association. *Diagnostic and Statistical Manual of Mental Disorders*. 4th edn, text rev. Washington, DC: American Psychiatric Association; 2000.

46. Glazer GM, Dickson RA. Clozapine reduces violence and

persistent aggression in schizophrenia. *J. Clin. Psychiatry*. 1998; **59**(Suppl 3): 8–14.

47. Spina E, Avenoso A, Facciol`a G, *et al*. Relationship between plasma concentrations of clozapine and norclozapine and therapeutic response in patients with schizophrenia resistant to conventional neuroleptics. *Psychopharmacology (Berl.)*. 2000; **148**(1): 83–89.

48. Humbert-Claude M, Davenas E, Gbahou F, Vincent L, Arrang JM. Involvement of histamine receptors in the atypical antipsychotic profile of clozapine: a reassessment in vitro and in vivo. *Psychopharmacology (Berl.)*. 2012; **220**(1): 225–241.

49. Stahl SM. *Psychopharmacology of Antipsychotics*. London: Martin Dunitz; 1999.

50. Harrison AA, Everitt BJ, Robbins TW. Central 5-HT depletion enhances impulsive responding without affecting the accuracy of attentional performance: interactions with dopaminergic mechanisms. *Psychopharmacology (Berl.)*. 1997; **133**(4): 329–342.

51. Vukhac K, Sankoorika EL, Yanyan Wang. Dopamine D2L receptor and age-related reduction in offensive aggression. *Neuroreport*. 2001; **12**(5): 1035–1038.

52. Wade TR, Wit HD, Richards JB. Effects of dopaminergic drugs on delayed reward as a measure of impulsive behaviour in rats. *Psychopharmacology (Berl.)*. 2000; **150**(1): 90–101.

53. Chotai J, Kullgren J, Åsberg M. CSF monoamine metabolites in relation to the diagnostic interview for borderline patients (DIB). *Neuropsychobiology*. 1998; **38**(4): 207–212.

54. Coccaro EF, Silk KR, ed. Neurotransmitter function in personality disorders. In: *Biology of Personality Disorders*.

Washington, DC: American Psychiatric Press; 1998: 1–25.

55. Friedel RO. Dopamine dysfunction in borderline personality disorder: a hypothesis. *Neuropsychopharmacology*. 2004; **29**(6): 1029–1039.

56. Adams DB. Brain mechanisms for offence, defence, and submission. *Behav. Brain Sci.* 1979; **2**(2): 201–213.

57. Berman ME, Tracy JI, Coccaro EF. The serotonin hypothesis of aggression revisited. *Clin. Psychol. Rev.* 1997; **17**(6): 651–665.

58. Brown GL. Aggression, suicide, and serotonin: relationships of CSF amine metabolites. *Am. J. Psychiatry*. 1982; **139**(6): 741–746.

59. de Boer FS, Koolhaas JM. 5-HT1A and 5-HT1B receptor agonists and aggression: a pharmacological challenge of the serotonin deficiency hypothesis. *Eur. J. Pharmacol.* 2005; **526**(1–3): 125–139.

60. Gowin JL, Swann AC, Moeller FG, Lane SD. Zolmitriptan and human aggression: interaction with alcohol. *Psychopharmacology (Berl.)*. 2010; **210**(4): 521–531.

61. Miczek KA, Fish EW, Joseph F, De Almeida RM. Social and neural determinants of aggressive behaviour: pharmacotherapeutic targets at serotonin, dopamine and γ-aminobutyric acid systems. *Psychopharmacology (Berl.)*. 2002; **163**(3): 434–458.

62. Moss HB, Yao JK, Panzak GL. Serotonergic responsivity and behavioral dimensions in antisocial personality disorder with substance abuse. *Biol. Psychiatry*. 1990; **28**(4): 325–338.

63. Constantino JN, Morris JA, Murphy DL. CSF 5-HIAA and family history of antisocial personality disorder in newborns. *Am. J. Psychiatry*. 1997; **154**(2): 1771–1773.

64. Krakowski M. Violence and serotonin: influence of impulse control, affect regulation, and social functioning. *J Neuropsychiatry Clin Neurosci.* 2003; **15**(3): 294–305.

65. Umukoro S, Aladeokin AC, Eduviere AT. Aggressive behavior: a comprehensive review of its neurochemical mechanisms and management. *Aggression and Violent Behavior.* 2012; **18**(2): 195–203.

66. Paris P. Antisocial and borderline personality disorders: two separate diagnoses or two aspects of the same psychopathology? *Compr. Psychiatry.* 1997; **38**(4): 237–242.

67. Bateman AW, Tyrer P. Psychological treatment for personality disorders. *Advances in Psychiatric Treatment.* 2004; **10**(5): 378–388.

68. Bellino S, Paradiso E, Bogetto F. Efficacy and tolerability of pharmacotherapies for borderline personality disorder. *CNS Drugs.* 2008; **22**(8): 671–692.

69. Nelson KJ, Schulz CS. Treatment advances in borderline personality disorder. *Psychiatric Annals.* 2012; **42**(2): 59–64.

70. Dolan M. Psychopathic personality in young people. *Advances in Psychiatric Treatment.* 2004; **10**(6): 466–473.

71. Hare RD. Psychopathy, affect and behaviour. In: Cooke DJ, Forth AE, Hare RD, eds. *Psychopathy: Theory, Research and Implications for Society.* Dordrecht, the Netherlands: Springer; 1998: 105–137.

72. Salekin RT, Rogers R, Sewell KW. A review and meta-analysis of the Psychopathy Checklist and Psychopathy Checklist-Revised: predictive validity of dangerousness. *Clinical Psychology: Science and Practice.* 1996; **3**(3): 203–215.

73. Buckholtz JW, Treadway MT, Cowan RL, *et al.* Mesolimbic dopamine reward system hypersensitivity in individuals with psychopathic traits. *Nat. Neurosci.* 2010; **13**(4): 419–421.

74. Dolan MC, Anderson IM. The relationship between serotonergic function and the Psychopathy Checklist: Screening Version. *J. Psychopharmacol.* 2003; **17**(2): 216–222.

75. Soderstrom H, Blennow K, Sjodin AK, Forsman A. New evidence for an association between the CSF HVA:5-HIAA ratio and psychopathic traits. *J. Neurol. Neurosurg. Psychiatry.* 2003; **74**(7): 918–921.

76. Barkataki I, Kumar V, Das M, Taylor P, Sharma T. Volumetric structural brain abnormalities in men with schizophrenia or antisocial personality disorder. *Behav. Brain Res.* 2006; **169**(2): 239–247.

77. Kumari V, Das M, Taylor PJ, *et al.* Neural and behavioural responses to threat in men with a history of serious violence and schizophrenia or antisocial personality disorder. *Schizoph. Res.* 2009; **110**(1–3): 47–58.

78. Yang Y, Raine R. Prefrontal structural and functional brain imaging findings in antisocial, violent, and psychopathic individuals: a meta-analysis. *Psychiatry Res.* 2009; **174**(2): 81–88.

79. Chopra HD, Beatson JA. Psychotic symptoms in borderline personality disorder. *Am. J. Psychiatry.* 1986; **143**(12): 1605–1607.

80. Kendal T, Pilling S, Tyrer P, *et al.* Guidelines: Borderline and Antisocial Personality Disorders: Summary of NICE Guidance. *BMJ.* 2009; **338**(7689): 293–295.

81. Volavka J, Citrome L. Atypical antipsychotics in the treatment of the persistently aggressive psychotic patient: methodological concerns. *Schizophr. Res.* 1999; **35** (Suppl): S23–S33.

Chapter

19

Augmentation of clozapine with amisulpride: an effective therapeutic strategy for violent treatment-resistant schizophrenia patients in a UK high-security hospital

James E. Hotham, Patrick J. D. Simpson, Rosalie S. Brooman-White, Amlan Basu, Callum C. Ross, Sharon A. Humphreys, Fintan Larkin, Nitin Gupta, and Mrigendra Das

Introduction

Clozapine is an atypical antipsychotic with actions on multiple neurotransmitter systems [1]. It is one of the few agents that have been shown to improve symptoms in patients with treatment-resistant schizophrenia and is a drug of choice, with response rates between 30% and 60% [2,3]. However, its associated side effects can be severe [4].

The potential benefit for patients who are unresponsive to clozapine alone has been sought through augmentation of its effect with other pharmacological agents [5]. This is relatively common clinical practice [6–9]; however, the evidence base behind polypharmacy is limited [10,11]. Research to date has augmented clozapine treatment with antipsychotics [5,12], antidepressants [13–16], mood stabilizers [17–20], and glutamatergic agents [21,22]. Antipsychotics used for augmentation of clozapine are often selected based on the theory that they have alternative mechanisms of action to clozapine. A number of promising small studies that have augmented clozapine with amisulpride, a selective D2 antagonist, have shown clinical improvement in patients on combination therapy versus those on clozapine alone [23–27].

Amisulpride is not approved by the Food and Drug Administration for use in the United States, but it is used in Europe (France, Germany, Italy, Switzerland, Russia, United Kingdom), Israel, India, New Zealand, and Australia to treat psychosis and schizophrenia.

A subgroup of patients with schizophrenia presents with violence [28]. In fact, men with schizophrenia have a significantly increased rate of violent offending compared with men who suffer from non-schizophrenic mental disorders [29]. Given that schizophrenia has a significant relationship with violence, specific treatments to manage this violence may be as important as those to manage the illness [30]. Clozapine has been shown to have a desirable anti-aggressive effect in this population [31–33]. For violent patients within the subgroup who do not respond to clozapine monotherapy, there is no published literature to support the use of clozapine augmentation strategies.

Here we present a case series of patients with schizophrenia who were treated in a high-security hospital and who have a history of serious violence. High-security hospitals look after mentally disordered offenders who pose the highest risk of violence to others. We report the cases of six patients from this subgroup who were treated with clozapine augmented with amisulpride.

Methods

At the time of writing of this case series, eight patients were receiving augmentation of clozapine with amisulpride in the hospital. Of these, six patients were included for this retrospective case series, as they were able to provide informed consent, and the remaining two were deemed to lack the capacity to provide consent by their treating psychiatrists. The remaining

Violence in Psychiatry, ed. Katherine D. Warburton and Stephen M. Stahl. Published by Cambridge University Press. © Cambridge University Press 2016.

six patients did not have any history of learning disability, brain injury, epilepsy, or concurrent substance abuse. These patients are detained in a high-security hospital under the Mental Health Act 1983 (England and Wales). Patients had a median age of 33.5 years. Five patients were suffering from schizophrenia and one from schizoaffective disorder that was treatment-resistant (as per treatment-resistant schizophrenia criteria [2]). These diagnoses were made clinically by the treating consultant. Before amisulpride treatment was initiated, all patients had already received a mean clozapine dosage of 525 mg per day (range 400 mg to 600 mg per day) for at least 4.1 months (range 4.1 months to 13 years and 4 months, median 11.64 months), but were poorly treatment responsive. Clozapine serum levels noted prior to and after augmentation were in the therapeutic range for all patients. Doses of clozapine and amisulpride for each patient were recorded. Any changes in these doses and any concurrent medications, including changes after augmentation, were noted. Combined treatment duration ranged from 1.2 months to 3 years and 9.5 months (median 11.87 months). During the combined treatment period, the mean dosage for amisulpride was 667 mg per day, ranging from 400 mg to 1000 mg per day.

Clinical Global Impression (CGI) scores [34] were formulated retrospectively from clinical information for each patient by examining their illness severity before and after amisulpride augmentation, and also the degree of improvement and side effects while on this treatment. Patients were also asked for their subjective experience of their illness and side effects while taking clozapine and amisulpride combination therapy. The total duration of illness for each patient was also noted.

Case notes and information from the hospital's information recording system were reviewed for violent/aggressive incidents under the following subcategories: (1) verbal aggression, (2) aggression against property, and (3) aggression against people. The case notes were also reviewed for episodes of seclusion and self-harm, as well as positive factors such as engagement in occupational therapy (OT), vocational therapy, and psychological therapies. Formal risk assessments (HCR-20 [35] and the hospital's high-risk assessment) were reviewed to gauge change in risk status, and moves to lower- or higher-dependency wards were noted. Admission reports were examined for patients' index offenses. This information was used

to measure levels of aggression prior to augmentation and since augmentation commenced.

We examined metabolic parameters, where these were available, using the latest value prior to and after initiation of augmentation, including BMI (body mass index), total cholesterol:HDL ratio, and blood glucose levels.

Results
Symptom improvement
Of the six patients, three had a global improvement score of "very much improved," one had a score of "much improved," and two had a score of "minimally improved." The severity of illness decreased for all patients, although to variable degrees (Table 19.1).

Clozapine and norclozapine serum levels, PRN medication
Data were available for pre- and post-amisulpride clozapine and norclozapine levels and PRN medication where applicable (Table 19.1).

Improvement in violence
All patients' risk of violence and aggression to others was reduced following treatment with amisulpride and clozapine, as quantified by percentage reduction in the 90 days pre-amisulpride augmentation and most recent 90 days (where applicable) after augmentation on various parameters (Table 19.2). This risk reduction was generally associated with clinical improvement in symptoms. However, in three cases this reduction in aggression was greater than their overall clinical improvement. This is demonstrated further in individual patient case reports.

Metabolic parameters
One patient's BMI increased from 31.4 to 37.4, but other metabolic parameters appeared to be largely unaffected in all patients (Table 19.3).

Patient case reports
Patient A was referred for treatment in a high-security setting following multiple assaults driven by delusions in a medium-security unit (MSU). Until two months after initiation of augmentation, he remained in long-term segregation (LTS) due to his high risk of assaulting others. During this time, he

Table 19.1 Illness characteristics and medication details

Patient	Age	Duration of illness (years)	Length of current admission in HSH (months)	Duration of preaugmentation clozapine treatment (months)	Duration of augmentation so far	Original clozapine dose	Current clozapine dose	Concurrent medication	PRN medication	Amisulpride dose	Clozapine, norclozapine level (mg/l) Pre	Clozapine, norclozapine level (mg/l) Post	Severity of illness preaugmentation	Severity of illness present
A	40–44	18	23.8	8.55	7.46	550	600**	-		800	0.37, 0.19	0.72, 0.28	4	3
B	30–34	11	30.5	13.71	1.22	500	500	Sertraline	Promethazine 50 mg/day	800	1.14, 0.37	0.81, 0.32	6	4
C	25–29	4	24.1	4.11	18.58	575	575	Valproate, zopiclone	Chlorpromazine 200 mg/day	600	0.37, 0.18	0.45, 0.23	5	4
D	35–39	15	44.2	27.81	16.27	400	300	-		400	0.74, 0.39	0.67, 0.37	5	2
E	40–44	17	45.5	159.75	42.90	600	750	Valproate, sertraline		1000	0.87, 0.26	0.88, 0.24	7	5
F	20–24	7	8.7	9.57	6.90	525	400	-		400	0.46, 0.33	0.46, 0.48	5	3

Notes: HSH=High-security hospital. CGI=Clinical Global Improvement. CGI Severity of illness: 1 = normal, not at all ill; 2=borderline mentally ill; 3=mildly ill; 4=moderately ill; 5=markedly ill; 6=severely ill; 7=among the most extremely ill patients; 0=not assessed.

Table 19.2 Change in measures of aggression after augmentation with amisulpride

Patient	Age	Verbal aggression[a]	Aggression against property[a]	Aggression against others[a]	Self-harm	Risk of violence to others[b]	Dependency
				Violence			
A	40–44	70	100	50	100	↓	=
B	30–34	50	100	50	100	↓	=
C	25–29	20	100	80	n/a	↓	=
D	35–39	=	=	=	n/a	↓	↓
E	40–44	50	=	100	n/a	↓	↓
F	20–24	=	=	100	n/a	↓	↓*

Notes: ↓ – Reduction; = – no change; n/a – not applicable; ↓* – awaiting move to lower dependency ward.
[a] Percentage reduction.
[b] As assessed by HCR-20.

Table 19.3 Metabolic parameters before and after augmentation with amisulpride

Patient	BMI	Glucose	Total cholesterol: HDL ratio	Side effect profile	BMI	Glucose	Total cholesterol: HDL ratio	Side effect profile
	Pre-Augmentation				**Present**			
A	33	5.0	4.8	Sedation, hypersalivation.	33	5.2	4.6	nc
B	35	6.0	10	Occasional hypersalivation	33	4.9	10.9	nc
C	39	5.2	3.8	Sedation	37	4.7	-	Sedation, weight gain, joint stiffness
D	31	-	5	Weight gain, sedation, hypersalivation, constipation	37	-	5.4	Weight gain, sedation, hypersalivation, constipation, raised prolactin
E	32	-	-	None	33	7.6	4.6	None
F	26	-	-	Hypersalivation	47	4.1	5.4	nc

Notes: BMI=Body Mass Index; HDL=high density lipoprotein; nc=no change.

self-harmed and damaged property, including smashing his TV, and made several threats to assault staff. Following the augmentation strategy, his socialization time on the ward out of LTS has been increased. While he has made threats to assault, he now denies thoughts or intentions of harming others. He is also now engaging in off-ward activities and psychological therapies, and is awaiting a move from high dependency to an assertive rehabilitation ward. Before treatment, patient A was classified as moderately ill, and he is now considered only mildly ill. His side effects of sialorrhea and sedation do not significantly interfere with function.

Patient B was admitted to the high-security hospital following incidents of setting fires, absconding, and multiple assaults on staff, all driven by psychotic symptoms. This included one serious assault, wherein the victim required hospitalization. In the months leading up to augmentation, he exhibited multiple episodes of violence, verbal aggression, and self-harm. The self-harm was severe, including a suicide attempt that required medical attention for broken bones. He also made a serious assault on a member of staff and was being nursed continuously in LTS. Once augmentation was initiated, he was able to engage in ward activities; his aggression was generally improved, and self-harm ceased. He made one assault on another patient, requiring LTS to be resumed. Before augmentation, patient B was severely ill and is now considered only moderately ill; he is still psychotic, and his side effects of sedation and sialorrhea have not worsened.

Patient C was admitted to high-security facilities following his index offence of robbery and assault and his consistently aggressive behavior toward staff while in prison, which was linked to paranoid delusions. He also has a history of extensive property damage and arson, and has a high risk of harm to others. Since initiation of augmentation therapy, he has had his escort requirements reduced, been taken off the high-risk register, and been given more grounds privileges. He has had only one incident of verbal aggression, one incident of aggression against property, and one episode of seclusion. His engagement with OT is generally improving. After treatment, his mental state is minimally improved, and he is now considered moderately ill. His side effects of sialorrhea and sedation are no worse and do not significantly interfere with function.

Patient D was admitted to the high-security hospital following an index offence of homicide, which was driven by delusional symptoms. He has a long history of violence prior to this offense. Since admission, he has not been violent and his behavior has remained nonviolent throughout the addition of amisulpride to his treatment regimen. The reduction in his risk of violence has facilitated a move from a high-dependency ward to a low-dependency one. He has recently been engaging well with OT and vocational activities; his improvement has allowed his dose of clozapine to be reduced. Patient D was classified as markedly ill before beginning amisulpride, and now he is considered borderline mentally ill, with his main symptom being lack of insight. His side effects do not significantly interfere with function.

Patient E has an index offence of homicide, which was driven by delusional symptoms, and a long

history of violence, with seven reports of assault prior to his index offense, despite being prescribed clozapine in the community. He also has a history of weapon use, and he posed grave and immediate risk to others in MSU. Since augmentation, he has been attending off-ward activities, including education, asking for a ward job, and attending all scheduled therapy sessions. He is being assessed for group cognitive behavioral therapy (CBT). He has made one threat, but there have been no violent events and he has moved to a lower-dependency unit. Patient E was one of the most severely ill patients in the hospital when he was first admitted. Since starting amisulpride, he has been much improved without side effects. He is still markedly ill, but is happy with his current medication and does not report any side effects.

Patient F has a history of violence prior to admission to the high-security hospital. At his previous MSU, he committed a series of assaults, including his index offense of wounding with intent. He was placed on the high-risk register due to his risk of harm to others. His behavior and mental state have been exemplary since admission; he has been able to be removed from the high-risk register, and has transferred to medium security. His illness is very much improved; he has gone from being markedly ill to only mildly ill while following augmentation therapy and has had no side effects.

Discussion

We report a case series of six forensic patients who suffer from treatment-resistant schizophrenia or schizoaffective disorder, with a history of extreme violence, who are being treated in a high-security hospital. These patients were treated with clozapine that was subsequently augmented with amisulpride because of a lack of clinical efficacy of clozapine alone.

All six of the patients showed clinical improvement in symptoms with the amisulpride augmentation regimen and also a reduction in their risk of violence to others. Five of the six patients had a reduction in number of violent/aggressive incidents. Three of the six patients were eligible to move to lower-dependency wards. Two of the patients who had a presentation of self-harming behavior showed a reduction in this. The dose of clozapine prescribed was reduced for two patients and increased for two patients. All patients showed an improvement in engagement in occupational, vocational, and/or psychological work. Metabolic parameters (where available) were largely unchanged, except for one patient who had an increase in BMI. Side effects were reported as unchanged or improved in five of the six patients. To our knowledge, this is the first report of this combination treatment having a positive effect on reducing aggressive behavior and risk of violence in schizophrenia patients.

Strategies for augmentation of clozapine

Our findings are largely in keeping with previous studies that have investigated augmentation of clozapine with amisulpride or sulpiride. Sulpiride is an atypical antipsychotic that is closely related to amisulpride. Small, randomized, controlled trials (RCTs), open studies, and retrospective studies have demonstrated this effect, but there have been no large RCTs in this area to date. These trials all demonstrated a reduction in positive and negative symptoms [23–25]. In a single-blinded RCT, amisulpride was found to be a superior augmenting agent to quetiapine [36], and in other studies, augmentation with amisulpride allowed the prescribed clozapine dose to be reduced [26,27,37]. Our findings were in keeping with studies that found that this treatment combination did not increase side effects [27,37].

There have also been promising results in studies using other pharmacological agents to augment the actions of clozapine. Ziprasidone, risperidone, and aripiprazole have some evidence base to suggest that they may be effective augmenters of clozapine [38,39,41]. A meta-analysis [40] of clozapine augmentation with a second antipsychotic from 14 randomized, placebo-controlled, double-blind studies that showed augmentation conferred a small benefit over placebo. Some of our patients were taking valproate concurrently with amisulpride and clozapine (initiated before amisulpride augmentation). Mood stabilizers have also been investigated as augmenting agents with clozapine, but the evidence is both limited and mixed [5,42].

Rationale for augmentation of clozapine with amisulpride

Clozapine has a low D2 affinity and is possibly more selective of the mesolimbic system, resulting in fewer extra-pyramidal side effects (EPS). As well as having a low affinity, it also appears to have a faster dissociation time at D2 receptors, which may allow endogenous D2 to bind to the receptors more easily despite the antagonism [43]. This may contribute to the reduced side effect profile. Clozapine also acts at many other receptors, such as serotonin 5HT-2A receptors. Unfortunately, up to 70% of treatment-resistant patients are also poorly responsive to clozapine [2].

Amisulpride is a selective D2 and D3 antagonist [44,45], which appears to have little activity in the striatum and is instead selective for the mesolimbic system, thus causing fewer EPS [46]. It also seems to have effects on 5HT-7 receptors [47], as well as presynaptic autoreceptors, which may be important in modulating endogenous dopamine production [48]. Amisulpride does not affect the pharmacodynamics of clozapine metabolism [42]. Similarly, clozapine does not alter serum levels of amisulpride [49]. The most popular theory explaining the efficacy of amisulpride as an augmenting agent with clozapine is that the receptor profiles of the two drugs are complementary. It is possible that in clozapine nonresponders, the levels of the D2 receptor blockade cannot be met by clozapine alone [43]. Studies have shown that the levels of the D2 blockade need to be high, around 80%, for significant response [50,51]. In these patients who do not respond to clozapine monotherapy, the selective action of amisulpride in the mesolimbic system may allow the D2 blockade to reach these therapeutic levels. The D3-blocking effect of amisulpride may also be important.

Treating violent and aggressive behavior

Violent behavior is uncommon among schizophrenia sufferers in the community [52]. However, it remains a significant problem among patients in a forensic setting who tend to have severe illnesses that are poorly responsive to standard pharmacological therapy. Our six patients from this subgroup were all considered an extremely high risk of harm to others, such that they were admitted to conditions of high security. Studies which have included randomized controlled trials have demonstrated that aggressive treatment-resistant patients initiate fewer aggressive and violent incidents when treated with clozapine [31,32,53]. This is thought to be due to clozapine's wide receptor profile which includes dopamine and 5-HT receptors, which are implicated in the neurochemistry of aggression [54,55].

Our patients were all taking clozapine for at least 17 weeks (median: 11.64 months) prior to the addition of amisulpride with minimal change in their risk of aggression and violence toward others. Following addition of amisulpride to their treatment regimens, all patients were assessed as having a greatly reduced risk of violent and aggressive behavior. It is unlikely that the risk reduction in these patients is due to a late effect of clozapine, as several studies have proposed that 3–6 months of clozapine treatment is sufficient to assess response to this medication [56–59].

There are various possible reasons for the reduced risk of violence in these patients. First, it is possible that their aggressive behavior was reduced secondary to an overall clinical improvement in their illness on both amisulpride and clozapine. In one study, 40% of violent patients retrospectively reported that at least one violent incident had been motivated by a concurrent delusion [60]. However, the authors concluded that overall, violent incidents were probably not motivated by concurrent delusions. Two of our cases both committed a homicide based on their delusional beliefs, and so a reduction in their positive symptoms would reduce their risk of similar violent incidents in the future. It has been reported that the lower levels of aggression seen with clozapine monotherapy are associated with a reduction in positive symptoms [61]. However, for three of our subjects, risk of violence to others has reduced disproportionately to their clinical improvement. Other studies have suggested that aggressive behavior is not tightly coupled to severity of illness [52,62]. It is also considered that violence is often a separate dimension of the schizophrenia illness, and executive functioning can predict treatment response. However, clozapine retains its anti-aggressive benefits in those with lower cognitive functioning [63].

This area warrants further research to establish firmly whether clozapine and also clozapine augmentation with amisulpride have a specific anti-aggressive effect in excess of their antipsychotic efficacy. Our results show a reduction in aggressive behaviors for most patients and improvement in engagement for all patients following augmentation with amisulpride compared with their clozapine monotherapy.

Important considerations

However, there are limitations in extrapolating from our data to a wider setting. The retrospective nature of this case series, lack of objective rating scales, and the small sample size limit our ability to draw firm conclusions from our data. Research exploring pharmacotherapy with forensic psychiatric patients is a difficult area to conduct, as subjects who are enrolled in RCTs are not representative of the most difficult-to-manage patients found in secure units [64]. Retrospective analysis has allowed us to take a naturalistic approach, demonstrating more clearly how this augmentation strategy may be advantageous on an individual patient basis in a high-security hospital setting. It is also very difficult to quantify the beneficial effects of patient engagement with occupational therapy and psychological therapy sessions, which all these patients attended to some degree over the course of treatment post-augmentation, and this may well have contributed to their improvement.

However, there are also advantages to our approach. We were able to access large volumes of historical data for all patients. Also, due to these subjects being inpatients in a high-security setting, there are no issues with concurrent substance misuse and lack of compliance with medications. All patients were fully compliant with the amisulpride/clozapine combination therapy, and only two patients reported a worsening of their side effects. No new concurrent medication was prescribed to any patients after initiation of amisulpride.

Patients who are treatment-resistant are often also highly symptomatic, requiring long periods of hospital care [65]. This care often requires a disproportionately high amount of the total cost of schizophrenia treatment [66]. Patients with a history of schizophrenia and violence in the forensic setting are associated with higher treatment costs. Strategies to bring about improvement in this subgroup of patients in their symptoms and violence would be of immense cost benefit to health services.

Conclusion

Clozapine is an antipsychotic of choice for treating patients with treatment-resistant schizophrenia. However, a significant proportion of patients do not respond to clozapine alone, and other agents have been added to augment the response to clozapine. We report our experience of augmentation of clozapine with amisulpride in violent treatment-resistant patients in a high-security hospital.

We have found that in all of these patients with clozapine-unresponsive schizophrenia, amisulpride augmentation of clozapine treatment had a clinical benefit and reduced episodes of violence and risk of violence. This is the first time that the combination of clozapine and amisulpride has been reported to have an anti-aggressive effect in patients who had previously been very violent. Further research would better determine the beneficial effects of this augmentation strategy on violent patients with treatment-resistant schizophrenia.

Disclosures

The authors do not have anything to disclose.

References

1. Fakra E, Azorin JM. Clozapine for the treatment of schizophrenia. *Expert Opin. Pharmacother.* 2012; **13**(13): 1923–1935.

2. Kane J, Honigfeld G, Singer J, Meltzer H. Clozapine for the treatment-resistant schizophrenic: a double-blind comparison with chlorpromazine. *Arch. Gen. Psychiatry.* 1988; **45**(9): 789–796.

3. Rosenheck R, Cramer J, Xu W, *et al.* A comparison of clozapine and haloperidol in hospitalized patients with refractory schizophrenia. *N. Engl. J. Med.* 1997; **337**(12): 809–815.

4. Baldessarini RJ, Frankenburg FR. Clozapine—a novel antipsychotic agent. *N. Engl. J. Med.* 1991; **324**(11): 746–754.

5. Porcelli S, Balzarro B, Serretti A. Clozapine resistance: augmentation strategies. *Eur. Neuropsychopharmacol.* 2012; **22**(3): 165–182.

6. Stahl SM. Antipsychotic polypharmacy, part 1: therapeutic option or dirty little secret? *J. Clin. Psychiatry.* 1999; **60**(7): 425–426.

7. Stahl SM. Antipsychotic polypharmacy: evidence based or eminence based? *Acta Psychiatr. Scand.* 2002; **106**(5): 321–322.

8. Stahl SM. Antipsychotic polypharmacy: never say never, but never say always. *Acta Psychiatr. Scand.* 2012; **125**(5): 349–351.

9. Stahl SM. Emerging guidelines for the use of antipsychotic polypharmacy. *Rev. Psiquiatr. Salud Ment.* 2013; **6**(3): 97–100.

10. Pai NB, Laidlaw M, Vella SC. Augmentation of clozapine with another pharmacological agent: treatment for refractory schizophrenia in the "real world." *Acta Psychiatr. Scand.* 2012; **126**(1): 40–46.

11. Zink M, Englisch S, Meyer-Lindenberg A. Polypharmacy in schizophrenia. *Curr. Opin. Psychiatry.* 2010; **23**(2): 103–111.

12. Correll CU, Rummel-Kluge C, Corves C, *et al.* Antipsychotic combinations vs monotherapy in schizophrenia: a meta-analysis of randomized controlled trials. *Schizophr. Bull.* 2009; **35**(2): 443–457.

13. Buchanan RW, Kirkpatrick B, Bryant N, *et al.* Fluoxetine augmentation of clozapine treatment in patients with schizophrenia. *Am. J. Psychiatry.* 1996; **153**(12): 1625–1627.

14. Wetzel H, Anghelescu I, Szegedi A, *et al.* Pharmacokinetic interactions of clozapine with selective serotonin reuptake inhibitors: differential effects of fluvoxamine and paroxetine in a prospective study. *J. Clin. Psychopharmacol.* 1998; **18**(1): 2–9.

15. Berk M, Gama CS, Sundram S, *et al.* Mirtazapine add-on therapy in the treatment of schizophrenia with atypical antipsychotics: a double-blind, randomised, placebo-controlled clinical trial. *Hum. Psychopharmacol.* 2009; **24**(3): 233–238.

16. Zoccali R, Muscatello MR, Cedro C, *et al.* The effect of mirtazapine augmentation of clozapine in the treatment of negative symptoms of schizophrenia: a double-blind, placebo-controlled study. *Int. Clin. Psychopharmacol.* 2004; **19**(2): 71–76.

17. Tiihonen J, Hallikainen T, Ryynänen OP, *et al.* Lamotrigine in treatment-resistant schizophrenia: a randomized placebo-controlled crossover trial. *Biol. Psychiatry.* 2003; **54**(11): 1241–1248.

18. Goff DC, Keefe R, Citrome L, *et al.* Lamotrigine as add-on therapy in schizophrenia: results of 2 placebo-controlled trials. *J. Clin. Psychopharmacol.* 2007; **27**(6): 582–589.

19. Muscatello MR, Bruno A, Pandolfo G, *et al.* Topiramate augmentation of clozapine in schizophrenia: a double-blind, placebo-controlled study. *J. Psychopharmacol.* 2011; **25**(5): 667–674.

20. Small JG, Klapper MH, Malloy FW, Steadman TM. Tolerability and efficacy of clozapine combined with lithium in schizophrenia and schizoaffective disorder. *J. Clin. Psychopharmacol.* 2003; **23**(3): 223–228.

21. Evins AE, Fitzgerald SM, Wine L, *et al.* Placebo-controlled trial of glycine added to clozapine in schizophrenia. *Am. J. Psychiatry.* 2000; **157**(5): 826–828.

22. Heresco-Levy U, Javitt DC, Ermilov M, *et al.* Efficacy of high-dose glycine in the treatment of enduring negative symptoms of schizophrenia. *Arch. Gen. Psychiatry.* 1999; **56**(1): 29–36.

23. Assion HJ, Reinbold H, Lemanski S, *et al.* Amisulpride augmentation in patients with schizophrenia partially responsive or unresponsive to clozapine: a randomized, double-blind, placebo-controlled trial. *Pharmacopsychiatry.* 2008; **41**(1): 24–28.

24. Shiloh R, Zemishlany Z, Aizenberg D, *et al.* Sulpiride augmentation in people with schizophrenia partially responsive to clozapine: a double-blind, placebo-controlled study. *Br. J. Psychiatry.* 1997; **171**: 569–573.

25. Munro J, Matthiasson P, Osborne S, *et al.* Amisulpride augmentation of clozapine: an open non-randomized study in patients with schizophrenia partially responsive to clozapine. *Acta Psychiatr. Scand.* 2004; **110**(4): 292–298.

26. Zink M, Knopf U, Henn FA, Thome J. Combination of clozapine and amisulpride in treatment-resistant schizophrenia —case reports and review of the literature. *Pharmacopsychiatry.* 2004; **37**(1): 26–31.

27. Kämpf P, Agelink MW, Naber D. Augmentation of clozapine with amisulpride: a promising therapeutic approach to refractory schizophrenic symptoms. *Pharmacopsychiatry.* 2005; **38**(1): 39–40.

28. Walsh E, Buchanan A, Fahy T. Violence and schizophrenia: examining the evidence. *Br. J. Psychiatry.* 2002; **180**: 490–495.

29. Wessely S. The Camberwell Study of Crime and Schizophrenia. *Soc. Psychiatry Psychiatr. Epidemiol.* 1998; **33**(Suppl 1): S24–S28.

30. Taylor PJ, Estroff SE. Schizophrenia and violence. In: Hirsch FR, Weinberger DR, eds. *Schizophrenia*, 2nd edn. Oxford, UK: Blackwell Science Ltd.; 2007; 30: 591–612.

31. Citrome L, Volavka J, Czobor P, *et al.* Effects of clozapine, olanzapine, risperidone, and haloperidol on hostility among patients with schizophrenia. *Psychiatric Services.* 2001; **52**(11): 1510–1514.

32. Krakowski MI, Czobor P, Citrome L, *et al.* Atypical antipsychotic agents in the treatment of violent patients with schizophrenia and schizoaffective disorder. *Arch. Gen. Psychiatry.* 2006; **63**(6): 622–629.

33. Frogley C, Taylor D, Dickens G, Picchioni M. A systematic review of the evidence of clozapine's anti-aggressive effects. *Int. J. Neuropsychopharmacol.* 2012; **15**(9): 1351–1371.

34. Guy W. The Clinical Global Impression Scale. In: Guy W, ed. *ECDEU Assessment Manual for Psychopharmacology* –Rev. edn. Rockville, MD: US Department of Health, Education and Welfare, ADAMHA, MIMH Psychopharmacology Research Branch; 1976: 218–222.

35. Webster C, Douglas K, Eaves D, Hart S. *HCR-20: Assessing Risk for Violence.* Version 2. Burnaby, BC, Canada: Mental Health, Law and Policy Institute, Simon Fraser University.

36. Genç Y, Taner E, Candansayar S. Comparison of clozapine-amisulpride and clozapine-quetiapine combinations for patients with schizophrenia who are partially responsive to clozapine: a single-blind randomized study. *Adv. Ther.* 2007; **24**(1): 1–13.

37. Ziegenbein M, Sieberer M, Kuenzel HE, Kropp S. Augmentation of clozapine with amisulpride in patients with treatment-resistant schizophrenia: an open clinical study. *German Journal of Psychiatry.* 2006; **9**(1): 17–21.

38. Zink M, Kuwilsky A, Krumm B, Dressing H. Efficacy and tolerability of ziprasidone versus risperidone as augmentation in patients partially responsive to clozapine: a randomised controlled clinical trial. *J. Psychopharmacol.* 2009; **23**(3): 305–314.

39. Kuwilsky A, Krumm B, Englisch S, *et al.* Long-term efficacy and tolerability of clozapine combined with ziprasidone or risperidone. *Pharmacopsychiatry.* 2010; **43**(6): 216–220.

40. Taylor DM, Smith L. Augmentation of clozapine with a second antipsychotic—a meta-analysis of randomized, placebo-controlled studies. *Acta Psychiatr. Scand.* 2009; **119**(6): 419–425.

41. Chang JS, Ahn YM, Park HJ, *et al.* Aripiprazole augmentation in clozapine-treated patients with refractory schizophrenia: an 8-week, randomized, double-blind, placebo-controlled trial. *J. Clin. Psychiatry.* 2008; **69**(5): 720–731.

42. Sommer IE, Begemann MJ, Temmerman A, Leucht S. Pharmacological augmentation strategies for schizophrenia patients with insufficient response to clozapine: a quantitative literature review. *Schizophr. Bull.* 2012; **38**(5): 1003–1011.

43. Vauquelin G, Bostoen S, Vanderheyden P, Seeman P. Clozapine, atypical antipsychotics, and the benefits of fast-off D2 dopamine receptor antagonism. *Naunyn Schmiedebergs Arch. Pharmacol.* 2012; **385**(4): 337–372.

44. Leucht S. Amisulpride a selective dopamine antagonist and atypical antipsychotic: results of a meta-analysis of randomized controlled trials. *Int. J. Neuropsychopharmacol.* 2004; **7**(Suppl 1): S15–S20.

45. Scatton B, Claustre Y, Cudennec A, *et al.* Amisulpride: from animal pharmacology to therapeutic action. *Int. Clin. Psychopharmacol.* 1997; **12**(Suppl 2): S29–S36.

46. Vernaleken I, Siessmeier T, Buchholz HG, *et al.* High striatal

occupancy of D2-like dopamine
receptors by amisulpride in the
brain of patients with
schizophrenia. *Int.
J. Neuropsychopharmacol.* 2004;
7(4): 421–430.

47. Abbas AI, Hedlund PB, Huang
XP, *et al.* Amisulpride is a potent
5-HT7 antagonist: relevance for
antidepressant actions in vivo.
Psychopharmacology (Berl.). 2009;
205(1): 119–128.

48. Perrault G, Depoortere R, Morel
E, *et al.* Psychopharmacological
profile of amisulpride: an
antipsychotic drug with
presynaptic D2/D3 dopamine
receptor antagonist activity and
limbic selectivity. *J. Pharmacol.
Exp. Ther.* 1997; **280**(1): 73–82.

49. Bowskill SV, Patel MX, Handley
SA, Flanagan RJ. Plasma
amisulpride in relation to
prescribed dose, clozapine
augmentation, and other factors:
data from a therapeutic drug
monitoring service, 2002–2010.
Hum. Psychopharmacol. 2012;
27(5): 507–513.

50. Nordström AL, Farde L, Halldin
C. High 5-HT2 receptor
occupancy in clozapine treated
patients demonstrated by PET.
Psychopharmacology (Berl.). 1993;
110(3): 365–367.

51. Kapur S, Zipursky RB, Remington
G. Clinical and theoretical
implications of 5-HT2 and D2
receptor occupancy of clozapine,
risperidone, and olanzapine in
schizophrenia. *Am. J. Psychiatry.*
1999; **156**(2): 286–293.

52. Buckley P, Bartell J, Donenwirth
K, *et al.* Violence and
schizophrenia: clozapine as a

specific antiaggressive agent. *Bull.
Am. Acad. Psychiatry Law.* 1995;
23(4): 607–611.

53. Wilson WH. Clinical review of
clozapine treatment in a state
hospital. *Hosp. Community
Psychiatry.* 1992; **43**(7): 700–703.

54. Umukoro S, Aladeokin AC,
Eduviere AT. Aggressive behavior:
a comprehensive review of its
neurochemical mechanisms and
management. *Aggression and
Violent Behavior.* 2013; **18**(2):
195–203.

55. Nelson RJ, Trainor BC. Neural
mechanisms of aggression. *Nat.
Rev. Neurosci.* 2007; **8**(7):
536–546.

56. Lieberman JA, Safferman AZ,
Pollack S, *et al.* Clinical effects of
clozapine in chronic
schizophrenia: response to
treatment and predictors of
outcome. *Am. J. Psychiatry.* 1994;
151(12): 1744–1752.

57. Fabrazzo M, La Pia S, Monteleone
P, *et al.* Is the time course of
clozapine response correlated to
the time course of clozapine
plasma levels? A one-year
prospective study in drug-
resistant patients with
schizophrenia.
Neuropsychopharmacology. 2002;
27(6): 1050–1055.

58. Schulte PF. What is an adequate
trial with clozapine? *Clin.
Pharmacokinet.* 2003; **42**(7):
607–618.

59. Wilson WH. Time required for
initial improvement during
clozapine treatment of refractory
schizophrenia. *Am. J. Psychiatry.*
1996; **157**(7): 951–952.

60. Junginger J, Parks-Levy J,
McGuire L. Delusions and
symptom-consistent violence.
Psychiatr. Serv. 1998; **49**(2):
218–220.

61. Nolan KA, Volavka J, Czobor P,
et al. Aggression and
psychopathology in treatment-
resistant inpatients with
schizophrenia and schizoaffective
disorder. *J. Psychiatr. Res.* 2005;
39(1): 109–115.

62. Volavka J, Zito JM, Vitrai J,
Czobor P. Clozapine effects on
hostility and aggression in
schizophrenia. *J. Clin.
Psychopharmacol.* 1993; **13**(4):
287–288.

63. Krakowski MI, Czobor P.
Executive function predicts
response to antiaggression
treatment in schizophrenia: a
randomized controlled trial. *J.
Clin. Psychiatry.* 2012; **73**(1):
74–80.

64. Volavka J, Citrome L. Atypical
antipsychotics in the treatment of
the persistently aggressive
psychotic patient: methodological
concerns. *Schizophr. Res.* 1999;
35(Suppl): S23–S33.

65. McGlashan TH. A selective
review of recent North
American long-term followup
studies of schizophrenia.
Schizophr. Bull. 1988; **14**(4):
515–542.

66. Revicki DA, Luce BR,
Weschler JM, Brown RE,
Adler MA. Cost effectiveness
of clozapine for treatment-
resistant schizophrenic
patients. *Hosp. Community
Psychiatry.* 1990; **41**(8):
850–854.

Chapter

20

The psychopharmacology of violence: making sensible decisions

Leslie Citrome and Jan Volavka

Introduction

Violent behavior associated with mental disorders is a common reason for admission to a psychiatric inpatient unit. Once hospitalized, patients may continue to be intermittently agitated and have persistent aggressive behaviors, preventing their discharge back into the community.

The pharmacological management of agitated, aggressive, and violent behavior can be conceptualized as having two parts: acute and preventative. Acute treatment options are plentiful and generally efficacious. Preventative treatment aims to decrease the frequency and intensity of future acute episodes of agitated, aggressive, and violent behavior, and although effective therapeutic options do exist, they are far from being "one size fits all," and are highly dependent on the root causes of the dangerous behaviors. With few exceptions, most of the clinically relevant research in the longer-term management of violence has been conducted in psychotic individuals with schizophrenia.

Definitions and Scales

Agitation (excessive motor or verbal activity) can further escalate into aggressive behavior. Agitation can be associated with a number of conditions, including schizophrenia and bipolar disorder. Acute agitation in its severest forms is a medical emergency that requires immediate intervention to alleviate personal distress and to prevent harm to the individual and/or others.

Specific rating scales have been developed to measure agitation, such as the single-item Behavioral Activity Rating Scale (BARS) [1]. Also commonly used in the development of anti-agitation agents is the

Positive and Negative Syndrome Scale (PANSS) Excited Component (EC), or "PEC," which consists of the five PANSS items considered relevant in this regard: excitement, hostility, tension, uncooperativeness, and poor impulse control [2]. The PEC and BARS have been successfully used as the primary outcome measures to garner regulatory approval for several agents for the indication of agitation associated with schizophrenia and/or bipolar mania.

Aggressive behaviors can be verbal, against objects, against self, or against other persons. Physical aggression against other persons is frequently called violence. Aggressive behaviors have been assessed in research using questionnaires such as the Overt Aggression Scale (OAS) [3]. In clinical settings with acutely ill psychiatric patients, the Brøset Violence Checklist (BVC) can be used to predict inpatient violence in the short-term [4]; this instrument assesses the presence or absence of behaviors or states frequently observed before a violent incident, including confusion/disorientation, irritability, and threats. The goal of longer-term treatment is to minimize the future occurrence of aggressive behaviors. There are no agents specifically approved for aggression or violence per se. However, there is a substantial body of research examining these longer-term treatment options.

Of special note, the PANSS item of "hostility" is also used to measure effect of interventions over time but is loosely defined as "verbal and nonverbal expressions of anger and resentment, including sarcasm, passive-aggressive behavior, verbal abuse, and assaultiveness" [5]. Rated on a scale of 1 (absent) to 7 (extreme), mild hostility (a rating of 3) is defined as follows: "The patient shows indirect or restrained communication of anger, such as sarcasm, disrespect, hostile expressions and occasional irritability." More serious behaviors are not captured until the higher end of the scale.

Agitation

In addition to the early offering of medications, acute interventions that target agitation ordinarily also involve environmental and behavioral approaches, discussed elsewhere [6]. Goals include calming the agitated patient as rapidly as possible, decreasing the likelihood of harm to self or others, allowing the taking place of diagnostic tests and procedures, attenuating psychosis, and decreasing the need for seclusion or restraint (a time where staff and patient injury can occur). The induction of sleep is not desirable when evaluating a patient; sedation that necessitates constant observation and assistance in toileting places an excessive burden on staff time [7].

Diagnostic considerations center on ruling out somatic causes of the change in mental status; somatic causes may preclude the use of antipsychotic medication. An example would be acute withdrawal from alcohol or benzodiazepines where the preferred medication intervention would be a benzodiazepine such as lorazepam. This is not a trivial consideration, as it is estimated that approximately half of all patients with schizophrenia have a comorbid drug or alcohol abuse problem [8]. More unusual, but problematic, would be the presence of an underlying metabolic, toxic, or infectious process resulting in agitated behavior in a person otherwise well-known to the provider as a person with a chronic psychotic disorder.

Medication approaches usually involve drugs and formulations that have a rapid onset of action. This usually means that the therapeutic agent has a short Tmax and high Cmax; this often, but not always, requires parenteral administration. Interventions that have a high response rate for inducing calm without oversedation or other problematic adverse effects are desirable. Interventions that are easy to use, and for which clinicians have experience with, are often reached for first – even though patient acceptability may not be optimal. Commonly used in emergency departments to treat acute agitation are the intramuscular (IM) formulations of haloperidol or lorazepam, or the combination of both agents, often in the same syringe. This combination may be more efficacious and faster acting than haloperidol or lorazepam alone, and

may be associated with fewer problems with extrapyramidal symptoms and akathisia than haloperidol alone [9]. However, it is unlikely that this regimen would be used as a long-term treatment option, given the availability of better-tolerated second-generation antipsychotics. Moreover, it is not desirable to chronically administer benzodiazepines because of problems of physiological tolerance, risk of withdrawal, and no or little effect on the core symptoms of psychosis [7]. Table 20.1 provides an outline of additional considerations for haloperidol and lorazepam, and for the alternative agents discussed below.

The second-generation antipsychotics ziprasidone, olanzapine, and aripiprazole are available in short-acting intramuscular formulations. They are US Food and Drug Administration (FDA)-approved for the indication of agitation associated with schizophrenia (all three) and agitation associated with bipolar mania (olanzapine and aripiprazole). Akathisia and dystonia can be avoided by using these agents rather than haloperidol, and all three agents allow for smooth transition to long-term oral therapy, as tested in IM-to-oral transition studies [10–14].

Ziprasidone IM

There are two pivotal studies, each comparing a therapeutic dose of ziprasidone vs. 2 mg [15,16]. There appears to be a dose response with 20 mg IM being superior to 10 mg IM, as measured by change in BARS scores [17], where the number needed to treat (NNT) for response vs. 2 mg at 2 hours after injection was 4 for 10 mg and 2 for 20 mg. NNT for response for the pooled doses (10 mg and 20 mg) was 3. Somnolence, nausea, and dizziness were more common with 20 mg than with 10 mg or placebo [18].

Olanzapine IM

The short-acting IM formulation was evaluated in four randomized, double-blind placebo and active comparator studies in patients with schizophrenia [19,20], bipolar mania [21], and dementia [22] (not FDA-approved for this indication). Superior onset of efficacy to haloperidol IM and lorazepam IM was observed with no adverse event significantly more frequent for IM olanzapine vs. IM haloperidol or IM lorazepam. The optimal dose is 10 mg (2.5 to 5.0 mg for vulnerable patients, e.g., elderly). NNT for response vs. placebo as measured by the PEC at 2 hours after injection is 3 [17].

Table 20.1 Psychopharmacology of acute agitation—current options

Agent	Typical dose (mg)	Half-life (hours)	Advantages	Disadvantages	Comments
Lorazepam (intramuscular)	0.5–2.0	10–20	Treats underlying alcohol or sedative withdrawal	Respiratory depression, disinhibition, or paradoxical reactions	In contrast to most other benzodiazepines, lorazepam is readily absorbed when given intramuscularly, has a short half-life, and has no active metabolites. The oral formulation is not recommended for prolonged use because of tolerance, withdrawal, and no/little effect on core symptoms of psychosis.
Haloperidol (intramuscular)	0.5–7.5	12–36	Treats underlying psychosis	Acute dystonia, akathisia; will not treat underlying alcohol withdrawal	Continued use of the oral formulation of haloperidol is generally suboptimal, especially if anticholinergic medications (e.g., benztropine) are required.
Aripiprazole (intramuscular)	9.75	75	Favorable EPS profile; antipsychotic effect over time	If parenteral benzodiazepine therapy is deemed necessary in addition to aripiprazole injection treatment, patients should be monitored for excessive sedation and for orthostatic hypotension; will not treat underlying alcohol withdrawal	Aripiprazole differs from other available second-generation antipsychotics in that it is a partial agonist at the dopamine D2 receptor. Aripiprazole is also available in a long-acting injectable formulation.
Olanzapine (intramuscular)	10	34–38	Superior to haloperidol (schizophrenia)and lorazepam (bipolar disorder) in clinical trials; favorable EPS profile; antipsychotic effect over time	Do not co-administer with lorazepam; will not treat underlying alcohol withdrawal	Continued use can be associated with weight gain and metabolic abnormalities. Olanzapine is also available in a long-acting injectable formulation.
Ziprasidone (intramuscular)	10–20	2.2–3.4	Favorable EPS profile; antipsychotic effect over time	Label warning for prolongation of the QTc interval; caution in patients with impaired renal function because the cyclodextrin excipient is cleared by renal filtration; will not treat underlying alcohol withdrawal	Ziprasidone has a favorable weight/metabolic profile compared with olanzapine. The oral formulation of ziprasidone must be taken with food in order to achieve adequate bioavailability.

Table 20.1 (cont.)

Agent	Typical dose (mg)	Half-life (hours)	Advantages	Disadvantages	Comments
Loxapine (inhaled)	10	8	Favorable EPS profile	Bronchospasm; will not treat underlying alcohol withdrawal	A Risk Evaluation and Mitigation Strategies (REMS) program is in place (see text). Loxapine is a first-generation antipsychotic that currently sees little use.
Asenapine (sublingual)	10	24	Favorable EPS profile	Distorted or unpleasant taste and numbing of the tongue reported in product labeling; will not treat underlying alcohol withdrawal.	Must not be taken with food or liquids. In contrast to commercially available orally disintegrating tablets of olanzapine, risperidone, or aripiprazole, only orally disintegrating tablets of asenapine are absorbed in the oral mucosa.

Aripiprazole IM

The short-acting IM formulation was evaluated in four randomized, double-blind placebo and active comparator studies in schizophrenia [23,24], bipolar mania [25], and dementia [26] (not FDA-approved for this indication). The optimal dose is 9.75 mg (5.25 mg for vulnerable patients, e.g., elderly). The NNT for response vs. placebo as measured by the PEC at 2 hours after injection is 5, which although is not as favorable as for ziprasidone (NNT 3) or olanzapine (NNT 3), is similar to that observed with haloperidol IM or lorazepam IM from pooled data (NNT 4), with 95% confidence intervals that overlap [17].

Inhaled loxapine

This product received approval in 2013 for the acute treatment of agitation associated with schizophrenia or bipolar I disorder in adults. Inhaled loxapine was evaluated in three double-blind, placebo-controlled, randomized trials in patients with schizophrenia [27,28] and bipolar mania [29]. It is the first nonparenteral agent approved for such a purpose, and potentially represents a less intrusive and stigmatizing means of delivering an anti-agitation agent. The optimal dose is 10 mg. Efficacy was noted as early as 10 minutes post-administration, which was the earliest time point measured. NNT for response for 10 mg vs. placebo at 2 hours after administration as measured by the PEC in

the Phase III studies was 4 for patients with schizophrenia and 3 for patients with bipolar mania [30,31]. In the USA, the recommended dose is 10 mg with only a single dose within a 24-hour period permitted. At the present time, inhaled loxapine can be administered only by a healthcare professional in an enrolled healthcare facility. Because of the risk of bronchospasm, a Risk Evaluation and Mitigation Strategies (REMS) program is in place, and prior to administering inhaled loxapine, patients must be screened for a history of pulmonary disease and examined by chest auscultation for respiratory abnormalities such as wheezing. After administration, patients are required to be monitored for signs and symptoms of bronchospasm at least every 15 minutes for at least 1 hour.

Sublingual asenapine

Asenapine is a second-generation antipsychotic indicated for the treatment of schizophrenia, and for the acute treatment of manic or mixed episodes associated with bipolar I disorder [32]. The only available formulation of asenapine is as an orally disintegrating tablet. In contrast to the orally disintegrating tablets of olanzapine, risperidone, and aripiprazole, asenapine is administered sublingually and is absorbed in the oral mucosa, bypassing first-pass metabolism [33]. In a double-blind, placebo-controlled, randomized study of agitated adults presenting for treatment in an emergency department, sublingual asenapine 10 mg was efficacious in the treatment of agitation with an effect size comparable to that observed in prior studies of intramuscular antipsychotics [34]. NNT for response vs. placebo as measured by the PEC at 2 hours after administration was 3. At the present time, asenapine does not have regulatory approval for this indication, but the relative ease of use merits further consideration.

What do guidelines say?

For psychosis-driven agitation in a patient with a known psychiatric disorder (e.g., schizophrenia, schizoaffective disorder, bipolar disorder), current guidelines for the management of agitation recommend that antipsychotics be used instead of benzodiazepines because antipsychotics address the underlying psychosis [35]. In addition, second-generation antipsychotics with data supporting their use in acute treatment of agitation are preferred over haloperidol and other standard neuroleptics administered either alone or with an adjunctive medication.

Persistent Aggressive Behavior

Persistent aggressive behavior may be related to psychosis, psychopathy, impulsivity, co-occurring substance or alcohol use, cognitive impairments, or underlying somatic conditions. Adverse drug reactions such as akathisia can be subtle and are often missed. Thus effective treatment approaches can vary considerably depending on the specific characteristics of the individual being treated [36].

Patients with schizophrenia who are aggressive can exhibit greater severity of positive symptoms than nonaggressive patients, as observed experimentally using the PANSS [37].

Psychopathy can also be a predictor of violence and recidivism in offenders and is usually associated with "instrumental aggression" (i.e., aggression that is planned and goal-directed) [38]. Psychopathy, as defined by an arrogant/deceitful interpersonal style, deficient affective experience, and impulsive/irresponsible behavioral style [39], can be measured using a specially designed checklist, and persons with schizophrenia who are violent score significantly higher on this checklist than those who are not violent [38].

Impulsivity can further complicate a clinical picture. Substances/conditions (alcohol, attention deficit disorder, traumatic brain injury) that diminish behavioral inhibition are linked with increased aggression. Violent subjects make more impulsive errors on experimental tasks and score higher on self-ratings of impulsivity [36]. Impulsive or "affective" aggression is ordinarily unplanned, unprovoked, or out of proportion to the provocation ("hairtrigger" response), and there is often subsequent remorse.

When using an assault interview checklist to attempt to tease out psychotic, psychopathic, and impulsive factors among psychiatric inpatients who were involved in aggressive incidents, it was apparent that multiple factors are often present in a single event, and that individuals sometimes assault for different reasons at different times [40]. This heterogeneity renders treatment of aggression challenging. Although hallucinations, delusions, and psychotic misinterpretation can be treated with antipsychotics, impulsivity is more difficult to control despite best efforts with adjunctive anticonvulsants, and psychopathy has no known effective pharmacological treatment.

Within this context, oral antipsychotics that were used for acute treatment in an individual are logical choices for maintenance treatment. It is useful to have multiple formulations, including long-acting injectables [41]. If aggressivity persists, there is a limited array of evidence-based pharmacological interventions, of which clozapine has the most support.

Clozapine

A specific anti-aggressive effect was first demonstrated in a retrospective analysis of data that were collected among 223 inpatients where reductions in the Brief Psychiatric Rating Scale hostility item score were statistically independent of changes in conceptual disorganization, suspiciousness, hallucinatory behavior, and unusual thought content [42]. Subsequently, two randomized, double-blind, controlled trials demonstrated this effect as well. The first was a study of 157 hospitalized patients with schizophrenia or schizoaffective disorder and a history of suboptimal treatment response randomized to receive clozapine, olanzapine, risperidone, or haloperidol for 14 weeks [43]. The PANSS hostility item scores of patients taking clozapine demonstrated significantly greater improvement than those of patients taking haloperidol or risperidone, and this effect was independent of the antipsychotic effect of clozapine on other rating scale items that reflect delusional thinking, a formal thought disorder, or hallucinations and independent of sedation. In the same study, clozapine also evidenced superiority regarding reduction of number and severity of incidents of overt aggression [44]. Confirming these findings were the results of a double-blind, 12-week study of 110 hospitalized patients with schizophrenia selected because they exhibited violent behaviors and where subjects randomized to clozapine had greater reductions compared to olanzapine and haloperidol in the number and severity of physical assaults [45]. Olanzapine was also superior to haloperidol in reducing the number and severity of aggressive incidents on these measures. These effects were independent of antipsychotic effects as measured by the PANSS.

Clozapine, although potentially a life-saving treatment, can also be life-threatening [46]. Because of clozapine's risk for agranulocytosis, patients receiving clozapine require enrollment in a registry, and frequent white blood cell count monitoring is required. Other safety concerns include myocarditis, seizures, and weight gain/metabolic abnormalities. Nonetheless, despite clozapine's perceived dangerousness, data on control of aggressive behavior make this antipsychotic a compelling choice for many patients with schizophrenia. Moreover, although clozapine was initially approved for treatment-resistant schizophrenia, clozapine subsequently received approval for reduction in the risk of recurrent suicidal behavior in schizophrenia or schizoaffective disorders.

Olanzapine

Support for the use of olanzapine for aggressive behavior has emerged from the randomized controlled study described above [45], and through post-hoc analyses of two large effectiveness trials, EUFEST [47] for patients in their early phase of their illness, and CATIE [48], for more chronically ill patients with schizophrenia. Additional post-hoc analyses for olanzapine included a published report where olanzapine was superior to haloperidol on measures of agitation, but selectivity of effect was not reported [49]. The long-term use of olanzapine must involve close monitoring of weight and metabolic variables.

Other second-generation antipsychotics

Limited information is available supporting the use of risperidone, quetiapine, ziprasidone, and aripiprazole,

as reported in post-hoc analyses examining anti-hostility effects [50].

Augmentation strategies

Augmentation strategies where non-antipsychotic medications are added to an antipsychotic in order to reduce the frequency of aggressive or violent behavior are also used, but the evidence base is mixed [51]. For example, although the use of adjunctive valproate is commonly encountered [52], presumably for its potential effect on hostility or impulsivity, no significant differences between risperidone monotherapy vs. combination treatment with risperidone and valproate were observed on any of the rating scale outcomes among patients with schizophrenia and hostile behavior who were enrolled in a small ($N = 33$), 8-week, open-label, randomized controlled trial [53]. In a Cochrane review of antiepileptics for aggression and associated impulsivity [54], valproate was superior to placebo for outpatient men with recurrent impulsive aggression, for impulsively aggressive adults with Cluster B personality disorders, and for youths with conduct disorder, but not for children and adolescents with pervasive developmental disorder.

Although primarily tested in patients with organic brain disease, beta adrenergic blockers, such as propranolol, metoprolol, nadolol, and pindolol, represent another category of potentially useful augmenting agents in patients with schizophrenia. This is supported by case reports, as well as specifically by double-blind, placebo-controlled trials of adjunctive nadolol [55,56] and a double-blind, cross-over study of adjunctive pindolol [57].

Conclusions

Acutely managing agitation is relatively straightforward, and there are several options, many of them FDA-approved, from which to choose. Second-generation antipsychotics are preferred over older agents because of their superior acute tolerability profile; the risk of acute dystonia and akathisia is considerably less than with haloperidol. Prevention of future episodes of agitation is more complex and is dependent on the root cause of the persistent aggressive behavior. This can be difficult to determine, as multiple factors are often present in a single event, and individuals sometimes assault for different reasons at different times. Presently, the best option for a specific antihostility medication is clozapine, followed by olanzapine. Both of these agents require careful monitoring for weight and metabolic abnormalities, with clozapine also requiring monitoring for potential untoward effects on the production of neutrophils and on heart muscle. Although the real-world extent of use of agents such as adjunctive valproate in patients with schizophrenia is not justified given the weakness of the supportive evidence, time-limited "N = 1" trials in individual persons remain a reasonable option in the face of failure of other strategies.

Disclosures

This review was written without any external financial or editorial support. In the past 12 months, L. Citrome was a consultant for, has received honoraria from, owns a small number of shares of common stock in, or has engaged in collaborative research supported by the following: Alexza, Alkermes, AstraZeneca, Bristol-Myers Squibb, Eli Lilly, Envivo, Forest, Genentech, Janssen, Lundbeck, Merck, Mylan, Novartis, Noven, Otsuka, Pfizer, Reckitt Benckiser, Reviva, Shire, Sunovion, and Takeda. J. Volavka has nothing to disclose.

References

1. Swift RH, Harrigan EP, Cappelleri JC, Kramer D, Chandler LP. Validation of the behavioural activity rating scale (BARS): a novel measure of activity in agitated patients. *J. Psychiatr. Res.* 2002; **36**(2): 87–95.

2. Lindenmayer JP, Brown E, Baker RW, *et al.* An excitement subscale of the Positive and Negative Syndrome Scale. *Schizophr. Res.* 2004; **68**(2–3): 331–337.

3. Yudofsky SC, Silver JM, Jackson W, Endicott J, Williams D. The Overt Aggression Scale for the objective rating of verbal and physical aggression. *Am. J. Psychiatry.* 1986; **143**(1): 35–39.

4. Björkdahl A, Olsson D, Palmstierna T. Nurses' short-term prediction of violence in acute psychiatric intensive care. *Acta Psychiatr. Scand.* 2006; **113**(3): 224–229.

5. Kay SR, Opler LA, Fiszbein A. *Positive and Negative Syndrome Scale Manual.* North Tonawanda, NY: Multi-Health Systems; 2000.

6. Citrome L, Green L. The dangerous agitated patient: what to do right now. *Postgrad. Med.* 1990; **87**(2): 231–236.

7. Citrome L. Agitation III: pharmacologic treatment of agitation. In: Glick RL, Berlin JS, Fishkind A, Zeller S, eds. *Emergency Psychiatry: Principles and Practice.* Baltimore, MD: Lippincott Williams & Wilkins, Wolters Kluwer Health; 2008: 137–147.

8. Regier DA, Farmer ME, Rae DS, *et al.* Comorbidity of mental disorders with alcohol and other drug abuse: results from the Epidemiologic Catchment Area (ECA) Study. *JAMA.* 1990; **264**(19): 2511–2518.

9. Battaglia J, Moss S, Rush J, *et al.* Haloperidol, lorazepam, or both for psychotic agitation? A multicenter, prospective, double-blind, emergency department study. *Am. J. Emerg. Med.* 1997; **15**(4): 335–340.

10. Brook S, Lucey JV, Gunn KP. Intramuscular ziprasidone compared with intramuscular haloperidol in the treatment of acute psychosis: Ziprasidone I.M. Study Group. *J. Clin. Psychiatry.* 2000; **61**(12): 933–941.

11. Daniel DG, Zimbroff DL, Swift RH, Harrigan EP. The tolerability of intramuscular ziprasidone and haloperidol treatment and the transition to oral therapy. *Int. Clin. Psychopharmacol.* 2004; **19**(1): 9–15.

12. Brook S, Walden J, Benattia I, Siu CO, Romano SJ. Ziprasidone and haloperidol in the treatment of acute exacerbation of schizophrenia and schizoaffective disorder: comparison of intramuscular and oral formulations in a 6-week, randomized, blinded-assessment study. *Psychopharmacology (Berl.).* 2005; **178**(4): 514–523.

13. Wright P, Meehan K, Birkett M, *et al.* A comparison of the efficacy and safety of olanzapine versus haloperidol during transition from intramuscular to oral therapy. *Clin. Ther.* 2003; **25**(5): 1420–1428.

14. Andrezina R, Marcus RN, Oren DA, *et al.* Intramuscular aripiprazole or haloperidol and transition to oral therapy in patients with agitation associated with schizophrenia: sub-analysis of a double-blind study. *Curr. Med. Res. Opin.* 2006; **22**(11): 2209–2219.

15. Lesem MD, Zajecka JM, Swift RH, Reeves KR, Harrigan EP. Intramuscular ziprasidone, 2 mg versus 10 mg, in the short-term management of agitated psychotic patients. *J. Clin. Psychiatry.* 2001; **62**(1): 12–18.

16. Daniel DG, Potkin SG, Reeves KR, Swift RH, Harrigan EP. Intramuscular (IM) ziprasidone 20 mg is effective in reducing acute agitation associated with psychosis: a double-blind, randomized trial. *Psychopharmacology (Berl.).* 2001; **155**(2): 128–134.

17. Citrome L. Comparison of intramuscular ziprasidone, olanzapine, or aripiprazole for

agitation: a quantitative review of efficacy and safety. *J. Clin. Psychiatry.* 2007; **68**(12): 1876–1885.

18. Pfizer Inc. Geodon: US package insert for Geodon (ziprasidone HCl) capsules and Geodon (ziprasidone mesylate) injection for intramuscular use. September 2013. http://labeling.pfizer.com/ ShowLabeling.aspx?id=584. Accessed December 2, 2013.

19. Wright P, Birkett M, David SR, *et al.* Double-blind, placebo-controlled comparison of intramuscular olanzapine and intramuscular haloperidol in the treatment of acute agitation in schizophrenia. *Am. J. Psychiatry.* 2001; **158**(7): 1149–1151.

20. Breier A, Meehan K, Birkett M, *et al.* A double-blind, placebo-controlled dose–response comparison of intramuscular olanzapine and haloperidol in the treatment of acute agitation in schizophrenia. *Arch. Gen. Psychiatry.* 2002; **59**(5): 441–448.

21. Meehan K, Zhang F, David S, *et al.* A double-blind, randomized comparison of the efficacy and safety of intramuscular injections of olanzapine, lorazepam, or placebo in treating acutely agitated patients diagnosed with bipolar mania. *J. Clin. Psychopharmacol.* 2001; **21**(4): 389–397.

22. Meehan KM, Wang H, David SR, *et al.* Comparison of rapidly acting intramuscular olanzapine, lorazepam, and placebo: a double-blind, randomized study in acutely agitated patients with dementia. *Neuropsychopharmacology.* 2002; **26**(4): 494–504.

23. Andrezina R, Josiassen RC, Marcus RN, *et al.* Intramuscular aripiprazole for the treatment of acute agitation in patients with schizophrenia or schizoaffective disorder: a double-blind, placebo-controlled comparison

with intramuscular haloperidol. *Psychopharmacology (Berl.).* 2006; **188**(3): 281–292

24. Tran-Johnson TK, Sack DA, Marcus RN, *et al.* Efficacy and safety of intramuscular aripiprazole in patients with acute agitation: a randomized, double-blind, placebo-controlled trial. *J. Clin. Psychiatry.* 2007; **68**(1): 111–119.

25. Zimbroff DL, Marcus RN, Manos G, *et al.* Management of acute agitation in patients with bipolar disorder: efficacy and safety of intramuscular aripiprazole. *J. Clin. Psychopharmacol.* 2007; **27**(2): 171–176.

26. Rappaport SA, Marcus RN, Manos G, McQuade RD, Oren DA. A randomized, double-blind, placebo-controlled tolerability study of intramuscular aripiprazole in acutely agitated patients with Alzheimer's, vascular, or mixed dementia. *J. Am. Med. Dir. Assoc.* 2009; **10**(1): 21–27.

27. Allen MH, Feifel D, Lesem MD, *et al.* Efficacy and safety of loxapine for inhalation in the treatment of agitation in patients with schizophrenia: a randomized, double-blind, placebo-controlled trial. *J. Clin. Psychiatry.* 2011; **72**(10): 1313–1321.

28. Lesem MD, Tran-Johnson TK, Riesenberg RA, *et al.* Rapid acute treatment of agitation in individuals with schizophrenia: multicentre, randomised, placebo-controlled study of inhaled loxapine. *Br. J. Psychiatry.* 2011; **198**(1): 51–58.

29. Kwentus J, Riesenberg RA, Marandi M, *et al.* Rapid acute treatment of agitation in patients with bipolar I disorder: a multicenter, randomized, placebo-controlled clinical trial with inhaled loxapine. *Bipolar Disord.* 2012; **14**(1): 31–40.

30. Citrome L. Inhaled loxapine for agitation revisited: focus on effect

sizes from 2 Phase III randomised controlled trials in persons with schizophrenia or bipolar disorder. *Int. J. Clin. Pract.* 2012; **66**(3): 318–325.

31. Citrome L. Addressing the need for rapid treatment of agitation in schizophrenia and bipolar disorder: focus on inhaled loxapine as an alternative to injectable agents. *Ther. Clin. Risk Manag.* 2013; **9**: 235–245.

32. Merck & Co., Inc. Saphris: US package insert for Saphris (asenapine) sublingual tablets. March 2013. http://www.merck .com/product/usa/pi_circulars/s/ saphris/saphris_pi.pdf. Accessed December 2, 2013.

33. Citrome L. Asenapine for schizophrenia and bipolar disorder: a review of the efficacy and safety profile for this newly approved sublingually absorbed second-generation antipsychotic. *Int. J. Clin. Pract.* 2009; **63**(12): 1762–1784.

34. Pratts M, Citrome L, Grant W, Leso L, Opler LA. A single-dose, randomized, double-blind, placebo-controlled trial of sublingual asenapine for acute agitation. *Acta Psychiatrica Scand.* 2014 Jul; **130**(1): 61–68.

35. Wilson MP, Pepper D, Currier GW, Holloman GH Jr, Feifel D. The psychopharmacology of agitation: consensus statement of the American Association for Emergency Psychiatry Project Beta Psychopharmacology Workgroup. *West. J. Emerg. Med.* 2012; **13**(1): 26–34.

36. Volavka J, Citrome L. Heterogeneity of violence in schizophrenia and implications for long-term treatment. *Int. J. Clin. Pract.* 2008; **62**(8): 1237–1245.

37. Nolan KA, Volavka J, Czobor P, *et al.* Aggression and psychopathology in treatment-resistant inpatients with schizophrenia and schizoaffective

disorder. *J. Psychiatr. Res.* 2005; **39**(1): 109–115.

38. Nolan KA, Volavka J, Mohr P, Czobor P. Psychopathy and violent behavior among patients with schizophrenia or schizoaffective disorder. *Psychiatr. Serv.* 1999; **50**(6): 787–792.

39. Cooke DJ, Michie C. Refining the construct of psychopathy: towards a hierarchical model. *Psychol. Assess.* 2001; **13**(2): 171–188.

40. Nolan KA, Czobor P, Roy BB, *et al.* Characteristics of assaultive behavior among psychiatric inpatients. *Psychiatr. Serv.* 2003; **54**(7): 1012–1016.

41. Citrome L. New second-generation long-acting injectable antipsychotics for the treatment of schizophrenia. *Expert Rev. Neurother.* 2013; **13**(7): 767–783.

42. Volavka J, Zito JM, Vitrai J, Czobor P. Clozapine effects on hostility and aggression in schizophrenia. *J. Clin. Psychopharmacol.* 1993; **13**(4): 287–289.

43. Citrome L, Volavka J, Czobor P, *et al.* Effects of clozapine, olanzapine, risperidone, and haloperidol on hostility among patients with schizophrenia. *Psychiatr. Serv.* 2001; **52**(11): 1510–1514.

44. Volavka J, Czobor P, Nolan K, *et al.* Overt aggression and psychotic symptoms in patients with schizophrenia treated with clozapine, olanzapine, risperidone, or haloperidol. *J. Clin. Psychopharmacol.* 2004; **24**(2): 225–228.

45. Krakowski MI, Czobor P, Citrome L, Bark N, Cooper TB. Atypical antipsychotic agents in the treatment of violent patients with schizophrenia and schizoaffective disorder. *Arch. Gen. Psychiatry.* 2006; **63**(6): 622–629.

46. Citrome L. Clozapine for schizophrenia: life-threatening or life-saving treatment? *Current Psychiatry.* 2009; **8**(12): 56–63.

47. Volavka J, Czobor P, Derks EM, *et al.* EUFEST Study Group. Efficacy of antipsychotic drugs against hostility in the European First-Episode Schizophrenia Trial (EUFEST). *J. Clin. Psychiatry.* 2011; **72**(7): 955–961.

48. Volavka J, Czobor P, Citrome L, Van Dorn RA. Effectiveness of antipsychotic drugs against hostility in patients with schizophrenia in the Clinical Antipsychotic Trials of Intervention Effectiveness (CATIE) study. *CNS Spectr.* 2014; **0**(5): 374–381. DOI: http://dx.doi.org/10.1017/S1092852913000849

49. Kinon BJ, Roychowdhury SM, Milton DR, Hill AL. Effective resolution with olanzapine of acute presentation of behavioral agitation and positive psychotic symptoms in schizophrenia. *J. Clin. Psychiatry.* 2001; **62**(Suppl 2): 17–21.

50. Citrome L, Volavka J. Pharmacological management of acute and persistent aggression in forensic psychiatry settings. *CNS Drugs.* 2011; **25**(12): 1009–1021.

51. Citrome L. Adjunctive lithium and anticonvulsants for the treatment of schizophrenia: what is the evidence? *Expert Rev. Neurother.* 2009; **9**(1): 55–71.

52. Citrome L, Levine J, Allingham B. Changes in use of valproate and other mood stabilizers for patients with schizophrenia from 1994 to 1998. *Psychiatr. Serv.* 2000; **51**(5): 634–638.

53. Citrome L, Shope CB, Nolan KA, Czobor P, Volavka J. Risperidone alone versus risperidone plus valproate in the treatment of patients with schizophrenia and hostility. *Int. Clin. Psychopharmacol.* 2007; **22**(6): 356–362.

54. Huband N, Ferriter M, Nathan R, Jones H. Antiepileptics for aggression and associated impulsivity. *Cochrane Database Syst. Rev.* 2010;(**2**): CD003499.

55. Ratey JJ, Sorgi P, O'Driscoll GA, *et al.* Nadolol to treat aggression and psychiatric symptomatology in chronic psychiatric inpatients: a double-blind, placebo-controlled study. *J. Clin. Psychiatry.* 1992; **53**(2): 41–46.

56. Alpert M, Allan ER, Citrome L, *et al.* A double-blind, placebo-controlled study of adjunctive nadolol in the management of violent psychiatric patients. *Psychopharmacol. Bull.* 1990; **26**(3): 367–371.

57. Caspi N, Modai I, Barak P, *et al.* Pindolol augmentation in aggressive schizophrenic patients: a double-blind crossover randomized study. *Int. Clin. Psychopharmacol.* 2001; **16**(2): 111–115.

Treating the violent patient with psychosis or impulsivity utilizing antipsychotic polypharmacy and high-dose monotherapy

Debbi A. Morrissette and Stephen M. Stahl

Introduction

Guidelines for treating schizophrenia with antipsychotics are well known, but when patients with psychosis and violent behavior fail to respond to standard treatments or continue to exhibit violent behavior despite control of psychosis, there is little consensus on what to do (Figure 21.1) [1]. Here we review the neurobiological rationale as well as evidence- and practice-based treatment strategies that utilize dosing of antipsychotics above the range normally recommended in published treatment guidelines, as well as the somewhat controversial practice of combining two antipsychotics for addressing psychotic and impulsive violence in patients with schizophrenia who fail to respond adequately to standard treatment.

Evaluation of Violence and Treatment of Comorbidities Before Going Beyond the Guidelines

Patients with schizophrenia who exhibit violent behavior in inpatient settings should first be treated according to published guidelines for all patients with schizophrenia, including a series of monotherapies with atypical antipsychotics and a trial of clozapine (Figure 21.1) [1]. If a patient with schizophrenia continues to exhibit violent behavior, that violence should be categorized as psychotic, impulsive, or predatory; predatory behavior is not an appropriate target for antipsychotic treatment, but psychotic and impulsive violence can be [2,3]. Most violent acts in forensic and state hospital settings (where patients mostly suffer from psychotic disorders) are impulsive, with predatory violence and psychotic violence being less frequent [4–9]. Psychotic violence is

hypothetically linked to excessive neuronal activity in the mesolimbic dopamine pathway, and can often, but not always, be successfully treated with standard antipsychotic monotherapies, including clozapine [10–13]. Impulsive violence is also common in psychotic patients in forensic and state hospital settings, even after positive symptoms of psychosis have been controlled with standard antipsychotic treatment [14–16]. Impulsive violence is hypothetically linked to an imbalance between "top-down" cortical inhibitory controls and "bottom-up" impulsive drives, and, empirically, high dosing and polypharmacy can reduce these behaviors in some patients who respond inadequately to standard treatments [2,11,12,17–19]. However, before considering high dosing or polypharmacy for schizophrenic patients with psychotic or impulsive violence who have failed to respond adequately to standard antipsychotic treatments, it is important to treat and stabilize any coexisting cognitive dysfunction or substance abuse issues [5,7,20–27].

Treatment of Violence and Aggression: Attaining Sufficient Dopamine D2 Receptor Occupancy

Neuroimaging studies have repeatedly shown that blockade of at least 60% of D2 receptors by antipsychotic treatment is necessary in order to reduce psychosis [10,11,28]. At greater than 80% occupancy of D2 receptors, the threshold for extrapyramidal symptoms (EPS) is reached in many patients. Thus, antipsychotics at standard doses aim to achieve between 60%–80% D2 receptor occupancy (Figure 21.2) [28–31]. Data indicate that obtaining sufficient D2 receptor occupancy and achieving the downstream therapeutic effects of D2 receptor blockade

Violence in Psychiatry, ed. Katherine D. Warburton and Stephen M. Stahl. Published by Cambridge University Press.
© Cambridge University Press 2016.

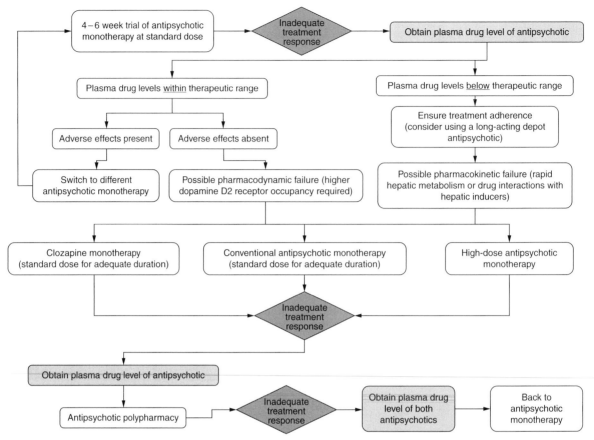

Figure 21.1 Antipsychotic treatment algorithm. Following several unsuccessful atypical antipsychotic monotherapy trials, a trial with a conventional antipsychotic or with clozapine is recommended. High-dose monotherapy may also be considered for such treatment-resistant patients. Antipsychotic polypharmacy is recommended only after antipsychotic monotherapy has failed. Note that throughout the treatment algorithm, monitoring of plasma drug levels of each antipsychotic is critical when determining the next course of action.

by an antipsychotic often take more than 6 weeks to manifest [32,33]. In fact, it may be necessary to treat schizophrenia with an antipsychotic for as long as 1–2 years before a significant improvement in psychotic symptoms is evident, although this may not be practical in forensic settings where violent behavior must be controlled [34–37]. Additionally, there are some data to suggest that nonresponse to an antipsychotic after 4 weeks of treatment predicts nonresponse at 12 weeks [38]. In this particular study by Stentebjerg-Olesen *et al.*, patients who were early treatment responders had a significantly greater chance of being treatment-responsive at 12 weeks compared to early treatment nonresponders [38]. However, we do wish to point out that over one-third of patients who were considered early treatment nonresponders did ultimately respond to treatment by week 12 [38].

Pharmacokinetic failure, treatment resistance, and violence

When a patient with schizophrenia who exhibits either psychotic or impulsive violence fails to respond to standard doses of antipsychotic monotherapy of adequate duration and with adherence to treatment, this can be due to either pharmacokinetic failure or pharmacodynamic failure [29]. Pharmacokinetic interactions describe the effects of a biological system on a medication and include rapid metabolization, cytochrome P450 polymorphisms, poor absorption (e.g., due to gastric bypass), and interactions with other medications/substances. In the case of pharmacokinetic failure, plasma drug levels do not reach adequate levels (and therefore D2 receptor occupancy is less than 60%) despite standard antipsychotic doses

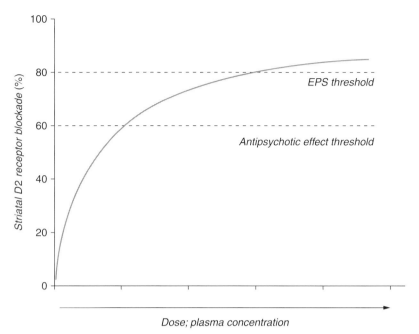

Figure 21.2 Dopamine D2 receptor occupancy. Antipsychotic blockade of at least 60% of D2 receptors in the striatum is necessary to ameliorate psychotic symptoms. However, when 80% or more of D2 receptors are blocked, extrapyramidal symptoms (EPS) are likely to occur. Standard doses of atypical antipsychotics are based on achieving 60% D2 receptor occupancy without exceeding the 80% EPS threshold. Note that the slope of the curve flattens out with increasing dose; that is, at higher doses, large increases in dose are needed to obtain substantial increases in D2 receptor occupancy.

(Figure 21.3A). Often, pharmacokinetic failure presents as a lack of both therapeutic and adverse effects at standard antipsychotic doses. Therapeutic drug monitoring is essential for determining if a pharmacokinetic issue or treatment nonadherence underlies treatment nonresponse; in these cases, plasma drug levels will be lower than expected [18,39]. Solutions to pharmacokinetic failure include increasing the antipsychotic dose to achieve sufficient plasma levels, switching to a different antipsychotic monotherapy (such as one with a sublingual or intramuscular formulation), instituting antipsychotic polypharmacy, or simply taking the antipsychotic with food [17].

Pharmacodynamic failure, treatment resistance, and violence

Pharmacodynamic interactions describe how antipsychotics impact biological systems once they occupy 60%–80% of D2 dopamine receptors. Pharmacodynamic failure occurs when there is a lack of therapeutic response despite attaining adequate plasma drug levels (Figure 21.3B) [29]. Why some patients do not respond to the usual degree of D2 receptor occupancy remains a quandary, but can include insensitive D2 receptors, or even supersensitive D2 receptors, where increasing doses of antipsychotics may be necessary in order to reduce psychotic

symptoms [40–42]. Interestingly, several factors, including substance abuse, can increase dopamine supersensitivity [42]. These treatment-resistant patients may present with excessive psychotic symptoms and violence leading to institutionalization in forensic settings. For these individuals, it may be necessary to use treatment strategies (including high-dose antipsychotic monotherapy and antipsychotic polypharmacy) aimed at greater than 80% D2 receptor occupancy in order to relieve psychotic symptoms (Figure 21.1) [17,29].

Heroic treatment strategies such as high-dose monotherapy or antipsychotic polypharmacy may not be necessary for typical patients with schizophrenia included in clinical research studies and for which the evidence in the literature is generated. In fact, most clinical trial data do not show any superior benefit from using high-dose monotherapy or antipsychotic polypharmacy for such patients [36,37]. Those patients with pharmacodynamic or pharmacokinetic failures and who may require bold treatment measures are often treatment-resistant to standard doses of a single drug and present with violent or aggressive behaviors [18]. Unfortunately, these patients (who are the most likely candidates for high-dose antipsychotic monotherapy or antipsychotic polypharmacy) are excluded from clinical trials because they are too psychotic, too substance-abusing,

223

(a)

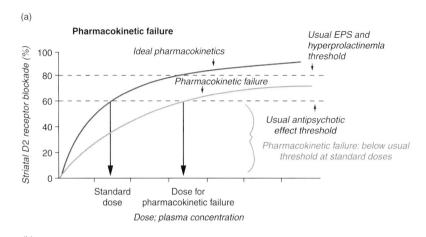

(b)

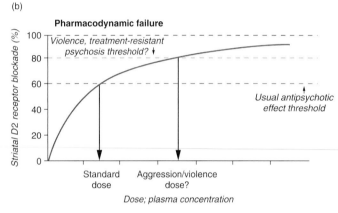

Figure 21.3 Pharmacokinetic and pharmacodynamic failures. The failure of a patient to respond to antipsychotic treatment may be due to either pharmacokinetic or pharmacodynamic failure. (A) Pharmacokinetic failure occurs in cases in which the therapeutic threshold (~60% D2 occupancy) is not achieved despite dosing at standard therapeutic levels. (B) Pharmacodynamic failure occurs in cases in which occupancy of greater than 80% of D2 receptors may be required before therapeutic effects are achieved. Pharmacodynamic failure therefore alters antipsychotics' threshold for therapeutic effects and may be quite prevalent in patients with psychotic or impulsive aggression.

too aggressive, or too treatment-resistant to meet inclusion criteria or give informed consent [29,43,44]. Thus, it is not surprising that many (but not all) of the published clinical trial data have failed to find any clear benefit of antipsychotic polypharmacy or high-dose monotherapy over standard therapeutic doses of a single antipsychotic. It may therefore be difficult for the prescribing clinician to know the best strategy to optimize care for treatment-resistant, violent, or aggressive patients given the paucity of studies that include the patients who require it. However, most studies that investigate the actual use of high antipsychotic dosing (including high dosing that results from combining two antipsychotics) find that those patients for whom high dosing is used are often the most treatment-resistant, aggressive, or otherwise difficult-to-treat cases, and that clinicians who utilize high-dosing strategies are often those with the most clinical experience [45–53].

These data suggest that currently available guidelines fall short for many patients in real-world clinical practice, especially in forensic and state hospital inpatient settings or for outpatients on compulsory treatment orders [45]. These same patients may exhibit psychotic or impulsive violence, and there is substantial practice-based evidence for the use of treatment measures including high-dose monotherapy and antipsychotic polypharmacy [36,37]. Most guidelines for the treatment of schizophrenia advocate several trials of antipsychotic monotherapy (using both first- and second-generation agents), followed by a trial of clozapine, and either do not advocate antipsychotic polypharmacy or reserve it for only the most difficult cases (Figure 21.1) [46,48]. A trial of clozapine is a critical, yet often bypassed, step, since there is an abundance of data that shows the superior efficacy of clozapine for treatment-resistant patients as well as for the amelioration of aggression [46,48,54,55]. Even so, as many as 40% of patients may experience only partial or no response to clozapine [56]. While adherence to these published guidelines is likely the best course of action for the majority of patients, what is the clinician to do when a patient is persistently psychotic and possibly aggressive following several standard-dose monotherapies and an unsuccessful trial of clozapine? In the following sections, we offer guidance and recommendations for using high-dose antipsychotic monotherapy and antipsychotic polypharmacy based on practice-based evidence involving patients who are chronically violent or aggressive and for whom standard guidelines typically fall short (Figure 21.1).

Antipsychotic Polypharmacy

Although data supporting the use of antipsychotic polypharmacy (the simultaneous use of two antipsychotics) are somewhat limited, this practice is very common in psychiatry; as many as 30% of patients receive antipsychotic polypharmacy [57,58]. In fact, despite several guidelines recommending that polypharmacy should only be used as a last resort (following failure of several monotherapies and a trial of clozapine), many clinicians attempt polypharmacy as the rule, rather than the exception [18,47]. Alarmingly, a recent study showed that as many as one-quarter of patients are not treated using prescribing pathways that are consistent with treatment guidelines, with up to 65% receiving antipsychotic polypharmacy as their first antipsychotic treatment [55]. Such prescribing practices appear to have led to some backlash, with calls and efforts to reduce antipsychotic polypharmacy, including several articles authored by ourselves [47,59–65]. We advocate here that published treatment guidelines should be adhered to, and will likely be effective for the majority of patients [1]. Recent studies have shown that as many as two-thirds of patients treated with antipsychotic polypharmacy can be successfully switched to monotherapy, supporting the notion that antipsychotic polypharmacy may not be necessary for the majority of patients [58,66]. The study by Essock et al. [58] in particular showed that not only did patients who were switched from polypharmacy to monotherapy have no worsening of symptoms or increased hospitalization, but many also had reversal of the metabolic effects that were presumably due to antipsychotic polypharmacy. However, it is important to note that polypharmacy was necessary for symptom management in one-third of all patients in the Essock et al. study. Also, although many studies have failed to show a benefit of antipsychotic polypharmacy over standard-

dose monotherapy, more recent investigations do show some evidence for the benefit of combining antipsychotics [48,67,68]. Notably, in line with our previous assertion that time may itself be like a drug, there is some evidence to suggest that treatment with antipsychotic polypharmacy must be continued for at least 10 weeks before a significant therapeutic effect is seen [35,67]. Together, these data support the notion that a subpopulation of patients, likely including those who are treatment-resistant or violent, may require treatment measures such as antipsychotic polypharmacy [18]. Resorting to antipsychotic polypharmacy is probably not necessary for most patients and should be reserved for those patients for whom several antipsychotic monotherapy trials have failed and a trial with clozapine is unsuccessful or cannot be attempted.

Antipsychotic polypharmacy is often employed as a method for increasing dopamine D2 receptor occupancy, but also may be used to recruit additional properties of antipsychotics in order to treat non-positive symptoms such as depression and anxiety [47,67]. Atypical antipsychotics bind to a variety of receptors, some of which are hypothesized to have therapeutic benefit [10]. Indeed the recruitment of various serotonergic and noradrenergic receptors may help to normalize the aberrant neurotransmission associated with violence and aggression [69–71]. For example, increasing serotonergic neurotransmission in the prefrontal cortex (PFC) may, in theory, improve top-down cortical control of the limbic system and thereby improve impulsive aggression [10,11,15,69].

Unfortunately, each atypical antipsychotic also binds to receptors associated with increased risk of intolerable effects (e.g., sedation), so using two antipsychotics simultaneously can increase the side effect burden. A recent study by Langle et al. [57] suggested that patients with schizophrenia on antipsychotic polypharmacy have a worse clinical course compared to those on monotherapy. However, it is unclear if worse clinical outcome was caused by antipsychotic polypharmacy or if it is simply a matter of more treatment-resistant or otherwise difficult patients being the most likely to require more extreme treatment measures such as polypharmacy. Earlier studies also suggested that antipsychotic polypharmacy was associated with increased mortality; however, subsequent studies do not support this idea, and, in fact, a more recent analysis suggests that antipsychotic polypharmacy may actually be associated with reduced mortality as well as fewer psychiatric hospitalizations [51,53,72,73].

If polypharmacy is attempted, antipsychotics should be combined in a rational manner, based on the binding profiles of each antipsychotic for various receptors [48,54]. The logic of combining two antipsychotics should take into account not only the desired boost in D2 antagonism, but also the potential therapeutic and adverse effects of recruiting additional non-dopamine receptors. Combinations of antipsychotics that have similar side effect profiles should be avoided, and potential interactions of antipsychotics should be considered, especially with respect to the cytochrome P450 system [48,74]. Interestingly, antipsychotic polypharmacy may actually be preferable as a way to increase D2 receptor occupancy while avoiding particular adverse effects that may occur with high-dose monotherapy [47,54]. For example, a recent study showed that the addition of aripiprazole to clozapine treatment resulted in a reduction in clozapine-induced cardiometabolic effects [75]. Although this particular study did not show improvement in symptoms (measured using the Positive and Negative Symptom Scale [PANSS]) using a combination of clozapine and aripiprazole, other studies of clozapine and aripiprazole have found some symptom improvement [72,76]. It is also important to note that combining aripiprazole with a non-clozapine antipsychotic may actually worsen symptoms of psychosis due to actions of aripiprazole as a partial agonist with high binding affinity for D2 receptors [54].

Antipsychotic combinations that include clozapine have the most evidence for efficacy [48,67]. When clozapine is not an option, most clinicians who utilize antipsychotic polypharmacy appear to prefer a second-generation antipsychotic (SGA) in combination with a first-generation antipsychotic (FGA), and there are some data to support this [56,67]. Often the rationale for antipsychotic polypharmacy involves combining an antipsychotic with relatively weak binding affinity for D2 receptors (such as clozapine or olanzapine) with an antipsychotic that binds more strongly to D2 receptors (such as sulpiride or amisulpride); in this way D2 receptor occupancy can be maximized while taking advantage of the vast molecular non-D2 binding affinities inherent to many SGAs [47,56].

The rationale for attempting polypharmacy should be carefully documented, along with any therapeutic or side effects that occur. Throughout the course of treatment, plasma levels of both antipsychotics should be monitored in order to ensure treatment adherence and rule out pharmacokinetic issues.

High-Dose Monotherapy

High-dose monotherapy is another strategy for increasing D2 receptor occupancy, although this strategy may also increase the risk of intolerable side effects (notably EPS and akathisia) and, as with antipsychotic polypharmacy, can be associated with substantially higher medication costs, especially for newer agents, than standard dose monotherapy. As with all off-label practices, dosing of antipsychotics above standard therapeutic levels warrants informed consent and increased monitoring of the patient. As the pharmacodynamic and pharmacokinetic characteristics vary from patient to patient, it is virtually impossible to predict what daily dose will be needed in order to achieve an antipsychotic effect [77]. Antipsychotic dosing should be started at the low FDA-approved dose and then titrated upward accordingly until therapeutic efficacy or intolerable side effects occur; thus antipsychotic plasma levels should be continuously monitored as the dose is escalated [78]. The standard dose ranges for atypical antipsychotics and special considerations for high dosing are summarized in Table 21.1. In the following sections, we review the art and science of prescribing each of the FDA-approved atypical antipsychotics at high doses. As antipsychotics are dosed at a level that blocks 60%–80% of D2 receptors (with the exception of clozapine), it is important to note that any receptor binding that is stronger than that of D2 receptors will also be occupied at levels greater than 60% and will likely cause additional therapeutic and adverse effects [10]. It is essential to keep the relative receptor binding affinities in mind when dosing an atypical antipsychotic at higher-than-usual levels to attain >80% occupancy of D2 receptors, so that potential effects of binding to receptors other than D2 can be anticipated and monitored.

Clozapine

Clozapine is not recommended as a first-line treatment strategy due to the risk for serious adverse effects, most notably agranulocytosis; however, in patients who have failed several first-line atypical

Table 21.1 High-dose considerations for atypical antipsychotics

Medication	Usual dose range (mg/day)*	Recommended plasma levels (ng/mL)**	Considerations for high dosing
Clozapine	300–450	350–600	Maximum dose is usually 900 mg/day. Doses above 550 mg/day may require concomitant anticonvulsant administration to reduce the chance of a seizure
Risperidone	2–8	20–60	FDA-approved up to 16 mg/day. Very high doses usually not tolerated
Paliperidone	3–6	20–60	Maximum dose is generally 12 mg/day
Olanzapine	10–20	20–80	Some forensic settings up to 90 mg/day
Quetiapine	400–800	100–500	Some forensic settings up to 1800 mg/day
Ziprasidone	40–200	50–200	Must be taken with food. Positron emission tomography (PET) data support > 120 mg/day. Some forensic settings up to 360 mg/day may be appropriate
Aripiprazole	15–30	150–500	Higher doses usually not more effective and possibly less effective
Iloperidone	12–24	5–10	High dosing not well-studied and may be limited due to risk of orthostatic hypotension
Asenapine	10–20	2–5	High dosing not well-studied
Lurasidone	40–160	>70***	Must be taken with food. Nightly administration may improve tolerability. High dosing not well-studied, but some patients may benefit from doses up to 160 mg/day

* Based on oral formulation in adults.
** Based on recommendations from the AGNP Therapeutic Drug Monitoring consensus guidelines [83].
*** From Potkin *et al.* [84]

antipsychotic monotherapies, a trial of clozapine is warranted. Clozapine has been well-documented for treatment-resistant patients and those who are violent or aggressive, and is therefore recommended for such patients [6,79]. Interestingly, the anti-aggressive effects of clozapine are somewhat independent of its ability to improve positive symptoms [7]. Usual doses of clozapine (plasma levels of 400–600 ng/ml) actually bind less than 60%–80% of dopamine D2 receptors; however, clozapine often has antipsychotic effects at 20%–67% D2 occupancy, suggesting that the antipsychotic effects of clozapine go beyond its ability to block D2 receptors [31]. This is not surprising given the vast molecular binding profile of clozapine. Clozapine has relatively weak affinity for dopamine D2 receptors compared to its affinity for many other receptors, including histaminic H1, adrenergic alpha-1, serotonin 5HT2B, and muscarinic M1 receptors, as well as a host of other receptors. Owing to

these high binding affinities for receptors other than D2, high dosing of clozapine may cause sedation (due to antagonism of M1, H1, and alpha-1 receptors), hypersalivation and constipation (due to antagonism of M1), cardiometabolic issues (due to antagonism of H1 and 5HT2C receptors, as well as the hypothesized receptor "X"), and seizures (mechanism unknown) [34]. A meta-analysis by Davis and Chen [43] showed that patients with high plasma levels of clozapine responded more frequently than those with low plasma levels, indicating that doses above 400 mg/day may be required by many patients. Titration of clozapine to high doses should be done by increasing the dose every 5–7 days [29,43].

Risperidone/paliperidone

Risperidone and its active metabolite paliperidone have similar receptor binding profiles, with relatively strong affinity for dopamine D2 receptors. In the "average" patient, dosing of risperidone at 2–4mg/day is associated with 70%–80% D2 receptor occupancy and is rarely useful at doses above 8 mg/day [30,34]. Both risperidone and paliperidone are associated with increased risk of EPS in a dose-dependent manner, so care must be exercised when increasing the dose of these agents [43]. Titration of risperidone or paliperidone to high doses should be executed by increasing the dose every 5–7 days [29]. One pharmacokinetic difference between paliperidone and risperidone is that paliperidone is not metabolized in the liver so has less chance of drug–drug interactions or effects from cytochrome P450 polymorphisms [34]. Paliperidone may also be more tolerable, with less sedation and fewer EPS, and should be dosed higher than risperidone [34]. Both of these agents are also available as long-acting depot formulations, so an alternative strategy for achieving high D2 receptor occupancy would be to simultaneously use the depot formulation along with its oral counterpart.

Olanzapine

Olanzapine is perhaps the most well-studied atypical antipsychotic in terms of its use at high doses [59]. The risk of EPS is minimal, even at high doses of olanzapine; however, among the atypical antipsychotics, olanzapine carries one of the greatest risks for cardiometabolic effects due to its strong binding affinity for histaminic H1 and serotonin 5HT2C receptors [34]. Olanzapine has also been shown to improve both cognitive and aggressive behavior in patients with schizophrenia [7]. Doses of olanzapine between 10–20 mg/day often correspond to 60%–80% D2 receptor occupancy, but at plasma levels above 700–800 ng/ml, olanzapine is associated with QTc prolongation [31,34,39]. Several studies have indicated that olanzapine may be most effective at higher doses (40–60 mg/day) and may be useful in treatment-resistant violent patients in forensic settings at doses as high as 90 mg/day [39,47,59,78]. Olanzapine titration to higher doses should take place with dose escalation every 5–7 days [29]. Olanzapine is also available in a long-acting depot formulation that can be supplemented with oral olanzapine to achieve high D2 receptor occupancy.

Quetiapine

Quetiapine is available as both immediate release (IR) and extended release (XR) formulations. Quetiapine binds dopamine D2 receptors with relatively weak affinity; it has far greater affinity for many other receptors, including histaminic H1, adrenergic alpha-1, and serotonin 5HT2C receptors, as well as the norepinephrine transporter (NET). Because of this binding profile, high doses of at least 800 mg/day are usually required for quetiapine to have antipsychotic effects. Quetiapine has a very low risk of EPS associated with it, even at high doses, but is associated with a moderate risk for sedation and metabolic syndrome due to its high binding affinity for H1 and 5HT2C receptors. Most literature suggests that 1200 mg/day is no more effective than 600 mg/day, but anecdotal use in forensic settings of doses up to 1800 mg/day may be effective in violent patients who tolerate but do not respond to lower doses [34,43,78]. Titration of quetiapine usually involves daily dose increases, but the dose should be increased at a slower rate when exceeding 800 mg/day [34,67].

Ziprasidone

Ziprasidone has a fairly high binding affinity for dopamine D2 receptors, surpassed only by its affinity for serotonin 5HT2A and 5HT1B receptors. Ziprasidone is associated with virtually no risk of metabolic effects, and earlier concerns about QTc prolongation have not been supported [34]. Importantly, ziprasidone must be taken with food in order to optimize its absorption. There are data to suggest that higher doses of ziprasidone may be most effective, and doses as high as 360 mg/day have been reported [34,39,47,78]. For titration of ziprasidone to high doses, daily increases in dose can be done [29].

Aripiprazole

Aripiprazole is a unique member of the approved atypical antipsychotics. Rather than dopamine D2 receptor antagonism, it acts as a partial agonist at D2 receptors. What this partial agonism means is that in the presence of a full D2 receptor agonist (e.g., dopamine), aripiprazole will act as an antagonist at D2 receptors; however, in the presence of a D2 receptor antagonist (e.g., another antipsychotic), aripiprazole will act more as a D2 receptor agonist [34]. Owing to this partial agonism and its very high binding affinity for D2 receptors, aripiprazole may actually be less effective for psychosis at higher doses and may reduce the effectiveness of another antipsychotic if an attempt at polypharmacy is made [34].

Aripiprazole is not associated with significant risks for sedation, EPS, or metabolic syndrome, but it may cause akathisia in some patients. Although the initial titration of aripiprazole can be rapid, dose increases after a steady state has been reached should be done every 10–14 days [29].

Asenapine, iloperidone, and lurasidone

Asenapine, iloperidone, and lurasidone are the newest atypical antipsychotics on the market, so less is known regarding their use at high doses. When looking to use a high-dose strategy, it would be prudent to first try a high-dose trial of one of the older atypical antipsychotics that have more clinical experience.

Asenapine has moderate binding affinity for dopamine D2 receptors and is usually not associated with increased risk for EPS or metabolic syndrome. Asenapine is available only as a sublingual formulation, and therefore it may be a good option for patients who have pharmacokinetic failures in response to other antipsychotics due to hepatic metabolism or poor absorption [34]. Doses as high as 30–40 mg/day can be used but must be administered 10 mg at a time given at least 1 hour apart. The titration of asenapine should be done by increasing the dose every 5–7 days [29].

Iloperidone is most distinguished by its high binding affinity for adrenergic alpha-1 receptors. Due to this binding property, iloperidone is associated with a high risk of orthostatic hypotension and sedation, so it must be titrated slowly and is not recommended for use at high doses [34].

Lurasidone is the newest antipsychotic approved for use in the United States. It has moderately high binding affinity for dopamine D2 receptors but is most notable for its antagonism of serotonin 5HT7 receptors. Lurasidone is approved up to 160 mg/day and, importantly, lurasidone should be taken with food to optimize absorption [34]. Although the original trials on lurasidone suggested that side effect risk increased with higher dosing, recent data indicate that administration of lurasidone in the evening may minimize the risk of adverse side effects [80].

Conclusion

Heroic treatment measures aimed at achieving adequate D2 receptor occupancy may be effective for the treatment of psychotic or impulsive, but not predatory, violence in patients with psychotic illness such as schizophrenia. One strategy for using such intrepid treatment measures, either antipsychotic polypharmacy or high-dose monotherapy, involves combining a long-acting depot formulation with an oral antipsychotic [47,81]. For example, depot risperidone can be combined with oral risperidone (high-dose monotherapy) or with oral clozapine (antipsychotic polypharmacy). Numerous FGAs and SGAs are available as long-acting depots, providing a variety treatment options. If either a high-dose monotherapy or antipsychotic polypharmacy treatment strategy is attempted, the importance of therapeutic blood monitoring cannot be overstated. In addition to obtaining therapeutic blood levels for any antipsychotic given, it is critical to define therapeutic endpoints and discontinue a treatment strategy should adverse effects become evident or if clinical efficacy is not achieved. Increasing D2 receptor occupancy can lead to the development of EPS that necessitate the use of anticholinergic medications, which may exacerbate cognitive impairment [50]. Given the connection between cognitive deficits and aggression, such a treatment strategy may actually worsen violent and aggressive behaviors, and caution is warranted [51,82].

If either heroic measure of antipsychotic polypharmacy or high-dose monotherapy is successful in a treatment-resistant, violent patient, it may be tempting to simply continue with the successful treatment regimen. However, it is recommended that an attempt be made to switch the patient to more conventional antipsychotic therapy [2]. Documented decompensation upon discontinuing antipsychotic polypharmacy or high-dose monotherapy provides substantial evidence that the patient is a part of the subpopulation who requires heroic treatment measures.

Disclosures

Debbi Morrissette does not have anything to disclose. Stephen Stahl's disclosure information: Stephen M. Stahl, MD, PhD is an Adjunct Professor of Psychiatry at the University of California, San Diego School of Medicine, Honorary Visiting Senior Fellow at the University of Cambridge, UK and Director of Psychopharmacology for California Department of State Hospitals. Over the past 12 months (March 2013 – April 2014) Dr. Stahl has served as a Consultant for Astra Zeneca, Avanir, Biomarin, Envivo, Forest, Jazz,

Lundbeck, Neuronetics, Noveida, Orexigen, Otsuka, PamLabs, Servier, Shire, Sunovion, Taisho, Takeda and Trius; he is a board member of RCT Logic and GenoMind; on the Speakers Bureau for Astra Zeneca, Janssen, Otsuka, Sunovion and Takeda and he has received research and/or grant support from AssureX, Eli Lilly, EnVivo, Janssen, JayMac, Jazz, Lundbeck, Mylan, Neuronetics, Novartis, Otsuka, Pamlabs, Pfizer, Roche, Shire, Sunovion, Takeda, Teva and Valeant.

References

1. Stahl SM, Morrissette DA, Citrome L, et al. "Meta-guidelines" for the management of patients with schizophrenia. *CNS Spectr.* 2013; **18**(3): 150–162.

2. Stahl SM. Emerging guidelines for the use of antipsychotic polypharmacy. *Rev. Psiquiatr. Salud Ment.* 2013; **6**(3): 97–100.

3. Citrome L, Volavka J. Pharmacological management of acute and persistent aggression in forensic psychiatry settings. *CNS Drugs.* 2011; **25**(12): 1009–1021.

4. Warburton K. The new mission of forensic mental health systems: managing violence as a medical syndrome in an environment that balances treatment and safety. *CNS Spectr.* 2014; **0**(5): 368–373.

5. Nolan KA, Czobor P, Roy BB, et al. Characteristics of assaultive behavior among psychiatric inpatients. *Psychiatr. Serv.* 2003; **54**(7): 1012–1016.

6. Volavka J, Citrome L. Heterogeneity of violence in schizophrenia and implications for long-term treatment. *Int. J. Clin. Pract.* 2008; **62** (8): 1237–1245.

7. Volavka J, Citrome L. Pathways to aggression in schizophrenia affect results of treatment. *Schizophr. Bull.* 2011; **37**(5): 921–929.

8. Swanson JW, Swartz MS, Van Dorn RA, et al. Comparison of antipsychotic medication effects on reducing violence in people with schizophrenia. *Br. J. Psychiatry.* 2008; **193**(1): 37–43.

9. Quanbeck CD, McDermott BE, Lam J, et al. Categorization of aggressive acts committed by chronically assaultive state hospital patients. *Psychiatr. Serv.* 2007; **58**(4): 521–528.

10. Stahl SM. *Stahl's Essential Psychopharmacology*, 4th edn. New York: Cambridge University Press; 2013.

11. Stahl SM, Morrissette DA. *Stahl's Illustrated Violence: Neural Circuits, Genetics, and Treatment.* New York: Cambridge University Press; 2014.

12. Siever LJ. Neurobiology of aggression and violence. *Am. J. Psychiatry.* 2008; **165**(4): 429–442.

13. Frogley C, Taylor D, Dickens G, Picchioni M. A systematic review of the evidence of clozapine's anti-aggressive effects. *Int. J. Neuropsychopharmacol.* 2012; **15**(9): 1351–1371.

14. Coccaro EF, McCloskey MS, Fitzgerald DA, Phan KL. Amygdala and orbitofrontal reactivity to social threat in individuals with impulsive aggression. *Biol. Psychiatry.* 2007; **62**(2): 168–178.

15. Coccaro EF, Sripada CS, Yanowitch RN, Phan KL. Corticolimbic function in impulsive aggressive behavior. *Biol. Psychiatry.* 2011; **69**(12): 1153–1159.

16. Bobes J, Fillat O, Arango C. Violence among schizophrenia out-patients compliant with medication: prevalence and associated factors. *Acta Psychiatr. Scand.* 2009; **119**(3): 218–225.

17. Meyer J. A rational approach to employing high plasma levels of antipsychotics for violence associated with schizophrenia: case vignettes. *CNS Spectr.* 2014; **19**(5): 432–438. DOI: http://dx.doi.org/10.1017/S1092852914000236.

18. Stahl SM. Antipsychotic polypharmacy: never say never, but never say always. *Acta Psychiatr. Scand.* 2012; **125**(5): 349–351.

19. Pavlov KA, Chistiakov DA, Chekhonin VP. Genetic determinants of aggression and impulsivity in humans. *J. Appl. Genet.* 2012; **53**(1): 61–82.

20. Fazel S, Grann M, Langstrom N. What is the role of epidemiology for forensic psychiatry? *Crim. Behav. Ment. Health.* 2009; **19**(5): 281–285.

21. Fazel S, Gulati G, Linsell L, Geddes JR, Grann M. Schizophrenia and violence: systematic review and meta-analysis. *PLoS Med.* 2009; **6** (8): e1000120.

22. Fazel S, Langstrom N, Hjern A, Grann M, Lichtenstein P. Schizophrenia, substance abuse, and violent crime. *JAMA.* 2009; **301**(19): 2016–2023.

23. Topiwala A, Fazel S. The pharmacological management of violence in schizophrenia: a structured review. *Expert Rev. Neurother.* 2011; **11**(1): 53–63.

24. Krakowski MI, Czobor P. Executive function predicts response to antiaggression treatment in schizophrenia: a randomized controlled trial. *J. Clin. Psychiatry.* 2012; **73**(1): 74–80.

25. Krakowski MI, Czobor P, Nolan KA. Atypical antipsychotics, neurocognitive deficits, and aggression in schizophrenic patients. *J. Clin. Psychopharmacol.* 2008; **28**(5): 485–493.

26. Singh JP, Grann M, Fazel S. A comparative study of violence risk assessment tools: a systematic review and metaregression analysis of 68 studies involving 25,980 participants. *Clin. Psychol. Rev.* 2011; **31**(3): 499–513.

27. Song H, Min SK. Aggressive behavior model in schizophrenic patients. *Psychiatry Res.* 2009; **167**(1–2): 58–65.

28. Uchida H, Takeuchi H, Graff-Guerrero A, *et al.* Dopamine D2 receptor occupancy and clinical effects: a systematic review and pooled analysis. *J. Clin. Psychopharmacol.* 2011; **31**(4): 497–502.

29. Correll CU. From receptor pharmacology to improved outcomes: individualising the selection, dosing, and switching of antipsychotics. *Eur. Psychiatry.* 2010; **25**(Suppl 2): S12–S21.

30. Nord M, Farde L. Antipsychotic occupancy of dopamine receptors in schizophrenia. *CNS Neurosci. Ther.* 2011; **17**(2): 97–103.

31. Uchida H, Takeuchi H, Graff-Guerrero A, *et al.* Predicting dopamine D receptor occupancy from plasma levels of antipsychotic drugs: a systematic review and pooled analysis. *J. Clin. Psychopharmacol.* 2011; **31**(3): 318–325.

32. Stauffer V, Case M, Kollack-Walker S, *et al.* Trajectories of response to treatment with atypical antipsychotic medication in patients with schizophrenia pooled from 6 double-blind, randomized clinical trials. *Schizophr. Res.* 2011; **130**(1–3): 11–19.

33. Robinson DG, Woerner MG, Alvir JM, *et al.* Predictors of treatment response from a first episode of schizophrenia or schizoaffective disorder. *Am. J. Psychiatry.* 1999; **156**(4): 544–549.

34. Stahl SM. *Stahl's Essential Psychopharmacology*, 3rd edn. New York: Cambridge University Press; 2008.

35. Morrissette DA, Stahl SM. Optimizing outcomes in schizophrenia: long-acting depots and long-term treatment. *CNS Spectr.* 2012; **17** (Suppl 1): 10–21.

36. Ritsner MS, ed. *Polypharmacy in Psychiatric Practice, Volume I: Multiple Medication Use Strategies.* New York: Springer Verlag; 2013.

37. Ritsner MS, ed. *Polypharmacy in Psychiatric Practice, Volume II: Use of Polypharmacy in the "Real World".* New York: Springer Verlag; 2013.

38. Stentebjerg-Olesen M, Jeppesen P, Pagsberg AK, *et al.* Early nonresponse determined by the Clinical Global Impressions scale predicts poorer outcomes in youth with schizophrenia spectrum disorders naturalistically treated with second-generation antipsychotics. *J. Child Adolesc. Psychopharmacol.* 2013; **23**(10): 665–675.

39. Mauri MC, Volonteri LS, Colasanti A, *et al.* Clinical pharmacokinetics of atypical antipsychotics: a critical review of the relationship between plasma concentrations and clinical response. *Clin. Pharmacokinet.* 2007; **46**(5): 359–388.

40. Remington G, Kapur S. Antipsychotic dosing: how much but also how often? *Schizophr. Bull.* 2010; **36**(5): 900–903.

41. Samaha AN, Seeman P, Stewart J, Rajabi H, Kapur S. "Breakthrough" dopamine supersensitivity during ongoing antipsychotic treatment leads to treatment failure over time. *J. Neurosci.* 2007; **27**(11): 2979–2986.

42. Seeman P. Dopamine D2 receptors as treatment targets in schizophrenia. *Clin. Schizophr. Relat. Psychoses.* 2010; **4**(1): 56–73.

43. Davis JM, Chen N. Dose response and dose equivalence of antipsychotics. *J. Clin. Psychopharmacol.* 2004; **24**(2): 192–208.

44. Krakowski MI, Kunz M, Czobor P, Volavka J. Long-term high-dose neuroleptic treatment: who gets it and why? *Hosp. Community Psychiatry.* 1993; **44**(7): 640–644.

45. Gisev N, Bell JS, Chen TF. Factors associated with antipsychotic polypharmacy and high-dose antipsychotics among individuals receiving compulsory treatment in the community. *J. Clin. Psychopharmacol.* 2014; **34**(3): 307–312.

46. Roh D, Chang JG, Kim CH, *et al.* Antipsychotic polypharmacy and high-dose prescription in schizophrenia: a 5-year comparison. *Aust. N. Z. J. Psychiatry.* 2014; **48**(1): 52–60.

47. Barnes TR, Paton C. Antipsychotic polypharmacy in schizophrenia: benefits and risks. *CNS Drugs.* 2011; **25**(5): 383–399.

48. Fleischhacker WW, Uchida H. Critical review of antipsychotic polypharmacy in the treatment of schizophrenia. *Int. J. Neuropsychopharmacol.* 2014; **17**(7): 1083–1093.

49. Fujita J, Nishida A, Sakata M, Noda T, Ito H. Excessive dosing and polypharmacy of antipsychotics caused by prorenata in agitated patients with schizophrenia. *Psychiatry Clin. Neurosci.* 2013; **67**(5): 345–351.

50. Gallego JA, Bonetti J, Zhang J, Kane JM, Correll CU. Prevalence and correlates of antipsychotic polypharmacy: a systematic review and meta-regression of global and regional trends from the 1970s to 2009. *Schizophr. Res.* 2012; **138**(1): 18–28.

51. Lochmann van Bennekom MWH, Gijsman HJ, Zitman FG. Antipsychotic polypharmacy in psychotic disorders: a critical review of neurobiology, efficacy, tolerability and cost effectiveness. *J. Psychopharmacol.* 2013; **27**(4): 327–336.

52. Sagud M, Vuksan-Cusa B, Zivkovic M, *et al.* Antipsychotics: to combine or not to combine? *Psychiatr. Danub.* 2013; **25**(3): 306–310.

53. Suokas JT, Suvisaari JM, Haukka J, Korhonen P, Tiihonen J. Description of long-term polypharmacy among schizophrenia outpatients. *Soc. Psychiatry Psychiatr. Epidemiol.* 2013; **48**(4): 631–638.

54. Freudenreich O, Goff DC. Antipsychotic combination therapy in schizophrenia: a review of efficacy and risks of current combinations. *Acta Psychiatr. Scand.* 2002; **106**(5): 323–330.

55. Goren JL, Meterko M, Williams S, *et al.* Antipsychotic prescribing pathways, polypharmacy, and clozapine use in treatment of schizophrenia. *Psychiatr. Serv.* 2013; **64**(6): 527–533.

56. Englisch S, Zink M. Treatment-resistant schizophrenia: evidence-based strategies. *Mens Sana Monogr.* 2012; **10**(1): 20–32.

57. Langle G, Steinert T, Weiser P, *et al.* Effects of polypharmacy on outcome in patients with schizophrenia in routine psychiatric treatment. *Acta Psychiatr. Scand.* 2012; **125**(5): 372–381.

58. Essock SM, Schooler NR, Stroup TS, *et al.* Effectiveness of switching from antipsychotic polypharmacy to monotherapy. *Am. J. Psychiatry.* 2011; **168**(7): 702–708.

59. Stahl SM, Grady MM. A critical review of atypical antipsychotic utilization: comparing monotherapy with polypharmacy and augmentation. *Curr. Med. Chem.* 2004; **11**(3): 313–327.

60. Stahl SM. Focus on antipsychotic polypharmacy: evidence-based prescribing or prescribing-based evidence? *Int. J. Neuropsychopharmacol.* 2004; **7**(2): 113–116.

61. Stahl SM. Antipsychotic polypharmacy: evidence based or eminence based? *Acta Psychiatr. Scand.* 2002; **106**(5): 321–322.

62. Stahl SM. Antipsychotic polypharmacy: squandering precious resources? *J. Clin. Psychiatry.* 2002; **63**(2): 93–94.

63. Stahl SM. Antipsychotic polypharmacy, part 2: tips on use and misuse. *J. Clin. Psychiatry.* 1999; **60**(8): 506–507.

64. Stahl SM. Antipsychotic polypharmacy, part 1: therapeutic option or dirty little secret? *J. Clin. Psychiatry.* 1999; **60**(7): 425–426.

65. Stahl SM. "Awakening" from schizophrenia: intramolecular polypharmacy and the atypical antipsychotics. *J. Clin. Psychiatry.* 1997; **58**(9): 381–382.

66. Suzuki T, Uchida H, Tanaka KF, *et al.* Revising polypharmacy to a single antipsychotic regimen for patients with chronic schizophrenia. *Int. J. Neuropsychopharmacol.* 2004; **7**(2): 133–142.

67. Correll CU, Rummel-Kluge C, Corves C, Kane JM, Leucht S. Antipsychotic combinations vs monotherapy in schizophrenia: a meta-analysis of randomized controlled trials. *Schizophr. Bull.* 2009; **35**(2): 443–457.

68. Iasevoli F, Buonaguro EF, Marconi M, *et al.* Efficacy and clinical determinants of antipsychotic polypharmacy in psychotic patients experiencing an acute relapse and admitted to hospital stay: results from a cross-sectional and a subsequent longitudinal pilot study. *ISRN Pharmacology.* 2014; **2014**: 762127.

69. Coccaro EF. Intermittent explosive disorder as a disorder of impulsive aggression for DSM-5. *Am. J. Psychiatry.* 2012; **169**(6): 577–588.

70. Rosell DR, Thompson JL, Slifstein M, *et al.* Increased serotonin 2A receptor availability in the orbitofrontal cortex of physically aggressive personality disordered patients. *Biol. Psychiatry.* 2010; **67**(12): 1154–1162.

71. Winstanley CA, Theobald DE, Dalley JW, Glennon JC, Robbins TW. 5-HT2A and 5-HT2C receptor antagonists have opposing effects on a measure of impulsivity: interactions with global 5-HT depletion. *Psychopharmacology (Berl.).* 2004; **176**(3–4): 376–385.

72. Englisch S, Zink M. Combined antipsychotic treatment involving clozapine and aripiprazole. *Prog. Neuropsychopharmacol. Biol. Psychiatry.* 2008; **32**(6): 1386–1392.

73. Katona L, Czobor P. Bitter I. Real-world effectiveness of antipsychotic monotherapy vs. polypharmacy in schizophrenia: to switch or to combine? A nationwide study in Hungary. *Schizophr. Res.* 2014; **152**(1): 246–254.

74. Ballon J, Stroup TS. Polypharmacy for schizophrenia. *Curr. Opin. Psychiatry.* 2013; **26**(2): 208–213.

75. Fleischhacker WW, Heikkinen ME, Olie JP, *et al.* Effects of adjunctive treatment with aripiprazole on body weight and clinical efficacy in schizophrenia patients treated with clozapine: a randomized, double-blind, placebo-controlled trial. *Int. J. Neuropsychopharmacol.* 2010; **13**(8): 1115–1125.

76. Chang JS, Ahn YM, Park HJ, *et al.* Aripiprazole augmentation in

clozapine-treated patients with refractory schizophrenia: an 8-week, randomized, double-blind, placebo-controlled trial. *J. Clin. Psychiatry.* 2008; **69**(5): 720–731.

77. Thompson C. The use of high-dose antipsychotic medication. *Br. J. Psychiatry.* 1994; **164**(4): 448–458.

78. Schwartz TL, Stahl SM. Treatment strategies for dosing the second generation antipsychotics. *CNS Neurosci. Ther.* 2011; **17**(2): 110–117.

79. Volavka J, Czobor P, Nolan K, *et al.* Overt aggression and psychotic symptoms in patients with schizophrenia treated with clozapine, olanzapine, risperidone, or haloperidol. *J. Clin. Psychopharmacol.* 2004; **24** (2): 225–228.

80. Kantrowitz JT, Citrome L. Lurasidone for schizophrenia: what's different? *Expert Rev. Neurother.* 2012; **12**(3): 265–273.

81. Aggarwal NK, Sernyak MJ, Rosenheck RA. Prevalence of concomitant oral antipsychotic drug use among patients treated with long-acting, intramuscular, antipsychotic medications. *J. Clin. Psychopharmacol.* 2012; **32**(3): 323–328.

82. Elie D, Poirier M, Chianetta J, *et al.* Cognitive effects of antipsychotic dosage and polypharmacy: a study with the BACS in patients with schizophrenia and schizoaffective disorder. *J. Psychopharmacol.* 2010; **24**(7): 1037–1044.

83. Hiemke C, Baumann P, Bergemann N, *et al.* AGNP consensus guidelines for therapeutic drug monitoring in psychiatry: update 2011. *Pharmacopsychiatry.* 2011; **44**(6): 195–235.

84. Potkin SG, Keator DB, Kesler-West ML, *et al.* D2 receptor occupancy following lurasidone treatment in patients with schizophrenia or schizoaffective disorder. *CNS Spectr.* 2014; **19**(2): 176–181.

Chapter 22

A rational approach to employing high plasma levels of antipsychotics for violence associated with schizophrenia: case vignettes

Jonathan M. Meyer

Introduction

Enthusiasm for routine use of high-dose antipsychotic therapy waned in the 1980s due to tolerability concerns and the absence of evidence to support superior efficacy compared with more traditional approaches [1,2]. By the early 1990s, prior to the widespread availability of second-generation antipsychotics, extended use of high-dose antipsychotic treatment was often relegated to long-term inpatient settings populated by severely ill, violent patients with schizophrenia [3]. The improved neurological adverse effect profile with second-generation antipsychotics combined with data demonstrating clozapine's unique efficacy for persistent violence in patients with schizophrenia [4] provided a valid rationale for limiting the use of high doses of potent dopamine D_2 antagonists [5]. Nonetheless, high-dose antipsychotic prescribing persists in inpatient settings despite consensus recommendations [6] and efforts to curtail this practice [7]. The Royal College of Psychiatrists (RCP) consensus statement succinctly summarizes a rational view of high-dose antipsychotics.

> On the basis of current evidence, high-dose prescribing, either with a single agent or combined antipsychotics, should rarely be used and then only for a time-limited trial in treatment-resistant schizophrenia after all evidence-based approaches have been shown to be unsuccessful or inappropriate [6].

Unlike acute inpatient settings, forensic psychiatric facilities are more likely to contain significant numbers of treatment-resistant or violent schizophrenia patients whose care demands the use of high plasma level antipsychotic strategies due to pharmacodynamic response failure at lower dosages despite therapeutic antipsychotic levels. In this sense, we are making a clear distinction between those who achieve expected plasma antipsychotic levels but fail to respond as opposed to patients treated with known cytochrome P450 (CYP) or p-glycoprotein (PGP) inducers such as carbamazepine [8], or who possess biological variants (e.g., CYP 2D6 ultrarapid metabolizers) [9] that require high dosages to achieve therapeutic drug levels. As will be discussed below, the use of plasma antipsychotic levels is crucial to ascertaining whether the high dosages used are indeed resulting in high plasma drug levels or whether nonresponse is due to kinetic failure.

The biological hypothesis for pharmacodynamic nonresponders revolves around the concept that some schizophrenia patients require $\geq 80\%$ D_2 receptor blockade for efficacy. Because antipsychotic D_2 receptor occupancy curves flatten out considerably around 80%, large increases in plasma antipsychotic levels are required to realize small increases in receptor occupancy [10]. For example, tripling the plasma olanzapine level from 50 ng/ml to 150 ng/ml changes D_2 receptor occupancy from just below 80% to a value close to 83% [10].

In the absence of modern clinical guidelines for high plasma level antipsychotic therapy, the following practice-based treatment principles have been developed by the California Department of State Hospitals (DSH) Psychopharmacology Resource Network for the use of antipsychotics in schizophrenia patients with psychotic or impulsive violence in whom the need for high antipsychotic dosages is not primarily to overcome the impact of CYP or PGP induction or rapid drug metabolism. These are not strategies for the management of routine nonviolent community patients, nor do these principles apply to the use of antipsychotics in psychotic patients who may have

Violence in Psychiatry, ed. Katherine D. Warburton and Stephen M. Stahl. Published by Cambridge University Press.
© Cambridge University Press 2016.

severe or profound intellectual disability due to the limited clinical experience and literature in this area, or for control of violence driven by sociopathic or predatory behavior, or psychopathy.

Principles

(1) Clozapine has the best evidence for violence reduction in patients with schizophrenia independent of its impact on psychotic symptom severity.

(2) High plasma level antipsychotic therapy may be considered in violent schizophrenia patients prior to a clozapine trial in the following circumstances:

   (a) failure of routine clinical doses of medium/potent D_2 antagonists;

   (b) and, the absence of dose limiting adverse effects, particularly extrapyramidal side effects (EPS) or akathisia.

(3) High plasma level antipsychotic therapy can be used for violent schizophrenia patients who refuse or have failed a clozapine trial and who did not exhibit dose limiting adverse effects during routine antipsychotic exposure.

(4) Antipsychotic treatment should be carefully titrated until one of two well-defined clinical endpoints are reached: clinical response or intolerability.

   (a) Treatment trials should not be routinely terminated on the basis of daily dose or high plasma levels: certain patients may both require and tolerate high doses and high plasma levels of D_2 antagonists.

   (b) A small subset of schizophrenia patients exhibits enormous tolerance for D_2 antagonism without EPS or akathisia. While not an absolute rule, consideration can be given for terminating a medication trial for futility with any of the following plasma levels: haloperidol $\gg$ 30 ng/ml, fluphenazine $\gg$ 4.0 ng/ml, or olanzapine $\gg$ 200 ng/ml.

The first principle was derived from open-label experience [4] and data from a randomized, double-blind, 12-week, parallel-group trial in which clozapine demonstrated superiority to olanzapine and haloperidol for the treatment of violent schizophrenia patients, especially in those with low cognitive function, and without statistical separation between the medication arms for symptom reduction [11,12].

Olanzapine was also superior to haloperidol for some measures of aggression [11]. The second principle emerged from two clinical realities: (1) certain individuals may fail to evince adverse effects for kinetic or adherence reasons, and thus are deprived of an adequate antipsychotic trial [13]; (2) there is an enormous range in antipsychotic tolerability [14]. Principle 3 may be viewed as a corollary of the first two principles, and reiterates the RCP position regarding the appropriate use of high-dose antipsychotics in a treatment algorithm.

The use of plasma antipsychotic levels as noted in Principle 4 is critical to documenting the antipsychotic trial and guiding treatment decisions. While older literature often used the term high-dose treatment as synonymous with a high level of antipsychotic exposure, this is clearly not the case and engenders significant confusion. Most antipsychotics undergo significant phase I metabolism through the CYP system, with intestinal absorption (and central nervous system penetration across the blood–brain barrier) influenced by antipsychotic affinity for the efflux transporter PGP [8]. The concurrent use of potent PGP and CYP 3A4 inducers, such as carbamazepine, phenytoin, rifampin, efavirenz, or nevirapine, lower antipsychotic levels significantly, ranging from 16% for asenapine [15] and 35%–37% for ziprasidone or paliperidone (due to their limited phase I metabolism) [8] to 50% for haloperidol, fluphenazine, olanzapine, and risperidone [8], and a 70%–80% reduction for aripiprazole, quetiapine [8], and lurasidone [16]. Valproate in some reports has also been associated with reductions in plasma levels of olanzapine [17] and clozapine [18], although the mechanism and extent of the effect on other agents is not well defined. The use of any of these inducers, and possibly valproate, will often result in subtherapeutic plasma antipsychotic levels for most agents and inadequate response unless markedly higher antipsychotic doses are employed, or the patient can be switched from potent inducers such as carbamazepine to those with lower (e.g., valproate) or no propensity (e.g., lithium) to induce antipsychotic metabolism. It should be anticipated at the outset of treatment that the use of potent inducers with most antipsychotics may result in kinetic failures, underscoring the need to obtain antipsychotic plasma levels. Several reviews provide a good resource for correlations between threshold plasma antipsychotic levels and response for haloperidol [19], fluphenazine [20], and olanzapine [21], and

Table 22.1 Therapeutic plasma antipsychotic ranges for selected agents and plasma levels associated with 80% dopamine D_2 receptor occupancy

Drug	Minimum threshold for response	Tolerability threshold	Estimated plasma level associated with 80% D_2 occupancy
Haloperidol	3 ng/ml [19]	18 ng/ml [19]	2.0 ng/ml [33]
Haloperidol (LAI)*	3 ng/ml [34]	15 ng/ml [34]	2.4 ng/ml [35]
Fluphenazine	1.0 ng/ml [36]	2.7 ng/ml [36]	No published data
Fluphenazine (LAI)	0.8 ng/ml [37]	2.7 ng/ml [36]	No published data
Risperidone active moiety** (oral)	Poorly defined	Poorly defined	47 ng/ml [10]
Risperidone active moiety (LAI)	Poorly defined	Poorly defined	45 ng/ml [22,38]
Olanzapine (oral)	23.2 ng/ml [21]	176 ng/ml [27]	70 ng/ml [10]
Olanzapine (LAI)	No published data	No published data	78 ng/ml [23]

* LAI = long-acting injectable.
** Active moiety = risperidone+9-OH risperidone.

for plasma levels of risperidone and olanzapine with central D_2 occupancy [10,22,23] (Table 22.1). These correlations between antipsychotic plasma levels and D_2 occupancy hold for both oral and the comparable long-acting injectable forms [22,23]. The abundance of clinical data for haloperidol, fluphenazine, and olanzapine that provides therapeutic ranges makes these antipsychotics ideal candidates for treatment decisions guided by therapeutic drug monitoring. Such correlations have generally not been found consistently with risperidone [24]. It should be noted that D_2 occupancy data are from normal volunteers or stable schizophrenia patients, and not from violent forensic populations.

A clinically occult source of kinetic failure for some schizophrenia patients prescribed antipsychotics metabolized via CYP 2D6 relates to duplication of the genes encoding CYP 2D6. The net result of these extra copies is greater enzyme production and increased 2D6 clinical activity [9]. While relatively uncommon in white northern Europeans (3%), the prevalence of these 2D6 ultrarapid metabolizers (UM) is 10%–29% in populations from northeastern Africa (e.g., Ethiopia) and geographically proximate parts of the Middle East (e.g., Saudi Arabia) [9]. Although genetic testing exists for CYP polymorphisms, it is not routinely employed due to expense or lack of local availability, so this effect is difficult to anticipate in those who are not clear descendants of individuals from areas with high 2D6 UM prevalence. In the absence

of genetic testing, one might infer the presence of UM status in those who are on antipsychotics metabolized via 2D6 in whom adherence issues have been ruled out (e.g., by use of long-acting injectable antipsychotics), and plasma levels are significantly below what might be expected for the degree of medication exposure [25].

At a minimum, the use of plasma antipsychotic levels thus helps avoid treatment failure due to known or unrecognized kinetic issues [26]. As will be illustrated in Case 1, Principle 4a enunciates the proposition that some patients may require high plasma antipsychotic levels for response – levels that might be outside of the reported therapeutic reference range. When no clinical evidence exists for adverse effects, this fact must be documented before further dose titration is pursued if the clinical endpoint (violence reduction) has not been met. Aside from clozapine, few antipsychotics have robust data on response and tolerability, including haloperidol, fluphenazine, and olanzapine (Table 22.1) [27,28]. While tolerability may decrease significantly for plasma fluphenazine levels > 2.0 ng/ml [20] (Figure 22.1), haloperidol levels > 12 ng/ml [29] (Figure 22.2), or olanzapine levels > 100 ng/ml [27], the absence of EPS/akathisia or other significant adverse effects despite higher plasma levels is an indication that the patient might reasonably be tried at a higher dosage, especially if clozapine is not an option or the patient is a clozapine failure.

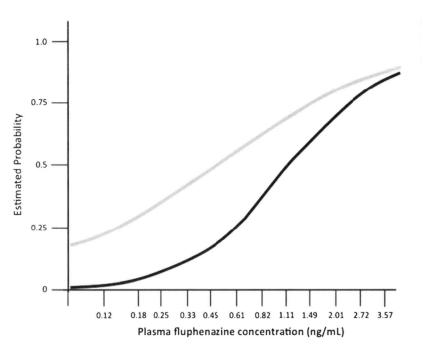

Figure 22.1 Relationship between plasma fluphenazine levels and estimated probability of improvement (gray line) and disabling side effects (black line) [20].

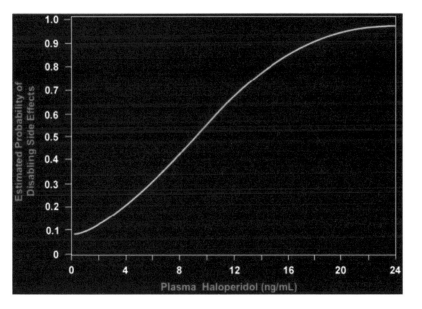

Figure 22.2 The relationship between plasma haloperidol and the estimated probability of disabling side effects [20].

It should be acknowledged that there are rare circumstances in which schizophrenia patients may exhibit no threshold for neurological adverse effects. The data in Table 22.2 are from a trifluo-perazine titration study in which 10 male patients with schizophrenia were started on trifluoperazine 15 mg/d (equivalent to 6 mg haloperidol) without antiparkinsonian treatment, and advanced by 10 mg per week until they reached a predefined level of neurological adverse effects [14]. Subject 5 remained in the titration arm for over 36 weeks, achieving a daily trifluoperazine dose of 480 mg, yet had the

Table 22.2 Outcomes in an escalating trifluoperazine dose protocol [14]

Patient	Age (years)	Length of hospitalization (years)	Maximum daily trifluoperazine dose (mg)	Degree of psychiatric improvement*	Maximum neurological rating	Weight change (lbs)
1	35	16	30	–	3.0	–5
2	52	31	150	–	1.2	5
3	52	27	100	0	1.5	–3
4	23	6	220	+	1.1	25
5	30	11	480	+	0.4	30
6	41	23	100	±	1.1	10
7	51	14	20	+	3.1	10
8	57	16	30	+++	2.0	12
9	42	11	40	±	2.0	12
10	55	32	60	+	2.0	6
Mean	43.8	18.7	123		1.74	10.2

* Interpretation of psychiatric symptom change: – =no improvement with later worsening; 0 = no improvement; ± = mild improvement with later worsening; + = mild improvement; + + = moderate improvement; + + + = marked improvement.

lowest neurological side effect rating among the subjects in this study despite obvious evidence of significant drug exposure (weight gain). In such individuals, an antipsychotic trial may be terminated for futility (Principle 4b), although no definite guidelines exist. Clinical experience within the DSH system has yielded very few responders at fluphenazine levels significantly greater than 4.0 ng/ml, haloperidol levels above 30 ng/ml, and olanzapine levels above 200 ng/ml.

The principles listed above do not cover details such as the rapidity of titration or duration for any dosage, as these parameters are often dictated by clinical acuity. Recent analyses of industry-sponsored schizophrenia trials do indicate that, with respect to symptom reduction, the absence of any treatment effect after 2 weeks predicts nonresponse at week 6, and should prompt reconsideration of the treatment approach [30]. In many instances, the response to the lack of improvement will include documentation of plasma levels and consideration of dose increases when tolerability is not yet an issue. In patients who have failed high doses of high-potency first-generation antipsychotics with supporting plasma level data, olanzapine is an option for those who cannot or will not take clozapine, bearing in mind its inferiority to clozapine [11].

Case 1: A High-Dose Responder: Plasma Level Guided High-Dose Antipsychotic Therapy

The patient is a 50-year-old African-American female with a diagnosis of schizophrenia, and multiple medical problems including type 2 diabetes mellitus (DM), who was admitted to a forensic psychiatric hospital following a conviction for manslaughter. Owing to ongoing assaultiveness and suicidality, she was started on clozapine with significant clinical response, but also the development of poorly controlled DM, necessitating the withdrawal of clozapine therapy. Trials of other atypical antipsychotics at high dosages proved ineffective in managing her psychotic symptoms and violence, so the decision was made to embark on a course of high-dose haloperidol therapy, given her prior tolerance for lower dosages. Over several months, the patient was titrated to a daily dose of 45 mg with a marked reduction in psychotic symptoms, requirements for PRN medications, and acts of aggression toward herself and others. Neither EPS nor akathisia were evident, and she was not maintained on routine antiparkinsonian medication. A new psychiatrist assumed the patient's care and obtained a plasma haloperidol level of 29.5 ng/ml. Alarmed that this greatly exceeded the laboratory reference range (5–12 ng/ml), the haloperidol dose was decreased to 20 mg/d (plasma level 8.1 ng/ml). Over the next month, the patient deteriorated, started to refuse routine medication, and required numerous PRN medications for stability. The haloperidol dose was increased to 30 mg for several months, but the patient was frequently assaultive despite this dose increase and the addition of adjunctive lithium and lamotrigine. Another psychiatrist agreed to assume the patient's care, but the patient continued to intermittently refuse oral haloperidol, primarily for delusional reasons. The patient was convinced to try fluphenazine in lieu of haloperidol, and titrated to 20mg/d with a trough plasma level of 0.7 ng/ml, but limited clinical improvement. To increase the plasma level and also to limit any confounding issues related to adherence, fluphenazine decanoate was started at 25mg every 2 weeks, oral fluphenazine was tapered off, and the depot dose increased over ensuing months to 100mg every 2 weeks. With moderate improvement on this regimen and the absence of EPS and akathisia, the psychiatrist chose to supplement fluphenazine decanoate with oral fluphenazine 15 mg with marked reduction in psychosis and complete resolution of aggressive acts. The plasma fluphenazine level on this combination was in the range 3.0–3.2 ng/ml.

Commentary

Although a plasma haloperidol level of 29.5 ng/ml would be intolerable for the vast majority of patients, this patient clearly demonstrated both a requirement of, and tolerability for, a very high level of D_2 blockade, with significant clinical deterioration at lower antipsychotic levels. The latest treating psychiatrist correctly recognized the clinical situation and convinced the patient to try a similar medication to haloperidol, fluphenazine. The patient's response to a second high potency first-generation antipsychotic at extremely high plasma levels is consistent with the prior clinical history. The lack of significant adverse effects also supports continued fluphenazine treatment with dosages required to maintain a plasma fluphenazine level ≥ 3.0 ng/ml.

Case 2: High-Dose Failure: The Value of Plasma Levels

The patient is a 29-year-old Latino with a diagnosis of schizophrenia, who was admitted to a forensic psychiatric hospital after being found incompetent to stand trial on numerous charges including assault with a deadly weapon, criminal threats, and arson of an inhabited structure. The court commitment included an involuntary medication order in the case of treatment refusal. The patient was admitted to the hospital from custody on a combination of oral olanzapine 40 mg at bedtime and divalproex 1000 mg twice per day, but extent of adherence was unknown, and he was grossly psychotic in the admission suite, requiring intramuscular medications to control agitation. The medication combination started in jail was continued with good adherence, as documented by trough plasma olanzapine levels of 73 ng/ml and 79 ng/ml and therapeutic serum valproate levels, but on hospital day 12, the patient engaged in an unprovoked assault on a peer with serious injury, and required seclusion and restraints.

Given the severity of the assault, the ongoing significant level of psychotic symptoms, and records from a prior hospitalization that this patient tolerated oral haloperidol doses of 20 mg/d or more, a decision was made to load the patient on haloperidol decanoate while continuing olanzapine and divalproex at prior dosages. The most aggressive depot haloperidol load permissible in DSH facilities is 300mg weekly for three doses; this regimen is designed to mimic plasma levels achievable with 30 mg/d of oral haloperidol [28]. This dosing equivalency is an extrapolation of prior loading studies demonstrating that, after three weekly injections of haloperidol decanoate 100 mg, mean plasma haloperidol concentrations from the depot were comparable to 10 mg/d of oral haloperidol (7.95 ± 4.94 ng/ml vs. 7.79 ± 4.79 ng/ml) [31]. The three loading injections of 300 mg were administered in weekly intervals without evidence of adverse effects. Of note, a plasma haloperidol level obtained 1 week after the last loading injection (i.e., at T_{Max}) was 6.4 ng/ml. An assault occurred two days after the third loading injection, but the patient was subsequently free from assaultive behavior and continued to show no evidence of EPS or akathisia. However, his psychotic symptoms appeared to worsen slightly in the week prior to the scheduled maintenance depot dose, so haloperidol decanoate 300 mg was administered

22 days after the last loading injection. A haloperidol level obtained 4 days later was 2.8 ng/ml. The following week, this patient was again involved in a serious unprovoked assault that necessitated seclusion and restraints. A psychopharmacology consultation was obtained to assist with management. Based on the unexpectedly low plasma haloperidol levels obtained despite aggressive loading, it was concluded that this patient's inadequate response to haloperidol was a kinetic failure, but one that might not be easily overcome without the administration of extremely high weekly or biweekly injections of haloperidol decanoate – doses that would be unlikely to be continued outside of the forensic setting due to unfamiliarity with the rationale for a high-dose regimen in this patient. As this patient manifested expected plasma levels from oral olanzapine, a high-dose strategy for this medication was recommended, noting that doses of 60–80mg/d might be required to achieve plasma levels in the 100–150 ng/ml range, levels associated with 80%–85% D_2 occupancy.

Commentary

In the absence of plasma haloperidol levels, one might conclude that this patient was one of the unusual individuals who does not experience EPS or akathisia, and is likely a pharmacodynamic failure of haloperidol treatment. As noted above, an expected haloperidol level after three weekly loading doses of 100mg haloperidol decanoate is approximately 7 ng/ml [31]. The fact that this patient's haloperidol level 1 week after his third 300mg dose was 6.4 ng/ml was critical

to the conclusion that this patient was a kinetic failure, and most likely was an ultrarapid metabolizer for medications such as haloperidol that utilize cytochrome P450 (CYP) 2D6 [32], but not for those metabolized via CYP 1A2 (e.g., olanzapine) based on plasma olanzapine levels.

Conclusions

For treatment-resistant and violent patients with schizophrenia, there are limited therapeutic options, with clozapine and high antipsychotic plasma levels having the greatest evidence base. High plasma level antipsychotic therapy thus remains a viable strategy when employed in a rational manner as enumerated by the principles above. The appropriate use of plasma antipsychotic levels is central to the management of high-dose antipsychotic regimens, but must be complemented by documentation of changes in target symptoms and tolerability. Ongoing tolerability without efficacy represents a failure to achieve one of two firm clinical endpoints, and provides a sound basis for continued dose advancement despite what might be considered supratherapeutic plasma levels for average patients with schizophrenia.

Disclosures

Jonathan M. Meyer discloses the following: BMS, speaker, speaker's fee; Genetech, speaker, speaker's fee; Genetech, advisor, honoraria; Otsuka, speaker, speaker's fee.

References

1. Bollini P, Andreani A, Colombo F, et al. High-dose neuroleptics: uncontrolled clinical practice confirms controlled clinical trials. *Br. J. Psychiatry.* 1984; **144**(1): 25–27.

2. Mackay AVP. High-dose antipsychotic medication. *Advances in Psychiatric Treatment.* 1994; **1**(1): 16–23.

3. Krakowski MI, Kunz M, Czobor P, Volavka J. Long-term high-dose neuroleptic treatment: who gets it and why? *Hosp. Community Psychiatry.* 1993; **44**(7): 640–644.

4. Frogley C, Taylor D, Dickens G, Picchioni M. A systematic review of the evidence of clozapine's anti-aggressive effects. *Int. J. Neuropsychopharmacol..* 2012; **15**(9): 1351–1371.

5. Volavka J, Czobor P, Nolan K, et al. Overt aggression and psychotic symptoms in patients with schizophrenia treated with clozapine, olanzapine, risperidone, or haloperidol. *J. Clin. Psychopharmacol.* 2004; **24**(2): 225–228.

6. Royal College of Psychiatrists. *Consensus Statement on High-Dose Antipsychotic Medication.* Council Report CR138. London: Royal College of Psychiatrists; 2006.

7. Paton C, Barnes TR, Cavanagh MR, Taylor D, Lelliott P; POMH-UK project team. High-dose and combination antipsychotic prescribing in acute adult wards in the UK: the challenges posed by p. r.n. prescribing. *Br. J. Psychiatry.* 2008; **192**(6): 435–439.

8. Meyer JM. Drug–drug interactions with antipsychotics. *CNS Spectr.* 2007; **12**(suppl 21): 6–9.

9. Kirchheiner J, Schmidt H, Tzvetkov M, et al.

Pharmacokinetics of codeine and its metabolite morphine in ultra-rapid metabolizers due to CYP2D6 duplication. *Pharmacogenomics J.* 2007; **7**(4): 257–265.

10. Uchida H, Takeuchi H, Graff-Guerrero A, *et al.* Predicting dopamine D2 receptor occupancy from plasma levels of antipsychotic drugs: a systematic review and pooled analysis. *J. Clin. Psychopharmacol.* 2011; **31**(3): 318–325.

11. Krakowski MI, Czobor P, Citrome L, Bark N, Cooper TB. Atypical antipsychotic agents in the treatment of violent patients with schizophrenia and schizoaffective disorder. *Arch. Gen. Psychiatry.* 2006; **63**(6): 622–629.

12. Krakowski MI, Czobor P, Nolan KA. Atypical antipsychotics, neurocognitive deficits, and aggression in schizophrenic patients. *J. Clin. Psychopharmacol.* 2008; **28**(5): 485–493.

13. Glick ID, Balon RJ, Ballon J, Rovine D. Teaching pearls from the lost art of psychopharmacology. *J. Psychiatr. Pract.* 2009; **15**(5): 423–426.

14. Simpson GM, Kunz-Bartholini E. Relationship of individual tolerance, behavior and phenothiazine produced extrapyramidal system disturbance. *Dis. Nerv. Syst.* 1968; **29**(4): 269–274.

15. Merck under license to Forest Pharmaceuticals. Saphris [package insert]. St. Louis, MO: Forest Pharmaceuticals, Inc.; 2014.

16. Sunovion Pharmaceuticals, Inc. Latuda [package insert]. Marlborough, MA: Sunovion Pharmaceuticals, Inc.; 2013.

17. Haslemo T, Olsen K, Lunde H, Molden E. Valproic acid significantly lowers serum concentrations of olanzapine – an interaction effect comparable with

smoking. *Ther. Drug Monit.* 2012; **34**(5): 512–517.

18. Longo LP, Salzman C. Valproic acid effects on serum concentrations of clozapine and norclozapine. *Am. J. Psychiatry.* 1995; **152**(4): 650.

19. Coryell W, Miller DD, Perry PJ. Haloperidol plasma levels and dose optimization. *Am. J. Psychiatry.* 1998; **155**(1): 48–53.

20. Midha KK, Hubbard JW, Marder SR, Marshall BD, Van Putten T. Impact of clinical pharmacokinetics on neuroleptic therapy in patients with schizophrenia. *J. Psychiatry. Neurosci.* 1994; **19**(4): 254–264.

21. Perry PJ, Lund BC, Sanger T, Beasley C. Olanzapine plasma concentrations and clinical response: acute phase results of the North American Olanzapine Trial. *J. Clin. Psychopharmacol.* 2001; **21**(1): 14–20.

22. Gefvert O, Eriksson B, Persson P, *et al.* Pharmacokinetics and D2 receptor occupancy of long-acting injectable risperidone (Risperdal Consta) in patients with schizophrenia. *Int. J. Neuropsychopharmacol.* 2005; **8**(1): 27–36.

23. Mamo D, Kapur S, Keshavan M, *et al.* D2 receptor occupancy of olanzapine pamoate depot using positron emission tomography: an open-label study in patients with schizophrenia. *Neuropsychopharmacology.* 2008; **33**(2): 298–304.

24. Seto K, Dumontet J, Ensom MH. Risperidone in schizophrenia: is there a role for therapeutic drug monitoring? *Ther Drug Monit.* 2011; **33**(3): 275–283.

25. Hiemke C, Baumann P, Bergemann N, *et al.* AGNP consensus guidelines for therapeutic drug monitoring in psychiatry: update 2011. *Pharmacopsychiatry.* 2011; **44**(6): 195–235.

26. Salzman C, Glick ID, Keshavan MS. The 7 sins of psychopharmacology. *J. Clin. Psychopharmacol.* 2010; **30**(6): 653–655.

27. Kelly DL, Richardson CM, Yu Y, Conley RR. Plasma concentrations of high-dose olanzapine in a double-blind crossover study. *Hum. Psychopharmacol.* 2006; **21**(6): 393–398.

28. Meyer JM. Understanding depot antipsychotics: an illustrated guide to kinetics. *CNS Spectr.* 2013; **18**(Suppl 1): 55–68.

29. Van Putten T, Marder SR, Mintz J, Poland RE. Haloperidol plasma levels and clinical response: a therapeutic window relationship. *Am. J. Psychiatry.* 1992; **149**(4): 500–505.

30. Stauffer V, Case M, Kollack-Walker S, *et al.* Trajectories of response to treatment with atypical antipsychotic medication in patients with schizophrenia pooled from 6 double-blind, randomized clinical trials. *Schizophr. Res.* 2011; **130**(1–3): 11–19.

31. Wei FC, Jann MW, Lin HN, Piao-Chien C, Chang WH. A practical loading dose method for converting schizophrenic patients from oral to depot haloperidol therapy. *J. Clin. Psychiatry.* 1996; **57**(7): 298–302.

32. Panagiotidis G, Arthur HW, Lindh JD, Dahl ML, Sjoqvist F. Depot haloperidol treatment in outpatients with schizophrenia on monotherapy: impact of CYP2D6 polymorphism on pharmacokinetics and treatment outcome. *Ther. Drug Monit.* 2007; **29**(4): 417–422.

33. Kapur S, Zipursky R, Roy P, *et al.* The relationship between D2 receptor occupancy and plasma levels on low dose oral haloperidol: a PET study. *Psychopharmacology (Berl.).* 1997; **131**(2): 148–152.

34. Ereshefsky L, Mascarenas CA. Comparison of the effects of different routes of antipsychotic administration on pharmacokinetics and pharmacodynamics. *J. Clin. Psychiatry.* 2003; **64**(Suppl 16): 18–23.

35. Nyberg S, Farde L, Halldin C, Dahl ML, Bertilsson L. D2 dopamine receptor occupancy during low-dose treatment with haloperidol decanoate.

Am. J. Psychiatry. 1995; **152**(2): 173–178.

36. Levinson DF, Simpson GM, Lo ES, *et al.* Fluphenazine plasma levels, dosage, efficacy, and side effects. *Am. J. Psychiatry.* 1995; **152**(5): 765–771.

37. Marder SR, Midha KK, Van Putten T, *et al.* Plasma levels of fluphenazine in patients receiving fluphenazine decanoate: relationship to clinical response.

Br. J. Psychiatry. 1991; **158**(5): 658–665.

38. Ikai S, Remington G, Suzuki T, *et al.* A cross-sectional study of plasma risperidone levels with risperidone long-acting injectable: implications for dopamine D2 receptor occupancy during maintenance treatment in schizophrenia. *J. Clin. Psychiatry.* 2012; **73**(8): 1147–1152.

Chapter

23

Illustrative cases to support the Cal-VAT guidelines

Laura J. Dardashti, Eric H. Schwartz, Jennifer A. O'Day, Michael W. Barsom, and George J. Proctor

Introduction

Forensic hospital systems contain a significant number of patients who engage in acts of violence. Persistent aggressive behavior may be due to insufficient treatment of the various origins of such violence, which can include, but are not limited to, psychotic aggression, impulsive aggression due to mood disorders, schizophrenia, personality disorders, trauma or ADHD, and predatory aggression due to personality disorders [1]. While psychotic violence is the least difficult to treat, it is also the least frequently occurring form of violence, with impulsive being both the most common and most difficult to treat [2,3]. A complicating factor in the treatment of the violent patient is that many acts of aggression may be multifactorial – that is, patients may be driven to act by more than one of the three characterized forms of violence. Conventional use of psychotropic medications is often insufficient in adequately controlling violence [4], or there is hesitation on the part of treating psychiatrists to use recommended treatments such as clozapine for those that are refractory [5]. This hesitation may be due to concerns about patient compliance with blood draws, lack of familiarity in use of the medication, discomfort with managing its potential side effects, and/or fear that the medication will be discontinued if the patient is transferred back to a correctional facility. Furthermore, forensic hospital settings are limited, in some cases, in providing the appropriate environmental milieu that may serve to mitigate violent acts.

The following is a series of seven cases that illustrate the various psychopharmacological, therapeutic, and environmental interventions discussed in the California State Hospital Violence Assessment and Treatment (Cal-VAT) guidelines [6] and employed to treat each patient's violence. All individuals were or are inpatients in smoke-free facilities with limited access to caffeinated beverages. These cases represent some of the most difficult-to-treat patients within the state hospital setting, but also provide hope for the provider in that, with aggressive and appropriate treatment, violence can be significantly reduced if not completely eliminated.

Case 1: Psychotic Violence Requiring High-Dose Antipsychotic Therapy

Description

The patient is a 44-year-old, African-American woman who was admitted to a forensic psychiatric hospital as incompetent to stand trial for alleged arson of an inhabited structure, battery, and exhibiting a deadly weapon. Upon admission, she was found to be argumentative and paranoid. Her risk for violence was elevated due to her irritability, sensitivity to provocation, and being easily angered when requests were denied. She also experienced auditory hallucinations of her name being whispered and visual hallucinations of snakes. She was an unreliable historian, and no records were available for review. Admission laboratory analyses were unremarkable, except for being hepatitis C positive. Her urine admission drug screen was negative, and she refused to have an electrocardiogram.

Despite several weeks of adherence to olanzapine 20 mg (increased to 40 mg) and mirtazapine 30 mg, she remained irritable, paranoid, and violent. She engaged in repeated verbal threats and occasional episodes of physical aggression, resulting in five-point restraints on one occasion, wrist-to-waist restraints on two occasions, and a period of one-to-one nursing

Violence in Psychiatry, ed. Katherine D. Warburton and Stephen M. Stahl. Published by Cambridge University Press.
© Cambridge University Press 2016.

observation. Mirtazapine was discontinued as it was deemed unnecessary and was possibly promoting irritability via enhancing norepinephrine release. It was difficult to determine whether the removal of mirtazapine had an appreciable effect on her irritability, since she had an increase in olanzapine to 50 mg at the same time. After steady state was established on a daily dose of 50 mg, her AM trough olanzapine plasma concentration was measured at 78 ng/ml. Olanzapine was then increased to 60 mg to achieve an increased olanzapine plasma concentration with an ultimate target plasma concentration greater than 100 ng/ml, if clinical response at lower concentrations was inadequate. After 11 days, she was no longer paranoid and reported that her auditory and visual hallucinations were gone; however no olanzapine level was obtained at the 60 mg dose. Clonazepam 1.5 mg and quetiapine 50 mg were added after several days on the increased olanzapine dose to assist with residual irritability and initial insomnia, respectively. Her cognitive ability to learn court-related material improved, although she would occasionally become loud and intrusive. Divalproex sodium, extended release, was initiated with the dose titrated to target her irritable and intrusive episodes. An AM trough valproic acid serum concentration of 72 mcg/ml was achieved while on a daily dose of 1500 mg, and she became calmer within 17 days of starting the medication. She was discharged and returned to court 3 months after admission. The prescribed medication regimen at discharge included olanzapine 50 mg daily, divalproex 1500 mg daily, clonazepam 1.5 mg daily, and quetiapine 50 mg each evening.

Commentary

A high dose of olanzapine helped to control this patient's psychosis and reduced the majority of her violence. The addition of divalproex was effective in alleviating her residual irritability and intrusiveness. Since some patients have shown tolerability and efficacy with higher-than-typical antipsychotic blood levels, correlating with D_2 receptor occupancy in the upper ranges of tolerability (80% and greater), it is possible that reaching the targeted olanzapine plasma concentration of 100 ng/ml would have avoided the need for additional medication [7]. In addition, the use of valproic acid or divalproex should target a plasma concentration of 80–120 mcg/ml to allow sufficient non-protein-bound valproic acid to have its optimal CNS effect [8].

An alternative explanation to the patient's responsiveness to divalproex and benefit from stopping mirtazapine, is that the patient suffered from a bipolar spectrum disorder. If a therapeutic trial of medication directed at signs and symptoms of a diagnosis lacks efficacy, revisiting the diagnostic formulation should be considered, in addition to efforts to augment the initial medication trial. Nevertheless, the patient's presentation and antipsychotic response to high-dose olanzapine appeared most consistent with her psychotic violence being driven by a schizophrenia spectrum disorder.

Case 2: Treatment-Resistant Psychotic Violence Responding to Clozapine
Description

The patient is a 48-year-old, Hispanic male with a longstanding history of schizophrenia who was admitted to a forensic psychiatric hospital as not guilty by reason of insanity for assaulting his board and care roommate due to his delusions. Prior to hospital admission, he had been taking fluphenazine decanoate 50 mg intramuscularly (IM) every 2 weeks, fluoxetine 20 mg daily, quetiapine 200 mg twice daily, and benztropine 1 mg twice daily. He had previously had trials of olanzapine, ziprasidone, quetiapine, divalproex, and lithium. His medical conditions included hepatitis C and an extensive history of substance abuse, including alcohol, cannabis, cocaine, inhalants, opiates, and methamphetamine.

Upon admission, he was unkempt, paranoid, and reported having command auditory hallucinations. Laboratory analysis was done at admission, and the following abnormalities were noted: platelets 103×10^3/ul (low); uric acid 7.5 mg/dl (high); ALT 49 u/l (high); AST 52 u/l (high); amylase 320 u/l (high); and hepatitis C RNA quantitative PCR 6.2 log IU (high). His lipase level was within normal limits, and amylase isoenzyme analysis revealed normal pancreatic amylase isoenzymes with elevated salivary isoenzymes. He was prescribed quetiapine 500 mg daily, fluphenazine decanoate 50 mg IM every 2 weeks, lithium carbonate 600 mg each evening, and temazepam 30 mg each evening. Quetiapine was increased to 800 mg daily after 14 days due to frequent episodes of psychomotor agitation in response to psychotic stimuli. Later, olanzapine 20 mg was added due to ongoing psychosis and agitation. His liver transaminase enzymes normalized, as did his amylase, within 30 days of admission. Despite continued low platelets, a trial of divalproex sodium (extended release) was initiated to augment the antipsychotic medication; however, tremor and transaminase elevations led to its discontinuation after one week. Lithium was stopped due to tremor, as well.

His episodic agitation and violence due to unremitting psychosis remained problematic. The daily dose of olanzapine was increased to 60 mg, 47 days after admission, and quetiapine was decreased to 200 mg daily. He remained intrusive (would stand over patients' beds at night and stand close to them during the day), would frequently curse loudly to himself and at staff without provocation, and would occasionally strike peers and staff. He had steady state plasma concentrations of fluphenazine 0.6 ng/ml and olanzapine >200 ng/ml with extrapyramidal side effects in the form of parkinsonism without akathisia or dystonia.

Owing to his treatment-resistant psychosis, his treating psychiatrist initiated a clozapine trial, as olanzapine and quetiapine were tapered and discontinued. Clozapine was titrated to a dose of 300 mg daily, resulting in a trough clozapine plasma concentration of 799 ng/m with mild sialorrhea. The patient's psychosis persisted. However, his cursing decreased, and he was no longer threatening and hitting others. After 8 weeks on the same dose of clozapine, his auditory hallucinations and visual hallucinations were substantially decreased. His clozapine plasma concentrations ranged from 688–850 ng/ml on the same dose, and the medication was well tolerated with episodes of violence remaining absent for over a year to date.

Commentary

This patient had a notably low fluphenazine plasma concentration (0.6 ng/ml) when measured at the hospital. When fluoxetine was discontinued upon admission, the fluphenazine metabolism was no longer inhibited via fluoxetine's influence on CYP2D6, leading to a decline in the fluphenazine plasma concentration of roughly 50%. Checking for this pharmacokinetic drug–drug interaction and measuring a baseline fluphenazine plasma concentration upon admission would have allowed maintenance of fluphenazine plasma concentrations within the therapeutic range. Nevertheless, this patient's psychosis persisted during antipsychotic trials both in the hospital and prior facility, leading to a clozapine trial. Clozapine has a superior response rate compared to other antipsychotics for treatment-resistant schizophrenia and shows efficacy in decreasing aggressive behavior independent of its antipsychotic properties [9-11].

Case 3: Impulsive Violence Requiring Control of Psychosis, Attention, and Psychosocial Skills

Description

The patient is a 51-year-old, African-American male who was admitted to a psychiatric forensic hospital after he was found not guilty by reason of insanity for attempted rape. After admission to the hospital, he was continued on oral haloperidol 10 mg twice daily and valproic acid 2000 mg each evening. Admission laboratory tests revealed normal chemistries and a negative urine drug screen. The electrocardiogram on admission showed nonspecific T wave abnormalities with a ventricular rate of 79 bpm and QT/QTc of 389/396 msec.

The patient had a history of ADHD with impulsiveness and aggression beginning in adolescence. His level of aggression in his youth led to criminal charges and institutionalization beginning at 14 years of age. Later in adolescence, he developed a psychotic illness with persecutory delusions that progressed into a schizophrenia-spectrum disorder. His clinical picture was complicated by the presence of borderline intellectual functioning. Previous medication trials included chlorpromazine, fluphenazine, loxapine, risperidone, paliperidone, paliperidone palmitate, olanzapine, quetiapine, thiothixene, fluoxetine, paroxetine, mirtazapine, lithium carbonate, valproic acid, lamotrigine, gabapentin, tiagabine, clonidine, and buspirone.

His history of treatment with a variety of antipsychotics and mood stabilizers in both monotherapy and polypharmacy resulted in a partial response at best, with his psychosis showing only a modest improvement in response to medication. However, his aggression and impulsivity persisted. Medications used in the course of his current hospitalization included olanzapine, fluphenazine decanoate, and lithium carbonate. Consistent with his prior history, his psychosis improved, but the agitation and impulsive aggression continued.

Once his psychosis was under moderate control, he was assigned a nursing staff member (Behavioral Change Agent, BCA) who would spend one shift daily working with the patient to assist him with the use of coping strategies other than aggression. The BCA would interface with other team members to provide greater consistency in the behavioral approach to the patient. The assigned nursing staff member (BCA) assisted the patient and his team in recognizing his triggers to violence that led to a modest reduction in threats, though his PRN medication use increased. Despite the use of the BCA, the patient continued to engage in violence against his treatment team. The addition of methylphenidate extended release (Concerta ER) appeared to improve his concentration and attention, and his BCA observed that the patient had an improved ability to implement use of his coping strategies. At that point, his medication regimen included olanzapine 50 mg each evening, divalproex (extended release) 2500 mg each evening (switched from lithium due to lithium-related tremors), fluphenazine decanoate 75 mg every 14 days, and methylphenidate extended release 54 mg daily.

He was enrolled in a multifaceted neurocognitive and social cognition training program for patients with psychiatric disorders and severe cognitive needs and challenges. The program was specifically designed to target aggression to self and others. His medication regimen remained stable, and he continued to have the services of the BCA while also attending the new aggression-reduction program. His use of PRN medications decreased from 78 in the 21 months prior to starting the program to a total of 8 in the 36 months while enrolled. His episodes of seclusion/restraint dropped to zero from a baseline of two occurrences per year. His aggressive acts showed a reduction from his average of 4.5 serious episodes per year to only one incident in the current year.

Commentary

Violence that persists after controlling the psychosis is predatory or impulsive. Since this patient's violence was impulsive, enhancing attention with a stimulant seemed to, indeed, improve attention, but this addition was not sufficient alone. Structured psychosocial and cognitive skills programs were required to obtain the most substantial reductions in violence [12-14].

Case 4: Predatory Violence Exceeding Security Capacity of Hospital Setting
Description

The patient is a 45-year-old, African-American male who was admitted to a forensic psychiatric hospital when he was 23-years-old after being found not guilty by reason of insanity for entering a home he believed he owned and threatening the homeowner with a knife.

Upon admission, the patient was disheveled, guarded, and reported persecutory delusions, ideas of reference, and thought broadcasting. He had several healed fractures from prior fights but no other medical conditions. Admission laboratory tests were unremarkable, showing values within normal limits.

His history of mental illness began at 16-years-old with his experience of auditory hallucinations. Characteristic signs and symptoms of his illness consisted of auditory hallucinations, persecutory delusions, grandiose delusions, disorganized thinking, disorganized behavior, social isolation, assaults, and sexually inappropriate behaviors. His course of illness had been complicated by substance abuse, including early adolescent use of alcohol, cannabis, and inhalants. Later in adolescence, he began abusing methamphetamine, psilocybin, and cocaine.

His psychosis improved early in the course of hospitalization. He was treated with haloperidol 10 mg twice daily (later, converted to haloperidol decanoate 200 mg IM every 28 days due to his refusal to take oral haloperidol), valproic acid 1500 mg twice daily (targeting his affective fluctuations, often in response to internal stimuli), clonazepam 1 mg twice daily (targeting his irritability), and trazodone 400 mg each evening (for insomnia). His auditory hallucinations disappeared, and he had significant improvement in the level of organization of his speech and behavior. He continued to experience some persecutory delusions with occasional ideas of reference that other people were talking about him when he passed them.

Despite the improvement in his psychosis, he made frequent threats toward staff and peers when his desires were not met. He was involved in several physical altercations with peers and assaulted a staff member early in his hospitalization. He also engaged in rules violations, such as gambling, smoking on the unit, collecting contraband items, and making sexually inappropriate remarks and gestures, such as masturbating in front of staff, touching female staff on the breasts and buttocks, and soliciting sexual favors from them. His level of violence increased during his hospitalization, such that he assaulted a peer with an object, striking him repeatedly in the head and face. Ten days later, he went on to attack several staff members, injuring two of them severely. He was convicted of assault and sent to serve a term in prison.

Upon his return to the forensic inpatient setting, he resumed many of the same behaviors, including rules violations, threats, and assaults. His psychotic symptoms remained well controlled; however, his disruptive behaviors and violence increased after the psychosis improved. The frequency and severity of his violence increased to the point that he required unit transfers approximately every 3 months. Several attempts were made to guide him toward more pro-social conduct, including skills building, anger management group participation, and the development of individualized behavior plans on various units. He was referred to the behavior specialist team that assisted in the development and implementation of his behavior plans. He showed an initial decrease in physically aggressive episodes per month (from eight to five, at one point). However, such improvements were short-lived.

Due to his persistent violence in the hospital setting, he was assessed by a forensic examiner for referral to a prison setting. The examiner noted that the patient had 33 incidents of threats, sexually inappropriate behavior, and violence over the 1 month period prior to his forensic evaluation. As a result, he was transferred to a prison setting, where he has been less violent and disruptive according to prison records.

Commentary

Controlling this patient's psychosis resulted in an increase of aggression and violence. The pattern of rules violations and lack of effort to engage in pro-social behaviors in the absence of psychosis pointed to predatory violence. After failing on multiple treatment units within the hospital, his behaviors were determined to exceed the security capacity of the hospital, necessitating a more secure setting to minimize the impact of his violence on those in his environment [15].

Case 5: Impulsive, Severe, Self-Injurious Behavior Responsive to Dialectical Behavioral and High-Dose Depot Neuroleptic Treatment

Description

The patient is a 49-year-old, Caucasian female who was admitted on a civil commitment to a forensic psychiatric hospital after recurrent community hospitalizations for self-injury and suicide attempts. Her diagnoses included recurrent major depressive disorder and borderline personality disorder. She also had a significant history of violence resulting in prior felony convictions for criminal threats and assault and battery on hospital staff and emergency personnel while in the community. Owing to her severe self-injurious and violent behavior, she required continuous 2:1 observation during a several-year-long stay at a previous state psychiatric hospital. In addition to her complicated and lengthy psychiatric history, she had multiple medical problems, including morbid obesity, metabolic syndrome, and large, self-inflicted wounds of the abdominal wall, inguinal area, and popliteal fossa.

Prior to her current hospitalization, she had had trials of atypical and typical antipsychotics, as well as mood stabilizers, anxiolytics, and antidepressants, all with reportedly little change in her impulsivity, suicidality, and aggression. On admission, she was prescribed chlorpromazine 50 mg twice a day, clonazepam 2 mg daily, and fluoxetine 60 mg daily along with lorazepam 2 mg PO or IM every 6 hours as needed for agitation or anxiety. Medications were adjusted over the next year to address ongoing aggressive and violent behaviors. Chlorpromazine was increased to 300 mg four times a day. Fluoxetine was increased to 80 mg daily, clonazepam was tapered off, and lamotrigine was added at doses up to 200 mg twice daily without noted side effects. Prior to that, she was given a brief trial of olanzapine 10 mg at bedtime.

Despite medication adjustments, she continued to have frequent periods of agitation and aggression toward others and herself. Her self-injurious behaviors included digging into already open wounds in her abdomen and inguinal areas. She would physically assault staff who attempted to stop her during her process of further enlarging her wounds as well as threaten to lacerate her femoral artery, which was easily accessible at that point. She continued to require continuous 2:1 observation and frequent PRN medications to treat her agitation and aggression as well as regular use of restraints to curb her dangerous behaviors.

The patient was transferred to a dialectical behavioral therapy (DBT) unit. Chlorpromazine and lamotrigine were tapered off, and fluphenazine decanoate was initiated and titrated up to 100 mg every 2 weeks to target her impulsive aggression. A long-acting injectable was chosen due to her history of medication nonadherence. Fluoxetine was discontinued in exchange for mirtazapine 30 mg nightly due to continued sleep complaints. Continuous use of wrist-to-waist restraints was implemented to decrease her compulsive self-injurious behaviors. Her observation level was able to be tapered down from a 2:1 to 1:1, and she was able to remain safe during periods off 1:1 observation and while out of wrist-to-waist restraints. Though remaining hospitalized, her high-risk behaviors were drastically reduced, including aggressive behaviors toward herself and others, and her wounds were able to begin to heal. She had a decreased need for restraints and PRN medication administration.

Commentary

The use of mirtazapine as an antidepressant was chosen for its 5HT2A antagonism. That antagonism serves to mitigate the risk of EPS/akathisia [16], which allowed fluphenazine to be more tolerable, given the patient's need for high therapeutic doses of neuroleptic agents to target her extreme impulsive aggression, which had been previously nonresponsive to alternative antipsychotic agents. Furthermore, adjunctive treatment with inpatient dialectical behavioral therapy and use of chronic wrist-to-waist restraints were critical and necessary in decreasing her impulsive aggressive behaviors.

Case 6: Impulsive and Predatory Violence Responding to Clozapine and Lithium

Description

The patient is a 21-year-old, Hispanic female who was re-hospitalized on a civil commitment to a forensic psychiatric hospital following a year-long incarceration for an organized assault on another patient during her previous hospitalization. The patient had a history of posttraumatic stress disorder, major depressive disorder, borderline personality disorder, and antisocial personality disorder, with at least 23 acute psychiatric hospitalizations beginning in her early teens and for depressive symptoms and self-injurious behavior. She had a known history of intense, unstable interpersonal relationships, identity disturbance, impulsivity, chronic feelings of emptiness, and difficulty controlling her anger. She would engage in parasuicidal and suicidal behaviors, such as cutting and tying ligatures around her neck, in response to her perceived abandonment by family members. She reported psychotic symptoms in the form of auditory hallucinations. Additionally she complained of nightmares and flashbacks of her childhood sexual abuse by caretakers while in the foster care system where she had been placed at a young age. Her physical medical history was significant for asthma.

Upon readmission, her medication regimen included citalopram 20 mg daily, valproic acid 500 mg twice daily, and quetiapine that was increased from 350 mg daily to 800 mg daily. However, her aggression toward herself and others persisted. Quetiapine was cross-titrated with olanzapine, but she continued to show episodes of aggression to self and unprovoked violence toward patients and staff, which also appeared predatory with evidence of planning and organization. In some of her violent incidents, she changed into more comfortable clothes prior to attacking, while other incidents of violence appeared impulsive, often reactive to her own feelings of agitation or her misinterpretation of interpersonal interactions. Her complaints of depressive symptoms, including thoughts of suicide and parasuicidal/suicidal gestures, continued and occasionally necessitated 1:1 observation. Additionally, she had insomnia and irritability with continued complaints of auditory hallucinations.

Due to her persistent violent behaviors, it was determined that she should be treated in a more secure setting to minimize the impact of her violence on those in her environment. She was transferred to a penal code unit within the hospital with the goal of the new environment shaping her behavior. The main difference between the civil and penal code units is the presence of higher functioning forensic patients who are less easily victimized, rather than any structural or security differences.

Upon transfer to the forensic setting, her medication regimen was changed. Olanzapine was discontinued, and treatment with quetiapine 600 mg (crushed) twice a day was resumed. Citalopram was continued, and valproic acid was discontinued due to her complaints of side effects and questionable efficacy. Treatment with prazosin for her nightmares was initiated; the dose was titrated up to 4 mg at bedtime, and the medication proved effective. After a 60-day period without aggression, she was transferred back to her prior unit in a nonforensic setting.

Upon transfer, her aggressive behavior resumed, necessitating the frequent use of restraints and seclusion, and leading to the addition of clozapine that was titrated up to 450 mg daily (AM trough level of 805 ng/ml at steady state) with concomitant taper and discontinuation of quetiapine. Lithium was also added to her medication regimen with the dose titrated up to 1200 mg daily (level of 0.3 mEq/l). In addition to these medications, the patient continued to be prescribed prazosin and citalopram. She was also started on levothyroxine 75 mcg daily for hypothyroidism and metformin 500 mg twice daily for pre-diabetes.

During the 5 months of gradual dose increases of clozapine and lithium, her acts of aggression diminished and her depressive symptoms improved. Prior to clozapine, she had 25 aggressive acts to others (14 toward peers and 11 toward staff) and 30 aggressive act to self (29 aggressive acts to self and 1 suicide attempt) over a 7-month period. After treatment with clozapine was initiated, she had three aggressive acts to others (two toward peers and one toward staff) and four aggressive acts to self and no suicide attempts over the remaining 9 months of her hospitalization. Two months after clozapine initiation, she began to actively participate in her work assignment three times a week without any problems. Three months after clozapine initiation, she demonstrated enough stability and improvement in her symptoms to be eligible to go on day passes and even home visits with her family without any behavior problems and began attending dialectical behavioral therapy (DBT) groups regularly. Her improvement resulted in her discharge from the hospital to a less secure setting with discharge medications of clozapine 450 mg daily, lithium 1200 mg daily, prazosin 4 mg at bedtime, and citalopram 40 mg daily.

Commentary

This patient showed decreased violence and improved behavior in response to placement among a higher functioning patient population, but this improvement was short-lived. While she had micro-psychotic symptoms characteristic of borderline personality disorder, her violence was consistent with having both predatory and impulsive elements. In response to the addition of clozapine at therapeutic levels and lithium at antidepressant augmentation levels, the patient had a marked decrease in her agitation and violence. Not only has clozapine been found to reduce aggression in patients with schizophrenia, but it has also been found to reduce violence in those with psychopathy [17]. Her reduction in self-harm/suicide attempts can be related to the beneficial effects of both clozapine and lithium [18,19].

Case 7: Treatment-Resistant Psychotic Violence Responding to Clozapine
Description

The patient is a 31-year-old, Caucasian male who was committed to a forensic psychiatric hospital with diagnoses of schizophrenia and antisocial personality disorder. The patient had a significant history of violence toward others, including assault with a deadly weapon and battery.

Initially upon hospitalization, he was noted to have prominent psychotic symptoms, including disorganized thought processes and behaviors and aggression attributed to persecutory delusions. The patient was treated with doses of haloperidol and olanzapine, which resulted in high plasma levels of these medications and a resultant significant reduction in psychotic symptoms over a period of 12 months. However, he continued to have episodes of impulsive aggression. He was unpredictable and easily angered, often rapidly escalating from calm to threatening with prominent psychomotor agitation. He was also verbally abusive and difficult to redirect with ongoing staff concerns over his behavior escalating into significant violence. This impulsive aggression precluded him from participating in group therapy sessions because of the risk of violence. However, these group therapy sessions were necessary for him to transition to an outpatient setting. For 9 months his medication regimen remained unchanged and included olanzapine 65 mg daily (olanzapine blood levels ranged from 119–161 ng/ml), haloperidol 40 mg daily (haloperidol blood levels ranged from 24–33 ng/ml), and mirtazapine 30 mg daily. He tolerated the antipsychotics without any extrapyramidal symptoms (EPS), and pertinent laboratory tests remained normal with no signs or symptoms of metabolic syndrome. He also had a 7-month trial of valproic acid at adequate serum values without impact on his impulsive aggression.

After 24 months of inpatient hospitalization, clozapine was started in an attempt to reduce his impulsive aggression. Over a period of 24 days, the dose of clozapine was titrated to 250 mg daily with a final clozapine plasma level of 188 ng/ml and norclozapine level of 109 ng/ml. Concurrently, olanzapine was crosstapered to 25 mg daily with a plan to ultimately discontinue it. Haloperidol was continued at 40 mg daily.

Throughout the clozapine titration, the treatment team noticed a significant change in his demeanor, as his volatility and unprovoked aggressive outbursts were eliminated. He was calm and respectful toward others without any threatening behaviors and with complete remission of his impulsive aggression. Six weeks after starting the clozapine titration and after a total of 25.5 months of inpatient hospitalization, he was successfully discharged to a forensic psychiatric outpatient setting on oral daily doses of clozapine 250 mg with a clozapine plasma level of 188 ng/ml, haloperidol 40 mg, and olanzapine 25 mg.

Commentary

This patient tolerated high plasma-level haloperidol and olanzapine therapy with a resultant decrease in psychotic disorganization, but his ability to move to a less restrictive level of care was hindered by continuing impulsive aggression. The impulsive aggression was ultimately eliminated after the initiation of treatment with clozapine. Psychopharmacological treatment assisted the patient in becoming mentally available for additional forms of psychosocial treatment.

Discussion

These cases serve to illustrate the various modalities employed in the treatment of the three types of violence. The utility of prescribing clozapine in the treatment of psychotic violence as well as impulsive and predatory types is elucidated, as many cases demonstrate its positive outcome. Psychiatrists often avoid prescribing clozapine because they lack experience and knowledge of the medication or they give far more weight to the risks over benefits of its use [5]. An underappreciated benefit of clozapine is its ability to reduce violence aside from its antipsychotic and sedative properties [10,20]. Awareness of clozapine's aggression-reducing properties may help to increase its use and ultimately lead to improved quality of lives for patients and improved overall safety of forensic mental health facilities. The initiation of treatment with clozapine for patients demonstrating impulsive aggression should be considered early in the course of treatment due to the demonstrated efficacy.

In the cases of predatory violence, placement of the patient in a more secure environment is critical in reducing acts of aggression [6], as well as in providing a more therapeutic environment for staff and other patients on the unit.

Other pharmacologic treatments employed included the use of high-dose antipsychotics, long-acting injectable antipsychotics, stimulants to enhance concentration, and mood stabilizers, particularly valproic acid and lithium. The use of these medications in conjunction with therapeutic modalities appropriate for the type of violence (i.e., DBT for impulsive violence associated with borderline personality disorder) appears to be particularly effective in further reducing aggressive acts and giving the patient the best chance of reducing violence relapse.

Disclosures

The authors do not have anything to disclose.

References

1. Dack C, Ross J, Papadopoulos C, Stewart D, Bowers L. A review and meta-analysis of the patient factors associated with psychiatric in-patient aggression. *Acta Psychiatr. Scand.* 2013; **127**(4): 255–268.

2. Nolan KA, Czobor P, Roy BB, *et al.* Characteristics of assaultive behavior among psychiatric inpatients. *Psychiatr. Serv.* 2003; **54**(7): 1012–1016.

3. Quanbeck CD, McDermott BE, Lam J, *et al.* Categorization of aggressive acts committed by chronically assaultive state hospital patients. *Psychiatr. Serv.* 2007; **58**(4): 521–528.

4. Morrissette DA, Stahl SM. Treating the violent patient with psychosis or impulsivity utilizing antipsychotic polypharmacy and high-dose monotherapy. *CNS Spectr.* 2014; **19**(5): 439–448.

5. Nielsen J, Dahm M, Lublin H, Taylor D. Psychiatrists' attitude towards and knowledge of clozapine treatment. *J. Psychopharmacol.* 2010; **24**(7): 965–971.

6. Stahl SM, Morrissette DA, Cummings M, *et al.* California State Hospital Violence Assessment and Treatment (Cal-VAT) guidelines. *CNS Spectr.* 2014; **19**(5): 449–465.

7. Kelly DL, Richardson CM, Yu Y, Conley RR. Plasma concentrations of high-dose olanzapine in a double-blind crossover study. *Hum. Psychopharmacol.* 2006; **21**(6): 393–398.

8. Hirschfeld RM, Allen MH, McEvoy JP, Keck PE Jr, Russell JM. Safety and tolerability of oral loading divalproex sodium in acutely manic bipolar patients. *J. Clin. Psychiatry.* 1999; **60**(12): 815–818.

9. Kane J, Honigfeld G, Singer J, Meltzer H. Clozapine for the treatment-resistant schizophrenic: a double-blind comparison with chlorpromazine. *Arch. Gen. Psychiatry.* 1988; **45**(9): 789–796.

10. Volavka J, Czobor P, Nolan K, *et al.* Overt aggression and psychotic symptoms in patients with schizophrenia treated with clozapine, olanzapine, risperidone, or haloperidol. *J. Clin. Psychopharmacol.* 2004; **24**(2): 225–228.

11. Frogley C, Taylor D, Dickens G, Picchioni M. A systematic review of the evidence of clozapine's anti-aggressive effects. *Int. J. Neuropsychopharmacol.* 2012; **15**(9): 1351–1371.

12. Shelton D, Sampl S, Kesten KL, Zhang W, Trestman RL. Treatment of impulsive aggression in correctional settings. *Behav. Sci. Law.* 2009; **27**(5): 787–800.

13. Heinrichs RW, Zakzanis KK. Neurocognitive deficit in schizophrenia: a quantitative review of the evidence. *Neuropsychology.* 1998; **12**(3): 426–445.

14. Keefe RS, Bilder RM, Harvey PD, *et al.* Baseline neurocognitive deficits in the CATIE schizophrenia trial. *Neuropsychopharmacology.* 2006; **31**(9): 2033–2046.

15. Kennedy HG. Therapeutic uses of security: mapping forensic mental health services by stratifying risk. *Advances in Psychiatric Treatment.* 2002; **8**(6): 433–443.

16. Hieber R, Dellenbaugh T, Nelson LA. Role of mirtazapine in the treatment of antipsychotic-induced akathisia. *Ann. Pharmacother.* 2008; **42**(6): 841–846.

17. Brown D, Larkin F, Sengupta S. Clozapine: an effective treatment for seriously violent and psychopathic men with antisocial personality disorder in a UK high-security hospital. *CNS Spectr.* 2014; **19**(5): 391–402.

18. Meltzer HY, Alphs L, Green AI, *et al.* Clozapine treatment for suicidality in schizophrenia: International Suicide Prevention Trial (InterSePT). *Arch. Gen. Psychiatry.* 2003; **60**(1): 82–91.

19. Baldessarini R, Tondo L, Davis P, *et al.* Decreased risk of suicides and attempts during long-term lithium treatment: a meta-analytic review. *Bipolar Disord.* 2006; **8**(5 Pt 2): 625–639.

20. Krakowski MI, Czobor P, Citrome L, Bark N, Cooper TB. Atypical antipsychotic agents in the treatment of violent patients with schizophrenia and schizoaffective disorder. *Arch. Gen. Psychiatry.* 2006; **63**(6): 622–629.

24

A new standard of care for forensic mental health treatment: prioritizing forensic intervention

Katherine D. Warburton

Introduction

Forensic populations are increasing; however, mental health treatment paradigms have not changed to accommodate this new population. The recovery principles that currently guide psychiatric delivery systems do not account for forensic environments, which are in themselves "settings in which self-determination is already strongly curtailed," nor do they answer the question of how a system designed to divert individuals from legal consequences based on their lack of competency or responsibility can at the same time be treated with a model that emphasizes full agency [1]. This leads to a paradox for forensic hospital systems that are simultaneously trying to meet treatment standards grounded in recovery philosophy while at the same time addressing the unique needs of a forensic population (see Table 24.1).

How Should State Hospitals Treat Forensic Patients? Is This an Unsolvable Problem?

There is a new forensic population housed in state hospital systems. Many of these state hospitals are older facilities that employ clinical policies developed during the reforms of the 1960s and 1970s. These "state" hospitals are often now referred to as "forensic hospitals," most often due to the changed patient population rather than any updated infrastructure or practice. In general, state hospital systems have multiple oversight mechanisms. Despite these strict monitoring practices, state/forensic hospitals can be plagued with problems, most notably inpatient violence, which frequently makes national headlines (sometimes international headlines), creating a treatment paradox in forensic psychiatry [2–20].

For example, a single week of national headlines in 2014 illustrates the current problems confronted by facilities that are trying to deliver humane mental health services to populations with high levels of inpatient violence. On one day, the Hartford Courant reported on the controversial placement of a patient found not guilty by reason of insanity, because he was held on bail at a correctional institution rather than returned to the state/forensic hospital where he had allegedly committed numerous serious assaults on patients and other staff. The patient was suing to return to the state/forensic hospital citing an entitlement to treatment [21]. At issue was his level of violence risk and the inability of the hospital to provide the same level of safety as the correctional setting. The following day, the Associated Press reported that four Hawaii State Hospital employees were suing the state due to the unsafe work environment created by assaultive psychiatric inpatients in their state hospital [22]. Later that same week, the Portland Press Herald reported on a controversy involving the allegedly punitive and controlling environment at the state/forensic hospital in Maine; in the same article, a psychiatrist on staff described the forensic unit as the most dangerous inpatient psychiatric unit that he had ever seen [23]. Thus, three state/forensic hospitals attempted to handle the same situation (uncontrollable violence in inpatient forensic populations) three different ways, and all three approaches were flawed, controversial, and worthy of media attention. This week was not an anomaly; the issue of inpatient violence, especially among forensic patients and especially in state/forensic hospitals, has been widely reported in the media over recent years [2–23]. This is

Violence in Psychiatry, ed. Katherine D. Warburton and Stephen M. Stahl. Published by Cambridge University Press.
© Cambridge University Press 2016.

Table 24.1 The forensic paradox

Recovery principles [55]	Forensic commitment criteria [56–59]
Recovery is person-driven. Self-determination and self-direction are the foundations for recovery as individuals define their own life goals and design their unique path(s) toward those goals. Individuals optimize their autonomy and independence to the greatest extent possible by leading, controlling, and exercising choice over the services and supports that assist their recovery and resilience. In so doing, they are empowered and provided the resources to make informed decisions, initiate recovery, build on their strengths, and gain or regain control over their lives.	The defendant is unable to understand the charges and/or does not have the ability to aid attorney in own defense. It must be clearly proved that, at the time of the committing of the act, the party accused was laboring under such a defect of reason, from disease of the mind, as not to know the nature and quality of the act he was doing; or, if he did know it, that he did not know he was doing what was wrong.
Recovery is holistic. Recovery encompasses an individual's whole life, including mind, body, spirit, and community. This includes addressing self-care practices, family, housing, employment, transportation, education, clinical treatment for mental disorders and substance use disorders, services and supports, primary healthcare, dental care, complementary and alternative services, faith, spirituality, creativity, social networks, and community participation. The array of services and supports available should be integrated and coordinated.	"Sexually violent predator" means a person who has been convicted of a sexually violent offense against one or more victims and who has a diagnosed mental disorder that makes the person a danger to the health and safety of others, in that it is likely that he or she will engage in sexually violent criminal behavior. As a result of the severe mental disorder, the prisoner represents a "substantial danger of physical harm to others."

confounding, because most state/forensic hospitals receive a extensive amount of external oversight from state, private, advocacy, and federal agencies. Tremendous resources are expended trying to meet the mandated conditions of what these various agencies define as the standard of care for inpatient psychiatric facilities.

Frequently, this includes implementation of recovery principles, recovery-based multifocal treatment planning, active treatment in the form of multiple hours of group therapy each week, and the development of treatment malls. However, most forensic patients are sent to state/forensic hospitals not to recover from their mental illness, but as a result of involvement in the criminal justice system. In many cases the recovery-based treatment planning and subsequent active treatment delivery do little to address the forensic or criminogenic needs of these patients, and failing to address these needs in lieu of comprehensive care based on recovery principles has the unintended effect of neglecting the most salient immediate clinical needs. Hence we have the continual cycle of violence, treatment disruption, and administrative changes in response to treatment and systemic failures that can be found in many state/forensic hospitals across the country.

Have state/forensic hospitals been handed an unsolvable problem, or is there a sweet spot between applied recovery principles and appropriate forensic treatment that will ensure that individuals with a combination of mental health and criminogenic needs will receive appropriate treatment in an appropriate environment? Is it time to develop new standards of care for forensic settings that prioritize the forensic and legal needs of these individuals?

Who Are Forensic Psychiatric Patients?

Broadly defined, forensic psychiatric patients are mental health patients who also have some involvement with the criminal justice system. Historically, the term "forensic patient" was used to describe a narrow class of individuals: those found "not guilty by reason of insanity" (NGRI) and those found "incompetent to stand trial" (IST). Adding to those traditional forensic commitments are inmates sentenced to correctional facilities (jails and prisons) who have mental illness; there is now a tremendous focus on the growing need for forensic psychiatric services in these settings [24,25]. Newer commitment types, such as sexually violent predators (individuals who have completed a prison term but are retained for treatment due to a nexus between a psychiatric disorder and their sexual predation) and individuals who have completed a prison term but who are committed because they pose a high risk of violence due to their psychiatric disorder (referred to as "mentally disordered offenders" in California) add further diversity to this growing population. There is even some suggestion that the term "forensic patient" should be expanded to include patients involuntarily committed by a civil court [26]. Anecdotal reports indicate an increasing level of criminal behavior and violence even in these "civil" commitments, perhaps due to the successful social movement that ensures that people who can be safely treated in the community are treated in the community, thereby increasing the concentration of violence in involuntary civil state hospital settings. Regardless, the fact that forensic treatment needs are growing, both in state psychiatric institutions as well as correctional environments, is clear [27–30]. The most well-supported explanation for this growth is the phenomenon of the "criminalization" of mentally ill populations. In short, this social trend began when mental health patients who would have been served in state institutions were instead deinstitutionalized. For a variety of reasons, most notably withdrawal of federal funding, these patients were not provided with adequate care or treatment in the community, and thus began drifting into illegal activities and arrest. Therefore, many forensic patients end up in correctional environments, while others are captured by mental health law and adjudicated to state mental hospitals [31–35]. There is evidence that this growing population has features of both mental illness and criminal thinking [36–41]. There is also evidence that forensic hospitals are no longer treating categorical diagnoses, but are instead treating violence, and this poses a challenge to these facilities [42,43].

The Current Standard of Care for State Hospitals Does Not Work for Forensic Populations

The definition of the term "standard of care" has much more of a legal basis than a medical one, but in general it can be summarized as how similarly qualified practitioners would have managed care under the same or similar circumstances [44]. Existing treatment standards

for psychiatric inpatients represent an entirely appropriate evolution of practice following the institutional abuses of the 1950s and 1960s. But they are not appropriate for violent forensic populations, precisely because circumstances have changed, including patient profiles and precipitants for hospitalization.

One historical English law test for the standard of care, the Bolam test, was ultimately rejected because it "allows the standard in law to be set subjectively by expert witnesses" in favor of the Bolitho decision that "standards proclaimed must be justified on a logical basis and must have considered the risks and benefits of competing options" [45]. Given the increasing struggles to safely and humanely treat the growing forensic population, examining the current standard of care from a perspective of logic and risk/benefit analysis is warranted. While there are multiple guidelines for treating psychiatric patients in public, private, and even in correctional settings, very little exists on treating forensic patients in state hospital settings, rendering mandates somewhat subjective [46–48]. For the forensic patients found not guilty by reason of insanity or incompetent to stand trial, guidelines tend to focus on initial evaluation rather than subsequent treatment of dangerousness, barriers to trial competency, and/or criminogenic needs.

Complicating the treatment of mental illness in the modern state/forensic psychiatric facility is the recognition that many forensic patients evidence both bona fide mental health symptoms and criminogenic thinking, contributing to what may be a new type of patient with new treatment needs [36–41]. As such, a standard of treatment designed to facilitate recovery in a civilly committed patient without concomitant criminal behaviors and/or criminal justice system involvement may not be effective for this new population. An examination of forensic commitment criteria indicates that most forensic commitment language can be translated into two primary discharge criteria: restoration of competence and/or the ability to be safely treated in the community. It is therefore logical that forensic treatment would be focused on restoration to competence and/or mitigation of violence risk, with an eye toward addressing learned criminogenic attitudes. However, as a carryover from the standards set for the older state hospital system, treatment is often not focused this way, but rather on reduction of symptoms of psychiatric disorders within a holistic framework of recovery concepts such as self-direction and autonomy. This is not to suggest that treating psychiatric disorders with a recovery framework is not important, but rather that for forensic patients, addressing their forensic commitment criteria and reducing criminal behavior, including violence, is more so. As such, the recovery approach in the state/forensic psychiatric hospital would be better seen as part of a continuum of care where the patient can be discharged to the community after violence mitigation is successful, for recovery in that setting [49].

For example, approximately 15%–20% of patients referred as incompetent to stand trial may actually be malingering to avoid adjudication [50,51]. For those individuals, screening for malingering and follow-up forensic evaluation should be the focus of treatment, rather than recovery from a mental illness that is feigned to begin with. For patients who evidence predatory aggression rooted in psychopathic characteristics, principles of self-direction are inappropriate and put other patients at risk. For patients who have been diverted from court or prison because they are not competent or not criminally responsible, the concept of autonomy can be difficult to reconcile.

It appears that the standard of care needs to be defined for these commitment types as well as other patients now confined to state/forensic facilities, including those serving criminal sentences and referred from prisons, those referred from prisons as a condition of parole, sex offenders, and even seriously ill and violent civilly committed individuals who are unable to be safely treated in the community [52].

Why a New Standard Will Matter

In current forensic treatment environments, uncontrolled inpatient violence interferes with patient and staff safety, as well as treatment delivery. Available interventions to control violence include seclusion and restraint, 1:1 observation, and PRN medications. Both seclusion and restraint, and PRN medication are heavily weighted toward psychotic violence, which is easier to predict and medicate, but far less common, than other types of inpatient aggression [53,54]. Prediction and prevention of inpatient aggression in a forensic setting is more appropriately done via violence risk assessment techniques and proper level of custodial security based on overall risk level, rather than "imminent" risk level based on antecedent behaviors that might not exist in the predatory or impulsive patient. Utilizing the presence of 1:1 observation is the practice of devoting one staff member to observe an individual who has been identified as potentially violent to others. In many cases, this practice provides that patient with a target, puts our level of care staff at unacceptable risk, and drives up overtime and workers' compensation costs. Additionally, outcomes measures such as symptom reduction and length of stay do not necessarily measure whether the forensic goals (competency, violence mitigation) have been met. Focusing care primarily on outdated emergency interventions and recovery-based treatment planning, rather than reduction of risk and restoration of competency, can result in the unintended consequence of delaying discharge and violating the major dimensions needed to support recovery principles, such as the need for a stable and safe place to live [55].

Conclusion

Evidence suggests that there is a new type of patient, and that we therefore need a new standard of treatment. Modern forensic treatment should not be primarily focused on recovery from a mental illness, but instead on reducing violence and meeting forensic discharge criteria in order to eventually return patients to recovery environments in the community.

Disclosures

The author does not have anything to disclose.

References

1. Pouncey CL, Lukens JM. Madness versus badness: the ethical tension between the recovery movement and forensic psychiatry. *Theor. Med. Bioeth.* 2010; **31**(1): 93–105.

2. Laurence E. Report into psychiatric ward killing exposes uncoordinated health system. AM with Chris Uhlmann. November 3, 2014. http://www.abc.net.au/am/content/2014/s4119995.htm.

3. Kalamazoo authorities seeking assault charges against psychiatric hospital workers. WKZO Kalamazoo. December 24, 2014.

4. Napa State Hospital psychiatric worker slain. *San Francisco Chronicle.* October 25, 2010. http://www.sfgate.com/health/article/Napa-State-Hospital-psychiatric-worker-slain-3248688.php

5. Treatment problems, fear found in state's high-security mental hospital, workers say. *Baltimore Sun.* November 7, 2011. http://articles.baltimoresun.com/2011-11-07/health/bs-hs-perkins-fear-20111107_1_patients-maximum-

securitypsychiatric-hospital-susan-sachs

6. Perkins patients can be the toughest to treat. *Baltimore Sun.* November 20, 2011. http://articles.baltimoresun.com/2011-11-20/health/bs-hs-perkins-treatment-20111120_1_perkins-patients-dangerous-patients-fewer-hospital-beds

7. Violence and fear in state mental hospitals on the rise nationally. *Baltimore Sun.* November 24, 2011. http://articles.baltimoresun.com/2011-11-24/news/bs-ed-perkins-20111124_1_donna-gross-perkins-patients-mentally-ill-patients

8. Our view: forensic patients swamp state mental hospital. *The Portland Press Herald.* August 25, 3013. http://www.pressherald.com/opinion/forensic-patients-swamp-state-mental-hospital_2013-08-25.html?pagenum5full

9. DHHS commissioner blames growth in court ordered patients for Riverview problems; urges passage of LePage's plan. WABI TV5. August 22, 2013.

10. ABC 15 investigation exposes a "shocking" level of violence at the Arizona State Hospital. ABC 15. August 9, 2013.

11. Violence at Texas mental hospitals on rise. United Press International. January 27, 2013. http://www.upi.com/Top_News/US/2013/01/27/Violence-at-Texas-mental-hospitals-on-rise/UPI-96021359313991/

12. Violence on the rise at Western State Hospital. Northwest Public Radio. May 3, 2012.

13. Patient violence jumps at state psychiatric hospitals. *Statesman.* January 26, 2013. http://www.statesman.com/news/news/local/patient-violence-jumps-at-state-psychiatric-hospit/nT7GH/

14. Assaults on staff are focus of scathing report at Catonsville Psychiatric Hospital. *Baltimore Sun.* March 2, 2013. http://www.baltimoresun.com/news/maryland/baltimore-county/catonsville/bs-md-co-spring-grove-report-20130302,0,7658971.story

15. Hegedus N. Danger at Mid-Hudson Psych: "I'm just waiting for a staff member to come out dead." *Times-Herald Record.* Undated. http://www.nyscopba.org/mid-hudson-psych-center-danger

16. State mental hospitals remain violent, despite gains in safety. *Los Angeles Times.* October 9, 2013. http://articles.latimes.com/2013/oct/09/local/la-me-mental-hospital-safety-20131010

17. Zimmerman M. Safety inspectors investigating violence at Hawaii State Hospital. *Hawaii Reporter.* December 5, 2013. http://www.Hawaiireporter.com/federal-safety-inspectors-investigating-violence-at-hawaii

18. Violence at California Mental Hospitals: "This is the norm." NPR. July 21, 2011.

19. Ontario mental health facility faces charges over worker safety violations. The Canadian Press. December 24, 2014. http://toronto.ctvnews.ca/ontario-mental-health-facility-faces-charges-over-worker-safety-violations-1.2161643

20. Canzano A. Daily attacks common at the Oregon State Hospital, some say. KATU.com. April 18, 2013. http://www.katu.com/news/investigators/Daily-attacks-common-at-the-Oregon-State-Hospital-employees-say-203717621.html

21. Griffen A. Too dangerous for psych hospital? Man acquitted for insanity now in prison after violent assaults. *Hartford Courant.* September 23, 2014. http://www.courant.com/news/connecticut/hc-anderson-cvh-court-hearing-advance-0924-2

22. Associated Press. Hawaii State Hospital employees sue over assaults. *Washington Post.* September 24, 2014. http://www.washingtontimes.com/news/2014/sep/24/hawaii-state-hospital-employees-sue-over-assaults/.

23. Lawlor J. At state-run Riverview, danger and dysfunction pervasive. *Portland Press Herald.* September 21, 2014. http://www.pressherald.com/2014/09/21/at-state-run-riverview-danger-and-dysfunction-pervasive/

24. Metzner JL, Dvoskin JA. Psychiatry in correctional settings. In: Simon RI, Gold LH, eds. *Textbook of Forensic Psychiatry.* American Psychiatric Publishing Inc. Washington DC; 2004: 377–391.

25. *Psychiatric Services in Jails and Prisons: A Task Force Report of the American Psychiatric Association.* Published by the American Psychiatric Association, Washington DC; 2000.

26. Bloom JD, Krishnan B, Lockey C. The majority of inpatient psychiatric beds should not be appropriated by the forensic system. *J. Am. Acad. Psychiatry Law.* 2008; **36**(4): 438–442.

27. Lamb HR, Weinberger LE. Persons with severe mental illness in jails and prisons: a review. *Psychiatr. Serv.* 1998; **49**(4): 483–492.

28. Fazel S, Seewald K. Severe mental illness in 33,588 prisoners worldwide: systematic review and meta-regression analysis. *Br. J. Psychiatry.* 2012; **200**(5): 364–373.

29. Torrey EF, Kennard AD, Eslinger D, *et al.* More mentally ill persons are in jails and prisons than hospitals: a survey of the states. Treatment Advocacy Center and National Sheriff's Association 2010. http://www.treatmentadvocacycenter.org/storage/documents/final_jails_v_hospitals_study.pdf.

30. Lutterman T. National Association of State Mental Health Program Directors

Research Institute Fiscal Year 2010 Revenues and Expenditure Study Results; 2012. http://media .wix.com/ugd/186708_c6beb 833346b45429322 cc4421d83aa1.pdf

31. Torrey EF. *American Psychosis: How the Federal Government Destroyed the Mental Illness Treatment System.* Oxford University Press, Oxford, UK; 2013.

32. Mundt AP, Chow WS, Arduino M, et al. Psychiatric hospital beds and prison populations in South America since 1990: does the Penrose hypothesis apply? *JAMA Psychiatry.* 2015; **72**(2): 112–118.

33. Abramson MF. The criminalization of mentally disordered behavior: possible side effect of a new mental health law. *Hosp. Community Psychiatry.* 1972; **23**(4): 101–105.

34. Swank GE, Winer D. Occurrence of psychiatric disorder in a county jail population. *Am. J. Psychiatry.* 1976; **133**(11): 1331–1333.

35. Sosowsky L. Crime and violence among mental patients reconsidered in view of the new legal relationship between the state and the mentally ill. *Am. J. Psychiatry.* 1978; **135**(1): 33–42.

36. Morgan RD, Fisher WH, Duan N, Mandracchia JT, Murray D. Prevalence of criminal thinking among state prison inmates with serious mental illness. *Law Hum. Behav.* 2010; **34**(4): 324–336.

37. Moran P, Hodgins S. The correlates of comorbid antisocial personality disorder in schizophrenia. *Schizophr. Bull.* 2004; **30**(4): 791–802.

38. Maghsoodloo S, Ghodousi A, Karimzadeh T. The relationship of antisocial personality disorder and history of conduct disorder with crime incidence in schizophrenia. *J. Res. Med. Sci.* 2012; **17**(6): 566–571.

39. Gross NR, Morgan RD. Understanding persons with mental illness who are and are not criminal justice involved: a comparison of criminal thinking and psychiatric symptoms. *Law Hum. Behav.* 2013; **37**(3): 175–186.

40. Wilson AB, Farkas K, Ishler KJ, et al. Criminal thinking styles among people with serious mental illness in jail. *Law Hum. Behav.* 2014; **38**(6): 592–601.

41. Wolff N, Morgan RD, Shi J, Huening J, Fisher WH. Thinking styles and emotional states of male and female prison inmates by mental disorder status. *Psychiatr. Serv.* 2011; **62**(12): 1485–1493.

42. Warburton K. The new mission of forensic mental health systems: managing violence as a medical syndrome in an environment that balances treatment and safety. *CNS Spectr.* 2014; **19**(5): 368–373.

43. Stahl SM. Deconstructing violence as a medical syndrome: mapping psychotic, impulsive, and predatory subtypes to malfunctioning brain circuits. *CNS Spectr.* 2014; **19**(5): 355–365.

44. Moffett P, Moore G. The standard of care: legal history and definitions: the bad and good news. *West. J. Emerg. Med.* 2011; **12**(1): 109–112.

45. Strauss DC, Thomas JM. What does the medical profession mean by the "standard of care?" *J. Clin. Oncol.* 2009; **27**(32): e192–e193.

46. Menzies RJ, Webster CD. Fixing forensic patients: psychiatry recommendations for treatment settings in pretrial detainees. *Behav. Sci. Law.* 1988; **6**(4): 453–478.

47. Zapf PA, Roesch R. Future directions in the restoration of competency to stand trial. *Current Directions in Psychological Science.* 2011; **20**(1): 43–47.

48. Scott CL. Commentary: a road map for research in restoration of competency to stand trial. *J. Am.*

Acad. Psychiatry Law. 2003; **31**(1): 36–43.

49. Parks J, Radke AQ, Haupt MB. *The Vital Role of State Psychiatric Hospitals.* National Association of State Mental Health Program Directors Medical Directors Council Technical Report. 2014. www.nasmhpd.org.

50. Vitacco MJ, Rogers R, Gabel J, Munizza J. An evaluation of malingering screens with competency to stand trial patients: a known-groups comparison. *Law Hum. Behav.* 2007; **31**(3): 249–260.

51. Rogers R, Salekin RT, Sewell KW, Goldstein A, Leonard K. A comparison of forensic and nonforensic malingerers: a prototypical analysis of explanatory models. *Law Hum. Behav.* 1998; **22**(4): 353–367.

52. Linhorst DM, Scott LP. Assaultive behavior in state psychiatric hospitals: differences between forensic and nonforensic patients. *J. Interpers. Violence.* 2004; **19**(8): 857–874.

53. Nolan KA, Czobor P, Roy BB, et al. Characteristics of assaultive behavior among psychiatric inpatients. *Psychiatr. Serv.* 2003; **54**(7): 1012–1016.

54. Quanbeck CD, McDermott BE, Lam J, et al. Categorization of aggressive acts committed by chronically assaultive state hospital patients. *Psychiatr. Serv.* 2007; **58**(4): 521–528.

55. Substance Abuse and Mental Health Services Administration. *SAMHSA's Working Definition of Recovery.* http://store .samhsa.gov/shin/content// PEP12-RECDEF/PEP12-RECDEF.pdf.

56. Dusky v. United States, 362 U.S. 402 (1960).

57. Re Daniel M'Naghten, 8 ER 718 (House of Lords, 1943).

58. California Welfare and Institution Code 6600 (a)1.

59. California Penal Code 2972 (e).

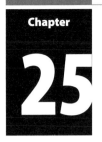

Forensic-focused treatment planning: a new standard for forensic mental health systems

Robert J. Schaufenbil, Stephen M. Stahl, Rebecca Kornbluh, and Katherine D. Warburton

"If you don't know where you are going, any road will get you there."
– *Lewis Carroll*

Introduction

The number of state hospital beds occupied by forensically committed psychiatric patients is rising, even as the overall number of state hospital beds continues to decline [1]. However, the standard treatment planning process for forensic psychiatric patients committed by the criminal justice system has not been reformulated to address the unique needs of this rapidly growing forensic population. The integration of forensic issues into the recovery movement has not been clearly articulated in the literature. A literature search (using the keywords treatment plan forensic, treatment plan inpatient psychiatry, multidisciplinary forensic treatment plan, recovery oriented treatment plan, forensically driven discharge criteria, and treatment goals forensic) produced few articles that explicitly and directly address the unique aspects of treatment planning for the forensic patient [2–5]. As most forensic state hospital admissions either target violence risk mitigation or trial incompetency, treatment planning should be focused on these two areas.

Treatment Planning for Violence Risk Mitigation

Most of the time, forensic patients lack the "medical necessity" justification that exists for community patients who are admitted for acute inpatient stays; for patients from a variety of commitments categories, such as Not Guilty by Reason of Insanity (NGRI)

or Mentally Disordered Offenders (MDO), hospitalization is based on a "likelihood" of violence, not an "imminent" danger. These patients, therefore, require a forensic risk evaluation that involves multiple static and dynamic factors, which range from previous violence to current negative attitudes to future exposure to destabilizers, in addition to more traditional clinical indicators such as positive symptoms [6,7]. Additionally, discharge is often dependent on the opinion of forensic evaluators and finders of fact, rather than the treatment team [8,9]. Treatment planning for individuals who are committed to a forensic hospital until they can be safely treated in the community should therefore focus upon violence risk assessment and mitigation, rather than multiple foci related to attainment of recovery, as the former approach hastens transfer to the next level of care, lessens risk to other patients and staff, and prevents the accumulation of further legal charges. In this respect, violence, conceptualized dimensionally as a specific syndrome with multiple etiologies, should be the focus of care.

Treatment Planning for Restoration of Trial Competence

Competency evaluations number in the tens of thousands per year [10,11], and anecdotal evidence suggests that the number of patients referred to state hospitals for restoration is rising. Research at the University of California–Davis indicates that patients determined to be incompetent can be separated into six groups [12] (see Table 25.1). Using this schema, the case formulation should focus on the primary barrier to competency, and discharge criteria should focus on the elimination of that barrier. Like the treatment of

Violence in Psychiatry, ed. Katherine D. Warburton and Stephen M. Stahl. Published by Cambridge University Press.
© Cambridge University Press 2016.

Table 25.1 Competency groups

1. Incompetent due to psychosis
2. Incompetent due to cognitive impairment
3. Malingering
4. Competence undermined due to language or cultural barriers
5. No substantial likelihood of regaining competence
6. Already trial competent

violence, incompetency should be viewed dimensionally and as the primary focus of forensic treatment for this commitment category.

A Forensic-Focused Treatment Planning Model

Forensic-focused treatment planning should target the legal reasons for admission and discharge based on the commitment-specific statutory language, and forensic interdisciplinary plans of care should focus on the factors that prevent discharge from a legal perspective. The goal of a forensic-focused treatment plan is thus to identify, organize, and track foci and treatment that specifically relate to either the barrier to competency, or the etiology and dynamic risk factors for violence, or in some cases both. While the forensic admission and discharge criteria should be the foundation for treatment planning, treatment should proceed with an understanding of the increasing complexity of the new forensic patient that results from the interplay between psychiatric illness, substance abuse, cognitive impairment, and criminogenic thinking. However, not all domains need to be addressed in every forensic patient; for example, a treatment plan that targets substance use in a patient found incompetent to stand trial may not be as critical as interventions focused on the primary barrier to competency.

There are three primary components to consider when developing a Forensic-Focused Treatment Plan.

(1) Forensic case formulation
(2) Forensically driven discharge criteria
(3) Forensic interdisciplinary plans of care

Each component is developed one at a time to generate the information sequentially needed to develop the next component on the list. First, information from the forensic case formulation is used to generate the forensically driven discharge criteria. Second, discharge criteria are used to generate the objectives

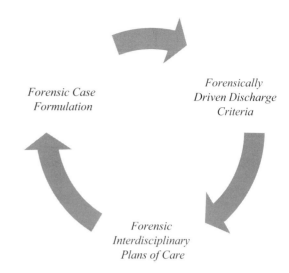

Forensic Case Formulation

Forensically Driven Discharge Criteria

Forensic Interdisciplinary Plans of Care

Figure 25.1 Forensic-focused treatment plan cycle.

and interventions that make up a forensic interdisciplinary plan of care (see Figure 25.1). Finally, the cycle continues such that information in all three components is updated on a regular basis as clinically indicated in order to continue progress toward discharge.

Forensic case formulation

Integrating forensic data into a case formulation can prove challenging, but there is some guidance in the literature [2–5,10–12]. In particular, the research literature supports the utility of structured risk assessment, etiology, and diachronicity as helpful components of a forensic case formulation [2,13,14].

For patients, such as those found "not guilty by reason of insanity" or classified as a "mentally disordered offender," whose sole discharge criterion is often simply the ability to be safely treated in the community, utilization of a structured clinical risk assessment that delineates risk factors into historical, clinical, and risk management domains can provide a useful framework [6]. An examination of past violence to determine the etiology (psychotic, impulsive, predatory) [13,14] allows for further refinement of the formulation. Recent guidelines for treatment based on etiology have been developed [15]. A critical component of a forensic case formulation, identified by Hart *et al.*, is the concept of diachronicity [2]. This means that the forensic case formulation includes

259

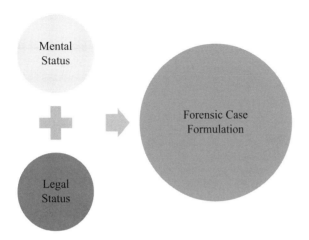

Figure 25.2 Forensic case formulation components.

Table 25.2 Statutory language for incompetent to stand trial

1. Patient will demonstrate adequate knowledge in the court proceedings.
2. Patient will demonstrate an ability to assist his or her attorney.

information from the patient's past and present, which generate predictions about the potential future clinical outcomes. The amount of historical information available to forensic clinicians in the form of documentation and evaluations completed during previous hospitalizations varies greatly from case to case, but a case formulation is incomplete and perhaps inaccurate without adequate historical information, especially related to past violence and criminal history. The reliability of information coming from patient self-report should be verified by collateral information whenever possible.

Patients who have been sent for competency restoration have met discharge criteria when they have sufficient present ability to consult with their lawyers with a reasonable degree of rational understanding and have a rational as well as factual understanding of the proceedings against them [16]. Therefore, there is utility in organizing case formulations for these patients into those categories identified by UC Davis, because it provides a focus for treatment on the primary barrier to competency (e.g., psychopharmacology intervention for a psychotic barrier to competency). For example, while issues related to substance use or a history of violence may be present, they do not represent a barrier to being discharged as competent, and ironically, incorporating multiple foci of treatment can prolong lengths of stay and ultimately impede upon constitutional rights [17]. The value of a forensic case formulation in these cases is to help clinicians determine what the barriers to regaining competency are and which treatments will be most effective in helping to quickly eliminate those barriers

(see Figure 25.2). Doing so will prioritize forensic outcomes such as restoration of trial competence or mitigation of violence risk as the first steps in a continuum of care that eventually leads to the patient's ability to resolve forensic issues and return to the community for recovery-oriented care.

Forensically driven discharge criteria

The term "discharge criteria" is somewhat of a misnomer, given that a forensic mental health system is only the first step along a continuum of care. Typically, discharge criteria are generated from the case formulation and directly influence the development of interdisciplinary plans of care. However, in the forensic setting, discharge criteria flow from the statutory language under which the patient is admitted. The case formulation should provide, primarily, an analysis of an individual's mental condition as it relates to that legal status. So the discharge criteria need to reflect resolution of the mental health/criminogenic dimensions that have bearing on the patient's legal status. Many stakeholders are involved in developing discharge criteria; however, unlike civil settings, it is ultimately the committing court that makes a decision regarding discharge. It is therefore suggested to design discharge criteria that speak directly to the statutory language (see Table 25.2) and are organized following the structure in the forensic case formulation.

Forensic interdisciplinary plans of care

The principles of good treatment planning apply to forensic plans. Kennedy [18] identifies several mechanics that are essential to treatment planning. Focus statements, objectives, and treatment interventions, developed by a multidisciplinary team of clinicians, should come together to form interdisciplinary plans of care, which serve as the functional components of a forensic-focused treatment plan. In treatment plans, focus statements should clearly articulate the problem. Whether it is medication noncompliance in a patient with psychotic aggression or a need to develop

Table 25.3 Forensic interdisciplinary plans of care

Focus statement:

The patient has been experiencing auditory command hallucinations for approximately the past 3 years. Patient currently experiences these hallucinations on a daily basis, which interfere with his concentration to the point where he cannot have a conversation with his attorney or follow court proceedings. Patient has a detailed history of noncompliance with medications and blood work.

Objectives:

1. Patient will take psychotropic medications as prescribed for 1 month.
2. Patient will cooperate with lab monitoring for 1 month.
3. Patient will alert treatment staff of adverse effects.
4. Patient will participate in twice-weekly medication education groups.
5. Patient will attend coping with symptoms groups.

Interventions:

1. The psychiatrist will prescribe psychotropic medications to reduce auditory hallucinations, and assess the efficacy of that medication at least weekly.
2. The psychiatrist will discuss with the patient the expected risks and benefits of each medication.
3. Staff will observe the patient to determine any warning signs of any adverse effects due to psychotropic medication.

prosocial thinking, a succinct focus statement is crucial to gaining understanding among all readers. Objectives that are behavioral, observable, and/or measurable ensure that forensic clinicians can appropriately track the patient's progress toward meeting desired outcomes. Attaching reasonable target dates to objectives provides a mechanism by which to establish the continued review of progress. Group, individual, and milieu treatment interventions are also important in establishing exactly what therapeutic modalities and strategies staff will provide in order to assist the patient in meeting their goals [18] (see Table 25.3).

Unlike civil treatment plans, forensic care plans should focus on mitigation of dynamic risk factors or elimination of the specific barrier to competency, depending on the commitment language.

Conclusions

No significant literature explicitly discusses the unique treatment planning needs for forensic psychiatry patients. Due to the increasing number of such forensic patients, there is a need for a new conceptual treatment planning model that takes into account the criminal justice requirements that must be met in order for patients to either be safely treated in the community or returned to court for trial. More research must be conducted on the efficacy of a model that incorporates a forensic viewpoint when assembling a case formulation, discharge criteria, and interdisciplinary plans of care for these patients.

Disclosures

Robert Schaufenbil, Rebecca Kornbluh, and Katherine Warburton do not have anything to disclose. Stephen M. Stahl, MD, PhD is an Adjunct Professor of Psychiatry at the University of California, San Diego School of Medicine, Honorary Visiting Senior Fellow at the University of Cambridge, UK and Director of Psychopharmacology for the California Department of State Hospitals. Dr. Stahl receives research support from Avanir, CeNeRx, Forest, Genomind, Lilly, Janssen, Mylan, Mylan Specialty, Otsuka, Pamlab, Servier, Shire, Sunovion, and Takeda; is a consultant/advisor to Avanir, BioMarin, Depomed, Forest, Genentech, Genomind, GlaxoSmithKline, Jazz, Merck, Navigant, Novartis, Noveida, Neuronetics, Orexigen, Otsuka, Pamlab, Reviva, Roche, Shire, Sunovion, Taisho, Teva, and Trius; is on the speakers bureaus of Arbor Scientia, Genomind, Janssen, Lilly, Pamlab, Pfizer, Sunovion, and Takeda; and is a board member at Genomind and RCT Logic.

References

1. Substance Abuse and Mental Health Services Administration. *Funding and Characteristics of State Mental Health Agencies, 2010.* http://www. aahd.us/wp-content/uploads/2012/12/FundingState MentalHealthAgencies2010.pdf.

2. Hart S, Sturmey P, Logan C, McMurran M. Forensic case formulation. *International Journal of Forensic Mental Health.* 2011; **10**(2): 118–126.

3. Hart SD, Logan C. Formulation of violence risk using evidence-based assessments: the structured professional judgment approach. In: Sturmey P, McMurran M, eds. *Forensic Case Formulation.* Hoboken, NJ: John Wiley; 2011: 83–106.

4. Moran MJ, Sweda MG, Fragala MR, Sasscer-Burgos J. The clinical application of risk assessment in the treatment-planning process. *International Journal of Offender Therapy and Comparative Criminology*. 2001; **45**(4): 421–435.

5. Davis DL. Treatment planning for the patient who is incompetent to stand trial. *Hosp Community Psychiatry*. 1985; **36**(3): 268–271.

6. Douglas KS, Hart SD, Webster CD, *et al. HCR-20V3: Assessing Risk of Violence—User Guide*. Burnaby, Canada: Mental Health, Law, and Policy, Institute, Simon Fraser University; 2013.

7. Hare RD. *Manual for the Revised Psychopathy Checklist*, 2nd edn. Toronto, Ontario, Canada: Multi-Health Systems; 2003.

8. Not Guilty By Reason Of Insanity, Cal. Penal Code § 1026.

9. Mentally Disordered Offender, Cal. Penal Code § 2972.

10. Skeem JL, Golding SL, Berge G, Cohn NB. Logic and reliability of evaluations of competence to stand trial. *Law Hum. Behav.* 1998; **22**(5): 519–547.

11. Fogel MH, Schiffman W, Mumley D, Tillbrook C, Grisso T. Ten year research update (2001–2010): evaluations for competence to stand trial (adjudicative competence). *Behav. Sci. Law.* 2013; **31**(2): 165–191.

12. McDermott BE, Warburton KD, Woofter C. The effectiveness of structured assessments in the detection of malingering. Presentation, The Royal Australian and New Zealand College of Psychiatrists, Section of Forensic Psychiatry, Prato, Italy, 2010.

13. Nolan KA, Czobor P, Roy BB, *et al.* Characteristics of assaultive behavior among psychiatric inpatients. *Psychiatr. Serv.* 2003; **54**(7): 1012–1016.

14. Quanbeck CD, McDermott BE, Lam J, *et al.* Categorization of aggressive acts committed by chronically assaultive state hospital patients. *Psychiatr. Serv.* 2007; **58**(4): 521–528.

15. Stahl SM, Morrissette DA, Cummings M, *et al.* California State Hospital Violence Assessment and Treatment (Cal-VAT) guidelines. *CNS Spectr.* 2014; **19**(5): 449–465.

16. Dusky v. United States, 362 U.S. 402 (1960).

17. US Cont. amend. VI.

18. Kennedy J. *Fundamentals of Psychiatric Treatment Planning*. Washington, DC: American Psychiatric Publishing, Inc.; 2003.

Chapter

26

Implementing an ecological approach to violence reduction at a forensic psychiatric hospital: approaches and lessons learned

Shannon M. Bader and Sean E. Evans

Introduction

For decades, violence and aggressive behavior have been identified as pressing issues facing institutional settings such as psychiatric hospitals and prisons. State psychiatric hospitals in California are no different. The California Department of State Hospitals (DSH) includes five hospitals that house an average of 5600 adult patients. During the 2013 calendar year, there were 3377 incidents of aggression perpetrated on other patients and 2596 incidents of aggression directed toward staff members. Approximately 3% of these assaults were sufficiently severe that the patient or staff member required medical treatment at an outside hospital or emergency room. Consistent with most existing research, attempts to reduce this rate of violence have typically involved medication algorithms or psychosocial methods to treat the aggressive patient. These various interventions stem from the view that violence is due to the psychiatric symptoms, characterlogical features, or behaviors of a disordered patient. The existing research highlights the necessity of a second generation of violence interventions. Specifically, this second-generation intervention would encompass a broader view and conceptualize inpatient aggression as an ecological problem that combines treatment for aggressive patients with environmental and situational interventions. In addition to treating the patient, environmental interventions treat the ward and treat the hospital in a way that mitigates violence and reduces opportunities for aggression.

Ecology is defined as the study of interactions between individual organisms as well as relationships between organisms and their physical surroundings.

This study includes the smallest bacteria living on a leaf to each individual tree to the entire forest. The connections between plants, animals, air, elevation, light, and a myriad of other factors are all analyzed as an integrated whole [1]. Moreover, small changes in an ecosystem can cascade into ramifications for all other species in an ecosystem. Previous theories of human behavior have also drawn from this broader ecological view. For example, Bronfenbrenner [2] coined the term "ecological systems theory" to describe how a child's development is influenced by his or her family and school, but also his or her neighborhood, cultural values, statewide economy, and country's political system. Aggression within hospitals, we argue, is related to patients' psychiatric symptoms as well as their interactions with other patients, staff members, the ward milieu, and hospital policies, similar to the delicate balance of ecosystems. After reviewing the existing research on the role of environment in hospital wards and hospitals, barriers to adopting an ecological approach are identified, and an example of one hospital's attempt to implement an ecological approach is described.

Literature Review

The environment of psychiatric hospitals involves numerous variables that have a relationship to aggression. Recent literature reviews on situational and environmental factors related to violence in an institutional setting found existing research support for a relationship between inpatient aggression rates and ward organization, patient populations, staff mixture, hospital management styles, and other environmental variables [3,4].

Violence in Psychiatry, ed. Katherine D. Warburton and Stephen M. Stahl. Published by Cambridge University Press.
© Cambridge University Press 2016.

For example, patients are often admitted onto a ward using a "one patient out, one patient in" system. Although this method maximizes hospital capacity, it does not allow analyses of the mixture of patients residing on that ward together. An ecological view would assess the ward as an ecosystem with a delicate balance. Cooke and Wozniak [5] argue that facilities without a systematic method to assess the potential violence of incoming patients and then adjust the mix of population on wards accordingly are at risk of greater violence. Specifically, age, diagnoses, and acuity of the patient population on a certain ward may all influence the rate of aggressive incidents. Research from prisons has demonstrated that younger prison populations have been associated with higher levels of violence, and a heterogeneous mix of ages within a housing unit has been shown to decrease rates of aggression [6,7]. Palmstierna *et al.* [8] found that an increased number of patients on a ward significantly increased aggressive behavior, especially for patients who were diagnosed with a psychotic spectrum disorder. These authors suggest that the coping and stress management needed to reduce feeling crowded may be compromised in individuals experiencing severe mental illness and result in the reported increased rate of violence in psychiatric hospitals. This finding also suggests that a mix of patient diagnoses on a ward may assist in lowering rates of aggression. Again, an ecological view would treat the individual patient's symptoms while simultaneously attempting to reduce aggression rates through management of the number and type of patients designated to live in close quarters.

In addition to the blend of patients, the staff members working are also a significant piece of the ecological system of a psychiatric ward. Numerous studies have found a relationship between staff member age or experience and aggression [9–14]. Some authors have suggested that a heterogeneous mix of staff members, both newly hired and those with extensive experience working together on the same shift, could reduce the rate of violence [15]. A hospital's inability to recruit and retain the appropriate number of qualified and motivated staff members increases the risk for violence [5]. As they state, under-staffing as well as high turnover and improperly trained staff lead to reduced morale and poor fidelity to risk-reducing policies or procedures. A ward with a chronically new or understaffed

workforce often results in a destabilized unit that is prone to increased violence. For example, recent analyses from one of the DSH hospitals over a 4-year period suggested that both the rate and severity of violent incidents increased when staff members were working an overtime shift. Out of all 5219 incidents at the one hospital, 43% ($N = 2260$) occurred when all regularly scheduled staff members were on duty and 57% ($N = 2959$) occurred with one or more staff working an overtime shift. The same pattern was seen with severe incidents; out of the 153 severe incidents, 37.9% ($N = 58$) occurred when all regularly scheduled staff members were on duty and 62.1% ($N = 95$) occurred when one or more overtime staff were present [16]. In addition to the number and experience of staff members present, numerous studies have identified that poor communication, patients reporting that they do not feel heard, and denial of privacy are related to aggressive acts [5,17]. The ecological view would argue that repeated training for all direct care staff, sufficient staffing, and progressive discipline for staff members who show a repetitive pattern of poor-quality relationships with patients are just as important as the medicine provided for patients to maintain a milieu environment that fosters psychiatric recovery and reduces or mitigates risk for violence.

Poor structure and organization on psychiatric wards has also been linked to increased violence [18–20]. Wards with lower rates of violence have been found to have consistent, reliable schedules and routines, clearly defined staff roles, a committed and active psychiatrist, trusting and calm relationships between staff members and patients, and therapeutic activities available. Wards with higher rates of violence have demonstrated haphazard or unreliable schedules and routines, poor teamwork and diffusion of responsibility, an uninvolved psychiatrist that was rarely present, a perception that the patients were dangerous and should be feared, little interaction between patients and staff members, and few opportunities for therapeutic activities [20]. The ward's structure, routine, and available treatment opportunities are happening around the patients and perhaps influencing the severity or frequency of psychiatric symptoms. A narrow focus on treating the patient's symptoms will miss the important interaction between the patient and the ward environment. Thinking in terms of ecology, unstructured psychiatric wards with poor interactions between staff and patients result in competition for scarce clinical resources, anxiety about when the next opportunity for a fresh air break may come, or concerns about whether the new unstable patients will be treated before they become aggressive toward you.

Extensive changes are not always needed to impact institutional violence, and often, small environmental changes have reduced violence. Baldwin [21] found a statistically significant reduction in physical violence when the furniture in the communal area was rearranged to promote social interaction between patients. After banning the sale of caffeinated drinks, but no other changes, one hospital saw a significant decline in aggressive acts [22]. The physical environment of a treatment ward may also influence the rates of aggression. For example, sensory overload, from excessive sound or noise, has been identified as a precipitant of violence [9,10].

Hospital management styles also appear to influence the rate of violence in institutional settings. Cooke and Wozniak [5] have suggested that poor information systems can increase a hospital's risk for aggression. Specifically, any procedures that limit staff members' ability to quickly access key information regarding a patient result in poor milieu management. If a patient is currently threatening and imminently aggressive, the development of an effective crisis plan to reduce risk is less likely without appropriate information. Hospital charts, signage, and computerized documents must be quickly accessible, clear, current, consistent, and provide risk-relevant information about patients and potential risk mitigation strategies. Reisig [23] argued that failure to resolve conflicts between administrators and level-of-care staff is related to poor staff morale, poor cooperation between staff members, and increased patient violence. Cooke and Wozniak [5] suggested that a negative organizational climate may have a poor commitment to managing violence and breed a tolerance for violence hospital-wide. Examples they provide include senior management rarely entering the units, no identified person assigned to violence management, incomplete or inaccurate written policies related to aggression, and acceptance of risky current practices as long as there was an appearance of calm.

As these existing studies reflect, aspects of ward organization as well as hospital decisions and policies influence the likelihood of violence. Consequently,

the second generation of intervention requires treatments that target individual patients, individual wards, and entire hospitals. Just as ecological interventions cannot focus on only one plant species without addressing the soil quality, air content, and water availability, patient aggression cannot be reduced without equal attention to the milieu structure and institutional processes happening simultaneously.

Implementation of an Ecological-Based Approach

Despite these findings, primary focus within psychiatric hospitals remains on treating aggressive patients. Indeed, clinicians are tasked with treating patients and making numerous treatment decisions on a daily basis.

Changes to treatments typically involve conversations between providers, the patient, and possibly family members or legal conservators. However, as long as the proposed treatment follows standard of care, there is typically little involvement from administrative leaders or personnel outside of the ward. The second generation of institutional risk management discussed here often requires an integrated approach between administration, clinicians, employee unions, patients' groups, and numerous members of the hospital support staff. The need for so many participants to meet, agree, and cooperate on changes is one of the crucial barriers to implementing an ecological invention for institutional violence. Table 26.1 lists other barriers to undertaking an ecological approach focused on the ward and the hospital. This table includes barriers due to legal or accreditation requirements, as well as barriers related to hospital culture. Just as each patient presents with a unique constellation of symptoms and social history, each ward and each hospital presents with varying treatment targets and distinctive strengths and weaknesses. Johnstone and Cooke [24] argue that any hospital attempting to address environmental and situational risk factors must complete an assessment of the symptoms, strengths, and social history of the institution before beginning to implement change.

One DSH hospital has attempted to adopt this ecological view by phasing out an existing risk management strategy, which had been devised by an outside agency, and implementing a new approach. Previously, a review meeting was scheduled after

Table 26.1 Potential barriers to implementing an ecological approach to institutional violence

- Ward staff and supervisors may have suggestions for safety but no effective way to voice them
- Executive leaders with no accountability for addressing recommendations with proposed changes
- Frequent changes in leadership, at the executive level and on the wards
- Practitioner training focused on new or established treatments for patients
- Employment culture that rewards status quo and does not encourage innovation or creativity.
- Fluctuating budgets and hesitance to spend funds now with no guarantee of future savings
- Prioritizing changes from outside accrediting and legal agencies, typically focused on patient care, patient rights, and maintaining standard of care to the exclusion of internally driven priorities
- Difficulty of creating a treatment environment that promotes safety, patient autonomy, and privacy
- Lack of agreed upon goals and priorities for the facility
- Concern about external criticism from the media, advocacy groups, or unions interfering with attempts to make changes
- Enduring belief that exposure to aggression is one expected pain of institutionalization

a patient had demonstrated a specified threshold of aggression. At the meeting, two clinical team members were asked to provide short background information about the patient before clinical supervisors and the medical director would discuss the patient's treatment and suggest potential changes to the medication regimen, type of group treatment, or other individualized treatment plans. Although the suggestions stemming from these meetings were often helpful, the meeting focused solely on the patient and the patient's presenting symptoms. With rare exception, the meeting did not include discussion or analysis of the patient's interaction with the treatment environment around him or her.

The new ecological approach continues to use a consultation-style meeting with clinical staff and clinical supervisors; however, there are crucial differences to the new meeting. First, the structure and time allocation of meeting immediately reflects the focus on an ecological view. Only one-third of the meeting is spent discussing the patient's risk factors for

aggression, current treatment response, and recommendations for changes to the treatment plan. Each meeting has an assigned facilitator, typically a clinical supervisor, who maintains the meeting structure and keeps the meeting on pace. The second third of the meeting focuses on the features of the ward that potentially escalate or increase the risk for aggression for this particular patient, as well as all other patients living on the ward. The facilitator ensures that this discussion remains neutral, constructive, and broader than the identified patient. The final third of the meeting is devoted to identifying hospital policies or procedures that interfere with building safer wards. Attendance at these new meetings is also broadly representative, and includes many additional key personnel. Instead of just two clinical team members, nurses, ward staff, and all clinicians working with the patient participate actively in the meeting to discuss the patient. These meetings also include participants not typically considered part of the treatment team. For example, attendance has also included hospital clergy members, patient's work assignment supervisors, forensic department staff members, the hospital librarian, health and safety officers, and maintenance staff. Anyone who may provide context, information, or solutions to interventions focused on the patient, the ward, and hospital is invited. Although the collaborative nature of meeting remains difficult when there are numerous attendees, the varied expertise is necessary. At a recent meeting, a staff member recommended adding a door to a small room where staff members reported feeling isolated and unsafe. The maintenance staff was able to describe the fire codes and propose alternatives to a door that would meet regulations and provide a safe barrier.

Perhaps most importantly, the tenor and tone of the new meetings is intentionally collaborative. Although envisioned to be supportive, the previous meetings often established a punitive interaction, with supervisors telling clinicians how to change their presumably flawed treatment plan after a patient was aggressive. The new meetings are established as an aid to the ward staff. Staff members are provided the opportunity to openly state the suggestions, frustrations, and concerns they may have kept to themselves or only previously discussed in the break room with colleagues. The facilitator prompts each portion of the meeting with reminders that all ideas and suggestions are welcome. In contrast to the previous meetings, these new ecological approach meetings have been requested by treatment teams prior to incidents of aggression as a preventative measure.

For each meeting, a designated staff member familiar with the philosophy behind the ecological approach takes notes about the factors identified as increasing risk for violence for the individual patient, the ward, and the hospital. These notes are compiled, and a list of recommendations is generated. Table 26.2 includes recommendations that have been proposed for patients, wards, and the hospital as a whole during these new meetings. The effectiveness of the new process comes after the recommendations have been generated. Administrators dedicated to reducing violence within the hospital prioritize the recommendations in the long-range planning for the hospital and delegate the implementation of new policies or procedures to key personnel [25].

As these new meetings have gained support from ward staff and administration, they have become even more ecological. Now, many meetings are held to discuss broader risk issues facing the hospital, instead of being based on any one patient. Specifically, recent meetings have focused on how to reduce the potential for aggression on a unit with many acutely ill patients or how to eliminate the entry of contraband items (such as drugs or currency) into the locked wards. These issues, which would have not been addressed at the previous type of meeting, are truly ecological in their intent to address risk for increased patient violence by targeting all types of risk, not just a single patient's symptoms.

Conclusion

Although adoption of these new consultation meetings reflects a commitment to an ecological approach, it remains merely an initial step to significant changes to hospital procedures. Collection of outcome measures, specifically surveys of staff members about their perceptions of the new meetings and assessments of how often recommendations generated at the meetings are addressed, is one of the next steps.

Despite the real barriers that make adoption of this ecological approach difficult, the existing research suggests that a narrow focus on patients' psychiatric symptoms is only part of the solution to reducing violence within hospitals. Indeed, hospitals cannot expect the complex patients admitted to

Table 26.2 Examples of recommendations based on an ecological approach

– Recommendations based on patient risk factors for violence

- Increase the number of body and locker searches to locate stolen property.
- Locate a suitable therapist from psychology or social work departments to begin individual therapy.
- Because of the patient's interest in music, identify any additional treatment groups utilizing music.
- Refer patient for an updated neuropsychological assessment.

– Recommendations based on ward risk factors for violence

- Investigate possibility of training ward staff on specialized treatment for patients with developmental disabilities.
- Request increased number of staff members during the morning shift.
- The current treatment team does not have a psychologist. Prioritize placement of any newly hired psychologist to this ward.
- Implement and strictly adhere to a schedule of fresh air breaks, access to the laundry room, and mail call.

– Recommendations based on facility-wide risk factors for violence

- Explore development of a specialized DBT unit.
- Analyze the current process for transferring patient from one ward to another and how to improve communication between the previous ward's treatment team and the new ward's clinicians.
- Eliminate patient access to the far southeast corner of the outside grounds area where visibility is reduced.
- Identify and provide leadership training for newly promoted nursing supervisors that includes positive communication and encouraging management styles, not just progressive discipline policies.

hospitals to recover and become well in polluted, toxic environments.

Disclosures

Shannon Bader and Sean Evans do not have anything to disclose.

References

1. Molles M. *Ecology: Concepts and Applications*. New York: McGraw Hill; 2012.

2. Bronfenbrenner U. Ecological systems theory. In: Bronfenbrenner U. ed. *Making Human Beings Human: Bioecological Perspectives on Human Development*. Thousand Oaks, CA: Sage Publications Ltd.; 2005: 106–173.

3. Gadon L, Johnstone L, Cooke D. Situational variables and institutional violence: a systematic review of the literature. *Clin. Psychol. Rev.* 2006; **26**(5): 515–534.

4. Welsh E, Bader S, Evans S. Situational variables related to aggression in institutional settings. *Aggression and Violent Behavior*. 2013; **18**(6): 792–796.

5. Cooke DJ, Wozniak E. PRISM applied to a critical incident review: a case study of the Glendairy prison riot and its aftermath in Barbados. *International Journal of Forensic Mental Health*. 2010; **9**(3): 159–172.

6. Ekland-Olson S, Barrick DM, Cohen LE. Prison overcrowding and disciplinary problems: an analysis of the Texas prison system. *Journal of Applied Behavioral Science*. 1983; **19**(2): 163–192.

7. Mabli J, Holley C, Patrick J, Walls J. Age and prison violence: increasing age heterogeneity as a violence-reducing strategy in prisons. *Criminal Justice and Behavior*. 1979; **6**(2): 175–186.

8. Palmstierna T, Huitfeldt B, Wistedt B. The relationship of crowding and aggressive behavior on a psychiatric intensive care unit. *Hosp. Community Psychiatry*. 1991; **42**(12): 1237–1240.

9. Flannery RB Jr, Hanson MA, Penk WE. Risk factors for psychiatric inpatient assaults on staff. *J. Ment. Health Adm.* 1994; **21**(1): 24–31.

10. Flannery RB, Staffieri A, Hildum S, Walker AP. The violence triad and common single precipitants to psychiatric patient assaults on staff: 16-year analysis of the Assaulted Staff Action Program. *Psychiatr. Q.* 2011; **82**(2): 85–93.

11. Davies W, Burgess PW. Prison officers' experience as a predictor of risk of attack: an analysis within the British prison system. *Med. Sci. Law*. 1988; **28**(2): 135–138.

12. Webster CD, Nicholls TD, Martin ML, Desmarais SL, Brink J. Short-Term Assessment of Risk and Treatability (START): the case for a new structured professional judgment scheme. *Behav. Sci. Law*. 2006; **24**(6): 747–766.

13. Hamadeh RR, Al Alaiwat B, Al Ansari A. Assaults and nonpatient-induced injuries among psychiatric nursing staff in Bahrain. *Issues Ment. Health Nurs*. 2003; **24**(4): 409–417.

14. Flannery RB Jr, White DL, Flannery GJ, Walker AP. Time of psychiatric patient assaults: fifteen-year analysis of the Assaulted Staff Action Program (ASAP). *Int. J. Emerg. Ment. Health*. 2007; **9**(2): 89–95.

15. Flannery RB Jr. Precipitants to psychiatric patient assaults on staff: review of empirical findings, 1990–2003, and risk management implications. *Psychiatr. Q.* 2005; **76**(4): 317–326.

16. Bader SM, Evans SE, Welsh E. Aggression among psychiatric inpatients: the relationship between time, place, victims and severity ratings. *J. Am. Psychiatr. Nurses Assoc.* 2014; **20**(3): 179–186.

17. Quanbeck CD, McDermott BE, Lam J, Eisenstark H, Sokolov G. Categorization of aggressive acts committed by chronically assaultive state hospital patients. *Psychiatr. Serv.* 2007; **58**(4): 521–528.

18. Flannery RB Jr, Hanson MA, Penk WE, Flannery GJ. Violence and the lax milieu? *Preliminary data. Psychiatr. Q.* 1996; **67**(1): 47–50.

19. Morrison E, Morman G, Bonner G, *et al*. Reducing staff injuries and violence in a forensic psychiatric setting. *Arch. Psychiatr. Nurs.* 2002; **16**(3): 108–117.

20. Katz P, Kirkland FR. Violence and social structure on mental hospital wards. *Psychiatry*. 1990; **53**(3): 262–277.

21. Baldwin S. Effects of furniture rearrangement on the atmosphere of wards in a maximum-security hospital. *Hosp. Community Psychiatry*. 1985; **36**(5): 525–528.

22. Zaslove MO, Beal M, McKinney RE. Changes in behaviors of inpatients after a ban on the sale of caffeinated drinks. *Hosp. Community Psychiatry*. 1991; **42**(1): 84–85.

23. Reisig MD. Administrative control and inmate homicide. *Homicide Studies*. 2002; **6**(1): 84–103.

24. Johnstone L, Cooke DJ. PRISM: a promising paradigm for assessing and managing institutional violence: findings from a multiple case study analysis of five Scottish prisons. *International Journal of Forensic Mental Health*. 2010; **9**(3): 180–191.

25. Braz R. Enterprise risk management: Part one: defining the concept, recognizing its value. *J. Healthc. Risk Manag.* 2005; **25**(4): 11–13.

Chapter

27

The appropriateness of treating psychopathic disorders

Alan R. Felthous

Introduction

Owing to their assaultive, destructive, and other anti-social acts, individuals with psychopathic disorders inflict untold harm on themselves, acquaintances, and strangers. The damage they inflict and the attempts at safe management by the criminal justice system amount to considerable economic cost to society. Yet the fatalistic conventional wisdom is that no treatment is effective for psychopathic disorders. From this perspective, efforts at treatment are counterproductive and a misuse of limited resources. Attempts to treat and cure the core defect of psychopathy may be futile in light of current medical and behavioral science.

Here the term "psychopathic disorders" is used with the same meaning as that in the comprehensive handbook on the topic [1,2]. The term follows "both taxonomical and dimensional approaches" and includes "diagnostic conditions characterized by antisocial behaviors," but not "all antisocial or criminal behaviors regardless whether a disorder exists." More specifically, psychopathic disorders include the Hare psychopathy concept and antisocial personality disorder (APD), as defined in the *Diagnostic and Statistical Manual of Mental Disorders* (DSM), now in the fifth edition (DSM-5) [3]. In identifying psychopathic disorders, most of the studies cited in this review relied on either a version of the Psychopathy Checklist or an edition of the DSM diagnostic manual.

The treatment of psychopathic disorders is not so much different from other chronic mental disorders, such as schizophrenia for example. The pathogenesis of the "core defect," if there is a single underlying defect, is neither fully understood nor curable by current therapeutic modalities. Yet with remarkable success, the more salient and disturbing symptoms of

schizophrenia are treated, often with substantial improvement in overall functioning. If, instead of seeking to eliminate or overcome the "core defect" of psychopathy, treatment were to target specific troublesome cognitive, emotional, or behavioral symptoms, enough improvement might be attained to make treatment appropriate and worth the effort.

Reviewers who address the effectiveness of treating psychopathic disorders typically compare outcomes to programmatic approaches. Programs are different, psychopathic disorders vary in characteristics and severity, and follow-up treatment upon completing a given program is often lacking. Unsurprising then, studies produce apparently contradictory results, and reviews result in uncertain conclusions. After a brief summary of reviews of treatment programs, this article's main focus is on evidence-based pharmacotherapy of the impulsive aggression of psychopathic disorders. To be noted is that outcome studies of treatment programs do not include pharmacotherapy of specific domains of psychopathy as part of the treatment and analysis of effectiveness.

The main focus here will then be on the pharmacotherapy of impulsive aggression, for which evidence-based effectiveness has been demonstrated even within the pathological context of a personality or psychopathic disorder. Whether impulsive aggression is a co-occurring condition (i.e., intermittent explosive disorder), a direct manifestation of the psychopathic disorder for which it is a diagnostic criterion, or a "domain" of the disorder may be more of a semantic or conceptual than a therapeutically practical distinction. At any rate, effective treatment ought not to be withheld because the patient also meets criteria for a psychopathic disorder, such as APD as delineated in (DSM-5) [3].

Violence in Psychiatry, ed. Katherine D. Warburton and Stephen M. Stahl. Published by Cambridge University Press.

Programmatic Treatment for Psychopathic Offenders

Whether a criminal offender's psychopathy is improved, worsened, or not affected by programmatic treatment remains unsettled. An attempt to categorize the non-pharmacotherapeutic approaches to treatment of personality and behaviorally disturbed criminal offenders in Canada and the United States showed the following approaches in use: the therapeutic community based on social learning, the token economy based on cognitive and/or behavioral therapy, and dialectic behavioral therapy [4]. Psychosocial rehabilitation programs reduce untoward behaviors while offenders remain in such intramural programs, i.e., while they are still incarcerated. Where psychosocial therapeutic services are continued after release from prison, limited evidence suggests diminished recidivism. Those with severe psychopathy, however, do not consistently show this benefit after release [4]. Conclusions from reviews that describe the nature of psychosocial rehabilitation programs must be tempered because reports of the methods and outcomes do not consistently describe the character pathology or measure the degree of psychopathy of the treated offenders. Moreover, descriptive reports of individual intramural psychosocial rehabilitation programs do not typically report continuing psychosocial programmatic or psychotherapeutic efforts in the community after offenders are released from prison [4].

Apart from the literature that describes psychosocial rehabilitation programs for criminal offenders, a few reviews include only studies that consistently measure the degree of psychopathy. From these reviews and individual studies themselves, the nature of the treatment is not consistently and adequately described, and follow-up treatment after release from the intramural program is neglected. Where the programs are described, they are so fundamentally different that any comparison is like that of the proverbial apples and oranges.

Two examples of frequently cited, but with substantially different treatments for psychopathic disorders, are the reports by Rice *et al.* [5] and by Skeem *et al.* [6], respectively. The study by Rice *et al.* suggested that psychopathy could be made worse by treatment. Theirs was a highly atypical therapeutic community program at the Social Therapy Unit in Pentaguishene, Canada. Recidivism was lower for nonpsychopathic subjects with Psychopathy Checklist – Revised (PCL-R) scores less than 25, in comparison with nontreated subjects. Psychopathic subjects, however, recidivated regardless whether or not they received treatment, and the rate of violent recidivism was higher for treated psychopathy but lower for nontreated psychopaths. This study would favor treatment in this therapeutic community program for nonpsychopathic offenders, but not psychopathic offenders.

In contrast, the study by Skeem *et al.* examined the effects of treatment, not in a corrections-based intramural therapeutic community program, but in a civil setting wherein subjects were provided standard psychiatric treatment as outpatients. Pharmacotherapy, presumably tailored for individualized treatment plans, was used but not described in this report. Results of this study, using different Psychopathy Checklist – Revised, Screening Version (PCL-SV) cutoff scores than the study by Rice *et al.*, indicated that subjects with "potentially psychopathic" personality disorders benefited from ordinary follow-up treatment in the community if such treatment consisted of a sufficient number of sessions. This study by itself does not contradict the assumption that severe psychopathy does not show improvement following treatment [7], but the effect of adequate follow-up treatment for severe psychopathy is not clarified by either of these two studies. Importantly, the two studies illustrate how different "treatment" is between studies that are compared to assess the amenability of psychopathic disorders to programmatic treatment.

Seto and Barbaree's [8] follow-up study of 224 sex offenders suggested that those who showed "good treatment behavior" while in the prison-based treatment program did not show diminished recidivism following release. Moreover, offenders who scored 15 or higher on the PLC-R and who demonstrated improved behavior during treatment were more likely to commit a serious offense. Together with the results by Rice *et al.* [5], their study suggests that the risk of recidivism can be increased as a result of treatment.

Two hypotheses are proffered to explain how treatment could worsen the psychopathic criminal behavior. The first is because psychopaths are prone to manipulate, they are able to appear improved during treatment without actually benefitting from treatment [9].

The "treatment-causes-harm" hypothesis suggests that psychopaths are only better armed to carry out their antisocial behavior as a result of treatment [10]. Citing programs that were associated with increased post-release criminal behavior, Hare [10] concluded that it was the insight orientation approach of these particular programs that contributed to the worsened outcome of those with elevated psychopathy. He did not conclude from this disappointing finding that psychopathy is immutable to any treatment.

When Looman et al. [11] attempted to replicate the study by Seto and Barbee [8], identifying psychopathy with a PCL-R cutoff of 25, they found that serious recidivism was related to psychopathy, but how well the subjects did during treatment did not affect their rates of serious recidivism. Similarly when Barbee [9] examined the sample of offenders from the Seto and Barbee study over a longer period of follow-up, he found that psychopathy remained a significant predictor of general and serious recidivism, but treatment behavior did not affect the rates of recidivism among psychopathic individuals, with 30 as the PCL-R cutoff.

In contrast, the review by Salekin et al. [12] found that three out of eight studies of adult subjects diagnosed with psychopathy showed treatment gains. Using a different method, D'Silva et al. [13] reviewed studies on the effectiveness of treatment programs in the treatment of psychopathy. They first attempted to identify all published and unpublished studies of treatment programs that diagnosed psychopathy by a high score on the PCL-R or a derivative measure. Four questions were used to evaluate the quality of each study. (1) Was an adequate control group included? (2) Did the treatment focus on "Hare psychopathy"? (3) Were the outcome variables adequate? (4) Was the follow-up study of adequate length? The authors concluded that none of these studies was acceptable, and that a negative relationship between treatment response and elevated PCL scores has not been demonstrated [13].

Reviews and individual studies taken together neither establish effective treatment for psychopathic disorders nor justify the conclusion that such disorders are untreatable. From reviews of outcome studies of treatment programs for psychopathic individuals, conclusions about what is and what is not effective treatment cannot be made. The treatment itself is not well described in the reviews or sometimes in the studies themselves [7]. If treatment is aimed at controlling and preventing offending behaviors, assessment and treatment of such behaviors by evidence-based treatment such as pharmacotherapy is not described; neither are measures of outpatient treatment or general relapse prevention following release from prison and from the in-service treatment program described, if such measures were attempted.

Impulsive Aggression in Psychopathic Disorders

It may well be that the core defect in psychopathy, if there is a single causal defect such as deficient capacity for empathy, is immutable to any pharmaceutical agent. Yet behaviors that are symptomatic of or co-occurring with psychopathic disorders are amenable to pharmacotherapy, and no less so because the individual is a psychopath. In this review, I use the term psychopathic disorders to include both Hare psychopathy [10,14,15] and also the APD of the DSM [3].

Physical aggression is one of the most serious manifestations and consequences of psychopathic disorders. Premeditated – also termed proactive, instrumental, and predatory – aggression appears to be most closely associated with psychopathic disorders [16–18]. A classification of aggression based on the degree of thought and emotion involved in each consists of four types: impulsive, spontaneous, compulsive, and premeditated [19]. Whether all four types are more commonly represented in psychopathic disorders remains to be determined empirically. If the spectrum of psychopathic disorders is extended to include the variously termed successful [20], creative, industrial [21], or corporate [22,23], then physical aggression is not such a pronounced manifestation of this latter condition for which there is no known pharmacotherapy. Premeditated aggression, i.e., the type that is conceptually most closely associated with psychopathic disorders, is not known to respond favorably to pharmacotherapy [24,25]. However, impulsive aggression, which also occurs with psychopathic disorders, is often controlled with evidence-based pharmacotherapy [26].

Although not completely defined, impulsive aggression corresponds to the following diagnostic criteria for APD in the DSM-5: "3. Impulsivity or failure to plan ahead; 4. Irritability and aggressiveness, as indicated by repeated physical fights or assaults" (p. 659) [3]. Likewise impulsive aggression corresponds to the following criteria for APD that are included in the "Alternative DSM-5 Model for Personality Disorders," which was added in the fifth edition: "4. Hostility (an aspect of Antagonism): Persistent or frequent angry feelings; anger or irritability in response to minor slights and insults, mean, nasty or revengeful behavior. 5. Impulsivity (an aspect of Disinhibition): Acting on the spur of the moment in response to immediate stimuli; acting on a momentary basis without a plan or consideration of outcomes; difficulty establishing or following plans" (p. 764) [3].

The psychological instruments for assessment of psychopathy developed by Hare [10] follow a dimensional rather than a categorical approach. The PCL-R is organized into a 2-part Factor Structure; Factor 1 represents affective and interpersonal components, and Factor 2 represents the more externalizing, socially deviant lifestyle of psychopathy. Within a superordinate 4-factor model – interpersonal, affective, lifestyle, and antisocial – impulsive aggression could support 2 factors in particular: "impulsive" under lifestyle and "poor behavioral controls" under antisocial. The PCL Youth Version (PCL-YV) uses the term "poor anger control" rather than "poor behavioral controls" [10].

Thus impulsive aggression supports criteria for APD under DSM-5, as well as factors of Hare psychopathy.

Primary Impulsive Aggression

Once impulsive aggression has been diagnosed, a determination must be made as to whether it is primary or secondary to another medical, neurological, or medical condition. If what is basically phenomenologically impulsive aggression is secondary to a mental disorder with known efficacious pharmacotherapy for the other mental disorder – schizophrenia, delusional disorder, bipolar disorder, or traumatic brain injury, for example – the impulsive aggression may well come under control with appropriate treatment of the primary mental disorder, the treatment of which has been discussed in several reviews [26–30]. Here we are interested in primary impulsive aggression, i.e., impulsive aggression that is not due to a mental disorder other than personality or psychopathic disorder.

Identification of primary impulsive aggression that co-occurs with a personality or psychopathic

disorder begs the question as to whether the impulsive aggression is secondary to the character pathology. Impulsive aggression in particular may distinguish the unsuccessful from the successful psychopath [21–23,31,32] and causes the unsuccessful psychopath to be preferentially subjected to arrest and incarceration. As shown above, aggressive behavior is a diagnostic criterion for APD and the conduct disorder in youth from which it evolves, as well as an element of the dimension of psychopathy described and measured by Hare [10,14,15].

Borderline personality disorder (BPD) is another Cluster B personality disorder for which impulsive and aggressive behavior can be diagnostic criteria [3]. Just as in APD or psychopathy, impulsive aggression can be a manifestation of BPD. However, the effect of divalproex in reducing impulsive aggression in BPD, an effect independent of that on the emotional dysregulation of BPD, led Hollander and colleagues [33–35] to conceptualize impulsive aggression as one of several "domains" of BPD.

A conceptualization of impulsive aggression as a domain of psychopathy may be equally justified and consistent with the dimensional approach in the second research criterion of APD [3]. If a dimension or domain is part of the disorder, then the disorder itself, BPD or APD, is being treated pharmacotherapeutically and efficaciously, even if the medication does not affect all symptoms of the disorder. Nonetheless, the distinction of primary impulsive disorder is useful, even if it is a manifestation of character pathology from which it is thought to be secondary. At the same time, the domain approach and the possibility of differential pharmacotherapeutic effects on impulsive aggression raise the possibility of different types of "primary impulsive aggression."

The Neurobiology of the Factor Domains of Psychopathy

Although relevant, it would be beyond the scope of this review to provide an update on the considerable literature on the childhood development, psychosocial evolution, and neurobiology of psychopathic disorders. For a more complete discussion of these and other dimensions of the etiology and pathogenesis of psychopathic disorders, the reader is referred to *The International Handbook of Psychopathic Disorders and the Law, Volume I: Diagnosis and Treatment* [36]. Some authors provide a translational approach to the theory and practice of the pharmacotherapy of aggressive behavior [37,38]. The emphasis in this review is more on empirical evidence for treatment efficacy than therapeutic mechanisms. Nonetheless, the potential theoretical importance of the prefrontal cortex, the orbital frontal cortex in particular, and the temporal lobes, especially the amygdala, may be of particular relevance to both psychopathy [39] and impulsive aggression. In controlling impulsive aggression, fluoxetine is a selective serotonin reuptake inhibitor (SSRI) with demonstrable effect on the prefrontal cortex; whereas certain anticonvulsants stabilize neurons of the amygdala in particular.

Two biological correlates of impulsive aggression are abnormally low amplitude of the P300 event-related potential and evidence of hyposerotonicity in the prefrontal cortex, both of which may pertain to the therapeutic effects of anti-impulsive aggressive agents (AIAAs). Phenytoin normalizes the low amplitude of P300 of impulsively aggressive subjects and reduces their aggression, but has no effect on the already normal amplitude of the P300 and premeditated aggressive episodes in subjects with antisocial personality disorder [24,25]. Evidence for hyposerotonicity in the prefrontal cortex, which has been shown to be associated with impulsive aggression [40], may be improved with SSRIs such as fluoxetine. Fluoxetine can reduce impulsive aggression, which in psychopathy corresponds to its impulsive–antisocial factor [41].

Suggesting a pathophysiological distinction between impulsive aggression and callousness are the differential degrees of 5-HT transporter (5-HTT) binding at different locations in the brain. Van de Giessen *et al.* [42] recently found a positive correlation between 5-HTT availability in the pregenual anterior cingulated cortex (pgACC) and callousness, whereas subjects with intermittent explosive disorder (IED) showed no differences in 5-HTT binding in comparison with controls. Therefore, while impulsive aggression is associated with hyposerotonicity, especially in the frontal cortex [40], the callousness domain of psychopathic disorders may also be related to aberrant serotonin availability, even if increased and in a different part of the brain.

Speculative to be sure, but perhaps future research will further clarify this possibility of specific abnormal serotonicity with callousness, which suggests a pharmacotherapeutic intervention for callousness as a trait that enables premeditated

aggression. For now, it is sufficient to recognize the amenability of impulsive aggression to pharmacotherapy, including the use of fluoxetine, an SSRI thought to ameliorate the hyposerotonicity of impulsive aggression.

Doland and Anderson [43] suggested that the construct of psychopathy is sufficiently complex that further investigation ought to examine the neurobiological correlates of each factor – impulsive–antisocial, arrogant/deceitful, and callous/remorseless, respectively – rather than the unified construct of the so-called prototypical psychopath. They anticipate, as does this author, that this more discerning approach will be more productive in studying the pharmacotherapy of psychopathic disorders. I maintain that the distinction between impulsive aggression, consistent with impulsive–antisocial conduct, and premeditated aggression, compatible with arrogant/deceitful and/or callous/remorseless trait factors, already informs the pharmacotherapy of psychopathic disorders, namely the pharmacotherapeutic target of impulsive but not premeditated aggression.

Pharmacotherapy of Aggression in Psychopathic Disorders

As in any patient, including patients with personality disorders and psychopathic disorders, pharmacotherapy should not be initiated until the nature of the aggression has been evaluated [26,44–46]. Although those with psychopathic disorders can show various types of untoward aggression, and premeditated or proactive aggression is thought to be the most characteristic of psychopathy, impulsive aggression also commonly occurs with psychopathic disorders. It is the physical aggressiveness of some antisocial or psychopathic disordered individuals that makes their condition so problematic and dangerous to others. In the prison studies by Barratt *et al.* [24,25], all aggressive subjects, both those with predominantly impulsive aggression and those with predominantly premeditated aggression, met the criteria for APD.

In general, those who meet the criteria for IED can be said to have impulsive aggression, but DSM-5 discourages the diagnosis and thereby the treatment of IED in those with APD by its exclusionary criterion. If "recurrent aggressive outbursts are not better explained by . . . e.g., antisocial personality disorder"

(p. 466) [3], then the diagnosis of IED is permissible. This exclusionary criterion would likely mislead many clinicians to avoid the diagnosis and treatment of IED in the context of an antisocial personality disorder. Yet the clinician, who is knowledgeable about the different types of aggression and their different amenabilities to pharmacotherapy, can provide effective pharmacotherapy for abnormal aggression that occurs with antisocial personality disorder without violating this exclusionary criterion.

We should note carefully the wording of this exclusion. It does not exclude the diagnosis of IED co-occurring with APD, but recurrent aggressive behavior that is better explained by APD. To the extent that premeditated or proactive aggressive behavior is more typical of APD and psychopathic disorders, premeditated aggression should not be diagnosed as IED and neither does it fit the description. Impulsive aggression, although often co-occurring with APD, is not thought to be such a specific manifestation of the core defect. We will not here resolve the question as to what extent IED or impulsive aggression is symptomatic of APD and psychopathic disorders versus a frequent, co-occurring condition. Suffice it to say that the diagnosis of impulsive aggression ought not be withheld because the individual is diagnosed with APD or psychopathy. An analogy can be made with substance use disorder (SUD), which occurs with such frequency in psychopathic disorders that it is considered part of the symptomatic constellation. Yet the diagnosis of SUD is made separately, and treatment and rehabilitation are not categorically withheld because of the psychopathic disorder.

What is more meaningful than the exclusionary criterion of DSM-5 is the empirical data from research on aggressive subjects with personality disorders. Where impulsive aggression is diagnosed, it has been found to be amenable to pharmacotherapy regardless of whether it co-occurs with a personality or psychopathic disorder. Fluoxetine has been shown to be effective in the treatment of impulsive aggression in individuals with personality disorders such as BPD [47], and phenytoin has controlled impulsive aggression in prisoners with APD [24,25]. Of decisive importance is the diagnosis of impulsive aggression and distinguishing impulsive from premeditated aggression. Premeditated aggression is singularly unresponsive to pharmacotherapy [24,25].

Here the concept of impulsive aggression is favored over IED, because the former is better grounded in drug trial research, is not confounded by the earlier exclusion of IED that is associated with generalized impulsivity, and, unlike the DSM criteria for IED, does not mislead clinicians away from the diagnosis simply because the condition co-occurs with APD [45]. Nonetheless, IED is impulsive aggression and should be treated accordingly.

Once impulsive aggression has been diagnosed, psychotherapy and/or pharmacotherapy can be initiated. Here the discussion is limited to pharmacotherapy and the selection of the most promising anti-impulsive aggressive agent (AIAA). Guidelines for selecting an efficacious AIAA begin with an accurate diagnosis of impulsive aggression [45] – a step that is not uncommonly overlooked in AIAA drug trials and literature reviews [44], and presumably in clinical practice. Assessment of impulsive aggression has been discussed previously [45], and so is not iterated here.

Selecting an AIAA

For optimal efficacy and safety, eight guidelines have been proffered by Felthous and Stanford [46] for selecting an AIAA for control of a patient's impulsive aggression. Although some of these guidelines would be prudent for the prescription of any psychotropic medication, they are especially important in the selection of an AIAA, none of which has been approved by the FDA for this indication.

Steps to follow in selecting an AIAA are as follows.

(1) Diagnose the condition as impulsive aggression.
(2) Identify the agents with evidence of efficacy by drug trials of satisfactory quality.
(3) Determine the risks of side effects for the individual patient.
(4) Determine the severity of the outbursts.
(5) Determine whether the patient has a co-occurring condition for which the AIAA is indicated.
(6) Obtain the patient's pharmacotherapeutic history.
(7) Determine if the AIAA is affordable and available to the patient.
(8) Determine how urgently the aggressive behavior must be brought under control [46].

Comment will be made on each of these factors, as the appropriateness of treating symptoms of psychopathic disorders depends on the logic of selecting the most appropriate AIAA.

The first two factors are of fundamental importance: identifying AIAAs that are efficacious and diagnosing impulsive aggression. In identifying efficacious AIAAs, two reports are especially useful. The meta-analysis by Jones *et al.* [48] that examined the efficacy of mood stabilizers in reducing impulsive aggression also took into account measures for ensuring the quality of these studies. This meta-analysis supported the efficacy of carbamazepine/oxcarbazepine, phenytoin, and lithium, but not valproate or levetiracetam [48]. In contrast to the negative finding concerning valproate, Hollander *et al.* [34,35] provided evidence of the efficacy of divalproex in controlling impulsive aggression within the context of Cluster B personality disorders and borderline personality disorder in particular [49].

Felthous and Stanford [46] reviewed 55 peer-reviewed studies on the pharmacotherapy of impulsive aggression. Of these, 23 satisfied inclusion criteria for quality placebo-controlled drug trials. Agents that were subjected to high-quality drug trials included the anticonvulsants carbamazepine, divalproex/valproate, levetiracetam, oxcarbazepine, and phenytoin; the mood stabilizer lithium; the antipsychotic haloperidol; the antidepressant fluoxetine; and the amphetamines d-amphetamine and pindolol. Only levetiracetam showed no efficacy [50]. Those AIAAs that have been shown to be efficacious in more than one high-quality study and therefore constituting the most appropriate selections for AIAA are carbamazepine/oxcarbazepine [51–53], divalproate/valproate [34,51,54], phenytoin [24,25], lithium [55–57], and fluoxetine [58,59].

Importantly, these drug trials concern the pharmacotherapy of impulsive aggression, not undefined aggression or disruptive behavior. Some algorithms have been developed for the treatment of aggression due to various mental disorders, but not impulsive aggression in particular [27–30]. Impulsive aggression is the type of aggression that is most likely to be subject to improvement with an AIAA. Impulsive aggression should not be neglected just because it occurs together with a psychopathic disorder, any more than one would neglect treatment of a primary mental disorder such as major depressive disorder that co-occurs with a psychopathic disorder. Of critical importance is the careful diagnosis of impulsive aggression and distinguishing it from premeditated aggression, which is also common in psychopathic disorders but is not improved with an AIAA.

Consideration of risks and side effects for the individual patient is especially important, as none of these agents is FDA approved for the treatment of impulsive aggression or IED. Severity of the outbursts will help to identify the aggression as high-frequency/low-intensity or low-frequency/high-intensity IED as detailed in DSM-5 [3]. Fluoxetine has been most studied with the former, and so would be a reasonable first choice in the treatment of less severe impulsive aggression.

Fluoxetine is more conveniently administered, as serum levels are not needed, and its side effect profile is favorable compared with other AIAAs. The patient may have co-occurring disorders that favor one or more AIAA over the other, phenytoin for seizure disorder for example, whereas levetiracetam would not have such a "2 for 1" advantage. Naturally the pharmacotherapeutic history should not be overlooked. One of the AIAAs might have been prescribed for another purpose but with concomitant reduction in aggressive behavior. Affordability is critical for medication compliance, and insurance may not always cover the best selection of an AIAA for impulsive aggression. Finally if the need to bring impulsive aggression under control is urgent, there is evidence that phenytoin may begin to take effect quickly [26,60].

Note that none of these considerations in selecting an AIAA pertains to whether or not the patient has a psychopathic disorder. The most important diagnostic question is whether the patient has impulsive aggression, which often but not always is found in psychopathic disorders.

Conclusions

Although the presence of a psychopathic disorder complicates and worsens the prognosis for successful treatment aimed at reducing general and violent recidivism, such a guarded outlook does not mean that treatment is necessarily inappropriate or without benefit. A potentially useful approach is to assess and treat particular domains of psychopathy for which treatment effectiveness has been demonstrated. The psychopathic individual's pattern of violent behavior, for example, can be evaluated. If his untoward aggression is predominantly impulsive, then a trial on an AIAA is indicated. Assessing the nature of an individual's aggression and considering an AIAA if he manifests predominantly impulsive aggression ought not to be neglected because he is diagnosed with a psychopathic disorder. This approach could inform programmatic treatment and outcome studies. Then outcome studies will advance our knowledge, not just about the appropriateness of treating psychopathic disorders, but about which treatments are effective for which domains of the disorder.

Disclosure

The author does not have anything to disclose.

References

1. Saß H, Felthous AR. Introduction to Volume 1. In: Felthous AR, Saß H, eds. *The International Handbook of Psychopathic Disorders and the Law, Volume I: Diagnosis and Treatment.* Chichester, UK: John Wiley and Sons, Ltd.; 2007: 1–5.

2. Saß H, Felthous AR. History and development of psychopathic disorders. In: Felthous AR, Saß H, eds. *The International Handbook of Psychopathic Disorders and the Law, Volume I: Diagnosis and Treatment.* Chichester, UK: John Wiley and Sons, Ltd.; 2007: 9–30.

3. American Psychiatric Association. *Diagnostic and Statistical Manual of Mental Disorders.* 5th edn. Washington, DC: Arlington, VA; 2013.

4. Felthous AR, Sass H. Behandlungsprogramme für Straftäter in den Vereinigten Staaten und Kanada. In: Kröber HL, Dölling D, Leygraf N, Sass H, eds. *Handbuch der Forensischen Psychiatrie, Band 3, Psychiatrische Kriminalprognose und Kriminaltherapie.* Darmstadt, Germany: Steinkoff; 2006: 390–412.

5. Rice ME, Harris GT, Cormier C. Evaluation of a maximum security therapeutic community for psychopaths and other mentally disordered offenders. *Law Hum. Behavior.* 1992; **16**(4): 399–412.

6. Skeem JL, Monahan J, Mulvey EP. Psychopathy, treatment and involvement, and subsequent violence among civil psychiatric patients. *Law Hum. Behavior.* 2002; **26**(6): 577–603.

7. Felthous AR. The "untreatability" of psychopathy and hospital commitment in the USA. *Int. J. Law Psychiatry.* 2011; **34**(6): 400–405.

8. Seto MC, Barbaree HE. Psychopathy, treatment behavior and sex offender recidivism. *J. Interpers. Violence.* 1999; **14**(12): 1235–1248.

9. Barbaree HE. Psychopathy, treatment behavior and recidivism: an extended follow-up of Seto and Barbaree. *J. Interpers. Violence.* 2005; **20**(9): 1115–1131.

10. Hare RD. Psychological instruments in the assessment of psychopathy. In: Felthous AR, Saß H, eds. *The International Handbook of Psychopathic Disorders and the Law, Volume I: Diagnosis and Treatment.* Chichester, UK: John Wiley and Sons, Ltd.; 2007: 41–67.

11. Looman J, Abracen J, Serin R, Marquis P. Psychopathy, treatment change and recidivism in high risk high need sexual offenders. *J. Interpers. Violence.* 2005; **20**(5): 549–568.

12. Salekin RT, Worley C, Grimes RD. Treatment of psychopathy: a review and brief introduction to the mental model approach for psychotherapy. *Behav. Sci. Law.* 2010; **28**(2): 235–266.

13. D'Silva K, Duggan D, McCarthy L. Does treatment really make psychopaths worse? A review of the evidence. *J. Personal. Disord.* 2004; **18**(2): 163–177.

14. Hare RD. *The Hare Psychopathy Checklist – Revised.* Toronto, Canada: Multi-Health Systems; 1991.

15. Hare RD. *Without Conscience: The Disturbing World of the Psychopaths Among Us.* New York: Guilford Press; 1998.

16. Cornell D, Warren J, Hawk G, *et al.* Psychopathy in instrumental and reactive offenders. *J. Consult. Clin. Psychol.* 1996; **64**(4): 783–790.

17. Patrick CJ. Emotional processes in psychopathy. In: Raine A, Sanmartin J, eds. *Violence and Psychopathy.* New York: Kluwer/ Plenum; 2001: 57–77.

18. Raine A, Yang Y. The neuroanatomical bases of psychopathy: a review of brain imaging findings. In: Patrick CJ, ed. *Handbook of Psychopathy.* New York: Guilford; 2006: 278–295.

19. Felthous AR. Schizophrenia and impulsive aggression: a heuristic inquiry with forensic and clinical implications. *Behav. Sci. Law.* 2008; **26**(6): 735–758.

20. Babiak P, Hare RD. *Snakes in Suits: When Psychopaths Go to Work.* New York: Harper-Collins; 2006.

21. Babiak P. When psychopaths go to work: a case study of an industrial psychopath. *Applied Psychology.* 1995; **44**(2): 171–188.

22. Babiak P. Psychopathic manipulation at work. In: Gacono CB, ed. *The Clinical and Forensic Assessment of Psychopathy: A Practitioner's Guide.* Mahwah, NJ: Erlbaum; 2000: 287–311.

23. Babiak P, Neumann CS, Hare RD. Corporate psychopathy: talking the walk. *Behav. Sci. Law.* 2010; **28**(2): 174–193.

24. Barratt ES, Standford MS, Felthous AR, Kent TA. The effects of phenytoin on impulsive and premeditated aggression: a controlled study. *J. Clin. Psychopharmacol.* 1997; **17**(5): 341–349.

25. Barratt ES, Stanford MS, Kent TA, Felthous A. Neurological and cognitive psychophysiological substrates of impulsive aggression. *Biol. Psychiatry.* 1997; **41**(10): 1045–1061.

26. Felthous AR. The pharmacotherapy of impulsive aggression. In: Thienhaus OJ, Piaski M, eds. *Correctional Psychiatry: Practice Guidelines and Strategies, Volume II.* Kingston, NJ: Civil Research Institute; 2013: 4-1-4-34.

27. Glancy GD, Knott TF. Part I: The psychopharmacology of long-term aggression—toward an evidence-based algorithm. *CPA Bulletin.* 2002; **34**(6).

28. Glancy GD, Knott TF. Part II: The psychopharmacology of long-term aggression—toward an evidence-based algorithm. *CPA Bulletin.* 2002; **34**(6).

29. Glancy GD, Knott TF. Part III: The psychopharmacology of long-term aggression—toward an evidence-based algorithm. *CPA Bulletin.* 2003; **35**(1): 18.

30. Moeller FG, Swann A. Pharmacotherapy of clinical aggression in individuals with psychopathic disorders. In: Felthous AR, Saß H, eds. *The International Handbook of Psychopathic Disorders and the Law, Volume I: Diagnosis and Treatment.* Chichester, UK: John Wiley & Sons, Ltd.; 2007: 397–416.

31. Babiak P. From darkness into the light: psychopathy in industrial and organizational psychology. In: Hervé H, Yville C, eds. *The Psychopath: Theory, Research and Practice.* Mahwah, NJ: Erlbaum; 2007: 411–428.

32. Gao Y, Raine A. Successful and unsuccessful psychopaths: a neurobiological model. *Behav. Sci. Law.* 2010; **28**(2): 194–210.

33. Taylor BP, Weiss M, Ferretti CJ, *et al.* Disruptive, impulse-control, and conduct disorders. In: Hales RE, Yudofsky SC, Roberts LW, eds. *American Psychiatric Publishing Textbook of Psychiatry*, 6th edn. Washington, DC: American Psychiatric Publishing; 2014: 703–734.

34. Hollander E, Tracy KA, Swann AC, *et al.* Divalproex in the treatment of impulsive aggression: efficacy in cluster B personality disorder. *Neuropsychopharmacology.* 2003; **28**(6): 1186–1197.

35. Hollander E, Swann AC, Coccaro EF, Jiang P, Smith TB. Impact of trait impulsivity and state aggression in divalproex versus placebo response in borderline personality disorder. *Am. J. Psychiatry.* 2005; **162**(3): 621–624.

36. Felthous AR, Saß H, eds. *The International Handbook of Psychopathic Disorders and the Law, Volume I: Diagnosis and Treatment.* Chichester, UK: John Wiley and Sons, Ltd.; 2007.

37. Comai S, Tau M, Gobbi G. The psychopharmacology of aggressive behavior: a translational approach. Part 1: Neurobiology. *J. Clin. Psychopharmacol.* 2012; **32**(1): 83–94.

38. Comai S, Tau M, Pavlovic Z, Gobbi G. The psychopharmacology of aggressive behavior: a translational approach. Part 2: Clinical studies using atypical antipsychotics, anticonvulsants, and lithium. *J. Clin. Psychopharmacol.* 2012; **32**(2): 237–260.

39. Blair JR. Neurobiological basis of psychopathy. *Br. J. Psychiatry.* 2003; **182**(1): 5–7.

40. Siever LJ, Buchsbaum MS, New AS, *et al.* D,l-fenfluramine response in impulsive personality disorder assessed with [18F] fluorodeoxyglucose positron emission tomography. *Neuropsychopharmacology.* 1999; **20**(5): 413–423.

41. Cooke DS, Mitchie C, Hart SD, Hare RD. Evaluating the Screening Version of the Hale Psychopathy Checklist—Revised (PCL-SV). *Psychol. Assess.* 1999; **11**(1): 3–13.

42. van de Giessen E, Rosell DR, Thompson JL, *et al.* Serotonin transporter availability in impulsive aggressive personality disordered patients: a PET study with [11C] DASB. *J. Psychiatr. Res.* 2014; **58**: 147–154.

43. Dolan MC, Anderson IM. The relationship between serotonergic function and the Psychopathy Checklist: Screening Version. *J. Psychopharmacol.* 2003; **17**(2): 216–222.

44. Felthous AR, Lake SL, Rundle BK, Stanford MS. Pharmacotherapy of impulsive aggression: a quality comparison of controlled studies. *J. Int. Law Psychiatry.* 2013; **36** (3–4): 258–263.

45. Felthous AR, Barratt ES. Impulsive aggression. In: Coccaro EF, ed. *Aggression: Psychiatric Assessment and Treatment.* New York: Marcel Dekker; 2003: 123–148.

46. Felthous AR, Stanford MS. A proposed algorithm for the pharmacotherapy of impulsive aggression. *J. Am. Acad. Psychiatry Law.* 2015; **43**(4): 456–467.

47. Coccaro EF, Kavoussi RJ. Fluoxetine and impulsive aggressive behavior in personality disordered subjects. *Arch. Gen. Psychiatry.* 1997; **54** (12): 1081–1088.

48. Jones RM, Arlidge J, Gilham S, *et al.* Efficacy of mood stabilizers in the treatment of impulsive or

repetitive aggression: systematic review and meta-analysis. *Br. J. Psychiatry.* 2011; **198**(2): 93–98.

49. Hollander E, Swann AC, Coccaro EF, Jiang P, Smith TB. Impact of trait impulsivity and state aggression on divalproex versus placebo response in borderline personality disorder. *Am. J. Psychiatry.* 2005; **162**(3): 621–624.

50. Mattes JA. Levetiracetam in patients with impulsive aggression: a double-blind, placebo-controlled trial. *J. Clin. Psychiatry.* 2008; **69**(2): 310–315.

51. Stanford MS, Helfritz LE, Conklin SM, *et al.* A comparison of anticonvulsants in the treatment of impulsive aggression. *Exp. Clin. Psychopharmacol.* 2005; **13**(1): 72–77.

52. Cueva JE, Overall JE, Small AM, *et al.* Carbamazepine in aggressive children with conduct disorder: a double-blind and placebo-controlled study. *J. Am. Acad. Child. Adolesc. Psychiatry.* 1996; **35**(4): 480–490.

53. Mattes JA. Oxcarbazepine in patients with impulsive aggression: a double-blind, placebo-controlled trial. *J. Clin. Psychopharmacol.* 2005; **25**(6): 575–579.

54. Donovan SJ, Stewart JW, Nunes EV, *et al.* Divalproex treatment for youth with explosive temper and mood lability: a double-blind, placebo-controlled crossover design. *Am. J. Psychiatry.* 2000; **157**(5): 818–820.

55. Campbell M, Adams PB, Small AM, *et al.* Lithium in hospitalized aggressive children with conduct disorder: a double-blind, placebo-controlled study. *J. Am. Acad. Child. Adolesc. Psychiatry.* 1995; **34**(4): 445–453.

56. Campbell M, Small AM, Green WH, *et al.* Behavioral efficacy of haloperidol and lithium carbonate: a comparison in hospitalized aggressive children with conduct disorder. *Arch Gen Psychiatry.* 1984; **41**(7): 650–656.

57. Sheard MH, Marini JL, Bridges CI, Wagner E. The effect of lithium on impulsive aggression behavior in man. *Am. J. Psychiatry.* 1976; **133**(12): 1409–1413.

58. Coccaro EF, Lee RJ, Kavoussi RJ. A double-blind randomized, placebo-controlled trial of fluoxetine in patients with intermittent explosive disorder. *J. Clin. Psychiatry.* 2009; **70**(5): 653–662.

59. Lee R, Kavoussi RJ, Coccaro EF. Placebo-controlled, randomized trial of fluoxetine in the treatment of aggression in male intimate partner abuse. *Int. Clin. Psychopharm.* 2008; **23**(6): 337–341.

60. Pritchard WS, Barratt ES, Faulk DM, Brandt ME, Bryant SG. Effects of phenytoin on N100 augmenting/reducing and late positive complex of the event related potential: a topographical analysis. *Neuropsychobiology.* 1986; **15**(3–4): 201–207.

Chapter

28 Psychosocial approaches to violence and aggression: contextually anchored and trauma-informed interventions

Deborah Horowitz, Margaret Guyer, and Kathy Sanders

Introduction

Across the United States, state mental health authorities are working to incorporate the voice of the person served into the mission and operating procedures of mental health services. The focus on providing trauma-informed, person-centered, recovery-focused (TPR) care has gone hand in hand with initiatives to reduce restraint and seclusion episodes in psychiatric hospitals. State inpatient psychiatric facilities have a special opportunity to facilitate recovery in a trauma-informed, person-centered way and to foster positive growth and change in individuals who have traditionally been underserved and are in acute and/or enduring phases of their illnesses. These facilities, with access to diverse, flexible resources and modalities of care, are a vital part of any integrated continuum of care [1].

Our mission as healthcare providers is to assist those seeking services to "turn pain into purpose" [2]. For those who express their pain through violence, our challenge is to help them transform that pain rather than meet it with the violence of restraint, seclusion, and coercion. Trauma engenders feelings of fear, anger, and shame, and violence is but one outward expression of those feelings. Violence, be it toward self or others, is multideterministic in nature, and as such requires interventions tailored to the individual and his or her own idiosyncratic behavioral expressions. Moreover, the episodes of violence in our inpatient psychiatric units jeopardize the healing environment necessary to provide effective treatment and to empower the person served to be an active participant in his or her recovery. Staff and the person served suffer when violence occurs in what should be an environment of hope and opportunity for healing

and change. As state mental health authorities across the country work to adopt TPR systems of care, implementation has often been met with anger and fear that these philosophical changes are at the expense of frontline staff members' ability to maintain safety for themselves and for those served [3]. The high rates of injury in behavioral healthcare settings, particularly among frontline staff, undermine the quality of the milieu and efficacy of the therapeutic alliance so necessary to recovery.

This article seeks to explore the ways in which TPR-informed psychosocial interventions can ameliorate the negative impact of violence for persons served and for staff (see Figure 28.1). The authors will discuss how, given this lens, comprehensive assessment is conducted and appropriate treatment engagement, including accurate choice of psychosocial interventions, are facilitated. We will utilize a threat assessment approach that is organized around the identification, assessment, and de-escalation of threatening situations and is grounded in the TPR paradigm. The authors will pay particular attention to those psychosocial interventions that ultimately result, not only in the absence of violent behavior, but in safety, hope, and healing for all.

Trauma-Informed Perspective

There is growing recognition that trauma is widespread, and that the experience of trauma has far-reaching effects on a person's physical and mental well-being. The Adverse Childhood Experience (ACE) Study, utilizing a 10-item survey, found a powerful relationship between the number of traumatic incidents individuals had experienced prior to the age of 18 and their developmental challenges and chronic

Components of Recovery

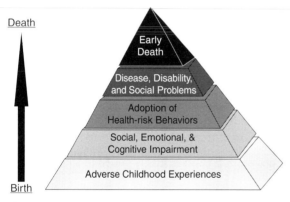

Figure 28.1 SAMHSA components and principles of recovery for individuals and organizations.

Death

Birth

Early
Death

Disease, Disability,
and Social Problems

Adoption of
Health-risk Behaviors

Social, Emotional, &
Cognitive Impairment

Adverse Childhood Experiences

Figure 28.2 Conceptual understanding of a common pathway from adverse childhood experiences through impairment, risky behaviors, and disease to premature mortality. Public domain from Centers for Disease Control.

Table 28.1 Correlation of public health and threat assessment prevention models

	Public health prevention model	Threat assessment prevention model
Primary	Institutional	Universal
Secondary	Structural	Identifying those at risk
Tertiary	Direct	Intervening in an act of violence

the innumerable effects of the traumas they have experienced (see Figure 28.2). Among people with severe mental illness, the sheer pervasiveness of trauma, estimated to be as high as 90%, is staggering and requires us to assume that trauma is a universal experience among people served on our state psychiatric inpatient units [5]. The implication is that more than 90% of persons served have suffered some form of significant pain, loss, and fear, often at the violent hands of another. Assessing and treating violence as a direct consequence of trauma is but the first step on that journey of recovery.

Assessment

Equally central to TPR is the observation that "violence is a process, not an act" [6]. In order to accurately address violent behavior for a particular individual, a wider lens is needed to assess and understand the context and risk for violence. The public health model of violence defines three levels of violence: organizational/institutional (e.g., stigma, discrimination); structural (e.g., unemployment, involuntary hospitalization); and direct (e.g., trauma) [7] (see Table 28.1). Violence is the synergistic culmination of individuals interacting with each other and the environment, each operating from their cultural affiliations and status within society overall, their relationships and trauma history, and their individual intrapsychic schemas [8]. Inpatient psychiatric units comprise miniature communities within which all three levels of violence (institutional, structural, and direct) are operating and relevant. A narrow focus on direct violence with little regard to the contributions of institutional and structural violence limits the efficacy of any intervention or treatment modality.

Within the field of violence risk assessment, the concept of threat assessment focuses on preventing

health conditions [4]. The items of the original ACE survey underscore that not only is trauma historical in nature, but it is also largely interpersonal, e.g., physical or sexual abuse at the hands of a family member or disrupted attachments due to parental death, incarceration, or substance abuse.

The TPR approach to treating violence starts with the recognition that the behaviors that lead to inpatient psychiatric care, e.g., violence to self or other, are a person's best attempt to communicate or mitigate violence within a community or institution. Threat assessment, consistent with the public health prevention model of violence, is organized into three levels of prevention: (1) primary (creating a community-wide climate that mitigates institutional violence and supports the commitment to nonviolence, (2) secondary (reducing structural violence by identifying and intervening with people at risk), and (3) tertiary (utilizing violence-specific interventions with people who are persistently violent).

Primary prevention at the culture of care level

The National Association of State Mental Health Program Directors (NASMHPD) has been the leader in emphasizing that the path to reducing violence on inpatient psychiatric units is to transform the authoritarian, controlling culture, which is too common among inpatient units, into a TPR culture [1,5]. NASMHPD clearly places the locus of change within the organizational culture, as the mechanism necessary to reduce violence and associated restraint and seclusion episodes [5]. A TPR culture of care may ameliorate the larger socioeconomic and cultural effects of institutional and structural violence, and thus reduce triggers for direct violence. Organizational expectations, values, and actions can influence the exhibition of challenging, aggressive, or violent behavior or they can encourage its prohibition. When a unit is motivated and committed to making changes, interventions are even more effective at reducing rates of violence. Fortunately, even when unit motivation is low, reduced violence rates are observed as a consequence of changes in the culture of care [3,9].

(1) Leadership commitment to TPR culture of care

In creating a TPR care delivery environment, the very process of culture change must reflect these principles across all organizational levels. Successful systems have engaged organizational leadership, frontline staff, and persons served in the process of direct change [3]. Staff supported in the pursuit of their own growth and development activities can foster this in others [10]. Also, those who are invested in the agency's mission are more likely to remain consistent with the interventions, modalities, and protocols associated with the overarching vision [5].

(2) Staff training

(a) Given the pervasiveness of trauma, one of the first steps in the promotion of TPR culture of care is staff training. Staff should receive training on the etiology and universality of trauma, trauma's neurobiological sequelae, and implications for the nature and timing of early intervention and de-escalation strategies [11,12].

(b) Since the therapeutic alliance is integral to recovery, recovery-based communication styles must be taught. Staff who utilize therapeutic approaches of compassion, empathy, and respect reduce violence motivated by fear, anger, and shame [13]. Training in low Expressed Emotion communication style, e.g., avoiding verbal and nonverbal criticism, hostility, or over-intrusive, paternalistic attitudes; using supportive and nonthreatening methods for limit-setting; and emphasizing positive rather than negative communications, has been associated with a reduction in rates of restraint and seclusion [3].

(c) Staff should be trained to respond to an individual who is experiencing distress in order to avert escalation and possible violence. Utilization of noncoercive de-escalation and crisis intervention techniques is associated with reduced violence and fewer episodes of restraint or seclusion [14–17].

(d) Safety, Hope, and Healing (SHH) is a model developed by the Massachusetts Department of Mental Health for training staff that assumes that trauma is pervasive and influences many aspects of human behavior including violence. SHH involves four key components: (1) knowing the individual, (2) knowing the environment, (3) knowing yourself, and (4) knowing society. Importantly, SHH empowers staff to understand their own histories, triggers, and risk factors, as well as those of persons served, as a vehicle for identifying and mitigating potentially dangerous situations. These tools enable staff to better understand, make meaning of, and predict violence, thereby increasing personal and organizational safety and fostering hope for both staff and persons served. This approach supports an individualized formulation and treatment plan for recognizing and responding to the contextual fluctuations in risk for violence, and allows for an accurate contextually based evaluation of historical, intrapsychic, and interpersonal factors at play in any given interaction at any given moment.

(3) Staff supervision and support

Staff members require ongoing training, supervision, and support in order to respond effectively to a person's level of distress. The intensity of people's need, despair, fear, shame, loneliness, or rage can be overwhelming, and may lead staff to recoil and distance themselves from their own intolerable feelings, which are often engendered by fear of professional inadequacy or fear for personal safety. Psychosocial interventions for staff include trauma-informed supervision, tertiary trauma and employee assistance services, and self-care and wellness activities that replenish staff and lead to higher work satisfaction. These interventions result in fewer negative encounters, including violence, as the result of staff compassion fatigue, vicarious trauma, and burnout [10].

(4) Modifying environmental factors

Violent incidents are lower on units where staff members have clear job descriptions and role expectations, and when staff are visibly present and actively engaged on the floor rather than sequestered in the nurses' station. The physical presence of unit and organizational leaders and predictable schedules filled with meaningful activities are associated with lower rates of violence [18].

(5) Systematic review of violent episodes

Systematic attention and review of past violent episodes have been associated with reductions in future violent episodes. Multidisciplinary consultation teams, with an eye toward reducing violence, consult on persons served who repeatedly exhibit challenging or unsafe behaviors, or who have had multiple episodes of seclusion or restraint. Formal debriefing of the involved persons served and staff is especially effective when a peer specialist participates in the

debriefing. The use of multidisciplinary feedback teams who review each violent incident for alternatives to restraint and seclusion decreases unwarranted restraint and seclusion episodes [3].

Secondary prevention at the culture of care level

In a TPR culture of care, secondary prevention efforts target the reduction of violence through identifying people at higher risk for violence, intervening to treat factors that increase vulnerability to violence, and monitoring risk status regularly and persistently over time. A comprehensive violence prevention assessment is ongoing and utilizes standardized measures; clinical observation; and collaboration, engagement, and empowerment with the person served [19,20]. Staff monitor both the universal indicators for potential escalation, as well as an individual's specific contextual triggers and indicators of escalating risk. When done in collaboration with the person served, this model proves to be more effective as individuals learn to accurately assess their own ongoing fluctuations in stress, triggers, and coping resources.

(1) Standardized assessment of universal risk factors

A person is most at risk for violent behavior in the first 3–4 days of admission [9,21]. A standardized violence risk assessment, e.g., the Brøset Violence Checklist, is most effective, given that the person served is new and not well known or understood by staff [22]. Systematic risk assessment upon admission can differentiate people at greatest risk for violent behavior [23]. Systematic and frequent risk monitoring (e.g., twice daily) during the first 3–4 days of a person's admission is associated with decreased rates of violent episodes [24,25].

The formalization of risk assessment procedures affects the culture of a unit in several intangible ways as well. Regular review of the risk assessments promotes more effective intra- and inter-team communication and treatment planning. Staff knowledge and attention to the universal indicators of violence risk is increased and the direct focus on early intervention supports the use of more effective strategies for de-escalation [9]. In one study, the number of severely aggressive incidents was unaffected; however, staff assessed these incidents as less severe, suggesting that systematic risk assessment increased staff's confidence in their ability to manage the risk for violence [16].

(2) Individualized formulations of violence risk

Traditional, systematic risk assessment is integral to violence prevention efforts, but must be supplemented with other modalities and types of assessment in order to increase efficacy. With TPR systems of care, violent behavior is conceptualized as a "message," be it to the self or others. In order to understand the meaning of a person's violent behavior, a multidisciplinary approach is necessary to uncover the connections between the individual, the situation at hand, the setting, and the target of the violence. Attention to the relevant institutional and structural violence a person is subject to further informs this formulation. It requires a more dynamic focus and "an investigative, skeptical, inquisitive mindset" [6].

(3) Therapeutic alliance

A powerful vehicle for preventing adverse events like violence is knowing the individual based on a nonstigmatizing therapeutic relationship built over time. Through this relationship, staff are aware of the meaningful aspects of an individual's history and are able to predict potential triggers, recognize early signs of difficulty, and utilize individual-specific interventions to avert escalation. Through this lens, the question becomes how to understand an individual's current presentation against the backdrop of "what happened to you?" rather than "what's wrong with you?" and shifts the paradigm even further to asking "what's strong in you?" [26]

(4) Collaborative monitoring

A person's risk status is fluid; it is not a static state. At any given moment, an individual's level of risk is specific to his/her present emotional state, motivational attributions, interpersonal reactivity, internal coping mechanisms, external sources of support, and the level of distress and hopelessness he/she is experiencing. Staff and persons served can utilize knowledge of the individualized formulation of violence risk to collaborate in the monitoring and early intervention process.

Psychosocial Interventions to Address Risk Factors Associated with Violence

Psychosocial interventions that address the underlying risk factors associated with risk for violence and foster a strength-based understanding of trauma are an essential component of secondary prevention of violence.

Treatment delivery in a TPR system of care is based on two core principles [27].

(1) Delivery of treatment reflects systemic awareness of the pervasiveness of trauma, the recognition of the impact of trauma on the individual, and an organizational responsiveness to that knowledge.

(2) Treatment includes an integrated continuum of trauma-specific modalities to address the immediate cognitive, somatic, and emotional distress experienced by the person served and to foster long-term hope and recovery.

Cognitive behavior therapy (CBT)

CBT is the most widely studied modality of psychotherapy in the field of violence prevention, although other forms, e.g., psychodynamic psychotherapy, are also effective [28]. Most CBT approaches emphasize the ability to (a) recognize internal and external triggers; (b) observe and manage one's cognitive and emotional responses; and (c) resolve interpersonal conflict and negotiate getting one's needs met. CBT helps the person served to recognize the power of his/her own thoughts, particularly interpersonal/relational triggers, cognitive distortions, and the possibility of alternative interpretations (see Table 28.2). As cognitions shift, people's associated feelings of inadequacy, inferiority, and hopelessness also shift, and the possibility of recovery increases. CBT components that address the psychological factors that underlie violence, including fear, anger, and shame, empower an individual to resume a self-regulated life course.

Sensory modulation interventions

More recently, there has been increased recognition that in order for most CBT to work, one must include attention to the body because people who are physiologically aroused have difficulty utilizing cognitive strategies [29]. People with mental illness are frequently less aware of their own physiological and sensory experiences [30]. Identifying sensory triggers and physiological reactivity are essential to any effort to understand the antecedents of a violent episode and

Table 28.2 Common cognitive behavioral treatment components*

Cognitive skills	Training on general thinking and decision-making skills such as to stop and think before acting, generate alternative solutions, evaluate consequences, and make decisions about appropriate behavior
Cognitive restructuring	Activities and exercises aimed at recognizing and modifying cognitive distortions and errors that trigger violence
Interpersonal problem solving	Training in problem-solving skills for dealing with interpersonal conflict and peer pressure
Social skills	Training in prosocial behaviors, interpreting social cues, taking other persons' feelings into account
Anger control	Training in techniques for identifying triggers and cues that arouse anger and maintaining self-control
Relapse prevention	Training on strategies to recognize and cope with high-risk situations and halt the relapse cycle before lapses turn into full relapses
Moral reasoning**	Activities designed to improve the ability to reason about right and wrong behavior and raise the level of moral development
Victim impact**	Activities aimed at getting people to consider the impact of their behavior on others

* Adapted from Lipsey *et al.* (2007) [43].
** Violence-specific interventions.

to develop person-specific strategies for early intervention and de-escalation. Teaching someone to recognize the changes in their own sensory experience enables them to more fully participate in the recovery process. Sensory modulation techniques allow for the creation of individualized tools to manage one's own physiological state. It is much easier for a person served to make their way in the world using personalized sensory tools under their conscious control than to rely on the presence of a staff member to do the same. Sensory modulation methods allow for

choice and empowerment and decrease the sense of shame associated with being "less than" or "dependent." Empowering someone to use sensory strategies to self-regulate their level of arousal promotes self-efficacy. Inpatient units have introduced "sensory rooms" that provide a calming space with avenues for soothing and arousing each sense [31].

Interventions based on the presenting emotions

Shame

Symptoms and behaviors that are triggered via a shame-based mechanism respond best to cognitive interventions within a "socio-ecological framework" [5]. Skill-based modalities that target the need for control, mastery, and meaningful purpose foster pride and self-respect. Cognitive restructuring and enhancing therapies, motivational interviewing, stress management, vocational training, community outreach, and access to housing and higher education all counteract the negative messages that persons served have experienced via institutional and structural violence (see Table 28.3).

Anger

For those violent behaviors that are intra- and inter-personal in nature with a primary expression in the form of anger or rage, effective treatments include individual psychotherapy, dialectical behavioral therapy (with its focus on mindfulness, distress tolerance, and affect regulation), group therapies, co-occurring addiction work, anger management, and psycho-education regarding the interplay of trauma and mental illness. Intra- and inter-personal therapies foster the ability of the individual to self-reflect and to regulate the level of social interactions desired with a corresponding increase in positive social connections, where previous ones may have been damaged or non-existent.

Fear

Symptoms and violent behaviors that are primarily fear-based with a large global somatic component, including dissociation or hyper-arousal, respond best to interventions that target the brainstem and have a direct impact on sensation. Sensory modulation techniques, including sensory kits, comfort rooms, trauma-informed yoga, grounding and centering skills, progressive muscle relaxation, diaphragmatic breathing, eye movement desensitization and reprocessing (EMDR), and gentle reprocessing, to name a

Table 28.3 Relationship between trauma-induced feelings and appropriate psychosocial interventions

Challenging emotions	Antidote emotions	Interventions	Examples
Fear	Compassion	Sensory modulation	Grounding, sensory kits, body-based therapies, trauma-informed yoga, muscle relaxation, breath work, EMDR
Anger	Empathy	Intra- and inter-personal therapies	DBT, individual therapy, group therapy, addiction work, anger management, mindfulness-based therapies
Shame	Pride	Skill mastery	CBT, cognitive enhancing therapy, stress management, motivational interviewing, skills training, vocational and educational training

EMDR = Eye Movement Desensitization and Reprocessing; DBT = dialectical behavior therapy; CBT = cognitive behavioral therapy

few, offer the fastest way to recalibrate the distorted fearful perceptions that lead to challenging, and even violent, behavior.

Tertiary Prevention

Treatments that address the underlying factors that give rise to violence are necessary but insufficient for the small minority of persons served (2%–6%) who engage in repeated episodes of violent behavior and are responsible for incidents of inpatient violence [32–34]. The increasing demands for state mental institutions to serve people with forensic-related service needs in the absence of increased resources exacerbate concerns about the relevance of TPR in the treatment of violence. While acknowledging that approximately 41% of states' inpatient psychiatric funds are spent on people admitted with forensic-related service needs [1], NASMHPD emphasizes that "all people served in state psychiatric hospitals [forensic or otherwise] should be considered in the process of recovery" [1]. Furthermore, while it is beyond the scope of this article to address the argument that persistent psychopathy in itself is a mental illness, there is burgeoning evidence that TPR is associated with violence reduction in forensic settings. Moreover, Skeem *et al.* [35] found that people with mental illness with high levels of psychopathy benefited as much from violence reduction treatments as people with mental illness without psychopathy.

Psychosocial interventions to address violence

Violence-specific interventions are necessary to decrease violence [36]. While the known interventions that directly target aggression in adults appear to be nascent, the evidence-based research on children and adolescents

who are aggressive provides a general direction from which we can extrapolate to our adult, long-stay, inpatient population. Closely examining all risk factors for violence from the level of physiological arousal to historical, motivational, interpersonal, environmental, cultural, and societal indicators within a TPR context provides the best opportunity to decrease violence and foster hope and healing for the persons we serve. There are some trends in the research base that support TPR as the necessary context for effectively addressing violence, particularly adolescent interventions [37,38].

- Theoretical model: treatments informed by a coherent theoretical model for understanding violence, its antecedents, and its consequences, and by clear principles that pervade the entire system of care are more likely to be effectively adopted [39].
- Multimodal and multifocused: treatments that utilize multiple modalities (e.g., individual, group, family), target multiple domains (e.g., emotion regulation, conflict resolution), and address larger system issues (e.g., identity and roles within the family and the larger community) had significant effect sizes in contrast to the effect sizes of interventions with a singular focus (e.g., a specific skill) [40]. CBT interventions that target anger control and interpersonal functioning show the most promise in reducing violent behavior [28,41–43].
- Skilled clinical workforce: a well-trained, skilled clinical workforce providing clear, compassionate treatment is effective in reducing violence [39]. The degree to which CBT is effectively implemented (e.g., rigor of staff training and supervision in CBT) is positively related to effect size [43].

The Mendota Juvenile Treatment Center (MJTC), located in a state psychiatric facility, is an example

285

of a residential treatment for persistently violent adolescents that is comprehensive, multimodal, and system-based, and that shares many of the features that characterize TPR. The adolescents and their behavior are conceptualized in the context of their places within larger social systems (family, peer, community, etc.). Treatment focuses on the individual's alienation from "conventional life," which is understood as a product of both how others view and react to the individual and the individual's aggressive disdain and rejection of others. Treatment is designed to change the nature of interactions and to expand the roles and identities available to the adolescent [39]. While the intervention includes skill training, the primary target is to increase the individual's openness and positive attitude to prosocial roles, identities, relationship dynamics, and life goals [44]. When immediate family members are not able to participate, the treatment team works to engage extended family members or community members who may offer support. The MJTC approach resonates with the focus on recovery in the mental health system: the recognition that an expanded sense of self and self in relation to others is necessary for people with mental illness to cope with their illness and build meaningful lives. Five years post-discharge from MJTC, youth were 34% less likely to be rearrested and 50% less likely to commit a violent crime compared to those who did not participate in the MJTC program [45].

Aggressive replacement therapy (ART) is a CBT violence reduction program that originated as a treatment for adolescents and has also been found to be effective in working with adults and people with mental illness [46–49]. ART is an intensive group treatment with multiple weekly sessions. Goldstein *et al.* [46] conceptualize violence as comprising affective, behavioral, and values components, and the ART treatment modules of emotion regulation, social skills, and moral reasoning address each of these aspects of violence, respectively. The moral reasoning component asks participants to discuss moral and ethical questions and promotes mentalization skills, including the ability to recognize and imagine another person's experience. ART is associated with reductions in felony recidivism [43,50].

Researchers at Children's Hospital in Boston have developed the RAGE-Control intervention, which recognizes the integral role of bodily focused interventions in the context of CBT and violence reduction. RAGE-Control is a video game that requires players to modulate their physiological arousal in order to play the game. Players who become physiologically hyperaroused effectively trigger the deactivation of their game control stick. The game settings are adjusted based on the individual's baseline arousal, and as the individual progresses, the settings can be set to present progressively more challenging goals of physiological modulation. Violence triggered by the need for power and control diminish as individuals master their own somatic processes and feel less at the mercy of their unregulated emotions. Preliminary data suggest that in conjunction with ACT, RAGE-Control may be associated with a decrease in violent episodes [51,52].

Putting It All Together

Traumatologist and consultant Donna Riemer, RN, PPMHN-BC, reported on the efforts of a treatment team to reduce violence on a maximum security forensic mental health hospital unit using a trauma-informed, sanctuary approach to (a) create cultural change in the milieu, (b) focus on consistent early interventions, and (c) develop working relationships between care providers and patients [53,54]. The most secure maximum security unit in Wisconsin's state mental health system was the setting in which the treatment team leaders worked together with persons served to create a significant culture change to effectively embrace a zero-tolerance for violence. Persons served by this unit included those with major mental illness, personality disorders, and alcohol and other drug abuse, as well as medical and developmental disabilities, and most had significant legal issues. In order to do this, both staff and persons served had to understand their beliefs about and approach to reducing violence and barriers to change. The development of consistent rules, definitions, and approaches to violence was established collaboratively. With that consistency in place, better tools for early intervention and de-escalation of violence could be created in partnership with the person served. Emphasis on identifying and managing stressors that lead to violent behavior allowed for creative adoption of self-calming and modulating activities that served not only to de-escalate situations but to create a true healing sanctuary. Many of these activities have been highlighted in our discussion of specific interventions, including breath work, grounding techniques, meditation, progressive relaxation, and groups learning these techniques. Mixed psychoeducation groups of staff and persons served, regarding nonviolent communication as a means of expressing oneself appropriately and getting needs met, facilitated the desired culture change and consistency in approaching violent episodes. Additionally, groups that addressed anger management, cognitive and emotional regulation, coping and problem-solving, and conflict resolution, as well as other prosocial skills that respect the rights and boundaries of others as a basis for a trauma-informed environment of care, were embraced by all [53]. Other changes incorporated included an emphasis on self-care and mutual support for the providers, as well as a robust debriefing process following all episodes of early intervention and de-escalation efforts.

The year-one results following the implementation of the culture change on this maximum security unit were striking. Compared to baseline episodes of violence from the year prior to the new approach, there was a 50% reduction in patient violence-related injuries, use of seclusion and restraint, emergency code calls, and complaints lodged by persons served [53]. Moreover, lost days due to staff injuries were reduced by 62%, and both staff and persons served reported an increase in feelings of safety [53].

Conclusion

The medical model for understanding violence by parsing violent behaviors into psychotic, predatory, or impulsive (developmental/medical/injury) serves us well in determining medical interventions [34]. There is a need to study and understand the history and experience of trauma in those with violent behaviors in order to provide evidence-based treatment and best practices for the treatment of individuals with aggressive and violent behavior. This will necessitate development of pilot programs that use trauma-informed approaches to violent behavior from primary, secondary, and tertiary prevention models. This comprehensive approach will serve both the individual and society at large. In that spirit, we call for primary prevention of violence in our society that supports community relationships, meaningful work, economic stability, and a trauma-informed perspective in all human service endeavors. More specifically, the organizational/ institutional commitment to a TPR orientation is crucial in the efficacy of any of the interventions discussed. In addition to the traditional

means of assessing risk for violence, using the public health model of violence as a lens helps us to better understand and ameliorate symptoms that result from institutional, structural, and direct violence. The dynamic nature of the individual, interpersonal, environmental, and cultural factors associated with the daily operations of the unit need to be assessed through the lens of primary and secondary violence prevention, which recognizes that the majority of people served have significant trauma histories. Once a compassionate, respectful, empathic, and empowering approach is embraced by leadership and staff, the work with the individual can proceed more effectively. Interventions used include a variety of cognitive–behavioral, interpersonal, and somatosensory therapies. These interventions, when effectively applied, result in more self-esteem, self-mastery, and self-control, and diminished behavioral violence. This is the hope for the future efficacy of treatment in our state mental hospitals that combines a rigorous medical model with environmental and psycho-social interventions.

We recognize that fiscal constraints will limit the implementation of this approach, which requires a better trained and supervised work force. The value of time with individuals served in our inpatient institutions is part of the cost of this TPR approach, which is founded on inter-personal engagement and training of both staff and persons served. It is imperative that this change start at the top, and institutional leaders embrace this perspective. Since all institutions have training as part of an ongoing requirement for quality service provision, these efforts can be retooled to develop new ways to train staff and increase the skills required for implementing these psychosocial interventions. More pilot studies are needed that include standardized violence/aggression assessment and monitoring tools, while applying a TPR approach to reducing violence. These studies will create the evidence base needed for systematic culture change for behavioral health integration throughout the healthcare delivery system, our communities, and families to create a nontraumatizing society.

Disclosures

The authors do not have anything to disclose.

Further Reading

To view supplementary material for this chapter, please visit http://dx.doi.org/10.1017/S1092852915000280.

References

1. Parks J, Radke AQ, Haupt MB. *The Vital Role of State Psychiatric Hospitals*. Alexandria, VA: National Association of State Mental Health Program Directors Medical Directors Council; 2014.

2. Colozzi E. *Creating Careers with Confidence in EOHSS*. Paper presented at the Aspiring Supervisor's Series, MA Executive Office of Health and Social Services, Westborough, MA, October 2014.

3. Espinosa L, Harris B, Frank J, *et al.* Milieu improvement in psychiatry using evidence-based practices: The long and winding road of culture change. *Arch. Psychiatr. Nurs.* 2015; **29**(4): 202–207. DOI: 10.1016/j.apnu.2014.08.004.

4. Anda RF, Felitti VJ, Walker J, *et al.* The enduring effects of abuse and related adverse experiences in childhood: a convergence of evidence from neurobiology and epidemiology. *Eur. Arch. Psychiatry Clin. Neurosci.* 2006; **256**(3): 174–186.

5. Substance Abuse and Mental Health Services Administration. *Trauma-Informed Care in Behavioral Health Services. Treatment Improvement Protocol (TIP) Series 57. HHS Publication No. (SMA) 13-4801*. Rockville, MD: Substance Abuse and Mental Health Services Administration; 2014.

6. Fein RA. *Behavioral Threat Assessment and Preventing Targeted Violence: History, Opportunity, Concerns*. Paper presented at Violence Risk and Threat Assessment: An Historic and Dynamic Perspective, Boston, MA, November 2014.

7. Gilligan J. *Violence: Our Deadly Epidemic and Its Causes.* New York: GP Putman's Sons; 1996.

8. Tremblay RE. The development of aggressive behaviour during childhood: what have we learned in the past century? *International Journal of Behavioral Development*. 2000; **24**(2): 129–141.

9. Abderhalden C, Needham I, Dassen T. *et al.* Structured risk assessment and violence in acute psychiatric wards: randomized controlled trial. *The British Journal of Psychiatry*. 2008; **193**(1): 44–50.

10. Figley CR. *Compassion Fatigue: Coping with Secondary Traumatic Stress Disorder in Those Who Treat the Traumatized*. New York: Routledge; 1995.

11. Fisher D. A professional's lived experience. Trauma Informed Training at Massachusetts Department of Mental Health, Worcester Recovery Center and Hospital, Worcester, Massachusetts, August 20, 2014.

12. Uram S. The neurobiology of trauma made simple. Trauma Informed Training at MA Department of Mental Health, Worcester Recovery Center and Hospital, Worcester, Massachusetts, August 20, 2014.

13. Huckshorn KH. Reducing seclusion and restraint in mental health settings: core strategies for prevention. *J. Psychosoc. Nurs. Ment. Health Serv.* 2004; **42**(9): 22–33.

14. Jambunathan J, Bellaire K. Evaluating staff use of crisis prevention intervention techniques: a pilot study. *Issues Ment. Health Nurs.* 1996; **17**(6): 541–558.

15. Richmond I, Trujillo D, Schmelzer J, Phillips S, Davis D. Least restrictive alternatives: do they really work? *J. Nurs. Care Qual.* 1996; **11**(1): 29–37.

16. Needham I, Abderhalden C, Meer R, *et al.* The effectiveness of two interventions in the management of patient violence in acute mental inpatient settings: Report on a pilot study. *J. Psychiatr. Ment.*

17. Richmond JS, Berlin JS, Fishkind AB, *et al.* Verbal de-escalation of the agitated patient: consensus statement of the American Association for Emergency Psychiatry Project BETA De-escalation Workgroup. *West. J. Emerg. Med.* 2012; **13**(1): 17–25.

18. Katz P, Kirkland FR. Violence and social structure on mental hospital wards. *Psychiatry*. 1990; **53**(3): 262–277.

19. McDermott BE, Holoyda BJ. Assessment of aggression in inpatient settings. *CNS Spectr.* 2014; **19**(5): 425–431.

20. Monahan J, Skeem JL. The evolution of violence risk assessment. *CNS Spectr.* 2014; **19**(5): 419–424.

21. McNeil DE, Binder RL, Greenfield TK. Predictors of violence in civilly committed acute psychiatric patient. *Am. J. Psychiatry.* 1988; **145**(8): 965–970.

22. Abderhalden C, Needham I, Miserez B, *et al.* Predicting inpatient violence in acute psychiatric wards using the Brøset-Violence-Checklist: a multicentre prospective cohort study. *J. Psychiatr. Ment. Health Nurs.* 2004; **11**(4): 422–427.

23. Newton VM, Elbogen EB, Brown CL, Snyder J, Barrick AL. Clinical decision-making about inpatient violence risk at admission to a public sector acute psychiatric hospital. *J. Am. Acad. Psychiatry Law.* 2012; **40**(2): 206–214.

24. McNiel DE, Binder RL. Predictive validity of judgments of dangerousness in emergency civil commitment. *Am. J. Psychiatry.* 1987; **144**(2): 197–200.

25. Grassi L, Peron L, Marangoni C, Zanchi P, Vanni A. Characteristics of violent behavior in acute psychiatric inpatients: a 5-year Italian study.

Acta Psychiatr. Scand. 2001; **104**(4): 273–279.

26. Sharp C. On becoming trauma informed. The National Council for Behavioral Health. www.thenationalcouncil.org/events-and-training/webinars/webinar-archive/. Relias Webinar, September 22, 2014.

27. Substance Abuse and Mental Health Services Administration. *SAMHSA's Concept of Trauma and Guidance for a Trauma-Informed Approach. HHS Publication No. (SMA) 14–4884.* Rockville, MD: Substance Abuse and Mental Health Services Administration; 2014.

28. Hockenhull JC, Whittington R, Leitner M, *et al.* A systematic review of prevention and intervention strategies for populations at high risk of engaging in violent behaviour: Update 2002–8. *Health Technol. Assess.* 2012; **16**(3): 1–152.

29. Linehan M. *The Cognitive Behavioral Treatment of Borderline Personality Disorder.* New York: Guilford Press; 1993.

30. Champagne T, Stromberg N. Sensory approaches in inpatient psychiatric settings: innovative alternatives to seclusion and restraint. *J. Psychosoc. Nurs. Ment. Health Serv.* 2004; **42**(9): 35–43.

31. LeBel J, Stromberg N, Duckworth K, *et al.* Child and adolescent inpatient restraint reduction: a state initiative to promote strength based care. *J. Am. Acad. Child. Adolesc. Psychiatry.* 2004; **43**(1): 37–45.

32. Rasmussen K, Levander S. Individual rather than situation characteristics predict violence in a maximum security hospital. *J. Interpers. Violence.* 1996; **11**(3): 376–390.

33. Polaschek DLL, Collie RM. Rehabilitating serious adult violent offenders: an empirical and theoretical stocktake.

Psychology, Crime and Law. 2004; **10**(3): 321–334.

34. Stahl S. Deconstructing violence as a medical syndrome: mapping psychotic, impulsive, and predatory subtypes to malfunctioning brain circuits. *CNS Spectr.* 2014; **19**(5): 357–365.

35. Skeem JL, Monahan JU, Mulvey EP. Psychopathy, treatment involvement, and subsequent violence among civil psychiatric patients. *Law Hum. Behav.* 2002; **26**(6): 577–603.

36. McGuire J. A review of effective interventions for reducing aggression and violence. *Phil. Trans. R. Soc. Lond. B Biol. Sci.* 2008; **363**(1503): 2577–2597.

37. Tate DC, Reppucci ND, Mulvey EP. Violent juvenile delinquents: treatment effectiveness and implications for future action. *Am. Psychol.* 1995; **50**(9): 777–781.

38. Eyberg S, Nelson M, Boggs S. Evidence-based psychosocial treatments for children and adolescents with disruptive behavior. *J. Clin. Child. Adolesc. Psychol.* 2008; **37**(1): 215–237.

39. Caldwell MF, VanRybroek G. Effective treatment programs for violent adolescents: programmatic challenges and promising features. *Aggression and Violent Behavior.* 2013; **18**(5): 571–578.

40. Garrido V, Morales LA. Serious (violent and chronic) juvenile offenders: A systematic review of treatment effectiveness in secure corrections. *Campbell Systematic Reviews.* 2007; **7**. DOI: 10.4073/csr.2007.7.

41. Renwick SJ, Black L, Ramm M, Novaco RW. Anger treatment with forensic hospital patients. *Legal and Criminological Psychology.* 1997; **2**(1): 103–116.

42. Frey REC, Weller J. Behavioural management of aggression

through teaching interpersonal skills. *Psychiatr. Serv.* 2000; **52**(5): 607–609.

43. Lipsey MW, Landeberger NA, Wilson SJ. Effects of cognitive behavioral programs for criminal offenders. *Campbell Systematic Reviews.* 2007; **6**. DOI: 10.4073/csr.2007.6.

44. Kornblum R. *Violence Prevention Through Movement and Pro-Social Skills.* Oklahoma City, OK: Wood and Barnes Publishing; 2002.

45. Caldwell MF. Treatment of adolescents with psychopathic features. In Kiehl KA, Sinnott-Armstrong WP, eds. *Handbook on Psychopathy and Law.* New York: Oxford University Press; 2013: 201–230.

46. Goldstein AP, Glick B, Rainer S. *Aggression Replacement Training.* Champaign, IL: Research Press; 1987.

47. Glick B, Gibbs JC. *Aggression Replacement Training®: A Comprehensive Intervention for Aggressive Youth*, 3rd edn. Champaign, IL: Research Press; 2011.

48. McGuire J, Clark D. A national dissemination program. In Goldstein AP, Nensen R, Daleflod RB, Kalt UM, eds. *New Perspective on Aggression Replacement Training.* Chichester, UK: Wiley; 2004: 139–150.

49. Hatcher RM, Palmer EJ, McGuire J, *et al.* Aggression replacement training with adult male offenders within community settings: a reconviction analysis. *Journal of Forensic Psychiatry and Psychology.* 2008; **19**(4): 517–532.

50. Barnoski R. *Washington State's Implementation of Aggression Replacement Training for Juvenile Offenders: Preliminary Findings.* Olympia, WA: The Evergreen State College, Washington State Institute for Public Policy; 2002.

51. Kahn J, Ducharme P, Travers B, Gonzalez-Heydrich J. Rage control: Regulate And Gain Emotional control. *Stud. Health Technol. Inform.* 2009; **149**: 335–343.

52. Ducharme P, Wharff E, Kahn J, Hutchinson Logan G. Augmenting anger control therapy with a videogame requiring emotional control: a pilot study on an inpatient psychiatric unit. *Adolescent Psychiatry*. 2012; **2**(4): 323–332.

53. Riemer D. Creating sanctuary: reducing violence in a maximum security forensic psychiatric hospital unit. *Forensic Nurses.* 2009; **15**(1): 302.

54. Bloom S. *Creating Sanctuary: Toward the Evolution of Sane Societies*. New York: Routledge; 1997.

Chapter

29

Comorbid mental illness and criminalness: implications for housing and treatment

Robert D. Morgan and Nicole R. Bartholomew

Introduction

The general public is misinformed about the relationship of mental illness to crime and violence, and believes that individuals with mental illness are dangerous [1,2]. It is not uncommon to see individuals with mental illness portrayed as violent, and violent acts are often attributed to mental illness. This happens in popular media (e.g., movies), as well as in news media following acts of violence such as the shootings in the Aurora, Colorado, movie theater and Sandy Hook Elementary School. In fact, following instances of violence, it seems almost inevitable that the mental health of a violent perpetrator is called into question by media outlets. This is in spite of the fact that media sources are notoriously unreliable with regard to reporting on the association of mental illness with violence [3,4]. The inaccurate link drawn by media outlets may be largely responsible for the "increase in the proportion of persons who associate persons with mental illness with dangerousness, violence, and unpredictability" (p. 39) [5]. Despite general misconceptions in the general public and media outlets regarding mental illness and violence, persons with mental illness (PMI) minimally contribute to overall rates of violence [6], and violent behavior in PMI is most common when other risk factors for violence are present (e.g., substance abuse, history of violence) [7].

In this chapter, we review the evidence regarding the association between mental illness and violence specifically, and mental illness and crime generally. The biopsychosocial factors that assist in differentiating which PMI will become violent and involved in crime will be discussed. Particular emphasis will be placed on the neurobiological underpinnings of violence, the role of criminal thinking (see Table 29.1), and the relationship between such antisocial cognitions

and mental illness. Additionally, housing considerations and treatment recommendations for criminal justice (CJ)-involved PMI are discussed.

Persons with Mental Illness, Violence, and Criminal Behavior

The relationship of mental illness to violence and crime is influenced by a complex interaction of

Table 29.1 Central eight risk factors for criminal behavior

Risk factor	Description
History of antisocial behavior	Early onset and continued involvement in antisocial activities
Antisocial personality traits	Impulsivity, deceitfulness, disregard of the rights of others, lack of remorse, failure to conform to social norms, aggressiveness
Criminal thinking	Maladaptive thought patterns that serve to increase and sustain one's propensity to engage in criminal behavior
Criminal associates	Peer group composed of individuals engaged in antisocial activities with a limited number of prosocial contacts
Substance abuse	Use of alcohol and/or other illicit substances
Family/marital problems	Poor or conflictual relationships with family and/or spouse
Poor work/school performance	Poor performance in the completion of work or school tasks; low work/school satisfaction
Lack of prosocial leisure activities	Few, if any, prosocial hobbies or interests

Violence in Psychiatry, ed. Katherine D. Warburton and Stephen M. Stahl. Published by Cambridge University Press.
© Cambridge University Press 2016.

neurobiological, social, and psychological factors that increase one's risk for violence and crime. At a neurobiological level, individuals who engage in violence and criminal behavior evidence structural and functional differences when compared to their nonviolent counterparts. Unfortunately, there is a dearth of research that has examined the neurobiological correlates of violence specifically in PMI populations; however, the available research utilizing non-PMI populations will be outlined to provide a general foundation for a discussion of biological factors associated with violence and crime.

Pardini et al. [8] conducted a study that utilized magnetic resonance imaging (MRI) to examine the volume of the amygdala (a structure of the limbic system involved in emotion) in a sample of 26-year-old males with varying histories of violence. The results indicated that males with lower amygdala volume evidenced more personality traits associated with psychopathy; reported more violent histories; and were more likely to evidence higher levels of aggression, violence, and psychopathy at a three-year follow-up [8]. Further, research utilizing functional MRI (fMRI) also indicated that individuals with higher levels of psychopathy evidenced reduced amygdala activity during moral reasoning tasks [9]. In addition to the amygdala, reduced activity in the anterior cingulate cortex (a structure implicated in impulsivity and behavioral inhibition) has been associated with future reoffending in a sample of prisoners [10].

Causal inferences regarding the role of neurological dysfunction and atrophy in violence are not possible from this body of correlational research; however, the findings still improve our understanding of violence. Collectively, the results suggest that one's propensity to engage in violent behavior, and likely crime, is associated with neurobiological dysfunction. A thorough review of the literature on the neuroanatomy of violence suggested that "empirical research provides support for the hypothesis that life-course persistent antisocial behavior is a neurological disorder that emerges in the transactions between individual vulnerabilities and environmental adversity" (p. 924) [11]. Consistent with the diathesis–stress model, research suggests that early childhood environmental stressors may impact brain development, and in turn may increase susceptibility to the onset of severe mental illness [12]. Knowing that, could it also be true that the same early childhood environmental stressors that alter the neurophysiology related to mental illness be the same (or similar) mechanism that elicits the onset of violent behavior?

Neurobiological mechanisms appear to offer a partial explanation for PMI who engage in criminal and violent behavior, but nonphysiological factors must also be considered to improve predictive and explanatory accuracy, as well as to identify treatment targets. Therefore, considering psychological and sociological factors provides a more holistic conceptualization of the link between mental illness and violence. Andrews and Bonta [13] identified eight risk factors, the "Central 8," that are the most significant predictors of criminal behavior (see Table 29.1). These risk factors are additive such that greater the number of risk factors experienced by an individual, the greater their propensity to engage in crime. It appears that criminal risk factors may differentially impact certain populations [14], and PMI may be disproportionately exposed to and affected by a greater number of criminal risk factors. Draine et al. [14] identified various environmental factors (e.g., homelessness, joblessness, antisocial peers), most of which are related to lower socioeconomic status, that are common to PMI and that predispose them to criminal risk. Notably, mental illness is not a central risk factor and has been found to be only minimally predictive of criminal behavior when not paired with at least one of the aforementioned criminal risk factors [15]. Prevalence of criminal risk factors for PMI is a plausible explanation for their CJ involvement, and has become an increasing focus of explanatory research.

A primary criminal risk factor of recent interest for CJ-involved PMI is antisocial cognitions or criminal thinking. Unlike prosocial individuals, people who engage in criminal behavior evidence thought patterns supportive of criminal actions [16]. Studies comparing inmates with and without mental illnesses in jail [17] and state penitentiaries [18,19] found that inmates with mental illness evidenced criminal thinking that was consistent with that of their nonmentally ill counterparts. Furthermore, criminal thinking has been shown to partially mediate the relationship between mental illness and institutional violence for incarcerated PMI [20]. Notably, meta-analytic studies have found that, with regard to violent offending, criminal history variables (e.g., previous violence or violent offending) are the best predictors of criminal behavior, with clinical variables (e.g., mental health diagnosis) being the least predictive [15,21]. Notably, Bonta *et al.* [15] found that offenders with severe mental illness were less likely to recidivate, generally or violently, as compared to their non-mentally ill counterparts, but this is in contrast to Douglas *et al.*'s [22] meta-analytic review that yielded an association between psychosis and violence. This suggests that criminal risk factors need to be considered, as they likely mediate the relationship between mental illness and violence (and likely crime). This is consistent with Skeem *et al.*'s [23] estimate that 9 in 10 PMI who become CJ-involved do so for reasons other than their mental illness. It appears that some CJ-involved PMI present with known features of criminal risk that increase their propensity to engage in crime and violence.

As previously noted, criminal thinking appears to be a general risk factor for crime committed by PMI [18,19,24], but may also contribute to an explanation of violence. Specifically, inmates with severe mental illness (i.e., schizophrenia or bipolar disorder), which are typically perceived to be more violent due to the presence of active symptoms [25], displayed higher levels of criminal thinking than those without mental illness and those with less severe mental illness (i.e., depression, posttraumatic stress disorder, and anxiety) [19]. Furthermore, criminal thinking is likely an important risk factor to be considered in noncorrectional settings.

Gross and Morgan [26] examined criminal thinking in a short-term, inpatient psychiatric sample with and without CJ involvement. Results indicated that inpatient PMI with CJ involvement present similarly to incarcerated PMI with regard to psychiatric symptomatology and criminal thinking. Therefore, the risk for violence and criminal behavior is relevant in a mental health setting, and not limited to correctional settings, for PMI with a history of violence or CJ involvement. The risk for dangerousness does not appear to be equal across PMI merely based on psychiatric features, as PMI without a history of CJ involvement were distinguished from incarcerated PMI by evidencing lower levels of criminal thinking and lower levels of psychiatric symptomatology directly related to criminal risk (i.e., antisocial personality disorder).

Furthermore, examining the presence of criminal thinking in community mental health samples has identified an association between criminal thinking and mental illness. Gross and Morgan [27] measured criminal thinking and psychiatric symptomatology in a sample of PMI enrolled in evidence-based community mental health treatment programs. Regardless of history of CJ involvement, linear regression analyses indicated a significant positive relationship between general criminal thinking and mental health symptomatology, such that as the number of symptoms experienced or symptom severity increased, so did the level of criminal thinking. Additionally, Bolanos *et al.* [28] recently examined other criminal risk factors (criminal associates; antisocial attitudes, behaviors, and personality traits; substance use; and childhood conduct disorder) in a sample of PMI with and without CJ involvements. Results indicated that, when compared to the non-CJ-involved PMI, CJ-involved PMI had a greater number of criminal associates, increased time spent with these associates, and higher scores on measures of criminal attitudes. Additionally, CJ-involved PMI evidenced greater substance use, a more extensive history of conduct problems, and a higher number of antisocial personality traits [28]. Collectively, these results appear conclusive regarding the clinical presentation of CJ-involved PMI in the mental health system and offenders with mental illness in corrections [29]. Specifically, the conceptualization of PMI with a history of violence and CJ involvements warrants a comorbid and integrative approach that holistically views the neurological, sociological, criminogenic (e.g., criminal thinking), and psychiatric problems experienced by the individual.

In summary, the empirical evidence outlined in this section suggests that PMI who engage in criminal behavior are, in fact, both criminals and mentally ill [18,26]. The presence of criminal risk factors, in addition to mental illness, better accounts for CJ involvement than mental illness alone.

Housing and Managing CJ-Involved PMI

Gross and Morgan [27] found that as criminal thinking increases, the number of lifetime arrests increases, but psychiatric hospitalizations decrease. This suggests that criminal thinking is more likely to result in illegal behavior (e.g., violence) than behavior that would indicate mental health decompensation (e.g., suicidality, poor self-care) and warrant hospitalization. This finding may also be attributed to the more easily detected symptoms of externalizing disorders (e.g., antisocial personality) versus internalized disorders (e.g., depression, anxiety) that are more apparent to outside observers. However, research has begun to posit that externalizing disorders precipitate and exacerbate internalizing disorders [30]. Consequently, the externalized behavior results in CJ involvement and subsequent incarceration with minimal judicial consideration of an alternative systemic response (e.g., placement in a mental health facility), especially if the PMI has engaged in violent behavior. Ideally, CJ and mental health systems would work collaboratively to ensure that PMI are housed in an environment that balances security, safety, and treatment; however, such coordinated teamwork is rarely a reality and varies greatly across states and jurisdictions. Creating an integrated CJ and mental health system is supported by findings that PMI are 3 times more likely to be incarcerated than admitted to a psychiatric facility [31,32], and correctional institutions have become the largest providers of mental health treatment in the United States [31].

The need for specialized housing in corrections is further supported by the disproportionate representation of PMI in the correctional system and subsequent healthcare demands placed on correctional institutions. Symptoms of mental illness are endorsed by inmates at an alarming rates, as 60.5% of jail inmates, 49.2% of state prison inmates, and 39.8% of federal inmates endorsed such symptoms [33]. Additionally, Steadman *et al.* [34] found that 14.5% of male and 31% of female offenders in jails met diagnostic criteria for a serious mental illness, while prevalence rates of severe mental illness in the general population are estimated to be less than 6% [35]. Mere presence of criminal justice involvement does not minimize the necessity of mental health treatment; rather, as discussed below (see Figure 29.1), it may exacerbate symptoms of mental illness. In fact, PMI with the greatest criminal risk in terms of criminal thinking also appear to evidence the greatest degree of psychiatric disturbance (i.e., symptom severity, number of symptoms experienced) [27].

Individuals high in criminal risk also likely require the most intensive mental health services, and they may be best managed and treated in a setting with an equal emphasis on mental health treatment and behavioral management. Therefore, having diversion opportunities (e.g., mental health court, inpatient treatment) or correctional staff and treatment programs that are equipped to provide treatment that addresses mental health and criminalness is imperative to improved

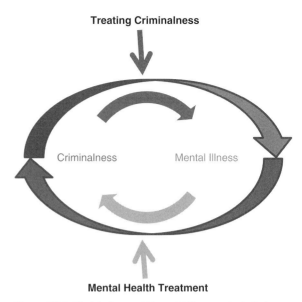

Treating Criminalness

Criminalness   Mental Illness

Mental Health Treatment

Figure 29.1 Model of comorbid mental illness and criminalness, and associated treatment needs.

outcomes for PMI and the community (e.g., safety, cost effectiveness). Although it seems preferable to have community resources to address the treatment needs of all PMI, most community-based mental health treatment programs do not integrate treatments designed to target criminalness [36,37], and the current reality is that correctional, forensic, and psychiatric facilities need to be prepared to treat these individuals.

PMI present many challenges to those responsible for managing the daily operations of correctional, forensic, and psychiatric institutions. The greatest concerns these facilities face include the security of the institution – emphasizing the safety of staff, inmates, and patients, and also members of the community.

Correctional facilities, specifically, are in the business of public safety, not psychiatric treatment. Although housing, managing, and treating PMI is not the mission of corrections, it is a necessity, but unfortunately, many correctional facilities are not equipped to handle the complex needs of this inmate population. Not only do they provide challenges regarding mental health treatment needs, but maintaining the safety of PMI within the correctional institution can be an added concern, as PMI inmates are at greater risk for victimization [38,39]. Furthermore, PMI may also be unable to conform their behavior to the rules and expectations of the institution. Thus, for their protection and management in the institution, PMI are often placed in disciplinary or administrative segregation [40]. Segregation includes placing inmates in a private cell (typically) with limited out of cell time (typically limited to 1 hour per day). This is problematic for PMI, in that such a placement impedes access to mental health services and hinders the ability of mental health treatment staff to provided needed care, and it has been argued that the housing itself is detrimental to the mental health of the inmate [40–42].

In spite of these concerns, systemic modifications in corrections may allow for a more effective balance between security and treatment without compromising safety. An example might be a correctional mental health program that designates a housing unit specifically for PMI and integrates a therapeutic milieu consistent with that in a psychiatric inpatient setting (e.g., treatment groups, behavioral modification strategies, community meetings, mental health staff, specially trained correctional staff). Although costly, such programming may not be any more expensive in the long term than placing inmates in segregation units ($75,000 per year per segregated inmate as opposed to $25,000 to keep an inmate in general population) [43] or psychiatric prisons.

In the same way that correctional facilities are challenged to meet the mental health needs of their population, mental health facilities may be challenged to meet the management issues of their CJ-involved population who exhibit violence toward self and others (staff and peers). PMI that are currently or have been historically involved in the CJ system are also housed in psychiatric units (including general psychiatric and forensic mental health facilities). For example, 54.3% of the sample in the study by Gross and Morgan [26] had been previously convicted of a criminal offense. The most common types of violence in inpatient mental health settings are impulse control-related and predatory violence [44,45], and rates of violence are highest for inpatients with criminal features (e.g., psychopathy) [46]. For the purposes of maintaining the safety of staff, patients, and community members, the setting (i.e., housing) in inpatient psychiatric facilities should be evaluated to ensure they meet the dual needs of this population, while effectively delivering mental health services and maintaining staff and patient safety.

Borrowing from penology, it has been recommended that psychiatric facilities decrease unit sizes, increase staff-to-patient ratios, and improve staff and patient visibility (and presence) in units and hallways to improve safety within the facility [47]; however, despite the plethora of research available that has led to recommendations for safer environments and facilities that house PMI, there is a lack of standardization between federal, state, and county mental health and correctional systems. Further, there is a dearth of research regarding the varying efforts across systems to manage the unique demands presented by the CJ-involved PMI population.

Given prison overcrowding and public costs associated with incarceration [48,49], attempts to more effectively intervene and serve CJ-involved PMI in less restrictive settings have led to the development of community-based management strategies. Programs of particular promise include community-based diversion programs (i.e., programs that utilize alternatives to incarceration) [23,50]. Examples of such programs include mental health or drug courts, specialized probation teams and officers, and outpatient mental health and criminal treatment programs where the individual resides in the community. Although the empirical support for community-based programs for PMI is mixed, with some showing success [51–54] and others failing to significantly impact CJ or mental health outcomes [55], one issue of continued concern is housing. Even empirically supported mental health and CJ interventions are not likely to be successful when housing remains unstable. As reported to the second author by a treatment provider, "It is very difficult to work on dual issues of mental health and criminalness when the client is complaining of bed bugs and random gunfire" (Kim Rosenzweig, personal communication, June 2014).

Housing is an essential consideration for the success of PMI in the community [56]. In fact, housing may be the single best predictor of community success [57], and therefore also a predictor of relapse. Specifically, without adequate and stable housing, successful community integration and PMI self-management will be thwarted [58]. Not surprisingly, homelessness is a primary predictor of relapse [59–61], as this aspect of social disadvantage that is prevalent among PMI contributes to exposure to criminal risk factors (e.g., substance abuse, criminal associates) [14]. PMI who are allowed to choose their housing, and who live in private, safe, and clean environments report a better quality of life [62], and such settings provide an environment conducive to service delivery and improved psychiatric outcomes [58]. Therefore, housing and management considerations are critical to the psychiatric and criminal recovery of CJ-involved PMI, whether they be housed in a correctional facility, mental health facility, or in the community.

Treatment Recommendations

In spite of recent advances in understanding the relationship of neurobiological mechanisms and criminal behavior, psychosocial interventions remain the current treatment of choice [63]. To be maximally beneficial, however, we submit that treatments should align with the etiological mechanisms of crime [18,64]. That is, the evidence is overwhelmingly clear that PMI with a history of violence and/or CJ involvement present with a complex set of co-occurring etiological factors that include biological, psychological, psychiatric, and social variables. Effective treatments must target this network of contributing factors.

The plethora of research on criminal risk with CJ-involved PMI summarized in this article clearly suggests that clinicians must conceptualize these individuals as having both mental illness and criminal proclivities. Although we do not yet know the intricacies and nature of this co-occurring relationship (an area ripe for future research), it seems reasonable to suggest that mental illness and criminalness feed each other in a continuous loop (see Figure 29.1). Negative outcomes in one domain (e.g., increased criminalness) negatively feed into and exacerbate outcomes in the other (e.g., increased psychiatric symptomatology) and vice versa. Thus, there is a complex interplay that includes bidirectionality within the criminal and mental health domains independently (untreated criminal risk results in increased criminal recidivism; untreated mental illness results in increased psychiatric recidivism) and multidirectionality across the two domains, in that decompensation in one results in complications and decompensation in the other domain. For example, PMI who display a greater number of criminal risk factors may have limited CJ contact until such time that situations associated with their mental illness bring them to the attention of law enforcement (e.g., criminal trespassing); however, upon law enforcement involvement, the individuals become defiant, resistant, and combative with officers resulting in a criminal offense. Thus, interventions need to break this cycle to reduce negative outcomes in both CJ and mental health domains.

In other words, we submit that, from a therapeutic perspective, mental illness and criminalness should be conceptualized as a self-propelling system, and that to treat one at the exclusion of the other is to facilitate change in only one domain. To enhance and improve criminal outcomes (e.g., reduced criminal recidivism, increased prosocial behavior) and psychiatric outcomes (e.g., reduced psychiatric recidivism, increased quality of life), interventions must be dually targeted to both domains.

Historically, tailoring treatments to the dual needs of CJ-involved PMI as outlined in Figure 29.1 has not been the treatment of choice. For example, Bewley and Morgan [65] surveyed correctional mental health professions that treat incarcerated PMI. Given the correctional setting of the mental health professional's work, it would seem likely that treatment efforts would be focused on reducing criminalness; however, results indicated that treatment providers considered mental illness recovery, personal growth, and improved institutional functioning to be more important treatment considerations than treating criminalness and preparing inmates for emotions management, criminogenic treatment needs, and community re-entry. Further, they reported spending significantly more therapeutic time on noncriminal mental health issues. In a meta-analytic review of current treatment efforts for CJ-involved PMI, it was discovered that only 8% of reviewed treatment studies targeted dual issues of mental illness and criminalness [63]. Thus, the model depicted in Figure 29.1 is not, from these authors' perspectives, particularly innovative or novel, but it emphasizes that it is imperative that treatment efforts be tailored to these co-occurring needs of CJ-involved PMI, which recent research suggests is not being done. In fact, we submit that the evidence of co-occurrence is so strong that it may be appropriate to consider any treatment program for CJ-involved PMI that is not concurrently targeting issues of mental illness and criminalness as professionally irresponsible.

Historically we have treated the mental health needs of CJ-involved PMI, resulting in positive psychiatric outcomes with no appreciable reductions in CJ outcomes (e.g., recidivism) [36,37]; however, less is known about treating criminalness in this unique psychiatric population. The treatment foci and corresponding interventions are one component of effective treatment, but the model that guides the delivery of the treatment may be just as important for addressing the criminalness of CJ-involved PMI. In other words, what models or strategies may be used to successfully intervene with this population?

Risk-Need-Responsivity (RNR) [66] is one model of service delivery, and is guided by three principles.

(1) The level of services should be matched to level of criminal risk (Risk principle).
(2) Services and treatment should target the dynamic (changeable) risks associated with criminal behavior (Need principle).
(3) Interventions should be tailored to match offender characteristics, such as cognitive abilities, learning styles, culture (Responsivity principle) [66].

Empirical evidence overwhelmingly supports the adherence to principles of RNR when intervening with offenders (see Andrews and Bonta [13] for a thorough review of this literature). In fact, interventions that adhere to the principles of RNR typically produce 10%–30% reductions in criminal recidivism [67]. The empirical support for RNR is such that it is widely accepted that the most effective rehabilitative programs adhere to the principles of RNR [68]. Given the empirical support of RNR, and the findings summarized above examining criminal risk in CJ-involved PMI, it stands to reason that interventions for this population must incorporate principles of RNR; however, as noted above, this has not typically been the case in practice [63,65]. For example, it was historically believed that simply enhancing mental health services to PMI in the community would result in reduced criminal activity (see for example Lamb and Bachrach [69], Lamb and Weinberger [70], and Teplin [71]), but we now know that treatment of mental health concerns fails to elicit change in criminal behavior [36,37]. Furthermore, when treating incarcerated PMI, treatment providers tend to place greater emphasis on basic mental health services (e.g., symptom management and stabilization) and personal growth, than on rehabilitative efforts, including principles of RNR, such as reducing criminal risk and preparing inmates for release [65]. This emphasis on mental health at the exclusion (or reduced emphasis) on criminalness is likely also true in mental health settings, such as forensic psychiatric units and general mental health practice. Given the current findings of the role of neuroanatomical abnormalities and criminal risk in PMI that become CJ-involved, such approaches are no longer recommended. It is time to provide services to CJ-involved PMI that target the

co-occurring needs of this population, that is, both mental illness and criminalness [18,71].

Results of two separate meta-analytic reviews support the benefit of targeting both mental illness and criminalness by demonstrating important improvements in both domains post-treatment. Specifically, mental health interventions for incarcerated offenders found significant treatment improvements for general mental health outcomes, to include reduced symptom distress, improved coping skills, and improved behavioral functioning [63,72]. Notably, however, interventions also appear to have an appreciable effect on criminal and psychiatric recidivism, complementary goals of interventions aimed at targeting offending, and mental illness needs. These meta-analyses also provide important insights into effective therapeutic strategies, including the use of homework and behavioral practice of new behaviors [63]. Also, continuity of services between institutions and community, some level of voluntariness in treatment participation, and not utilizing time-limited approaches [72] all produced more favorable outcomes.

Notably absent from these reviews were studies that targeted co-occurring issues of mental illness and crime. In fact, Morgan et al. [63] found only one study that examined the effectiveness of an enhanced assertive community treatment (ACT) treatment delivery model for reducing both criminal and psychiatric recidivism, and produced positive treatment effects for both ($d = 1.17$ for psychiatric recidivism and $d = 0.54$ for criminal recidivism; see Lamberti et al. [73]). These are significant findings, given that CJ-involved PMI present unique challenges, requiring service providers to treat both psychiatric symptoms and criminalness [74]. To enhance treatment options, Morgan et al. developed Changing Lives and Changing Outcomes: A Treatment Program for Justice Involved Persons with Mental Illness, a comprehensive intervention designed to target the dual issues of mental illness and criminal propensity [75]. Changing Lives and Changing Outcomes includes nine treatment modules that are uniquely tied to both mental illness and criminal risk. Results of preliminary program evaluations are promising, with evidence that participants generally learn the content and concepts presented [76], as well as clinically significant improvements over time (pre–post) on measures of psychiatric symptoms and psychopathology, and important aspects of criminal thinking [75]. Current efforts are examining effects on criminal recidivism and community re-entry.

The treatment summary discussed above reviews treatment gains with regard to PMI and general criminal behavior, but what about therapeutic interventions for PMI and violence? Special consideration for reducing one's risk for violence is especially important, as substance abuse in conjunction with poor medication compliance has been shown to lead to an increase in the risk for violent acting out among PMI [77,78].

Current approaches to treating violent offenders are based on social learning and social information processing theories [79–82], with little to no discourse on the role of neurobiology in the treatment process. The basic premise of these psychosocial approaches is that past violent behaviors have been learned (modeled) and reinforced. Not unexpectedly then, treatment efforts have aimed to reduce violence by teaching nonviolent alternatives or methods of responding. Specifically, treatment efforts typically seek to help participants increase awareness of triggers and develop skills of behavioral control, while also challenging antisocial attitudes (consistent with the Needs principle of RNR). Typical programs for reducing violence generally appear to be intensive in nature (recommended minimum of about 6 months), structured, and skills-based with an emphasis on modeling alternatives to violence. Such programs have proven to be quite successful. For example, an examination of a multimodal systemic intervention rooted in psychosocial and behavioral interventions, supplemented with psychopharmacology when warranted, resulted in significant behavioral improvements such as reduced disciplinary infractions, and reduced inmate–inmate and inmate–staff assaults [83]. Although this intervention is systemically based (and therefore quite costly), pure psychosocial interventions have also proven to be effective. A recently developed program, The Violence Reduction Program: A Treatment Program for Violence Prone Forensic Clients (VRP) [84], offers particular promise. The VRP includes three therapeutic phases: (1) learning about aggressive behaviors and readiness for change; (2) skill development to manage thoughts, feelings, and behaviors associated with violence; and (3) over-learning skills and relapse prevention. The intervention is not time-limited, so it allows participants to work at their own pace, and preliminary evaluations to date have resulted in reduced community violence, as well as institutional improvements including less restrictive housing placements and fewer institutional behavioral problems [82,85,86].

Recent gains in understanding neurobiological mechanisms that are associated with crime and violence offer promising areas of future research. Specifically, as research moves from correlational studies of this complex relationship to studies examining causal neurobiological mechanisms of crime and violence, the potential exists for a plethora of new treatment options. For example, if future studies advance beyond the findings summarized above to identify etiological markers, early detection of individuals at biological risk (beyond the Central 8 risk factors) becomes possible. As such developments occur, the breadth of treatment options significantly increases. At the very least, this will provide opportunities for early detection and intervention. Notably, intervening as early as 3 years of age can produce improved brain functioning and subsequent reductions in crime [87]. In fact, the earlier an intervention is delivered, the greater likelihood for a successful outcome [88]. As summarized by Miller [88], even simple physiological interventions, such as diet, can result in reduced criminalness and possibly violence. In other words, as Rainy noted, "Biology is not destiny. We can change the biological roots of crime and violence— there's no question about it" (as cited in Miller [88], p. 39).

Thus, the potential for more integrated interventions that holistically target the complex etiological mechanisms of crime exists.

Discussion

Mental illness, crime, and violence involve a complex interaction of neurobiological, social, and psychological/ sociological factors that are poorly understood by lay persons [1,2], and, in our opinion, professionals alike (see for example research by Bewley and Morgan [65]). Although historically, clinical practice emphasized the enhancement of mental health treatment to PMI to reduce CJ involvement, it is now clear that mental health treatment is insufficient for reducing crime and violence. Specifically, it is now clear that CJ-involved PMI present with criminal risk factors similar to offenders who are not mentally ill [15,17,19,28,29,43]. Given these findings, it is imperative that treatment efforts target co-occurring issues of mental illness and criminalness. Notably, psychosocial interventions offer significant potential for reducing criminal and psychiatric recidivism [43,68], and new programs are being developed that target these goals [56].

Of particular interest with regard to new research developments in CJ, forensic psychiatry, and forensic psychology are the findings by neuroscientists such as Pardini *et al.* [8] The use of MRIs to identify individuals at risk for future criminal activity, generally, and violence, specifically, presents numerous treatment possibilities. Specifically, findings that crime is associated with neurological dysfunction and atrophy opens new possibilities for interventions; however, more research, particularly research that allows for causal inferences, is needed to further advance our understanding and possible treatment options associated with neurobiological dysfunction. Until this is accomplished, increased efforts at improving the management of incarcerated PMI and housing situations for CJ-involved PMI in correctional institutions, psychiatric facilities, or the community are essential. Furthermore, current treatment efforts must not limit focus to treatment of mental illness, and must include efforts at reducing criminalness by implementing treatment strategies and models of intervention such as RNR.

In spite of the many significant gains that have produced enhanced understanding of the etiological and treatment needs of CJ-involved PMI, much work remains to be done. Future studies should continue with neuroimaging studies with PMI with and without criminal histories or comorbid antisocial traits. Specifically, future studies should aim to examine the etiology of neurobiological abnormalities and the role of environment in causing or exacerbating such abnormalities. Furthermore, although research has begun to demonstrate that psychosocial interventions can be effective for reducing both criminal and psychiatric recidivism, further research is warranted to identify effective treatment programs and the identification of best practices for reducing violence, crime, and psychiatric disturbance, while simultaneously improving quality of life when intervening with CJ involved PMI.

Disclosures

The authors do not have anything to disclose.

References

1. Pescosolido BA, Martin JK, Link BG, et al. American's Views of Mental Health and Illness at Century's End: Continuity and Change. Public Report on the MacArthur Mental Health Module, 1996 General Social Survey. Bloomington, IN: Indiana Consortium for Mental Health Services Research and Joseph P. Mailman School of Public Health, Columbia University; 2000.

2. Pescosolido BA, Monahan J, Link BG, Stueve A, Kikuzawa S. The public's view of the competence, dangerousness, and need for legal coercion of persons with mental health problems. *Am. J. Public Health.* 1999; **89**(9): 1339–1345.

3. Corrigan PW. *On the Stigma of Mental Illness: Practical Strategies for Research and Social Change.* Washington, DC: American Psychological Association; 2005.

4. Wahl OF. *Media Madness: Public Images of Mental Illness.* New Brunswick, NJ: Rutgers University Press; 1997.

5. Markowitz FE. Mental illness, crime, and violence: risk, context, and social control. *Aggression and Violent Behavior.* 2011; **16**(1): 36–44.

6. Institute of Medicine (US). Committee on Crossing the Quality Chasm, Adaptation to Mental Health, and Addictive Disorders. *Improving the Quality of Health Care for Mental and Substance-Use Conditions.* Washington, DC: National Academy Press; 2006.

7. Elbogen EB, Johnson SC. The intricate link between violence and mental disorder: results from the National Epidemiologic Survey on Alcohol and Related Conditions. *Arch. Gen. Psychiatry.* 2009; **66**(2): 152–161.

8. Pardini DA, Raine A, Erickson K, Loeber R. Lower amygdala volume in men is associated with childhood aggression, early psychopathic traits, and future violence. *Biol. Psychiatry.* 2014; **75**(1): 73–80.

9. Glenn AL, Raine A, Schug RA. The neural correlates of moral decision-making in psychopathy. *Mol. Psychiatry.* 2009; **14**(1): 5–6.

10. Aharoni E, Vincent GM, Harenski CL, et al. Neuroprediction of future rearrest. *Proc. Natl Acad. Sci. USA.* 2013; **110**(15): 6223–6228.

11. Fairchild G, van Goozen SHM, Calder AJ, Goodyer IM. Research review: evaluating and reformulating the developmental taxonomic theory of antisocial behavior. *J. Child Psychol. Psychiatry.* 2013; **54**(9): 924–940.

12. Teicher MH, Andersen SL, Polcari A, et al. The neurobiological consequences of early stress and childhood maltreatment. *Neurosci. Biobehav. Rev.* 2003; **27**(1–2): 33–44.

13. Andrews DA, Bonta J. *The Psychology of Criminal Conduct*, 5th edn. Cinicinnatti, OH: Anderson Publishing Co; 2010.

14. Draine J, Salzer MS, Culhane DP, Hadley TR. Role of social disadvantage in crime, joblessness, and homelessness among persons with serious mental illness. *Psychiatr. Serv.* 2002; **53**(5): 565–573.

15. Bonta J, Law M, Hanson K. The prediction of criminal and violent recidivism among mentally disordered offenders: a meta-analysis. *Psychol. Bull.* 1998; **123**(2): 123–142.

16. Yochelson S, Samenow SE. *The Criminal Personality. Volume I: A Profile for Change*. Northvale, NJ: Jason Aronson; 1976.

17. Wilson AB, Farkas K, Ishler K, *et al.* Criminal thinking styles among people with serious mental illness in jail. *Law Hum. Behav.* 2014; **38**(6): 592–601.

18. Morgan RD, Fisher WH, Duan N, Mandracchia JT, Murray D. Prevalence of criminal thinking among state prison inmates with serious mental illness. *Law Hum. Behav.* 2010; **34**(4): 324–336.

19. Wolff N, Morgan RD, Shi J, Fisher W, Huening J. Comparative analysis of thinking styles and emotional states of male and female inmates with and without mental disorders. *Psychiatric Services*, 2011; **62**: 1458–1493.

20. Walters GD. Criminal thinking as a mediator of the mental illness–prison violence relationship: a path analytic study and causal mediation analysis. *Psychol. Serv.* 2011; **8**(3): 189–199.

21. Phillips HK, Gray NS, MacCulloch SI, *et al.* Risk assessment in offenders with mental disorders relative efficacy of personal demographic, criminal history, and clinical variables. *J. Interpers. Violence.* 2005; **20**(7): 833–847.

22. Douglas KS, Guy LS, Hart SD. Psychosis as a risk factor for violence to others: a meta-analysis. *Psychol. Bull.* 2009; **135**(5): 679–706.

23. Skeem JL, Manchak S, Peterson JK. Correctional policy for offenders with mental illness. *Law Hum. Behav.* 2011; **35**(2): 110–126.

24. Carr WA, Rosenfeld B, Magyar M, Rotter M. An exploration of criminal thinking styles among civil psychiatric patients. *Criminal Behavior and Mental Health.* 2009; **19**(5): 334–346.

25. Fazel S, Gulati G, Linsell L, Geddes JR, Grann M. Schizophrenia and violence: systematic review and meta-analysis. *PLoS Medicine.* 2009; **6**(8): e1000120.

26. Gross NR, Morgan RD. Understanding persons with mental illness who are and are not criminal justice involved: a comparison of criminal thinking and psychiatric symptoms. *Law Hum. Behav.* 2013; **37**(3): 175–186.

27. Gross NR, Morgan RD. Criminal thinking in a community mental health sample: effects on treatment engagement, psychiatric recovery, and criminalness. Manuscript in preparation for publication. See: http://hdl.handle.net/2346/58919.

28. Bolanos A, Morgan RD, Mitchell S, Gabrowski K. Shared risk factors among persons with mental illness with or without involvement in the criminal justice system. Manuscript in preparation for publication.

29. Skeem JL, Winter E, Kennealy PJ, Eno Louden J, Tatar JR II. Offenders with mental illness have criminogenic needs, too: toward recidivism reduction. *Law and Hum. Behav.* 2014; **38**(3): 212–224.

30. Lilienfeld SO. Comorbidity between and within childhood externalizing and internalizing disorders: reflections and directions. *J. Abnorm. Child Psychol.* 2003; **31**(3): 285–291.

31. Abramsky S, Fellner J. *Ill Equipped: U.S. Prisons and Offenders with Mental Illness.* New York: Human Rights Watch; 2003.

32. Torrey EF, Kennard AD, Eslinger D, Lamb R, Pavle J. *More Mentally Ill Persons Are in Jails and Prisons than Hospitals: A Survey of the States.* Arlington, VA: Treatment Advocacy Center; 2010.

33. James DJ, Glaze LE. *Mental Health Problems of Prison and Jail Inmates. Bureau of Justice Statistics Special Report, NCJ 213600.* Washington, DC: Department of Justice; 2006.

34. Steadman HJ, Osher FC, Robbins PC, Case B, Samuels S. Prevalence of serious mental illness among jail inmates. *Psychiatr. Serv.* 2009; **60**(6): 761–765.

35. Kessler RC, Chiu WT, Demler O, Walters EE. Prevalence, severity, and comorbidity of twelve-month DSM-IV disorders in the National Comorbidity Survey Replication (NCS-R). *Arch. Gen. Psychiatry.* 2005; **62**(6): 617–627.

36. Calsyn RJ, Yonker RD, Lemming MR, Morse GA, Klinkenberg WD. Impact of assertive community treatment and client characteristics on criminal justice outcomes in dual disorder homeless individuals. *Criminal Behavior and Mental Health.* 2005; **15**(4): 236–248.

37. Morrissey J, Meyer P, Cuddeback G. Extending assertive community treatment to criminal justice settings: origins, current evidence, and future directions. *Community Ment. Health J.* 2007; **43**(5): 527–544.

38. Crisanti AS, Frueh BC. Risk of trauma exposure among persons with mental illness in jails and prisons: what do we really know? *Curr. Opin. Psychiatry.* 2011; **24**(5): 431–435.

39. Wolff N, Shi J, Blitz CL, Siegel J. Understanding sexual victimization inside prisons: factors that predict risk. *Criminology and Public Policy.* 2007; **6**(3): 535–564.

40. Metzner JL, Fellner J. Solitary confinement and mental illness in US prisons: a challenge for medical ethics. *Journal of the American Academy of Psychiatry and the Law Online.* 2010; **38**(1): 104–108.

41. Grassian S. Solitary confinement can cause severe psychiatric harm. *Long Term View.* 2010; 7(2): 15–19.

42. Haney C. Mental health issues in long-term solitary and "supermax" confinement. *Crime and Delinquency.* 2003; **49**(1): 124–156.

43. Bhalla AS. *Herman's House* [DVD]. Brooklyn, NY: Public Broadcast Station; 2012.

44. Nolan KA, Czobor P, Roy BB, *et al.* Characteristics of assaultive behavior among psychiatric inpatients. *Psychiatr. Serv.* 2003; **54**(7): 1012–1016.

45. Quanbeck CD, McDermott BE, Lam J, *et al.* Categorization of aggressive acts committed by chronically assaultive state hospital patients. *Psychiatr. Serv.* 2007; **58**(4): 521–528.

46. McDermott BE, Edens JF, Quanbeck CD, Busse D, Scott CL. Examining the role of static and dynamic risk factors in the prediction of inpatient violence: variable- and person-focused analyses. *Law Hum. Behav.* 2008; **32**(4): 325–338.

47. Warburton K. The new mission of forensic mental health systems: managing violence as a medical syndrome in an environment that balances treatment and safety. *CNS Spectr.* 2014; **32**(4): 325–338.

48. Haney C. Prison overcrowding. In Cutler BL, Zapf PA, eds. *APA Handbook of Forensic Psychology, Vol. 2: Criminal Investigation, Adjudication, and Sentencing Outcomes.* Washington, DC: American Psychological Association; 2015: 415–436.

49. Schmitt J, Warner K, Gupta S. *The High Budgetary Costs of Incarceration.* Washington, DC: Center for Economic and Policy Research; 2010.

50. Heilbrun K, DeMatteo D, Yasuhara K, *et al.* Community-based alternatives for justice-involved individuals with severe mental illness: Review of the relevant research. *Criminal Justice and Behavior.* 2012; **39**(4): 351–419.

51. Cosden M, Ellens JK, Schnell JL, Yamini-Diouf Y. Efficacy of mental health treatment court with assertive community treatment. *Behav. Sci. Law.* 2005; **23**(2): 199–214.

52. Herinckx HA, Swart SC, Ama SM, Dolezal CD, King S. Rearrest and linkage to mental health services among clients of the Clark County mental health court program. *Psychiatr. Serv.* 2005; **56**(7): 853–857.

53. Hiday V, Ray B. Arrests two years after exiting a well-established mental health court. *Psychiatr. Serv.* 2010; **61**(5): 463–468.

54. McNiel DE, Binder RL. Effectiveness of a mental health court in reducing criminal recidivism and violence. *Am. J. Psychiatry.* 2007; **164**(9): 1395–1403.

55. Skeem J, Manchak S, Vida S, Hart E. Probationers with mental disorder: what (really) works? Paper presented at the American Psychology and Law Society (AP-LS) 2009 Annual Conference, March 5, 2009–March 7, 2009; San Antonio, TX.

56. Stromwall LK, Hurdle D. Psychiatric rehabilitation: an empowerment-based approach to mental health services. *Health Soc. Work.* 2003; **28**(3): 206–213.

57. Corrigan PW, Mueser KT, Bond GR, Drake RE, Solomon P. *Principles and Practice of Psychiatric Rehabilitation: An Empirical Approach.* New York: Guilford Press; 2008.

58. Alverson H, Alverson M, Drake RE. An ethnographic study of the longitudinal course of substance abuse among people with severe mental illness. *Community Ment. Health J.* 2000; **36**(6): 557–569.

59. Appleby L, Desai P. Residential instability: a perspective on system imbalance. *Am. J. Orthopsychiatry.* 1987; **57**(4): 515–524.

60. Kushel MB, Vittinghoff E, Haas JS. Factors associated with the health care utilization of homeless persons. *JAMA.* 2001; **285**(2): 200–206.

61. Martell JV, Seitz RS, Harada JK, *et al.* Hospitalization in an urban homeless population: the Honolulu Urban Homeless Project. *Ann. Intern. Med.* 1992; **116** (4): 299–303.

62. O'Connell M, Rosenheck R, Kasprow W, Frisman L. An examination of fulfilled housing preferences and quality of life among homeless persons with mental illness and/or substance use disorders. *Journal of Behavioral Health Services and Research.* 2006; **33**(3): 354–365.

63. Morgan RD, Flora DB, Kroner DG, *et al.* Treating offenders with mental illness: a research synthesis. *Law Hum. Behav.* 2012; **36**(1): 37–50.

64. Moran P, Hodgins S. The correlates of comorbid antisocial personality disorder in schizophrenia. *Schizophr. Bull.* 2004; **30**(4): 791–802.

65. Bewley MT, Morgan RD. A national survey of mental health services available to offenders with

mental illness: who is doing what? *Law Hum. Behav.* 2011; **35**(5): 351–363.

66. Andrews DA, Bonta J, Hoge RD. Classification for effective rehabilitation: Rediscovering psychology. *Criminal Justice and Behavior.* 1990; **17**(1): 19–52.

67. Gendreau P, Goggin C. Treating criminal offenders. In Weiner IB, Otto RK, eds. *Handbook of Forensic Psychology.* Hoboken, NJ: John Wiley & Sons; 2014: 759–793.

68. Andrews DA, Bonta J. *Psychology of Criminal Conduct*, 4th edn. Cincinnati, OH: Anderson Publishing; 2006.

69. Lamb HR, Bachrach LL. Some perspectives on deinstitutionalization. *Psychiatr. Serv.* 2001; **52**(8): 1039–1045.

70. Lamb HR, Weinberger LE. Persons with severe mental illness in jails and prisons: a review. *Psychiatr. Serv.* 1998; **49**(4): 483–492.

71. Teplin LA. Criminalizing mental disorder: the comparative arrest rate of the mentally ill. *Am. Psychol.* 1984; **39**(7): 794–803.

72. Martin MS, Dorken SK, Wamboldt AD, Wooten SE. Stopping the revolving door: a meta-analysis on the effectiveness of interventions for criminally involved individuals with major mental disorders. *Law Hum. Behav.* 2012; **36**(1): 1–12.

73. Lamberti JS, Weisman RL, Schwarzkopf SB, *et al.* The mentally ill in jails and prisons: towards an integrated model of prevention. *Psychiatr. Q.* 2001; **72**(1): 63–77.

74. Hodgins S, Müller-Isberner R, Freese R, *et al.* A comparison of general adult and forensic patients

with schizophrenia living in the community. *International Journal of Forensic Mental Health.* 2007; **6**(1): 63–75.

75. Morgan RD, Kroner DG, Mills JF, Bauer R, Serna C. Treating justice involved persons with mental illness preliminary evaluation of a comprehensive treatment program. *Criminal Justice and Behavior.* 2014; **41**(7): 902–916.

76. Van Horn SA, Morgan RD. Mental health care in the justice system. In A. Wenzel, ed. *Encyclopedia of Abnormal and Clinical Psychology.* Thousand Oaks: Sage. In press.

77. Swartz MS, Swanson JW, Hiday VA, *et al.* Violence and severe mental illness: the effects of substance abuse and nonadherence to medication. *Am. J. Psychiatry.* 1998; **155**(2): 226–231.

78. Robbins PC, Monahan J, Silver E. Mental disorder, violence, and gender. *Law Hum. Behav.* 2003; **27**(6): 561–571.

79. Cortoni F, Nunes K, Latendresse M. *An Examination of the Effectiveness of the Violence Prevention Programme. Research Report No 178.* Ottawa, ON, Canada: Correctional Services of Canada; 2006.

80. Polaschek DLL, Dixon BG. The Violence Prevention Project: the development and evaluation of a treatment programme for violent offenders. *Psychology, Crime, and Law.* 2001; **7**(1–4): 1–27.

81. Serin RC, Preston DL. Managing and treating violent offenders. In Ashford JB, Sales BD, Reid W, eds. *Treating Adult and Juvenile Offenders with Special Needs.*

Washington, DC: American Psychological Association; 2001.

82. Wong SCP, Gordon A, Gu D. Assessment and treatment of violence prone forensic clients: an integrated approach. *Br. J. Psychiatry.* 2007; **190**(49): 66–74.

83. Wang EW, Owens RM, Long SA, Diamond PM, Smith JL. The effectiveness of rehabilitation of persistently violent male prisoners. *Int. J. Offender Ther. Comp. Criminol.* 2000; **44**(4): 505–514.

84. Wong S, Gordon A. The violence reduction program: a treatment program for violence prone forensic clients. *Psychology, Crime, and Law.* 2013; **19**(5–6): 461–475.

85. Di Placido C, Simon T, Witte T, Gu D, Wong SCP. Treatment of gang members can reduce recidivism and institutional misconduct. *Law Hum. Behav.* 2006; **30**(1): 93–114.

86. Wong SCP, Van der Veen S, Leis T, *et al.* Reintegrating seriously violent and personality disordered offenders from a super-maximum security institution into the general offender population. *Int. J. Offender Ther. Comp. Criminol.* 2005; **49**(4): 362–375.

87. Raine A, Mellingen K, Liu J, Venables P, Mednick SA. Effects of environmental enrichment at ages 3–5 years on schizotypal personality and antisocial behavior at ages 17 and 23 years. *Am. J. Psychiatry.* 2003; **160**(9): 1627–1635.

88. Miller A. The criminal mind. *Monitor on Psychology.* 2014; **45**(2): 39.

Chapter

30

Crime, violence, and behavioral health: collaborative community strategies for risk mitigation

Debra A. Pinals

The Relationship Between Violence, Crime, and Mental Illness

Violence in society is a public health problem that requires a broad-based approach to understand and diminish. Criminal recidivism is a separate construct, as not all crime is violent, and not all violence ends up criminalized. In the arena of mental health care, there are a number of hurdles that must be overcome with regard to notions of preventing violence and preventing the increased concentration of individuals with mental health and substance use disorders into the justice system. Media portrayals continually link violence with mental illness, which can make separating myth from reality difficult [1]. In a survey conducted during the aftermath of a tragic mass shooting in Newtown, Connecticut, nearly half of respondents reported beliefs that persons with mental illness are more dangerous than others [2].

There have been generations of research on the prevalence of violence and what proportion can be attributed to mental illness, with studies generally demonstrating that mental illness alone accounts for, at most, 3%–5% of violence in our society [3]. In one of the most methodologically sound studies of mental illness and violence, incidents of violence among persons with mental illness were not significantly different from a community sample when there was no substance use [4]. However, the presence of substance use increased the risk that an individual engaged in violence, and a greater proportion of individuals with mental illness also had substance use challenges [4]. Even with those findings, it is critical to recall that individuals with mental illness are more likely to be victims of crime [5]. Furthermore, substance use,

trauma histories, and a variety of factors other than mental illness are more likely variables that heighten the risk of violence than mental illness alone [6].

If one looks at the prevalence of criminality among persons with mental illness, one sees a further complicated picture. Studies have shown the high prevalence of criminal justice histories among public mental health populations. Fisher *et al.* [7], for example, examined a cohort of recipients of public mental health services over 10 years and found that about 28% had experienced at least one arrest, and that within that group, young adults aged 18 to 25 years of age had a 50% chance of one arrest during that period. In other analyses of that general data, odds of arrest for assault and battery on police officers were highest, with misdemeanor crimes against persons and property and crimes against public decency the next highest [8]. Felony behaviors (outside of the assault and battery on a police officer charges) were less common [8]. Swanson *et al.* [9] reviewed administrative records of individuals within a state mental health system with diagnoses of schizophrenia or bipolar disorder, and found that 1 in 4 individuals was involved with the justice system during a 2-year period.

The prevalence of mental illness and substance use disorders among criminal justice populations is also seen as higher than the general population [10]. This is a critical factor to consider, given the large numbers of people under correctional supervision in the United States. Data from the Bureau of Justice Statistics indicated that almost 7 million offenders were under some type of adult correctional system supervision at year end in 2012, including those incarcerated and out in the community under correctional

Violence in Psychiatry, ed. Katherine D. Warburton and Stephen M. Stahl. Published by Cambridge University Press.
© Cambridge University Press 2016.

supervision (with 1 in 50 adults supervised in the community on probation or parole compared to about 1 in every 108 adults who were incarcerated in prison or jail) [11].

Although these prevalence studies might point to mental illness as the key driving feature of justice involvement, other studies provide a more nuanced breakout of associated factors. Factors that heighten the risk of criminal recidivism among persons with mental illness seem to be similar to those that heighten the risk of recidivism among the general population, with one study showing that juvenile justice involvement and multiple prior incarcerations place people at greater risk of arrest than clinical factors [12]. In an analysis of criminal arrest patterns among persons with schizophrenia and psychotic disorders receiving public mental health services, comorbid antisocial personality disorder and substance use disorders seemed to significantly increase the risk for arrest, while among co-existing anxiety disorders, a diagnosis of posttraumatic stress disorder was more likely associated with a risk of arrest for violent crimes [13]. Other studies point to poverty, social disruptions, and inactivity associated with serious mental illness as factors that may produce higher rates of criminogenic need [14,15]. Furthermore, in a recent study examining offenders with mental illness and symptoms that directly preceded criminal behavior, symptoms of mental illness were infrequently the driving feature related to the criminal conduct (only 4%, 3%, and 10% of crimes related directly to symptoms of mental illness such as psychosis, depression, and bipolar disorder, respectively) compared to features such as antisocial traits [16].

The findings of these data point to an area for public health priority – mitigation and harm reduction that involves a variety of interventions in order to decrease criminal recidivism and decrease the incidence of violence. A focus on mental health symptom reduction alone will likely be insufficient to accomplish this. The field of research is pointing to more comprehensive strategies that involve multidimensional treatment planning and criminal justice supervision practices. Over the last several decades, in fact, collaborations between the criminal justice system and the systems providing for mental health and substance use services (i.e., behavioral health systems) have sprung up to address these issues among overlapping populations.

Bringing Justice and Mental Health Systems Together: Sequential Intercept Mapping

Mental health systems have not been static, and individuals who work in such systems may feel ill-prepared to deal with individuals at risk of harm to others and at risk of criminal conduct. Similarly, individuals who work with the justice system can feel at a loss with regard to the management of mental illness and substance use. Building a framework around decreasing the prevalence in the justice system of certain individuals with behavioral health disorders can be an important strategy to help organize initiatives [17].

One such model that has been widely promulgated is known as the Sequential Intercept model [18]. This model posits that the criminal justice system can be viewed along a continuum, from arrest to courts to re-entry from jails and prisons, and including when individuals are supervised in community settings by probation and/or parole. Within this continuum are points of potential interception, whereby an individual could be identified as having mental health difficulties that would be better addressed in the mental health service system. Once identified, such individuals could then be re-routed or diverted away from the criminal justice system and into treatment services, thereby reducing their risk of deeper criminal justice penetration.

Many jurisdictions have conducted Sequential Intercept Mapping workshops [19]. This activity allows for the behavioral health and criminal justice system staff in specific communities to learn about available programs and local connections to better manage the populations served across systems [20]. These mappings also provide opportunities to understand service gaps that may need to be addressed. Several practices are being promulgated that tie together the systems and services identified in such exercises (see Figure 30.1).

Police-based interventions

At the front-end early intercepts, there are evolving trends for police and community mental health providers to work together to achieve better outcomes, given that over many years it has been increasingly recognized that police may be first responders to increasing numbers of individuals with mental illness. Early research in this area referred to police as "street

---

Intercepts 1 and 2: Law Enforcement/Initial Detention and Court Hearings

- Crisis intervention teams
- Mental health specialists co-response with police
- Pre-arraignment diversion programs
- Post-arraignment pre-adjudication programs

Intercept 3: Jails and Court

- Programs involving conditions of release and alternatives to incarceration
- Specialty court dockets

Intercepts 4 and 5: Re-Entry and Community Corrections

- Specialized re-entry programs
- Specialized forensic assertive community treatment programs
- Specialized probation services

Figure 30.1 Examples of criminal justice and behavioral health collaborative strategies using a Sequential Intercept Mapping Framework [18,20].

corner psychiatrists" [21], and noted that police were often faced with problem solving and management decisions, or an option to arrest, during these encounters.

Specialized training for police, through Crisis Intervention Team (CIT) development, for example, has expanded to numerous communities across the United States. Available data suggest that when police are specifically trained to work with individuals with mental illness through Crisis Intervention Teams, fewer injuries result to those involved [22]. Although not specifically identified as a violence-prevention strategy, CIT was developed in Memphis, Tennessee, in the late 1980s after an individual with mental illness was shot and killed during an encounter with police [23]. As these CIT programs have developed, more research is demonstrating that police are better able to respond to individuals in crisis, and consider alternative dispositions [24], since part of the training involves gaining familiarity with local programs and services. Separate from CIT, other types of law enforcement and behavioral health partnerships, including co-response to scenes and protocols that provide for tight hand-off of case referrals, similarly work to avoid arrest and direct individuals into treatment.

Court-involved interventions

Specialty court sessions and other alternatives to incarceration (sometimes referred to as court-level jail diversion) have been expanding over recent years. The wave of specialty courts began with the first drug court, which was established in Miami-Dade County, Florida, in 1989, after local stakeholders began to feel that a remedy for the revolving door for individuals with substance use disorders could benefit from creative solutions [25]. As of 2012, over 2734 drug courts have been established [26]. Enthusiasm about the effectiveness of drug courts [27] spawned interest in a host of other specialty courts, including mental health courts, veterans courts, re-entry courts, co-occurring courts, courts for drunk driving offenses, homelessness courts, and the like.

The premise of each of these specialty courts is that a judicial leader partners with a "treatment team" composed of probation, usually adversarial parties (such as defense and prosecuting attorneys), plus treatment providers to bring together shared goals and common solutions for individuals before the court. The individual participant generally must agree to participate in the specialty court on a voluntary basis, recognizing that participation involves mandated activities, regular court appearances before the judge, with rewards and sanctions for adherence and non-adherence, respectively. Data continue to emerge demonstrating that these programs result in fewer jail days and improved outcomes [28,29].

In addition to specialty court sessions, court-based programs to provide alternative pathways out of traditional criminal case processing for individuals with co-occurring disorders have expanded (also referred to as jail-diversion programs or alternatives to incarceration). As more of these programs evolve, programs are targeting special populations, such as veterans [30]. The ability to work with these groups brings together a host of resources for those involved in the justice system that can help target public safety, behavioral health, and improved functioning.

Programs linked to re-entry and community correctional supervision

Specialized programs also bring together resources for individuals with co-occurring disorders who are re-entering communities after a period of incarceration in jails and prisons [31]. Critical Time Intervention, for example, is a time-limited, staged intervention that is designed to help link individuals with mental illness to services and enhance their engagement in community programs. Early studies showed promise with working with individuals with mental illness upon re-entry from jails and prisons [32]. Forensic Assertive Community Treatment is another type of program in which justice-involved individuals with mental illness are provided intensive wrap-around, community-based services that integrate criminal justice personnel and often receive referrals from criminal justice programs. Although more research is needed, this intervention has shown some positive results in preventing arrest and incarceration [33]. A more recent study examined these two types of programs and found that both represented differing strategies that worked to enhance engagement, though each has unique components that may link to different resources over time [34].

Integration of Conceptual Models into Programs to Reduce Violence and Criminal Risks

Collaborative behavioral health and justice programs and services will likely continue to be refined with their ongoing expansion as part of the fabric of community-based services. In order to utilize these interventions most beneficially, targeted populations and approaches continue to be developed. Steadman et al. [35], for example, noted that mental health courts reduce jail days and re-incarceration, but may be inherently more expensive overall, and thus from a fiscal perspective argued that it is critical to target the "right" services for the "right" people. With that in mind, this review turns next to specific guidance related to conceptual models that address criminal offender rehabilitation on an individualized level to achieve risk mitigation and decreased recidivism.

To begin with, it is important to note that criminal justice personnel view their roles from a different

perspective than behavioral health treatment providers. In particular, criminal justice personnel see their primary mission as enhancing public safety outcomes and adhering to court orders, whereas traditional behavioral health services have focused their overall mission on symptom reduction, recovery, and improved psychosocial functioning (see Figure 30.2). Indeed, actions related to treatment interventions and correctional supervision can be applied synergistically for justice-involved behavioral health populations in order to achieve the overarching goal of public safety [10].

Evolving concepts therefore involve taking apart an individual's risks and putting together treatment planning and correctional supervision planning that can enhance engagement and maximize benefit of treatment services, while focusing on mitigating public safety risks.

In the early 1990s, Andrews et al. [36] wrote about the classification of individuals for focused and effective criminal offender rehabilitation. Other models have also been promulgated, such as the Good Lives Model (see http://www.goodlivesmodel.com), to address offender rehabilitation [37]. For the purpose of this review, however, the model by Andrews et al. [36] is delineated. This model is quite commonly seen now in criminal justice programs. In this "risk–need–responsivity" (RNR) framework, individuals should be identified in accordance with their level of risk for reoffending, and with prioritization of treatments and specific interventions targeting those at highest risk [10,36]. Studies examining factors that lead to the greatest risk of criminal recidivism point to the "big 8" factors (with the first 4 being the most associated with risk):

1. Antisocial behavior
2. Antisocial personality patterns
3. Antisocial cognition
4. Antisocial associates
5. Family or marital relational disruptions
6. School and/or work difficulties
7. Leisure and/or recreation deficits
8. Substance misuse [13,38]

According to the RNR model, for each individual, criminogenic needs should also be targeted as the dynamic factors that can be modified to reduce the risk of reoffending. Finally, factors that create barriers to learning or to achieving success with the targeted intervention, or so-called "responsivity" factors, are

	Treatment	Correctional Supervision
Primary Goal	• Symptom reduction • Alleviation of suffering	• Public safety • Reduce criminal recidivism
Primary Duty	• To the patient	• To the public • To the court • To the correctional oversight body
Methodology	• Monitoring • Regular contact	• Monitoring • Regular contact • Cross verification through drug screens • Evidentiary hearings
Techniques	• Engagement • Occasional legal mandates • Linkages to services	• Legally mandated oversight • Requires engagement strategies to enhance compliance • Provides linkages to services
Protocols	• Standards of Care • Privacy rules	• Court orders • Terms of release • Communication not as constrained by privacy rules for adults in criminal justice settings

Figure 30.2 Sample treatment plan using approaches to address criminogenic risks and needs.

important to consider in aiming toward recidivism reduction. For example, an individual's cognitive deficits or ongoing depression might make it more difficult for him or her to adhere to probation terms, make appointments, and generally comply with court orders. An individual with these factors is at greater risk for difficulties, such as technical violations that can include new charges. A lack of system and provider awareness of and ability to accommodate the individual's responsivity can further compound the problem.

Treatment planning that addresses the central 8 risk/need factors and that also takes into account responsivity factors shows promise in reducing criminal recidivism. Figure 30.3 shows an example of a hypothetical treatment plan framed around RNR principles. This approach reflects desirable policy-level problem-solving efforts, given the aforementioned studies that point to the fact that recidivism among persons with mental illness may not be related as much to mental illness as to many of these other criminogenic risk factors [12,14,15]. Thus, although there remain countless questions that await further research, this area of treatment seems to offer an opportunity for augmentation of traditional behavioral health constructs to help address the problems of aggression and criminality among behavioral health populations.

Recidivism and Violence Risk Reduction in Practice

Traditional clinical violence risk assessment and risk management is an important practice for individuals in the behavioral health system who present concerns about public safety. Treatment planning traditionally includes a violence risk assessment approach of some type, which is targeted for the setting and for the purpose it is aiming to achieve [38]. Within an RNR framework, identification of the criminogenic risks and needs is a starting point that is focused on risk of criminal recidivism. There is a vast literature regarding instruments that might be used for screening for this risk that should serve as a reference point.

Once criminal recidivism risk (which is often thought of as a general public safety risk but may or may not involve a measure of violence) is established, the assessment of criminogenic needs helps to support treatment planning. In addition to focusing strongly on substance use treatment, practices related to psychotherapeutic techniques within correctional settings that have some evidence of efficacy could be helpful to consider [39]. Therapies, such as dialectical behavioral therapy, which is designed originally for individuals who engaged in frequent self-injury, have also shown positive results with correctional and forensic populations in reducing violence and criminal behavior [40].

Sample Treatment Plan with Recidivism Reduction Framework	
Antisocial behaviors	Frequent check ins, educational efforts to maximize understanding of consequences of behaviors, communication between probation and treatment provider; possible DBT to reduce violence and anger
Antisocial personality patterns	Reduced impulsivity through skills building, meditation, trauma-informed services, stress management, exercise
Antisocial cognitions	Evidence-based cognitive behavioral treatments that address antisocial thinking patterns
Antisocial peers	Provision of positive peer support services, support in changing negative social circles, engagement in community activities
Family/marital relationships	Exploration of relationship fractures, reparation where feasible, therapy, and support; education about restraining orders and legal mandates; partnership with probation to support adherence to such mandates
Employment/education	Linkages to vocational and educational support services, rewards for positive achievement
Leisure and recreation	Development of schedules for activities, community service, positive peer interactions related to social events
Substance use	Engagement in active treatment, medication assisted therapies as appropriate, monitoring through testing, planning for relapses, supportive groups such as AA, NA

Responsivity Factors (examples):

1. Mental health issues—Development of means to address symptoms of depression, anxiety, psychosis, etc. Pharmacological and therapeutic supports, including attention to negative symptoms and motivation to engage in treatment for the individual and the individual's support systems

2. Cultural factors—Development of means to maximize cultural competence among providers; help client help staff understand where culture plays a role in participation in programming

3. Cognitive factors—Utilization of testing to establish baseline; modification of programming to meet the client's needs; job aids, schedule aids, etc. to maximize adherence to correctional supervision

4. Trauma factors—Interventions to reduce social isolation, anxiety, irritability, hypervigilance, attachment deficits, limitations on the ability to develop trusting relationships- assist with relaxation strategies, reliable scheduled encounters, provide information and knowledge about plans and programs, foster person-centered planning to increase sense of self-control

Figure 30.3 Treatment and correctional supervision: similarities and differences.

Specific treatments involving cognitive behavioral techniques to address antisocial thinking may have promise for larger populations of behavioral health clients who cycle through the criminal justice system. These types of interventions have not traditionally been a part of general behavioral health services, though are more often seen in correctional settings.

Moral Reconation Therapy (MRT) [41,42] and Thinking for a Change [43], for example, have been utilized with some success in criminal justice populations. In fact, MRT began with a focus on individuals with substance use disorders who also had antisocial features.

Substance use presents as an identified criminogenic risk in and of itself. Mental illness fits into the

RNR framework not as one of the big 8 risk factors, but as part of what needs to be attended to with regard to responsivity. Osher *et al.* [10] lay out a criminogenic risk and behavioral health needs framework that targets interventions to the level of need in three main areas: criminogenic risk, substance use, and mental health. For a person with high criminogenic needs and low-level substance use or mental health needs, correctional supervision might be more intense and balanced by less intensive behavioral health treatments. In contrast, individuals who score low in criminogenic needs, but have high substance use treatment and mental health challenges, will require more intensive treatments, and perhaps less correctional monitoring and oversight.

One emerging manualized collaborative approach to such treatment is called MISSION-Criminal Justice. This approach combines several evidence-based practices and utilizes a case management and peer support model to target substance use, mental illness, and criminal recidivism, while taking into account the role of traumatic life experiences in behavioral responses [44,45]. Earlier versions of this model showed its utility among homeless veterans with co-occurring disorders [46], and preliminary administrative data in Massachusetts demonstrated its effectiveness in reducing re-incarceration, decreasing substance use, improving social connections, and helping individuals to stay engaged with mental health services.

In another innovative example, interventions have been developed that attend to the "culture of incarceration" [47]. A program designed to help individuals learn how to de-culturate from correctional settings, called Sensitizing Providers to the Effects of Correctional Incarceration on Treatment and Risk Management (SPECTRM), attempts to address staff readiness and client engagement as part of targeting responsivity factors in care [48]. Reentry After Prison (RAP) groups help clients learn about behaviors that may be adaptive in prison but are maladaptive upon re-entry, by using trauma-informed practices and cultural competence [47]. The application of these types of tools may be increasingly helpful in addressing the shared populations between criminal justice and behavioral health systems.

Recovery and Trauma-Informed Services

There is increased recognition of the critical importance of recovery concepts driving treatment that can help enhance engagement, improve individual lives, and potentially even impact recidivism. The concept of recovery is one that has grown exponentially from substance use delivery to mental health services.

The Substance Abuse and Mental Health Services Administration (SAMHSA) defines recovery as "a process of change through which individuals improve their health and wellness, live a self-directed life, and strive to reach their full potential" [49]. SAMHSA's principles of recovery include 10 factors:

1. Hope
2. Person-driven
3. Many pathways
4. Holistic
5. Peer support
6. Relational
7. Culture
8. Addresses trauma
9. Strengths/responsibility
10. Respect

These principles provide anchors that can each be examined in relation to how an individual may achieve positive outcomes and maintain a life with minimal criminal justice involvement. Principles of recovery do not offer excuses for misconduct, or lessen personal responsibility for violent or antisocial behavior. Some individuals receiving mental health services will have impaired mental capacities impacting cognition and conduct in specific circumstances, challenging notions of personal accountability. Nevertheless, if we frame our view of the majority of individuals with behavioral health conditions as responsible, productive individuals, it is important to keep in the forefront their strengths and resiliency factors to maximize positive outcomes.

Services that are trauma-informed and trauma-responsive provide the needed sensitivity to the realities of behavioral health and criminal justice populations. It is widely recognized that the prevalence of trauma in criminal justice populations is high [50]. Trauma can be a major factor in mental health [51], and this includes witnessing prior violence and experiencing physical and sexual abuse. Furthermore, as noted above, post-traumatic stress disorder and trauma histories can contribute to aggressive behavior [52,53]. Thus, trauma is a responsivity factor that plays a complicated multidirectional role in an individual's behavior and symptoms.

Enhancing trauma-sensitivity across systems and within treatment and across settings is therefore good practice. Here again, SAMHSA has recently offered some guidance that includes the "4 Rs" related to developing trauma responsive organizations, including (1) realization about trauma and how it can affect individuals and groups; (2) recognition of the signs of trauma; (3) responsiveness of the program or system to all persons involved by applying trauma-informed principles throughout; and (4) resistance of re-traumatization of clients and staff [54]. Beyond recognition of the individual's historical trauma exposure, it is also helpful to recognize how interactions across settings can themselves be traumatizing. Jails, prisons, and psychiatric hospitals, for example, are places where individuals are sent where they are less in control of aspects of their lives. Traumatizing circumstances, such as disruptions in social networks, exposure to high noise level, being surrounded by individuals with tragic life circumstances, or those with antisocial and even violent propensities, can be realities of these settings.

An individual who is receiving services but who has high levels of trauma-related anxiety, hypervigilance, and irritability, for example, may be at risk of acting out aggressively, leaving treatment providers in the difficult position of managing behavior that may pose public safety risks in the moment, and that may be frightening or jarring to staff. Behaviors that occur under stress might be reduced by de-escalation that recognizes a trauma-informed strategy to add to other prevention techniques (e.g., calm and respectful responses by staff, including responses that require setting limits, development of institutional cultures promoting respect and safety, and the development of safety and crisis intervention plans for individuals and the system). Training for staff and for persons served in the recognition of signs and symptoms of trauma-reactivity, de-escalation, and relaxation skills development, as well as referral to trauma-focused treatment when needed, can all be helpful, specific activities within "trauma-informed" services. Examination of an individual's natural support system may also yield some information that can be addressed with a trauma-responsive lens. As awareness of these issues evolves, correctional systems, community correctional supervision, specialty courts, and behavioral health systems have begun to examine how to develop more trauma-informed approaches in their work.

Peer Support

The concept of peer support is not a new one. With the establishment of Alcoholics Anonymous, the notion of a sponsor or a peer who was facing similar experiences in achieving sobriety was thought to be an important component of recovery. From there, recovery coaches and peers with lived experience have become increasingly common as part of a real behavioral health workforce. These individuals are seen as critical to aspects of recovery. Certification training programs assist them in their work and with services that are potentially reimbursable through Medicaid and other funds [55].

From a risk management lens, a positive peer network can be very helpful. Among the most recalcitrant problems with ongoing criminal activity is the association with antisocial peers. By bringing peers who have had similar life experiences to the forefront, individuals at risk for recidivism are able to see examples of hope, recovery, and positive prosocial development. Bringing positive peers with criminal justice backgrounds into the workforce can be difficult, given employment issues for individuals with criminal histories and sensitivity among criminal justice entities about negative peer associations. However, resources are available to assist systems in better establishing these roles, with guidance related to employment principles [56] as well as information showing the effectiveness of this type of peer support [57]. If engagement strategies are to be maximized, learning from successful individuals who have "been there and done that" can strengthen services with regard to recidivism. Over time, more research surrounding peer support as an intervention strategy will be important to help determine what factors in prosocial associations can help reduce the risk for specific violence and criminal recidivism among behavioral health consumers.

Conclusions

Individuals with mental health and substance use disorders who have criminal justice histories, and who may include a subset of individuals at risk of aggression or violence, warrant thoughtful attention to minimize criminal justice involvement and to reduce the risk of harm to others in their communities. Whether a person is identified through the behavioral health system, or through a police diversion program, specialty court, community supervision, or jail and prison re-entry service, treatment planning for this complex population should examine the key criminogenic risks and needs, as well as responsivity factors that can create barriers to positive outcomes. Trauma-informed approaches and peer support can foster engagement and ongoing connections to services and provide positive role modeling. The criminal justice behavioral health populations are often multiply stigmatized, and they face countless collateral consequences especially if they continue to recidivate. Multifaceted tools to address their needs are still maturing in the field, and ongoing research should be supported. Current efforts move beyond silos integrating criminal justice and behavioral health approaches. These share common goals of mitigating risks of violence and recidivism, while decreasing victimization, holding hope, and improving quality of life.

Disclosures

Debra Pinals does not have anything to disclose.

References

1. Whitley R, Bery S. Trends in newspaper coverage of mental illness in Canada: 2005–2010. *Can. J. Psychiatry*. 2013; **58**(2): 107–112.

2. Barry CL, McGinty EE, Vernick JS, Webster DW. After Newtown— public opinion on gun policy and mental illness. *N. Engl. J. Med.* 2013; **368**(12): 1077–1081.

3. Swanson JW. Mental disorder, substance abuse, and community violence: an epidemiological approach. In: Monahan J, Steadman H, eds. *Violence and Mental Disorder*. Chicago: University of Chicago Press; 1994: 101–136.

4. Steadman HJ, Mulvey EP, Monahan J, *et al*. Violence by people discharged from acute psychiatric inpatient facilities and by others in the same neighborhoods. *Arch. Gen. Psychiatry*. 1998; **55**(5): 393–401.

5. Teplin LA, McClelland GM, Abram KM, Weiner DA. Crime victimization in adults with severe mental illness: comparison with the national crime victimization survey. *Arch. Gen. Psychiatry*. 2005; **62**(8): 911–921.

6. Elbogen EB, Johnson SC. The intricate link between violence and mental disorder: results from the National Epidemiologic Survey on Alcohol and Related Conditions. *Arch. Gen. Psychiatry*. 2009; **66**(2): 152–161.

7. Fisher WH, Roy-Bujnowski KM, Grudzinskas AJ, *et al*. Patterns and prevalence of arrest in a statewide cohort of mental health care consumers. *Psychiatr. Serv.* 2006; **57**(11): 1623–1628.

8. Fisher WH, Simon L, Roy-Bujnowski K, *et al*. Risk of arrest among public mental health services recipients and the general public. *Psychiatr. Serv.* 2011; **62**(1): 67–72.

9. Swanson JW, Frisman LK, Robertson AG, *et al*. Costs of criminal justice involvement among persons with serious mental illness in Connecticut. *Psychiatr. Serv.* 2013; **64**(7): 630–637.

10. Osher F, D'Amora DA, Plotkin M, *et al*. *Adults with Behavioral Health Needs under Correctional Supervision: A Shared Framework for Reducing Recidivism and Promoting Recovery*. Criminal Justice/Mental Health Consensus Project; Council of State Governments Justice Center, 2012.

11. Glaze LE, Herberman EJ. Correctional populations in the United States, 2012. Bureau of Justice Statistics NCJ 243936, December 19, 2013. Available at http://www.bjs.gov/index.cfm?ty=pbdetail&iid=4843. Accessed October 11, 2014.

12. Fisher WH, Hartwell SW, Deng X, *et al*. Recidivism among released state prison inmates who received mental health treatment while incarcerated. *Crime & Delinquency*. 2014; **60**(6): 811–832.

13. McCabe PJ, Christopher PP, Druhn N, *et al*. Arrest types and co-occurring disorders in persons with schizophrenia or related psychoses. *J. Behav. Health Serv. Res.* 2012; **39**(3): 271–284.

14. Fisher WH, Silver E, Wolff N. Beyond criminalization: toward a criminologically informed framework for mental health policy and services research. *Adm. Policy Ment. Health*. 2006; **33**(5): 544–557.

15. Skeem JL, Manchak S, Peterson JK. Correctional policy for offenders with mental illness: creating a new paradigm for recidivism reduction. *Law Hum. Behav.* 2011; **35**(2): 110–126.

16. Peterson JK, Skeem J, Kennealy P, Bray B, Zvonkovic A. How often and how consistently do symptoms directly precede criminal behavior among offenders with mental illness? *Law Hum. Behav.* 2014; **38**(5): 439–449.

17. Pinals DA. Forensic services, public mental health policy, and financing: charting the course ahead. *J. Am. Acad. Psychiatry Law*. 2014; **42**(1): 7–19.

18. Munetz MR, Griffin PA. Use of the Sequential Intercept Model as an approach to decriminalization of people with serious mental

illness. *Psychiatr. Serv.* 2006; **57**(4): 544–549.

19. Blue-Howells JH, Clark SC, van den Berk-Clark C, McGuire JF. The U.S. Department of Veterans Affairs justice programs and the sequential intercept model: case examples in national dissemination of intervention for justice-involved veterans. *Psychol. Serv.* 2013; **10**(1): 48–53.

20. Sequential Intercept Mapping Delmar, NY: Substance Abuse and Mental Health Services Administration (SAMHSA) National GAINS Center, Policy Research Associates. Available at http://www.prainc.com/sequential-intercept-mapping/. Accessed October 11, 2014.

21. Teplin LA, Pruett NS. Police as streetcorner psychiatrist: managing the mentally ill. *Int. J. Law Psychiatry.* 1992; **15**(2): 139–156.

22. Reuland M, Schwarzfeld M, Draper L. Law enforcement responses to people with mental illness: a guide to research-informed policy and practice. New York: Council of State Governments Justice Center. 2009. Available at http://www.ojp.usdoj.gov/BJA/pdf/ CSG_le-research.pdf. Accessed May 27, 2013.

23. National Alliance on Mental Illness. CIT Toolkit. CIT Facts. Available at http://www.nami.org/Content/ContentGroups/Policy/CIT/CIT_Facts_4.11.12.pdf. Accessed October 10, 2014.

24. Canada KE, Angell B, Watson AC. Intervening at the entry point: differences in how CIT trained and non-CIT trained officers describe responding to mental health-related calls. *Community Ment. Health J.* 2012; **48**(6): 746–755.

25. Hora PF. Drug treatment courts in the twenty-first century: the evolution of the revolution in problem-solving courts. Ga. L. Rev. 2008; **42**: 717.

26. National Association of Drug Court Professionals Drug Court History. Available at http://www.nadcp.org/learn/what-are-drug-courts/drug-court-history. Accessed October 10, 2014.

27. National Association of Drug Court Professionals. Available at http://www.nadcp.org/nadcp-home/. Accessed October 10, 2014.

28. Goodale G, Callahan L, Steadman HJ. What can we say about mental health courts today? *Psychiatr. Serv.* 2013; **64**(4): 298–300.

29. Steadman HJ, Redlich A, Callahan L, et al. Effect of mental health courts on arrests and jail days: a multisite study. *Arch. Gen. Psychiatry.* 2011; **68**(2): 167–172.

30. Pinals DA. Veterans and the justice system: the next forensic frontier. *J. Am. Acad. Psychiatry Law.* 2010; **38**(2): 163–167.

31. Hoge SK, Buchanan AW, Kovasznay BM, Roskes EJ. *Outpatient Services for the Mentally Ill Involved in the Criminal Justice System: A Report of the Task Force on Outpatient Forensic Services.* American Psychiatric Association Resource Document; American Psychiatric Association, 2009.

32. Draine J, Herman DB. Critical time intervention for reentry from prison for persons with mental illness. *Psychiatr. Serv.* 2007; **58**(12): 1577–1581.

33. Lamberti JS, Weisman R, Faden DI. Forensic assertive community treatment: preventing incarceration of adults with severe mental illness. *Psychiatr. Serv.* 2004; **55**(11): 1285–1293.

34. Angell B, Matthews E, Barrenger S, Watson AC, Draine J. Engagement processes in model program for community reentry from prison for people with serious mental illness. *Int. J. Law Psychiatry.* 2014; **37**(5): 490–500.

35. Steadman HJ, Callahan L, Robbins PC, et al. Criminal justice and behavioral health care costs of mental health court participants: a six-year study. *Psychiatr. Serv.* 2014; **65**(9): 1100–1104.

36. Andrews DA, Bonta J, Hoge RD. Classification for effective rehabilitation: rediscovering psychology. *Criminal Justice and Behavior.* 1990; **17**(1): 19–52.

37. Whitehead PR, Ward T, Collie RM. Time for a change: applying the Good Lives Model of rehabilitation to a high-risk violent offender. *International Journal of Offender Therapy and Comparative Criminology.* 2007; **51**(5): 578–598.

38. Monahan J, Skeem JL. The evolution of violence risk assessment. *CNS Spectr.* 2014; **19**(5): 419–424.

39. Garvey K, Newring KAB, Parham RW, Pinals DA. The roles and limitations of evidence-based psychotherapy in correctional settings. In: Thienhaus OJ, Piasecki M, eds. *Correctional Psychiatry: Practice Guidelines and Strategies.* Vol. II. Kingston, NJ: Civic Research Institute; 2013.

40. Evershed S, Tennant A, Boomer D, et al. Practice-based outcomes for dialectical-behavioural therapy targeting anger and violence, with male forensic patients: a pragmatic and non-contemporaneous comparison. *Crim. Behav. Ment. Health.* 2003; **13**(3): 198–213.

41. Little GL, Robinson KD. Moral reconation therapy: a systematic step-by-step treatment system for treatment resistant clients. *Psychol. Rep.* 1988; **62**(1): 135–151.

42. Ferguson LM, Wormith JS. A meta-analysis of moral reconation therapy. *International Journal of Offender Therapy and*

Comparative Criminology. 2013; **57**(9): 1076–1106.

43. Golden L. Evaluation of the efficacy of a cognitive behavioral program for offenders on probation: thinking for a change. Available at: http://static.nicic .gov/Library/025057/default.html. Accessed October 28, 2014.

44. Pinals DA, Smelson D, Sawh L, *et al. Maintaining Independence and Sobriety Through Systems Integration and Outreach Networking—Criminal Justice Edition: Treatment Manual.* See: http://www.mission model.org.

45. Smelson D, Pinals DA, Sawh L, *et al. Maintaining Independence and Sobriety through Systems Integration and Outreach Networking—Criminal Justice Edition: Participant Workbook.* Available at http://www .missionmodel.org. Accessed October 10, 2014.

46. Smelson DA, Kline A, Kuhn J, *et al.* A wraparound treatment engagement intervention for homeless veterans with co-occurring disorders. *Psychol. Serv.* 2013; **10**(2): 161–167.

47. Rotter M, McQuistion HL, Broner N, Steinbacher M. Best practices: the impact of the incarceration culture on reentry for adults with mental illness: a training and

group treatment model. *Psychiatr. Serv.* 2005; **56**(3): 265–267.

48. Rotter M, Carr WA, Frischer K. The premise of criminalization and the promise of offender treatment. In Dlugacz HA, ed. *Reentry Planning for Offenders with Mental Disorders: Policy and Practice.* Kingston, NJ: Civic Research Institute; 2015.

49. Substance Abuse and Mental Health Services Administration 2015. SAMHSA's working definition of recovery. Available at: http://store.samhsa.gov/ product/SAMHSA-s-Working-Definition-of-Recovery/PEP12-RECDEF. Accessed October 1, 2014.

50. Miller NA, Najavits LM. Creating trauma-informed correctional care: a balance of goals and environment. *Eur. J. Psychotraumatol.* 2012; **3**. DOI: 10.3402/ejpt.v.20.17246.

51. van Nierop M, Viechtbauer W, Gunther N, *et al.* Childhood trauma is associated with a specific admixture of affective, anxiety, and psychosis symptoms cutting across traditional diagnostic boundaries. *Psychol. Med.* 2015; **45**(6): 1277–1288.

52. Barrett EL, Teesson M, Mills KL. Associations between substance use, posttraumatic stress disorder

and the perpetration of violence: a longitudinal investigation. *Addict. Behav.* 2014; **39**(6): 1075–1080.

53. Sarchiapone M, Carli V, Cuomo C, Marchetti M, Roy A. Association between childhood trauma and aggression in male prisoners. *Psychiatry Res.* 2009; **165**(1–2): 187–192.

54. Substance Abuse and Mental Health Services Administration. *SAMHSA's Concept of Trauma and Guidance for a Trauma-Informed Approach.* HHS Publication No. (SMA) 14–4884. Rockville, MD: Substance Abuse and Mental Health Services Administration, 2014.

55. Salzer MS, Schwenk E, Brusilovskiy E. Certified peer specialist roles and activities: results from a national survey. *Psychiatr. Serv.* 2010; **61**(5): 520–523.

56. Miller LD, Massaro J. *Overcoming Legal Impediments to Hiring Forensic Peer Specialists.* Delmar, NY: CMHS National GAINS Center; 2008.

57. Davidson L, Rowe M. *Peer Support Within Criminal Justice Settings: The Role of Forensic Peer Specialists.* Delmar, NY: CMHS National GAINS Center; 2008.

Chapter

31

New technologies in the management of risk and violence in forensic settings

John Tully, Thomas Fahy, and Fintan Larkin

Introduction

Novel technological interventions are increasingly used in mental health settings. Examples include mood monitoring by text messaging [1,2], cognitive behavior therapy by smartphone:apps" [3], and touchscreen technology in hospital settings [4]. Telepsychiatry, the practice of psychiatry over distances using information and communication technologies, has also continued to develop throughout the world, making use of new technologies [5–8]. In this article, we describe three novel technological strategies in use for the management of risk and violence in two forensic psychiatry settings in the United Kingdom: a medium secure service in London and Broadmoor high secure hospital.

Several studies evaluating technological interventions in psychiatry report encouraging results. Mood monitoring by text message in patients with bipolar disorder was shown to generate clinical data comparable to one-to-one interviews for monitoring of the condition [1]. A pilot study of a text message–based outreach program for patients with suicidal behaviors was accepted by patients who found it to have a positive preventive impact [2]. It also had several advantages such as lower cost and easier utilization compared to current post-acute care strategies. Another study showed reduced depressive symptoms using a mindfulness-based smartphone app intervention [3]. In a sample of 1308 consecutive inpatients and outpatients participating in a 2-week cognitive behavioral therapy group, daily self-report measures using touch-screen technology were effective in reducing symptoms for patients at risk of poor outcomes [4].

Forensic psychiatry services have been alert to these developments. Forensic services in the UK treat individuals with mental illness who have committed violent offences or are thought to be at especially high risk of doing so. Management of risk and violence is complex, and new cost-effective strategies to optimize outcomes for patients while reducing risk are of great interest to clinicians and service administrators. Inpatient services for these patients are provided through a network of high, medium, and low secure units [9].

The largest segment of UK forensic services are the medium secure units (MSUs), consisting of approximately 3500 beds in the UK [9]. MSUs are expensive services that combine high levels of physical and relational security with intensive medical, nursing, and psychological treatments. The medium secure forensic psychiatry service of the South London and Maudsley Foundation Trust (https://www.national.slam.nhs.uk/services/adult-services/forensic/) is a typical UK forensic service that aims to manage risk, reduce further offending, and support recovery throughout the patient's stay. There are eight wards, with varying levels of security. Admissions and intensive care wards offer enhanced physical, procedural, and relational security, while predischarge units offer a high level of independence with a lower level of security, increased access to community programs, and community outreach services, which foster the development of living skills before moving to independent settings in the community.

Broadmoor High Secure Hospital (http://www.wlmht.nhs.uk/bm/broadmoor-hospital/) is one of four high secure hospitals in the UK. People referred to high secure hospitals in the UK are detained under mental health legislation because they are thought to pose a "grave and immediate danger to the public" [9]. The hospitals treat people with mental illness and personality disorders who represent a high degree of risk to themselves or to others. There are

Violence in Psychiatry, ed. Katherine D. Warburton and Stephen M. Stahl. Published by Cambridge University Press.
© Cambridge University Press 2016.

approximately 210 patients, and the average stay is five years. Patients are transferred to conditions of lower security once the risks that they pose are diminished. The hospital provides a full range of therapeutic treatments that are tailored to each patient's individual needs, including assessment, specialist care, and rehabilitation.

Technologies for Management of Risk and Violence

Electronic monitoring by GPS tracking

Background

Use of the electronic devices to monitor the whereabouts of individuals is referred to in legal and scientific literature as "electronic monitoring" (EM). EM has been used for over three decades in criminal justice systems. Initial trials of EM included an experimental system used in 1964 to monitor parolees, with a one-way transmitter activated by repeater stations used to record an offender's location [10]. Early systems relying on radio frequency (RF) technology were cumbersome and required an offender to carry a heavy transmitter. The technological community responded by developing more advanced systems utilizing RF transmitters, and later, global positioning satellites (GPS). In the mid 1980s, in order to alleviate prison and jail crowding, a new system of EM was developed and refined. By 1987, 21 states were utilizing electronic monitoring to supervise offenders [10]. Initially, agencies viewed EM as a punishment and to reduce demand on prison places, rather than a means of preventing crime or aiding the rehabilitation of offenders, though these priorities have shifted in recent times [11].

There is some evidence to suggest that EM using GPS technology is superior to RF technology [11,12], and GPS-based systems have become more widely used. Since its introduction in the early 1990s by the US Department of Defense, GPS technology has become ubiquitous through use in mobile phones, laptop computers, and satellite navigation (satnav) devices. A GPS "tracking" device determines the precise location of a vehicle, person, or other asset to which it is attached. Some GPS systems store data within the GPS device for future review, known as "passive" tracking, while others send information on a regular basis to a centralized database via a modem within the device, known as "active" tracking.

Use of EM is on the increase, with more than 80,000 "tagging" orders made in the UK in 2010–2011, as both a community penalty and to monitor prisoners released early on home detention curfews [13]. However, the evidence for EM has failed to keep pace with increased use and development of technology. A recent report was critical of the lack of evidence for use of EM and for the slow progress made in converting to GPS-based systems [11]. Another report highlighted that despite widespread use in sex offender populations in the USA, the evidence base remains unconvincing [14]. A 2010 evaluation of EM in a large population of offenders [12] found that EM reduced the failure of community supervision by 31% compared to other forms of community supervision. The outcome measures were rates of absconding from supervision and revocations for technical violations, misdemeanor, or felony arrest. EM systems can offer additional functionality, such as secure continuous remote alcohol monitoring (SCRAM), which uses a device to monitor body sweat for alcohol levels, with alerts sent if alcohol is detected [15]. This technology is used in several corrections services in the USA [16]. A pilot project is underway in Scotland to evaluate the benefits of SCRAM in offenders sentenced to community orders or selected for early release from prison [17]. Recent studies by Dougherty and colleagues [18–20] have demonstrated the potential benefits of SCRAM, including complementing conventional behavioral interventions, such as contingency management, to help reduce alcohol consumption.

Limitations of EM

Since its inception, EM has been a focus of considerable empirical and philosophical debate. A recent overview of EM in sex offenders by Payne and DeMichele [14] highlighted five key potential problems: lack of empirical support, false sense of security, difficulties in community supervision, organizational issues, and legal issues. All of these factors need to be considered in applying EM to forensic psychiatric settings. Also referring to sex offender policies, including EM, Button et al. [21] have argued that research concerning public perceptions tends to be descriptive and largely atheoretical. The practical limitations of EM by tracking devices also need to be considered. While superior to radio frequency technology, GPS data are still reliant on a traceable signal. The signal is sometimes lost in our secure units, delaying leave. It is not traceable at all in other environments, such as underground trains or metal-lined secure transport vehicles. In December 2014, Steve Gordon, a high-risk sex offender in the USA who was required to wear a GPS tracking bracelet was charged with raping and murdering four women [22]. He had removed his bracelets and was unmonitored for nearly two weeks. However, information from his co-offender's EM tag confirmed his presence at the sites where victims disappeared. While the ankle straps used on our devices are reinforced and very difficult to remove, we have encountered one removal using cutting shears. In this instance, police returned the patient promptly upon having been informed of the most recent location of the device. Our devices also emit a security alert if there is an attempt to cut through the strap.

Electronic monitoring in a UK medium secure service (South London and Maudsley Trust)

Although patients may spend long periods in MSUs, the vast majority of patients will eventually be discharged to the community following periods of community leave, typically beginning with leave where the patient is accompanied by nursing staff and progressing to unescorted leave. During the predischarge period, there is a high risk of relapse and "leave violation," including "absconding" (when a patient on escorted leave escapes from the supervision of an escort) and "failure to return" (when a patient on unescorted leave is late or fails to return from arranged leave) [23]. In 2010, the forensic psychiatry service at our hospital reviewed security arrangements following a series of high-profile absconding incidents, one of which had a tragic outcome [24]. Subsequently, the service introduced a secure tracking device using GPS technology for electronic monitoring of patients on leave from the service as part of a comprehensive protocol for risk management and recovery. The device was used for patients in the initial stages of taking leave as part of their clinical pathway toward discharge to the community. It was envisioned that public protection could be enhanced by introducing a facility that would notify clinical staff immediately should any patient violate his or her leave conditions, or if patients did not return from leave at the agreed time. The device also provides the facility with the ability to identify the patient's location if he or she failed to return from leave or if they absconded from escorting staff.

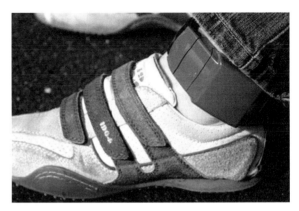

Figure 31.1 The "Buddi" GPS tracker. (See plate section for color version.)

The "Buddi" GPS tracker used by the service is an active tracking device. The following is an outline of how it operates.

- A security version of the device is attached to the patient's ankle with an individually measured lockable strap (Figure 31.1).
- The strap incorporates cabling to make the device nonremovable and optic fibers to provide anti-tamper alarms.
- Each patient using the system has his or her own allocated device.
- The device can be set with geographical parameters, known as "geo-fences" (Figure 31.2), which enable the creation of exclusion and inclusion zones – a common sanction in forensic patients.
- Information from each device is monitored by a security company, and breaches in agreed terms and conditions trigger a predetermined alert to relevant parties and a risk management plan.

The introduction of this technology proved controversial at local and national levels. In correspondence [25] to our recent editorial on the subject [26], one question of particular concern was that of consent. Patients are not obliged to wear the device without consent, with the exception of those high-risk patients requiring emergency hospital or court transfer. Patients are informed that use of electronic monitoring is optional. Permission for leave is risk assessed, and the benefits of EM in risk management are considered as a matter of routine. As we have pointed out, consent is a complex issue in psychiatry and may be defined in degrees, rather than as a binary concept [27]. We accept that patients' decisions about consent

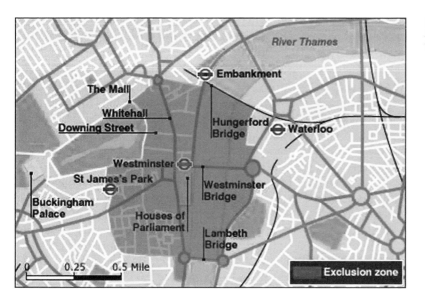

Figure 31.2 Example of an exclusion zone for a "geo-fence." (See plate section for color version.)

to EM are likely to be influenced by a wish to move more quickly toward leave and discharge.

This has parallels with consent to medication and engagement in psychotherapies and occupational activities, particularly in the forensic setting.

Ethical considerations must take account of possible benefits of EM, including potential increases in users' autonomy and acceleration of clinical progression through secure services and back to the community, as well as cost effectiveness of treatment programs. A research group was established to investigate quantitative and qualitative analysis of the impact of EM. Several projects are completed or nearing completion, and our research group aims to publish data on these projects in the near future. In the UK, GPS-based EM is currently being used by two other medium secure forensic units and for some individuals with severe neurodevelopmental disorders. Several psychiatric intensive care units are also investigating its potential use. It is anticipated that the next Code of Practice for the UK Mental Health Act will include specific guidance on the use of EM in detained patients.

Closed Circuit Television (CCTV)

Background

Closed circuit television (CCTV) is the use of video cameras to transmit a signal to a specific place, on a limited set of monitors. CCTV has become widespread in UK society, where it is estimated that there are now over 4 million CCTV cameras [28]. A major report into effectiveness of CCTV in the UK [29] suggested that the majority of the schemes evaluated did not reduce crime, nor did CCTV schemes make people feel safer or change their behavior. However, these conclusions were qualified in the same report as being too simplistic, pointing to the fact that mechanisms that increase recorded crime rates can work alongside those that reduce crime, cancelling each other out.

Use of CCTV in psychiatry was pioneered in 1953 by Tucker for mass therapy in California because of "the increasingly difficult situation of overcrowding and understaffing faced by most mental hospitals," and by Wittson for psychiatry education in Nebraska from 1955 [4]. In the UK, CCTV cameras have featured as a surveillance tool in mental health hospitals since 2002 [29] and have become commonplace in both general and psychiatric hospitals.

General and forensic psychiatric hospitals have identified several potential uses of CCTV. Many of these are practical considerations, such as monitoring of visits, protection of staff during searches, and easier monitoring of ward and patient areas where sightlines are suboptimal. CCTV can also assist robust prosecution of offending behaviors by patients or staff, and the review of serious incidents for training purposes. In this way, it can make both staff and patients safer, and act as a deterrent toward inappropriate practice by staff. This is particularly pertinent in the wake of a recent enquiry into abuse of vulnerable patients by staff in the UK [30].

CCTV can be used to monitor a range of more specific risks. For example, it may be employed in supervised confinement to monitor patient behavior more closely. Monitoring may be particularly difficult in the early stages of supervised confinement, when a severely unwell patient may be violent and hostile. In this way, risk of self-harm or injury can be minimized. Longitudinal assessment using CCTV may allow staff to get a clearer picture of the patient's level of agitation prior to face-to-face assessment. CCTV footage of disturbed or aggressive behavior could also be reviewed with a patient when he or she is relatively well, as part of overall treatment and planning.

Limitations of CCTV

Some research and development on CCTV in psychiatric settings has been undertaken, and comprehensive guidelines have been devised for its use [31]. However, very little research has assessed the impact of the cameras on patients and nursing practices. Desai [32] expressed concern about several aspects of the use of CCTV, including ethical considerations, the potential to distort the reality of what is happening in a ward environment, and reduction in face-to-face contact between staff and patients. In another article [28], the same author pointed to other potential negative consequences of CCTV, including "function creep" (applications for CCTV that did not feature in the original mandate), increased paranoia, and creation of a "panoptican" – an all-seeing eye reigning over staff and patients alike, as described by Foucault. A recent report was critical of use of CCTV in patients' bedrooms in an Irish psychiatric hospital without patients' consent [33].

Use of CCTV in a high secure hospital (Broadmoor)

Standard CCTV has been used routinely at Broadmoor Hospital for over a decade. There is extensive perimeter CCTV, which is part of the standard security measures for a high secure hospital. Recent years have seen the progression of its use. All higher dependency wards at Broadmoor hospital have CCTV covering communal areas (but not patients' bedrooms). Footage from CCTV cameras is used to support usual security protocols in real time. CCTV has also been used to provide evidence toward convictions for violent behavior. For practical reasons, such as the costs of storing large volumes of footage, footage is routinely kept for six weeks only. Should any

suspected offending be identified, that CCTV footage is stored longer for further potential use.

Requests can also be made to retain CCTV footage for other reasons, such as reflective practice and supervision. Footage has also been used in team reviews of particular incidents, as well as supervision of clinicians. High secure hospitals occasionally require planned responses from specially trained staff using shields, for example, to remove a weapon from a disturbed patient. These teams have been using handheld CCTV footage of their interventions for training and record-keeping purposes since 2012. In these ways, CCTV can be seen to aid risk management by securing prosecution of offending behaviors and for developing the skills of clinicians.

Body-worn video. Body-worn video (BWV; Figure 31.3) is a form of CCTV. Small cameras are attached to the front of the wearer. Sound can be recorded. Used by selected UK police force units since 2005 with a view to increasing both officer and civilian accountability, use of BWV by the police has become more widespread and will likely increase further in light of recent policing controversies in the United States [34]. In 2014, Broadmoor Hospital undertook the first trial of body-worn CCTV cameras in a UK hospital. One of the criticisms by patients in qualitative appraisal of the pre-existing CCTV system was the absence of sound recording, which they believed led to a lack of context when reviewing the visual images. BWV was introduced partly to address this issue, as well as to provide an extension of CCTV footage used for risk management in the unit.

The BWV device is not in constant use on the ward, nor is it in constant use when it is being worn.

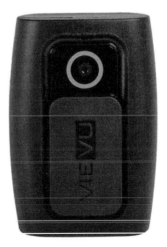

Figure 31.3 A body-worn video camera.

When on the ward, a member of nursing staff wears a small, clearly marked CCTV camera which is usually switched off, and has a red LED to clearly show when it is recording. It also records sound. To date, use of BWV has been judged as useful by staff members, who report a reduction in incidents when it is present. The overwhelming majority of patients supported its continued use, and the trial has been extended to other parts of the hospital.

Future potential use includes review of post-incident footage to assess the nature of the incident, quality of crisis management and contingency plans, and integration into patient clinical records to demonstrate both risk behaviors and examples of good coping skills. Qualitative and quantitative data on BWV and CCTV are being collected on an ongoing basis, with a view to publication in future articles.

Motion detector technology

Background

Motion detector or motion sensor technology refers to any instrument used to detect moving objects, particularly people. Several technologies are available, including passive infrared (PIR), microwave, ultrasonic, tomographic motion detector, and video camera software. A wide range of uses is possible, including computer game software (e.g., Wii and Xbox) and "smart lighting" systems for street, home, and office lighting. In healthcare settings, the potential applications are considerable. To date, motion sensor technology has been used in assisted rehabilitation [35], monitoring of cardiac and respiratory conditions [36], assistance of home living in the elderly and cognitively impaired [37,38], and monitoring of diabetes [39]. Personalized ambient monitoring (PAM) uses motion sensor (and other) technology, which is worn by patients in their homes, to collect physiological and environmental data. This information is then used to develop models of prodromal phases of illness, based on level of activity and physiological measures. Potential applications in mental health include monitoring of those with bipolar disorder, depression, schizophrenia, and dementia [40].

Use of motion detector technology in a high secure hospital

In forensic and general psychiatric hospitals, patients are usually subjected to regular checks during the night. This involves recording of a patient's breathing rate, heart rate, and oxygen saturation. These checks typically require light to properly visualize the patient and his or her breathing, leading to either patients being regularly woken up or checks regularly being poorly done, neither of which is acceptable.

To address this problem, Broadmoor Hospital has recently collaborated with a UK medical technology company (Oxehealth) to develop an adapted CCTV system that can work in total darkness and provide constant contactless monitoring, without the need for a patient to wear any monitoring equipment or physically co-operate with the process. This could prove extremely useful, as it means the patient does not have to be woken or disturbed at night. As well as the practical benefit to the patient of not having to be disturbed at night, this can aid risk management through improving therapeutic effect of appropriate sleep patterns.

The technology involved is twofold. First, the CCTV cameras employ infrared light to detect movement. This technology has been available for some time and is commonly used in night-time CCTV or night vision security cameras. Second, to process the information, Oxehealth developed a novel set of algorithms, known as Oxecam (Figure 31.4). The algorithms use techniques such as image-based photoplethysmography and movement tracking to extract information automatically from the camera data. No manual processing is required. The system can run continuously, gathering extended sections of monitoring data rather than spot-check measurements. If the latest measured data indicate a cause for concern, the system can raise an alarm automatically for staff to review the data and intervene if necessary. Bespoke hardware is not needed, as widely available cameras can be used. As well as monitoring patients in visible light (indoor lights or sunlight), the system can operate in total darkness by using invisible infrared illumination. This camera-based technology has been demonstrated in previous clinical studies involving adults undergoing hemodialysis [41] and pre-term infants in a neonatal intensive care unit [42]. The device currently being trialed can be placed in a ceiling, in secure CCTV housing.

Broadmoor Hospital is also currently piloting a separate system, which develops algorithms based on motion sensor data to identify prodromes of aggression and violent episodes. The device tracks the movement of every person on the ward. CCTV is not involved, and individuals are not identifiable.

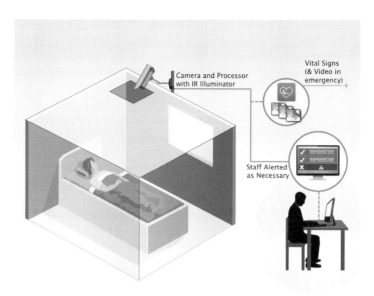

Figure 31.4 Oxecam system. (See plate section for color version.)

Alongside data on movement, data about the time, nature, and location of any significant incident that occurs on the ward are collected. Algorithms will be developed with the aim of identifying early warnings of patterns of movement that are known to precede significant clinical events, alerting staff when such patterns occur, and allowing a proactive approach to be taken to any developing situation.

Conclusions

New technologies offer a broad range of benefits in forensic psychiatry services. These include less restrictive options for patients, improved accountability of both staff and patients, less invasive testing, improved automated record keeping, and better assurance reporting.

A common theme of the developments described here is the use of technology to improve the completeness and accuracy of data used by clinicians to make decisions. In the complex interplay of risk management and patient recovery, such accuracy is vital. Another common thread is that each of these strategies supports and improves current clinical approaches rather than drastically changing them.

Some technologies are cost-neutral, or cost-saving, and for those that are not, the falling price and improving quality should reduce barriers to uptake.

Services that utilize technologies also need to be aware of limitations. EM may be seen as unduly restrictive by patients and advocates. Evidence for its use remains limited, and technical failures may render it ineffective in some cases. CCTV in psychiatric settings also lacks a robust evidence base, and concerns about reality distortion, "function creep," and impact on therapeutic relationships should be borne in mind. It is important that services retain the correct balance when deciding in what ways technological advances will be used, and in what ways they will not. It is vital that the types of technological innovations described in this article should be subject to thorough evaluation that addressed cost effectiveness, qualitative analysis of patients' attitudes, safety, and ethical considerations.

Disclosures

None of the authors has any commercial interests, nor conflicts of interest, actual nor implied, with any of the companies mentioned in this article.

References

1. Bopp JM, Miklowitz DJ, Goodwin GM, *et al*. The longitudinal course of bipolar disorder as revealed through weekly text messaging: a feasibility study. *Bipolar Disord*. 2010; **12**(3): 327–334.

2. Berrouiguet S, Gravey M, Le Galudec M, Alavi Z, Walter M. Post-acute crisis text messaging outreach for suicide prevention:

a pilot study. *Psychiatry Research.* 2014; **217**(3): 154–157.

3. Luxton DD, McCann RA, Bush NE, Mishkind MC, Reger GM. mHealth for mental health: integrating smartphone technology in behavioral healthcare. *Professional Psychology: Research and Practice.* 2011; **42**(6): 505–512.

4. Newnham EA, Doyle EL, Sng AA, Hooke GR, Page AC. Improving clinical outcomes in psychiatric care with touch-screen technology. *Psychol. Serv.* 2012; **9**(2): 221–223.

5. Mars M. Guest Editorial: telepsychiatry in Africa—a way forward? *African Journal of Psychiatry.* 2012; **15**(4): 215–217.

6. Shore JH. Telepsychiatry: videoconferencing in the delivery of psychiatric care. *Am. J. Psychiatry.* 2013; **170**(3): 256–262.

7. Miller TW, Burton DC, Hill K, *et al.* Telepsychiatry: critical dimensions for forensic services. *J. Am. Acad. Psychiatry Law.* 2005; **33**(4): 539–546.

8. Valdagno M, Goracci A, di Volo S, Fagiolini A. Telepsychiatry: new perspectives and open issues. *CNS Spectr.* 2014; **19**(6): 479–481.

9. Durcan G. *Pathways to Unlocking Secure Mental Health Care.* Centre for Mental Health; 2011. http://www.centreformentalhealth.org.uk/pdfs/Pathways_to_unlocking_secure_mental_health_care.pdf.

10. Button DM, DeMichele M, Payne BK. Using electronic monitoring to supervise sex offenders: legislative patterns and implications for community corrections officers. *Criminal Justice Policy Review.* 2009; **20**(4): 414–436.

11. Geoghegan R. *Future of Corrections: Exploring the Use of Electronic Monitoring.* Policy Exchange; 2012. http://www.policyexchange.org.uk/publications/category/item/future-of-corrections-exploring-the-use-of-electronic-monitoring.

12. Bales B, Mann K, Blomberg T, *et al. A Quantitative and Qualitative Assessment of Electronic Monitoring.* Florida State University, College of Criminology and Criminal Justice, Center for Criminology and Public Policy Research; 2010. https://www.ncjrs.gov/pdffiles1/nij/grants/230530.pdf.

13. Travis A, Hill A. Half of all tagged offenders break curfew rules, says report. *The Guardian.* June 14, 2012. http://www.theguardian.com/uk/2012/jun/14/half-tagged-offenders-break-curfew-rules.

14. Payne BK, DeMichele M. Sex offender policies: considering unanticipated consequences of GPS sex offender monitoring. *Aggression and Violent Behavior.* 2011; **16**(3): 177–187.

15. Litten RZ, Bradley AM, Moss HB. Alcohol biomarkers in applied settings: recent advances and future research opportunities. *Alcohol Clin. Exp. Res.* 2010; **34**(6): 955–967.

16. Barton B. *Secure Continuous Remote Alcohol Monitoring (SCRAM) Technology Evaluability Assessment.* Washington, DC: U.S. Department of Justice; 2009.

17. Fox A, Lockhart G. *From the Ground Up: Promising Criminal Justice Projects in the US and the UK.* London: Policy Exchange; 2011. http://www.policyexchange.org.uk/publications/category/item/from-the-ground-up-promising-criminal-justice-projects-in-the-us-and-the-uk.

18. Dougherty DM, Charles NE, Acheson A, *et al.* Comparing the detection of transdermal and breath alcohol concentrations during periods of alcohol consumption ranging from

moderate drinking to binge drinking. *Exp. Clin. Psychopharmacol.* 2012; **20**(5): 373–381.

19. Leffingwell TR, Cooney NJ, Murphy JG, *et al.* Continuous objective monitoring of alcohol use: twenty-first century measurement using transdermal sensors. *Alcohol Clin. Exp. Res.* 2013; **37**(1): 16–22.

20. Dougherty DM, Hill-Kapturczak N, Liang Y, *et al.* Use of continuous transdermal alcohol monitoring during a contingency management procedure to reduce excessive alcohol use. *Drug Alcohol Depend.* 2014; **142**: 301–306.

21. Button DM, Tewksbury R, Mustaine EE, Payne BK. Factors contributing to perceptions about policies regarding the electronic monitoring of sex offenders: the role of demographic characteristics, victimization experiences, and social disorganization. *Int. J. Offender Ther. Comp. Criminol.* 2013; **57**(1): 25–54.

22. Fohall E, St. John P. Sex offender had GPS bracelet removed and went unmonitored. *LA Times.* December 15, 2014.

23. Stewart D, Bowers L. Absconding and locking ward doors: evidence from the literature. *J. Psychiatr. Ment. Health Nurs.* 2011; **18**(1): 89–93.

24. France A. Escaped lag killed OAP for drug cash. *The Sun.* June, 16 2009.

25. Tully J, Hearn D, Fahy T. Authors' reply. *Br. J. Psychiatry.* 2014; **205**(2): 500–501.

26. Tully J, Hearn D, Fahy T. Can electronic monitoring (GPS 'tracking') enhance risk management in psychiatry? *Br. J. Psychiatry.* 2014; **205**(2): 83–85.

27. Konow J. Coercion and consent. *Journal of Institutional and*

Theoretical Economics JITE. 2014; **170**(1): 49–74.

28. Desai S. Violence and surveillance: some unintended consequences of CCTV monitoring within mental health hospital wards. *Surveillance & Society.* 2010; **8**(1): 84–92.

29. Gill M, Spriggs A. *Assessing the Impact of CCTV.* Home Office Research Study 292 London: Home Office Press; 2005.

30. Parish C. Winterbourne View hospital: the government's definitive response: Colin Parish summarises the Department of Health's final report on the neglect and abuse of patients with learning disabilities in a long-stay hospital. *Learning Disability Practice.* 2013; **16**(1): 32–35.

31. Warr J, Page M, Crossen-White H. *The Appropriate Use of CCTV Observation in a Secure Unit.* Bournemouth University; 2005. http://eprints.bournemouth.ac.uk/11684/.

32. Desai S. The new stars of CCTV: what is the purpose of monitoring patients in communal areas of psychiatric hospital wards, bedrooms and seclusion rooms? *Diversity in Health and Care.* 2009; **6**(1): 45–53.

33. Mental Health Commission. Department of Psychiatry, Connolly Hospital approved centre inspection report, 12 February 2013. Dublin: MHC;

2014. http://lenus.ie/hse/handle/10147/315270?locale=ga &language=ga.

34. Hermann P, Weiner R. Issues over police shooting in Ferguson lead push for officers and body cameras. *Washington Post.* December 2, 2014. http://www.washingtonpost.com/local/crime/issues-over-police-shooting-in-ferguson-lead-push-for-officers-and-body-cameras/2014/12/02/dedcb2d8-7a58-11e4-84d4-7c896b90abdc_story.html.

35. Jovanov E, Milenkovic A, Otto C, De Groen PC. A wireless body area network of intelligent motion sensors for computer assisted physical rehabilitation. *Journal of NeuroEngineering and Rehabilitation.* 2005; **2**(1): 6.

36. Lubecke OB, Ong PW, Lubecke VM. 10 GHz Doppler radar sensing of respiration and heart movement. In: *Bioengineering Conference, 2002: Proceedings of the IEEE 28th Annual Northeast.* IEEE; 2002; 55–56. http://ieeexplore.ieee.org/xpl/login.jsp?tp=&arnumber=9 99462&url=http%3A%2F%2Fieeexplore.ieee.org%2Fxpls%2Fabs_ all.jsp%3Farnumber%3D999462.

37. Demiris G, Oliver DP, Dickey G, Skubic M, Rantz M. Findings from a participatory evaluation of a smart home application for older adults. *Technol. Health Care.* 2008; **16**(2): 111–118.

38. Pollack ME. Intelligent technology for an aging population: the use of AI to assist elders with cognitive impairment. *AI Magazine.* 2005; **26**(2): 9.

39. Helal A, Cook DJ, Schmalz M. Smart home-based health platform for behavioral monitoring and alteration of diabetes patients. *J. Diabetes Sci. Technol.* 2009; **3**(1): 141–148.

40. Blum J, Magill E. M-psychiatry: sensor networks for psychiatric health monitoring. In *Proceedings of the 9th Annual Postgraduate Symposium on the Convergence of Telecommunications, Networking and Broadcasting (PGNET 2008).* 2008: 33–37. https://scholar.google.co.uk/scholar?q=M-psychiatry:+sensor+networks+for+psychiatric+health+monitoring.&hl=en&as_sdt=0&as_vis=1&oi=scholart&sa=X&ei=Xi81Vei3NIO1OqfagOAD&ved=0CCQQgQMwAA.

41. Tarassenko L, Villarroel M, Guazzi A, *et al.* Non-contact video-based vital sign monitoring using ambient light and auto-regressive models. *Physiol. Meas.* 2014; **35**(5): 807–831.

42. Villarroel M, Guazzi A, Jorge J, *et al.* Continuous non-contact vital sign monitoring in neonatal intensive care unit. *Healthcare Technology Letters.* 2014; **1**(3): 87–91.

Chapter

32

Risk reduction treatment of psychopathy and applications to mentally disordered offenders

Stephen C. P. Wong and Mark E. Olver

Introduction

Therapeutic nihilism on treating psychopathy is widespread, so much so that treatment is sometimes withheld predicated on the belief that nothing works or that treatment can cause harm. For example, a recent paper on the treatability of psychopathy stated that ". . . psychopathic disorders . . . are widely assumed to be untreatable conditions" and that "the absence of evidence based treatment efficacy for psychopathic disorders is a logical reason for not subjecting individuals with only a psychopathic disorder to involuntary hospitalization" (p. 400) [1]. The article was based on an award-winning lecture delivered at the annual meeting of the American Psychiatric Association. Despite such pessimism, recent advances in assessing psychopathy as well as offender risk assessment and rehabilitation have generated renewed optimism to re-conceptualize risk reduction-focused treatment for psychopathic offenders. Early treatment evaluation results are encouraging. A review and possible extension of this work to the treatment of mentally disordered offenders (MDOs) with schizophrenia, violence, and psychopathy are presented.

Psychopathy Assessment and Treatment: A Brief Overview

Psychopathy is a psychological construct generally characterized by a constellation of personality traits characterized by callous and remorseless manipulation of others, insincerity, and lying, as well as antisociality and criminal offending [2,3]. We use the term psychopath(y) to describe persons with a significant number of such characteristics. The present discussion on the treatment of psychopathy refers primarily to treatment to reduce the individual's risk of

violence and antisocial behaviors rather than to ameliorate the psychopathic personality traits and related psychopathologies.

The Psychopathy Checklist–Revised (PCL-R) [3], a 20-item construct rating scale, is a widely used assessment tool designed to assess some of the Clecklian features of psychopathy. The assessment and conceptualization of the construct of psychopathy using the PCL-R are not without its critics and controversies (see a review by Skeem *et al.*) [4], and other tools such as the Comprehensive Assessment of Psychopathic Personality [5] have been developed to assess psychopathy. The PCL-R was used as the operational definition of psychopathy in the present discussion because it has a broad empirical evidence base and it is also the most widely used. As such, we do know quite a lot "about the psychopathic offender as defined by the PCL-R" (p. 383) [6]. The PCL-R consists of two oblique factors: Factor 1 (F1), which measures the interpersonal and affective traits of psychopathy, and Factor 2 (F2), which measures the chronic antisocial behaviors and unstable lifestyle. F1 can be further subdivided into the Interpersonal (e.g., superficiality, grandiosity) and affective (e.g., callousness, lack of remorse) facets, while F2 can be subdivided into the lifestyle (e.g., irresponsibility, impulsivity) and antisocial (e.g., criminal versatility, early behavior problems) facets.

Despite the widespread therapeutic nihilism on treating psychopathy, there are, in fact, very few well-designed studies attesting to its treatment efficacy; that the literature is "short on quality and long on lore" is not an inappropriate characterization [7]. In a review of 74 studies of psychopathy treatment [8], only two studies using the same sample and operating a now completely discredited program [9,10] (also see next section) satisfied very basic criteria of an

Violence in Psychiatry, ed. Katherine D. Warburton and Stephen M. Stahl. Published by Cambridge University Press.
© Cambridge University Press 2016.

acceptable study design; a subsequent systematic review also pointed out the very poor state of the literature [11]. However, in a meta-analysis of 42 psychopathy treatment studies, the author identified some positive outcomes after making a number of methodological adjustments to compensate for the many methodologically flawed studies [12]. A subsequent updated meta-analysis [13] identified recent additions to the literature with better-designed studies with encouraging results [14,15]. There are still too few well-designed studies to draw firm conclusions on the efficacy of treating psychopaths. However, the absence of positive evidence does not mean that no treatment will work.

In an oft-quoted study [9], PCL-R–assessed psychopaths treated in a therapeutic community-type program in the 1950s recidivated violently more than a matched control group. This finding alone led to a widely held view that treatment could make psychopaths worse. The paradoxical finding is likely due to the use of totally inappropriate treatment regimes by the treatment providers. The regime was described as "... both idiosyncratic and extreme" [11] and "... would be considered to be unacceptable today" (p. 169), as it consisted of "... extreme measures such as nude marathon encounter sessions for 2 weeks, together with the use of drugs such as methedrine, LSD, scopolamine, and alcohol" (p. 168). Some program participants were allowed to operate the program and "prescribe" controlled medications to co-patients! Even the authors of the article concurred that the treatment regime "... is the wrong type of program for serious psychopathic offenders" [10]. Rather than asserting that treatment made psychopaths worse, a more appropriate conclusion to draw from the study is that the *wrong* treatment made psychopaths worse.

A Model for Risk Reduction Treatment of Psychopathy

Treatment progress can be facilitated by using an evidence-based or rationally derived conceptual framework together with appropriate safeguards to ensure treatment integrity; these basic notions were lacking in earlier treatment studies. A two-component (2-C) model has been proposed based on recent advances in the psychopathy assessment, offender risk assessment, and offender rehabilitation literatures [16–18]. The two components are the interpersonal component (C1), corresponding to the PCL-R F1 affective and interpersonal traits, and the criminogenic component (C2), corresponding to the PCL-R F2 dysfunctional lifestyle and antisociality, respectively. The model's main treatment objective is to reduce the risk of institutional and community violence and criminality.

Component 1

A growing body of research shows, perhaps counterintuitively, that the core PCL-R F1 affective and interpersonal personality traits, which underpin C1, are *not* predictive of violence or criminality. Dysfunctional lifestyle and antisociality features, or F2, which underpin C2, are significantly linked to violence and criminality. Two meta-analyses, one on violent nonsexual offenders [19] and one on sexual offenders [20], showed that F2, but not F1, predicted violent and sexually violent recidivism, respectively. Very similar findings were obtained in a number of studies of the predictive efficacy of F1 and F2 using different offender groups. These studies include a group of male Canadian aboriginal and non-aboriginal offenders [21], a group of male Canadian offenders followed up prospectively for 24 years [22], a group of male learning disabled offenders from Belgium [23], and a group of male and female forensic treatment patients and offenders (about 66%/34% respectively) from Sweden assessed with the PCL-Screening Version [24]. Further statistical analyses to determine the relative contributions of the four facets to predicting recidivism using eight international samples of male and female adults showed that "... the antisocial facet is the most trustworthy and powerful predictor of future recidivism on the PCL–R and PCL: SV" and "... to maximize the predictive power...we need the antisocial facet ... supported perhaps by the lifestyle facet and supplemented, on occasion, by the interpersonal and affective facets" (p. 556) [25]. A separate meta-analysis showed no interaction effects of F1 and F2 [26]. As F1 does not appear to predict violent reoffending, treatment aimed at changing F1, the core personality feature of psychopathy, is *not* expected to significantly impact future violence. However, F1 characteristics are closely linked to treatment interfering behaviors, such as poor treatment compliance and lack of motivation and engagement, as well as generally highly disruptive and manipulative behaviors during treatment [27–29]. Research has also reported high treatment drop-out rates for psychopaths [15,30–32]. Thus, behavioral manifestations of F1 traits in treatment must be closely and carefully managed to maintain motivation and engagement, to reduce drop-out, and to ensure program integrity. Violence reduction treatment should be directed at changing F2, rather than F1, characteristics; this is a key point, as it would seem intuitively obvious that to reduce one of the central concerns of the disorder–violence and anti-social behaviors, the psychopathic personality traits, essentially F1—should be the focus of treatment.

Component 2

Many of the PCL-R F2 dysfunctional lifestyle and antisociality features that underpin C2 are static and unchangeable (e.g., juvenile delinquency); a dynamic risk assessment tool can be used to identify equivalent dynamic or modifiable violence risk predictors to serve as the offender's treatment targets. Cognitive-behavioral treatment can then be used to modify affects, cognitions, and behaviors that cause or are

closely associated with the offender's violence and criminality to reduce the offender's risk of violence. A risk assessment tool such as the Violence Risk Scale (VRS) [33], with 20 dynamic risk factors, can be used to make such assessments. The VRS dynamic factors correlate strongly with F2 ($r = 0.80$) and can be used as a proxy measure of F2 [34].

Figure 32.1 features the titles of the 20 VRS dynamic factors/predictors (selected based on the extant literature on offender risk assessment) and the prevalence (%) of offenders in the sample with high (3) or moderately high (2) ratings on each of the factors, which then are the identified treatment targets. VRS dynamic factors are rated with a 4-point rating scale of 0, 1, 2, and 3; factors rated 2 or 3 indicate a moderate to substantial link to violence. One sample consists of 918 Canadian federal offenders, the majority with histories of violence, and the other consists of 65 PCL-R–rated (PCL-R≥30) psychopathic offenders (adapted from Wong and Gordon [33]). As expected, compared to the violent offender sample, the psychopathic sample has a much

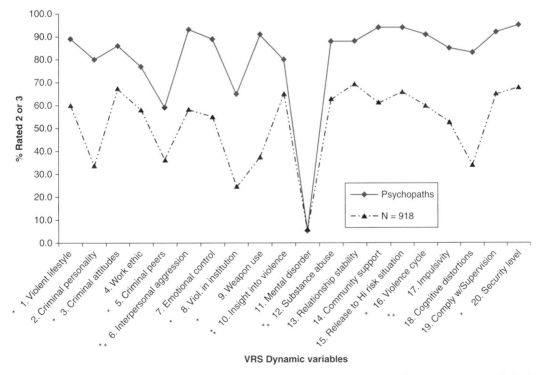

Figure 32.1 Risk profile assessed using 20 VRS dynamic factors. The sample of 918 is a male adult offender normative sample for the VRS (see Wong and Gordon [33]). The psychopathic sample was identified from an offender sample using PCL = R cutoff of 30. This figure was adapted from Wong and Gordon [33].

higher prevalence of all of the treatment targets except the mental disorder factor. The results suggested that psychopaths and violent offenders in general have qualitatively similar treatment targets, though the former showed a higher prevalence of almost all of them. The very low endorsement of the mental disorder factor results from both samples consisting of offenders whose violence is not attributable to diagnosed mental disorders; the converse should be the case for MDOs with violence associated with the disorder.

Recent research has shown that changes of the VRS dynamic factors assessed within a treatment program were associated with a subsequent reduction in violent reoffending post-release in the community among male high-risk PCL-R–assessed psychopathic offenders with no active psychotic symptoms [34,35]. Analogous results were obtained for psychopathic sexual offenders assessed using the Violence Risk Scale – Sexual Offender version (VRS-SO) [36] designed for sexual offenders [15,37]. The results suggest that the dynamic factors of the VRS and VRS-SO are modifiable and satisfy the criteria for causative dynamic factors [38]. Once the treatment targets are identified, risk reduction treatment can proceed.

The 2-C model is consistent with the generic and specific factors set forth by Livesley [39–41] for the treatment of personality disorders. The generic factor entails establishing therapeutic and supportive engagements between therapists and clients, vis-à-vis, the interpersonal C1 component, whereas the specific factor includes interventions that target the individual's specific problem areas, vis-à-vis, the criminogenic C2 component. The risk/need/ responsivity (RNR) principles are widely accepted as important principles to guide risk reduction treatment of offenders [42,43]. Higher-risk offenders should receive more intensive treatment (the Risk principle); treatment should be directed toward the person's criminogenic needs, that is, the causes or closely linked attributes of the criminal behaviors (the Need principle), and, treatment delivery should be tailored to the person's learning and response style such as the level of motivation, engagement, and intellectual abilities (the Responsivity principle). Risk and Need closely map onto C2, whereas Responsivity maps onto C1.

The 2-C model is also consistent with the National Institute of Health and Clinical Excellence (NICE, UK) guidelines for the treatment of antisocial

personality disorder including psychopathy [44]. The guidelines assert that persons with antisocial personality (including psychopathy) should not be excluded from any health or social care service because of their disorder or offending behaviors (p. 7). For reducing reoffending, the guidelines recommend the following: (1) using CBT group-based approaches, (2) adapting treatment to suit the individual, (3) monitoring treatment progress, and 4) providing appropriate staff training and support (pp. 16–18). Pharmacological interventions, however, should not be routinely used for the treatment of antisocial personality disorder or associated behaviors of aggression, anger, and impulsivity (p. 16).

Treatment programs with design and delivery similar to the 2-C model have produced positive outcome results. The Violence Reduction Program [45] and the Clearwater Sex Offender Programme [46–48] are two examples. During such treatment, offenders' criminogenic needs linked to sexual and nonsexual violence (F2), such as criminal attitudes and beliefs, sexually deviant interests, interpersonal aggression/ hostility, substance use, etc., are assessed and identified as possible treatment targets using the VRS/VRS-SO and clinical evaluations. Cognitive-behavioral group and/or individual interventions are used, if appropriate, in a structured but flexible manner to modify antisocial thoughts, feelings, and behaviors. Practice and generalization of socially appropriate behaviors to day-to-day living are very much encouraged and supported with ongoing close monitoring guided by what we referred to as Offence Analogue and Offence Reduction Behaviors (OAB and ORB, respectively) protocols [49]. OABs are the proxies of offending behaviors that manifest within an institutional context, and ORBs are the prosocial counterparts to replace the OABs in day-to-day functioning. Each VRS-identified treatment target should have corresponding OABs and ORBs. The here-and-now OABs are behaviors that treatment staff can focus on, and, using appropriate interventions, can assist offenders to learn to replace them with ORBs. To address F1-related issues, motivational and engagement work are emphasized throughout the program using, for example, motivational interviewing principles [50]. Intensive staff training to manage treatment-interfering behaviors and appropriate staff supervision and support are also important program components. The programs, about 8–9 months in duration, are suitable for both offenders with a significant history of nonsexual and sexual violence as well as for psychopathic offenders. The close integration of risk assessment and risk reduction treatment is essential in the program's implementation [51].

For MDOs with histories of violence, the 2-C model also can be used to guide risk reduction treatment once acute psychiatric symptoms are well managed, controlled, and carefully monitored and the person has regained a sufficient level of daily functioning to attend to risk reduction treatment requirements (see the next section).

Summary

The 2-C model is developed based on integrating the psychopathy assessment, risk assessment, and offender rehabilitation literatures to guide violence reduction treatment of high-risk and/or psychopathic offenders. Treatment should target the person's modifiable criminogenic features, analogous to F2 characteristics, which are identified using an appropriate dynamic risk assessment tool. Offenders can then learn, practice, and generalize offense-reducing thoughts, feelings, and behaviors to replace offense-producing behaviors in day-to-day functioning. Staff must closely monitor and manage treatment-interfering behaviors (linked to F1 features) to maintain treatment engagement and integrity. Treatment targeting F1 features, though intuitively appealing as they appear to target the most salient and obvious psychopathic personality traits, will unlikely reduce violence recidivism even if changes were successfully made, as these traits are *not* linked to future violence. Outcome evaluations of programs similar to the 2-C model have shown some positive results [15,16,35].

Psychopathy, Mental Disorder, and Violence

The majority of mentally ill persons are not violent. Among major mental disorders, psychosis has the closest link to violence. In a meta-analysis using 166 independent data sets, psychosis was associated with a 49%–68% increase in the odds of violence [52]. Again, most persons with psychosis are not violent. A recent systematic review and meta-analysis based on 110 eligible studies by Witt *et al.* [53] investigated static and dynamic predictors for aggression and violence among MDOs formally diagnosed with psychosis, the majority with schizophrenia (total $n = 45,533$ adults; 87.8% schizophrenia, 0.4% bipolar disorder, and 11.8% other psychoses). The sample base rate of violence was 18.5%. The strongest predictor for all aggression or serious violence was criminal history – a static predictor. The dynamic predictors were hostile behaviors, poor impulsive control, recent drug/alcohol misuse, lack of insight, and noncompliance with psychological therapies and medication; the predictors were essentially the same for aggression vs. severe violence as well as for inpatient vs. community or mixed settings, although the strengths of association varied. In Figure 32.1, the dynamic predictors identified for the MDOs with psychosis are marked with a double asterisk (**). The static criminal history predictors should have a number of likely underlying dynamic counterparts, such as violent (criminal) lifestyle, criminal attitude, criminal peers, violence (criminal) cycle, and so forth that are a part of the VRS dynamic factors marked in Figure 32.1 with a single asterisk (*). (For a more detailed discussion of this point, see Wong and Gordon [33].) The overlaps of dynamic violence predictors for the three groups are considerable (Figure 32.1), although the data were collected using very different methodologies. These findings are consistent with two meta-analyses, both showing criminological, rather than clinical, variables to be better predictors for violent and general recidivism for MDOs [54,55]. A recent study with MDOs and non-MDOs on parole also obtained very similar results [56]. Given the similarities in the risk factors for the three groups, it is possible that they share similar etiological pathways.

Developmental Trajectory of Schizophrenia

In the past two decades, the extant literature, including large longitudinal cohort studies, has identified three different types of MDOs with schizophrenia (MDO-S) with different developmental trajectories (types I, II, and III; see Hodgins [57] for a review). Type I or MDO-S early starters are those whose conduct problems start *before* their illnesses, with an onset around late adolescence or early adulthood. Their significant childhood conduct problems persist into adolescence and adulthood, often resulting in a record of quite diverse criminal behaviors. These Type I MDO-Ss share many similarities with life-course persistent antisocial offenders without mental illness [58]. The Type II MDO-S presents with no history of antisocial or aggressive behavior prior to illness onset (late onset), after which they repeatedly engage in many externalizing aggressive behaviors. Given their late onset, they generally accumulate fewer criminal convictions compared to the Type I. Of importance, a larger proportion of the Type II MDOs had been convicted of homicide than the Type I [59]. Type III MDOs with schizophrenia are likely men in their late thirties with no history of antisocial or aggressive behaviors who kill or try to kill someone who is likely their care provider. Many of the MDO-S cases in Witt et al.'s [53] study also had a significant criminal history, substance abuse problems, hostility, and impulsivity that were predictive of future violence – characteristics similar to the Type I MDO-S cases.

A separate study in Sweden investigated all men who underwent pretrial psychiatric assessments and were later convicted of violent offenses in a six-year period; 202 men were diagnosed with schizophrenia (the MDO-S cases), and 78 met PCL-R criteria for psychopathy without mental disorder [59]. Twenty-nine percent of the MDO-S obtained high scores on the PCL-R and they appear to be similar to non-mentally ill men with psychopathy. The high ratings of psychopathy are associated with earlier ages of first conviction for a criminal offense and more convictions among the men with schizophrenia, just as among men with no mental illness [59]. It is not unexpected that both MDO-S and non-MDOs who met PCL-R criteria would share similar criminological features, since high PCL-R ratings as well as the presence of antisocial personality disorder [60] would signal an early-onset and persistence of conduct problems, substance abuse, juvenile delinquency, criminal versatility, and so forth, essentially PCL-R F2 features.

Among MDOs with schizophrenia, those with higher PCL-R scores are more likely to be found among Type I early starters than Type II or Type III. We hypothesize that among MDO-S, the presence of high PCL-R scores is probably a proxy indication of life-course persistent antisocial behaviors, that is, a preponderance of PCL-R F2 features more so than F1 core psychopathic personality traits. In fact, it was

noted that in the non-offender population, few MDOs with schizophrenia have PCL-R ratings that satisfy the criteria for psychopathy, and characteristics such as glibness, superficial charm, promiscuity, and many short-term relationships (PCL-R items) are rarely observed among them [61]. It is also possible that the ratings of some PCL-R F1 items, such as shallow affect, lack of guilt or remorse, callous/lack of empathy, could be confounded by the presence of negative symptoms of schizophrenia, thus artificially inflating PCL-R scores. It remains to be seen what PCL-R composite and factor scores Type I MDOs would obtain should the ratings be made based only on their personality characteristics assessed prior to the onset of their illnesses.

If our hypothesis was correct and the relatively high ratings on the PCL-R among Type 1 are mainly due to the preponderance of F2 rather than F1 features, it would follow that risk reduction treatment of these MDOs should address their violence risk predictors (proxy of F2 features), not unlike the treatment of non-mentally ill offenders with psychopathy. A comprehensive risk assessment using an appropriate dynamic risk assessment tool should inform what risk factors are present that can be used as treatment targets; treatment delivery can be similarly guided by the proposed 2-C model. Assessing the possible presence and extent of F1 features would inform us of how best to manage the person to reduce the impact of treatment-interfering behaviors such as disruption of treatment group, staff splitting, etc.

Conclusion

Recent advances in the assessment of psychopathy, risk assessment, and offender rehabilitation have enabled the integration of these literatures to inform risk reduction treatment of psychopathy as illustrated by the recently developed two-component (2-C) treatment model for violence-prone psychopathic offenders. Parallel advances in the study of MDOs, in particular those with schizophrenia, have also shed light on their characteristics and possible etiology. This article reviewed the literature and extends the 2-C treatment model to mentally disordered offenders with schizophrenia, violence, and psychopathy with supporting evidence.

Disclosures

The authors do not have anything to disclose.

References

1. Felthous AR. The "untreatability" of psychopathy and hospital commitment in the USA. *Int. J. Law Psychiatry*. 2011; **34**(6): 400–405.

2. Cleckley H. *The Mask of Sanity*, 5th edn. St. Louis, MO: Mosby; 1976.

3. Hare RD. *The Hare Psychopathy Checklist–Revised*, 2nd edn. Toronto, ON: Multi-Health Systems, Inc.; 2003.

4. Skeem JL, Polaschek D, Patrick C, Lilienfeld SO. Psychopathic personality: bridging the gap between scientific evidence and public policy. *Psychological Science in the Public Interest*. 2011; **12**(3): 95–162.

5. Cooke DJ, Hart SD, Logan C, Michie C. Explicating the construct of psychopathy: development and validation of a conceptual model, the Comprehensive Assessment of Psychopathic Personality (CAPP). *International Journal of Forensic Mental Health*. 2012; **11**(4): 242–252.

6. MacDonald AW, Iacono WG. Toward an integrated perspective on the etiology on psychopathy. In: Patrick CJ, ed. *Handbook of Psychopathy*. New York: Guilford Press; 2006: 375–385.

7. Simourd DJ, Hoge RD. Criminal psychopathy: a risk-and-need perspective. *Criminal Justice and Behavior*. 2000; **27**(2): 256–272.

8. Wong S. Treatment of criminal psychopath. In: Hodgins S, Muller-Isberner R, eds. *Violence, Crime and Mentally Disordered Offenders: Concepts and Methods for Effective Treatment and Prevention*. London: Wiley; 2000: 81–106.

9. Rice ME, Harris GT, Cormier CA. An evaluation of a maximum security therapeutic community for psychopaths and other mentally disordered offenders. *Law and Human Behavior*. 1992; **16**(4): 399–412.

10. Rice M, Harris GT, Cormier CA. *Violent Recidivism Among Psychopaths and Nonpsychopaths Treated in a Therapeutic Community*. Penetanguishene, Ontario, Canada: Mental Health Centre; 1989.

11. D'Silva K, Duggan C, McCarthy L. Does treatment really make psychopaths worse? A review of the evidence. *J. Pers. Disord.* 2004; **18**(2): 163–177.

12. Salekin RT. Psychopathy and therapeutic pessimism: Clinical lore or clinical reality? *Clin. Psychol. Rev.* 2002; **22**(1): 79–112.

13. Salekin R, Worley C, Grimes RD. Treatment of psychopathy: a review and brief introduction to the mental model approach for psychopathy. *Behav. Sci. Law.* 2010; **28**(2): 235–266.

14. Bernstein DP, Nijman HLI, Karos K, *et al.* Schema therapy for forensic patients with personality disorders: design and preliminary findings of a multicenter randomized clinical trial in The Netherlands. *International Journal of Forensic Mental Health*. 2012; **11**(4): 312–324.

15. Olver ME, Wong SCP. Therapeutic responses of psychopathic sexual offenders: Treatment attrition, therapeutic change, and long term recidivism. *J. Consult. Clin. Psychol.* 2009; **77**(2): 328–336.

16. Wong SCP, Gordon A, Gu D, Lewis K, Olver ME. The effectiveness of violence reduction treatment for psychopathic offenders: empirical evidence and a treatment model. *International Journal of Forensic Mental Health*. 2012; **11**(4): 336–349.

17. McGuire J. A review of effective interventions for reducing aggression and violence. *Phil. Trans. R. Soc. Lond. B Biol. Sci.* 2008; **363**(1503): 2577–2597.

18. Wong SCP, Hare RD. *Guidelines for a Psychopathy Treatment Program*. Toronto, Canada: Multihealth Systems; 2005.

19. Yang M, Wong SCP, Coid J. The efficacy of violence prediction: A meta-analytic comparison of nine risk assessment instruments. *Psychol. Bull.* 2010; **136**(5): 740–767.

20. Hawes SW, Boccaccini MT, Murrie DC. Psychopathy and the combination of psychopathy and sexual deviance as predictors of sexual recidivism: meta-analytic findings using the Psychopathy Checklist–Revised. *Psychol. Assess.* 2013; **25**(1): 233–243.

21. Olver ME, Neumann CS, Wong SC, Hare RD. The structural and predictive properties of the Psychopathy Checklist–revised in Canadian aboriginal and non-aboriginal offenders. *Psychol. Assess.* 2013; **25**(1): 167–179.

22. Olver ME, Wong SCP. Short- and long-term recidivism prediction of the PCL-R and the effects of age: a 24-year follow-up. *Personal. Disord.* 2015; **6**(1): 97–105.

23. Pouls C, Jeandarme I. Psychopathy in offenders with intellectual disabilities: a comparison of the PCL-R and PCL-SV. *International Journal of Forensic Mental Health*. 2014; **13**(3): 207–216.

24. Douglas KS, Strand S, Belfrage H, Fransson G, Levander S. Reliability and validity evaluation of the Psychopathy Checklist: Screening Version (PCL-R: SV) in Swedish correctional and forensic psychiatric samples. *Assessment*. 2005; **12**(2): 145–161.

25. Walters GD, Wilson NJ, Glover AJ. Predicting recidivism with the Psychopathy Checklist: are factor score composites really necessary? *Psychol. Assess.* 2011; **23**(2): 552–557.

26. Kennealy PJ, Skeem JL, Walters GD, Camp J. Do core interpersonal and affective traits

of PCL-R psychopathy interact with antisocial behavior and disinhibition to predict violence? *Psychol. Assess.* 2010; **22**(3): 569–580.

27. Barbaree HE. Psychopathy, treatment behavior, and recidivism: an extended follow-up of Seto and Barbaree. *J. Interpers. Violence.* 2005; **20**(9): 1115–1131.

28. Hobson J, Shine J, Roberts R. How do psychopaths behave in a prison therapeutic community? *Psychology, Crime, & Law.* 2000; **6**(2): 139–154.

29. Hughes G, Hogue T, Hollin C, Champion H. First-stage evaluation of a treatment programme for personality disordered offenders. *Journal of Forensic Psychiatry.* 1997; **8**(3): 515–527.

30. Ogloff JRP, Wong S, Greenwood A. Treating criminal psychopaths in a therapeutic community program. *Behavioral Sciences and the Law.* 1990; **8**(2): 181–190.

31. Langton CM, Barbaree HE, Harkins L, Peacock EJ. Sex offenders' response to treatment and its association with recidivism as a function of psychopathy. *Sexual Abuse: A Journal of Research and Treatment.* 2006; **18**(1): 99–120.

32. Olver ME, Wong SCP. Predictors of sex offender treatment dropout: psychopathy, sex offender risk, and responsivity implications. *Psychology, Crime & Law.* 2011; **17**(5): 457–471.

33. Wong SCP, Gordon A. The validity and reliability of the Violence Risk Scale: a treatment friendly violence risk assessment scale. *Psychology, Public Policy and Law.* 2006; **12**(3): 279–309.

34. Lewis K1, Olver ME, Wong SCP. The Violence Risk Scale: predictive validity and linking changes in risk with violent recidivism in a sample of high risk offenders with psychopathic traits. *Assessment.* 2013; **20**(2): 150–164.

35. Olver M, Lewis K, Wong SCP. Risk reduction treatment of high-risk psychopathic offenders: the relationship of psychopathy and treatment change to violent recidivism. *Personality Disorder: Theory, Research and Treatment.* 2013; **4**(2): 160–167.

36. Wong S, Olver M, Nicholaichuk T, Gordon A. *Violence Risk Scale– Sexual Offender Version.* Saskatoon, Saskatchewan, Canada: University of Saskatchewan and Regional Psychiatric Centre; 2003–2009.

37. Olver ME, Wong SCP, Nicholaichuk TP, Gordon A. The validity and reliability of the Violence Risk Scale–Sexual Offender version: assessing sex offender risk and evaluating therapeutic change. *Psychol. Assess.* 2007; **19**(3): 318–329.

38. Kraemer HC, Kazdin AE, Offord DR, *et al.* Coming to terms with the terms of risk. *Arch. Gen. Psychiatry.* 1997; **54**(4): 337–343.

39. Livesley J. *Practical Management of Personality Disorder.* New York: Guilford Press; 2003.

40. Livesley J. Common elements of effective treatment. In: van Luyn B, Akhtar S, Livesley J, eds. *Severe Personality Disorder.* New York: Cambridge University Press; 2007: 211–239.

41. Livesley J. The relevance of an integrated approach to the treatment of personality disordered offenders. *Psychology, Crime & Law.* 2007; **13**(1): 27–46.

42. Andrews DA, Bonta J. *The Psychology of Criminal Conduct.* Cincinnati, OH: Anderson; 1994.

43. Andrews DA, Bonta J. *The Psychology of Criminal Conduct,* 5th edn. New Providence, NJ: LexisNexis; 2010.

44. National Institute of Clinical Excellence. *Antisocial Personality Disorder: Treatment, Management and Prevention.* London: National Collaborating Centre for Mental Health; 2009.

45. Wong SCP, Gordon A. The Violence Reduction Program: a treatment program for high risk violence prone offenders. *Psychology, Crime, & Law.* 2013; **19**(5–6): 461–475.

46. Nicholaichuk T, Gordon A, Gu D, Wong S. Outcome of an institutional sexual offender treatment program: a comparison between treated and matched untreated offenders. *Sexual Abuse: A Journal of Research and Treatment.* 2000; **12**(2): 137–153.

47. Olver M, Wong SCP, Nicholaichuk TP. Outcome evaluation of a high intensity inpatient sex offender treatment program. *Journal of Interpersonal Violence.* 2009; **24**(3): 522–536.

48. Olver M, Wong SCP. A description and research review of the Clearwater Sex Offender Treatment Programme. *Psychology, Crime & Law.* 2013; **19**(5–6): 477–492.

49. Gordon A, Wong SCP. Offense analogue behaviours as indicator of criminogenic need and treatment progress in custodial settings. In: Daffern M, Jones L, Shine J. eds. *Offence Paralleling Behaviour: An Individualized Approach to Offender Assessment and Treatment.* Chichester, UK: Wiley; 2010: 171–184.

50. Miller WR, Rollnick S. *Motivational Interviewing: Preparing People for Change,* 2nd edn. New York: Guildford; 2002.

51. Wong SCP, Gordon A, Gu D. The assessment and treatment of violence-prone forensic clients: an integrated approach. *Br. J. Psychiatry.* **190**(49): s66–s74.

52. Douglas KS, Guy LS, Hart SD. Psychosis as a risk factor for

violence to others: a meta-analysis. *Psychol. Bull.* 2009; **135**(5): 679–706.

53. Witt K, van dorn R, Fazel S. Risk factors for violence in psychosis: systematic review and meta-regression analysis of 110 studies. *PloS One.* 2013; **8**(2): e55942.

54. Bonta J, Law M, Hanson K. The prediction of criminal and violent recidivism among mentally disordered offenders: a meta-analysis. *Psychol. Bull.* 1998; **123**(2): 123–142.

55. Bonta J, Blais J, Wilson H. A theoretically informed meta-analysis of the risk for general and violent recidivism for mentally disordered offenders. *Aggression and Violent Behavior.* 2014; **19**(3): 278–287.

56. Skeem JL, Winter E, Kennealy PJ, Louden JE, Tatar JR 2nd. Offenders with mental illness have criminogenic needs, too: toward recidivism reduction. *Law Hum. Behav.* 2014; **38**(3): 212–224.

57. Hodgins S. Violent behaviour among people with schizophrenia: a framework for investigations of causes, and effective treatment, and prevention. *Phil. Trans. R. Soc. Lond. B Biol. Sci.* 2008; **363**(1503): 2505–2518.

58. Moffitt TE, Caspi A. Childhood predictors differentiate life-course persistent and adolescence-limited antisocial pathways among males and females. *Dev. Psychopathol.* 2001; **13**(2): 355–375.

59. Tengström A, Hodgins S, Grann M, Långström N, Kullgren G. Schizophrenia and criminal offending: the role of psychopathy and substance use disorders. *Criminal Justice and Behavior.* 2004; **31**(4): 367–391.

60. American Psychiatric Association. *Diagnostic and Statistical Manual of Mental Disorders*, 5th edn. Washington, DC: American Psychiatric Association; 2013.

61. Hodgins S, Côté G, Toupin J. Major mental disorder and crime: an etiological hypothesis. In: Cooke DJ, Forth AD, Hare RD, eds. *Psychopathy: Theory, Research, and Implications for Society.* Dordrecht, the Netherlands: Kluwer Academic; 1998: 231–256.

Index

Entries for tables, figures, and boxes are noted in bold typeface.